Imaging of Endometriosis: A Comparative Guide of US, MRI and Surgery

Isabelle Thomassin-Naggara
Editor

Imaging of Endometriosis: A Comparative Guide of US, MRI and Surgery

With Contributions by Pascal Rousset

Springer

Editor
Isabelle Thomassin-Naggara
Imageries Radiologiques et Interventionnelles
Spécialisées (IRIS)
Tenon Hospital, AP-HP,
Sorbonne Université
Paris, France

With Contributions by
Pascal Rousset
Department of Radiology
Lyon Sud University Hospital
Lyon, France

ISBN 978-3-031-82752-5 ISBN 978-3-031-82750-1 (eBook)
https://doi.org/10.1007/978-3-031-82750-1

This Springer imprint is published by the registered company Springer Nature Switzerland AG
The registered company address is: Gewerbestrasse 11, 6330 Cham, Switzerland

Contents

Part I Introduction

1 **Presentation of the Disease and Diagnostic Strategy** 3
Emile Darai and Isabelle Thomassin-Naggara

Part II Description of the Disease (US/MR/Surgical Correlation) (Radiologist/Surgeon)

2 **Peritoneal Endometriosis** 23
Elise Zareski, Aygline Paternostre, and Arnaud Fauconnier

3 **Adnexal Endometriosis. Typical Benign Endometriosis** 41
Sanja Stojanović, Vesna Kopitović, Luka Anđelić, Stevan Milatović, and Una Molnar

4 **Atypical Endometriosis and Malignant Transformation** 67
Helena Paixão and Teresa Margarida Cunha

5 **Anterocentral Compartment (Bladder, Round Ligament)** 87
Heng Zhang, Christine O. Menias, and Priyanka Jha

6 **Mediocentral Compartment: Torus Uterinum and Proximal Uterosacral Ligaments** 107
Adalgisa Guerra, Catarina Janicas, Marta Manso, and Inês Fortuna

7 **Mediocentral Compartment: Vaginal Endometriosis and Rectovaginal Septum** 123
Marie Florin and Yohann Dabi

8 **Mediocentral Compartment: Uterus: External Adenomyosis** 143
Rosemarie Forstner

9 **Posterocentral Compartment (Rectum)** 159
Pascal Rousset, Edouard Ruaux, Pierre-Adrien Bolze, Eddy Cotte, Isabelle Thomassin-Naggara, and François Golfier

10 Antero-, Medio-, and Posterolateral Compartments: Parametrium 187
Cyril Touboul, Isabelle Thomassin-Naggara, Yohann Dabi, Emile Darai, and Pascal Rousset

11 Lateral Deep Pelvic Endometriosis. Over Parietal Fascia: Nervous Locations 211
Luciana P. Chamié, Alice Brandão, and Izabela V. Pires Franco

12 Thoracic and Diaphragmatic Endometriosis 235
Aki Kido, Yuki Himoto, Toshihiro Ojima, and Tomoshi Tsuchiya

13 Extrapelvic Location: Abdominal Wall Endometriosis. Diagnostic and Interventional Imaging 243
Léo Razakamanantsoa and Milan Najdawi

Part III Technique and Reporting of the Different Imaging Techniques and Classifications

14 Techniques and Reporting of the Different Imaging Techniques and Classifications: Ultrasonography 263
Thierry Van den Bosch, Celine Bafort, and Dominique Van Schoubroeck

15 Techniques and Reporting of the Imaging Techniques and Classifications: MR Imaging 271
Isabelle Thomassin-Naggara, Rana Al Rouhban, and Lucia Manganaro

16 Technique and Reporting of the Imaging Techniques and Classifications: Laparoscopic Surgery 299
Adrien Crestani, Benjamin Merlot, and Horace Roman

Correction to: Techniques and Reporting of the Imaging Techniques and Classifications: MR Imaging C1
Isabelle Thomassin-Naggara, Rana Al Rouhban, and Lucia Manganaro

Part I

Introduction

1 Presentation of the Disease and Diagnostic Strategy

Emile Darai and Isabelle Thomassin-Naggara

1.1 Introduction

Endometriosis, defined by the presence of endometrium-like tissue outside the uterus (excluding adenomyosis), is thought to affect 2–10% of the female population, representing at least 190 million women worldwide [1, 2]. A recent French national study from 2011 to 2017 in women and girls aged 10 years and over, using comprehensive hospital discharge data, reported a crude incidence rate of 3.95/10,000 person-years [3]. Moreover from 2011 to 2017, the risk increased by 3.6% (95% CI: 0.6–6.8). This risk was geographically heterogeneous, suggesting the potential impact of environmental factors [3]. Endometriosis more frequently affects women of Philippine, Indian, Japanese, and Korean descent than the white population [4].

On one hand, the prevalence of endometriosis in the symptomatic population is reported to be 35%–50% [1]. On another hand, previous studies [1, 2, 5] have demonstrated that up to 80% of women with endometriosis exhibit a superficial peritoneal phenotype often ignored by imaging techniques. A superficial subtle lesion is named mild endometriosis [6]. In contrast, adnexal endometriosis and deep pelvic endometriosis exhibit more-aggressive behavior in some women with endometriosis and should be named endometriotic disease.

E. Darai (✉)
Gynecological and Obstetric Department, APHP Hopital Tenon, Sorbonne University, Paris, France
e-mail: emile.darai@aphp.fr

I. Thomassin-Naggara
Imageries Radiologiques et Interventionnelles Spécialisées (IRIS), Tenon Hospital, AP-HP, Sorbonne Université, Paris, France
e-mail: isabelle.thomassin@aphp.fr

1.2 Physiopathology

The physiopathology of endometriosis remains unknown [7, 8]. But a consensus has been reached on endometriosis as a multifactorial disease implicating the combined action of genetic, epigenetic, and environmental factors [9]. Endometriosis is an estrogen-dependent disease associated with the suppression of progesterone receptors [1]. Estrogen initiates the proliferation of the endometrial tissue and supports the growth of the endometrial glands before ovulation, preparing the endometrium for the action of progesterone. Estrogen and progesterone act by binding to their intracellular receptors, the estrogen receptor (ER) and progesterone receptor (PR), and members of the steroid/nuclear receptor (SR) superfamily [10]. Several abnormalities in the intracavitary endometrium and ectopic endometriotic tissue underlying endometriosis progression have been demonstrated: inflammation activated by excess estrogen biosynthesis,

I. Thomassin-Naggara (ed.), *Imaging of Endometriosis: A Comparative Guide of US, MRI and Surgery*, https://doi.org/10.1007/978-3-031-82750-1_1

defective differentiation due to progesterone resistance, the dysregulated differentiation of endometrial mesenchymal cells, and abnormal epigenetic factors. Among these, hypoxia and inflammation play important roles in the regulation of the steroidogenic pathway in the development of endometriosis [11, 12]. In endometriosis, progesterone and estrogen signaling are disrupted, commonly resulting in progesterone resistance and estrogen dominance [13].

Advances in technologies, candidate gene studies, gene association, and genome-wide association studies (GWASs) have been able to identify more than 30 candidate genes [14]. Moreover, 27 independent single-nucleotide polymorphisms (SNPs) are associated with endometriosis in GWASs, explaining over 5% of disease variances [15, 16]. However, the usefulness of these data for understanding the pathogenesis of endometriosis remains a matter of debate. Kennedy et al. suggested that the risk for first-degree relatives of women with severe endometriosis is six to nine times higher than that of unaffected women [17].

1.3 Symptoms

According to the 2022 ESHRE recommendations, endometriosis should be monitored not only in women with dysmenorrhea, pelvic pain, dyspareunia, dysuria, dyschezia, gastrointestinal symptoms such as diarrhea or constipation, rectorrhagia, and infertility but also in patients with less-specific signs, including back pain or chronic fatigue with the risk of overdiagnosis and overtreatment [18–20]. In addition, the lack of awareness of healthcare providers and the limited value of imaging techniques to diagnose all phenotypes of endometriosis (especially the superficial peritoneal endometriosis) contribute to delaying the diagnosis by an estimated 7–12 years, urging the use of new tools to assess the diagnosis. In this context, clinical history and pelvic examination raise the possibility of a diagnosis of endometriosis, but heterogeneity in clinical presentation, the high prevalence of asymptomatic endometriosis (2% to 50%), and the poor association between presenting symptoms and the severity of the disease contribute to difficulties in obtaining a reliable diagnosis of endometriosis on the sole basis of the presenting symptoms [21–23]. Indeed, in a prospective cross-sectional study, Tempest et al. assessed symptoms and nuclear magnetic resonance (NMR) spectroscopy–based metabolomics in 102 women before laparoscopic sterilization. Here, 12 women (11.7%) were incidentally diagnosed with endometriosis with a similar incidence of symptoms suggestive of endometriosis. Neither symptom, NMR, or both together could distinguish between patients with and without endometriosis [24].

1.4 Diagnostic Strategy

1.4.1 Questionaries

In this context of a lack of specificity in symptoms, many questionaries were developed to identify women with a high risk of endometriotic disease. Shafrir et al., comparing questionnaire-reported endometriosis with medical record notation from the Black Women's Health Study [25], found that patients who self-reported having endometriosis exhibited an accuracy of >70%, but this study also underlined the risk of misdiagnosis in about one-third of patients with symptoms suggestive of endometriosis. Bendifallah et al., using machine-learning algorithms (MLAs) in the diagnosis and screening of endometriosis, based on 16 key clinical and patient-based symptom features, reported respective sensitivity, specificity, F1-scores, and AUCs in the training and validation sets varying 0.82–1, 0–0.8, 0–0.88, and 0.5–0.89 and varying 0.91–0.95, 0.66–0.92, and 0.77–0.92, suggesting the potential relevance of an MLA as a self-evaluation tool to diagnose endometriosis [26]. Finally, in a case–control study including clinical symptoms and epidemiological data using a multiple regression model, Chapron et al. built two scoring systems. Score 1 is based on eight variables that aim to predict endometriosis (a family history of endometriosis, primary sterility, a BMI <22, and a short regular cycle (<28 j), and four Visual Analogic Scale (VAS) pain scores (i.e., dysmenorrhea ≥3 and deep/dyspareunia ≥6/gastrointestinal symptoms ≥5/urinary tract symptoms ≥1), with an AUC of 0.81 (95% CI: 79–83) and is validated on internal (C-index of 0.81) and external (C-index of 0.73) populations [27]. The authors determined three cutoff points: a score ≥25 with a specificity of 91%; a score <11 with a sensitivity of 91%; and a score ≥18, maximizing both sensitivity (73%) and specificity (75%). Score 2 avoided parameters that are subject to variations due to patient self-evaluations. According to five variables (a family history of endometriosis, primary sterility, a BMI <22, a short regular cycle (<28 j), Visual Analogic Scale (VAS) score for dysmenorrhea ≥3), on internal and external populations, score 2 had C-index values of 0.74 and 0.73, respectively, which did not support its use. The authors concluded that these scores may have high clinical value, allowing the selection of patients at a high risk of endometriosis with a cost-effective procedure that can readily be performed by patients themselves [27]. Conversely, Singh et al. evaluated the utility and impact of the painful periods screening tool (PPST) in improving healthcare delivery among patients with pelvic pain, aged between 18 and 55 years [28]. The PPST questionnaires were completed on the day of consultation and at 1–14 days after this clinic visit. Among the 1352 eligible patients, 1000 participants responded to both questionnaires. Severe pelvic/abdominal or lower back pain during menses was reported in 82.9% of patients. Moreover, 91.5% of participants reported that the PPST helped women to discuss their pain symptoms with healthcare providers (Table 1.1).

Other authors have underlined nonspecific types of symptoms, including gynecological and nongynecological conditions, making a timely diagnosis of endometriosis challenging and resulting in diagnostic delays of up to 10 years. In a real-world retrospective single-site [29], cross-sectional study of about 1000 women with surgically confirmed and/or clinically diagnosed endometriosis, the authors showed that more than half them had experienced chronic pelvic pain for ≥5 years and that the pain intensity was correlated with the number of prior physicians consulted. They concluded that the single-provider

Table 1.1 Endometriosis health profile-5 questionnaire

PART 1: DURING THE PAST 4 WEEKS, HOW OFTEN BECAUSE OF YOUR ENDOMETRIOSIS HAVE YOU…					
Please check whether you have ticked one box for each question before moving on to PART 2.	Never	Rarely	Sometimes	Often	Always
1. Found it difficult to walk because of the pain?					
2. Felt that symptoms are ruling your life?					
3. Had mood swings?					
4. Felt others do not understand what you are going through?					
5. Felt that your appearance has been affected?					
PART 2: DURING THE PAST 4 WEEKS, HOW OFTEN BECAUSE OF YOUR ENDOMETRIOSIS HAVE YOU…					
	Never	Rarely	Sometimes	Often	Always
A. Been unable to carry out duties at work because of the pain?					
B. Found looking after your child/children to be difficult?					
C. Felt worried about having sexual intercourse because of the pain?					
D. Felt that doctor(s) think your symptoms are all in your head?					
E. Felt frustrated because treatment is not working?					
F. Felt depressed at the possibility of not having children/more children?					

model of care was probably not adapted especially for women with nonmenstrual pelvic pain [29] and proposed alternative care models, including a multidisciplinary approach that has become a standard in France for women experiencing inefficacy during their medical treatment.

1.4.2 Role of Clinical Examination

Concerning physical examination, although an abnormal pelvic examination correlates with the presence of endometriosis on laparoscopy in 70% to 90% of cases [30], the differential diagnosis for most positive physical findings is wide. Furthermore, a normal clinical examination does not exclude endometriosis, because laparoscopically proven disease has been diagnosed in more than 50% of women with a clinically normal pelvic examination [31]. Recently, Roditis et al., in a retrospective study evaluating the ability of physical examination (PE), TVUS, and MRI alone and combined to diagnose deep pelvic endometriosis (DPE), demonstrated that the combination of PE, TVUS, and MRI was more accurate than each technique separately [32]. This improved accuracy was due mainly to the high sensitivity of MRI and to the high specificity of PE and TVUS, especially for vaginal endometriosis.

1.4.3 When to Use Different Imaging Techniques

Diagnosing endometriosis can be challenging due to its varied presentation and the fact that symptoms may mimic other conditions. The mean delay for the diagnosis of endometriosis is between 7 and 10 years in European countries. Various imaging techniques can aid in the diagnosis of endometriosis, each with its own strengths and limitations. Here are the different imaging techniques mentioned by Chat GPT for this issue: transvaginal ultrasound (TVUS), contrast-enhanced ultrasonography, magnetic resonance imaging, and laparoscopy.

Thus, these techniques are probably the most studied and detailed on the Internet. But is this list really accurate?

1.4.3.1 Laparoscopy

First, should we have to consider laparoscopy as a "diagnostic technique"? Historically and for many years recently, laparoscopy has been considered the only method to accurately diagnose pelvic endometriosis. In this setting, the former and most widely used classification for evaluating the disease is the American Society for Reproductive Medicine (ASRM) classification, which is a surgical classification that defines four stages of the disease, as follows, in its revised version: stage 1 (minimal); stage 2 (mild), including only peritoneal and ovarian locations; stage 3 (moderate), additionally including tubal lesions and Douglas pouch adhesions; and stage 4 (severe), which is used for describing deep pelvic endometriosis without taking into account the potential different impacts of the different DPE lesions.

Laparoscopy remains the best technique to diagnose superficial endometriosis given that other techniques have poor sensitivity values. It allows the direct visualization of endometrial implants, adhesions, and other pelvic abnormalities. Laparoscopy also enables tissue biopsy to confirm the diagnosis. However, it is an invasive procedure, requiring general anesthesia; it carries some risks; and the development of a salivary test [33] will probably dramatically decrease the indication of laparoscopy as a diagnostic tool.

1.4.3.2 Transvaginal Ultrasonography

TVUS is often the initial imaging modality used to evaluate pelvic pain and suspected endometriosis. It's relatively inexpensive and mini-invasive. Its sensitivity varies depending on the skill of the operator and the extent of disease involvement. It may offer improved resolution and better visualization of certain structures compared to other techniques, such as MR imaging.

The diagnostic performance of TVUS varies according to the type of locations: In 2016, Nisenblat et al. demonstrated in a Cochrane systematic review [34] that TVUS was as accurate as MRI or laparoscopy in diagnosing endometrioma, with a sensitivity of 0.93 (95% CI: 0.87–0.99) and a specificity of 0.96 (95% CI: 0.92–0.99). However, in that same paper, TVUS was shown to have lower sensitivity (0.79 (95% CI: 0.69–0.89)) than that of MRI in diagnosing deep pelvic endometriosis (0.94 (95% CI: 0.90–0.97)).

In a retrospective multicenter study involving 878 patients between 15 and 45 years old undergoing laparoscopy (LPS) for suspected endometriosis, Abrao et al. [35] evaluated transvaginal and transabdominal US (index test) to assess all sites of endometriosis according to the 2021 AAGL Endometriosis Classification. The AAGL-US and AAGL-LPS stages were concordant in 586 cases (66.7%) (weighted kappa [WK] 0.759; intraclass correlation = 0.906), with the highest agreement observed in patients with no endometriosis (n = 70, 75.3% concordance), AAGL-LPS stage 1 (104, 50.7%), and stage 4 disease (358, 88.2%). Endometriosis was most accurately diagnosed in the rectum/sigmoid (WK 0.862), bladder (WK 0.911), and ovaries (WK 0.835/0.795 for right/left, respectively) while being less diagnosed for superficial peritoneal (WK 0.442), tubal (WK 0.391 and 0.363 for right and left, respectively), and retrocervical/uterosacral ligament (WK 0.656) sites.

In a prospective study of 172 patients, Ros et al. [36] evaluated the accuracy of TVUS in diagnosing DPE involving uterosacral ligaments (USL), torus uterinum (TU), or posterior vaginal fornix (PVF) compared to laparoscopy. The global sensitivity and specificity of TVUS in diagnosing USL, TU, and/or PVF endometriosis were 92% and 87%, respectively. The accuracy, sensitivity, specificity, positive predictive value (PPV), negative predictive value (NPV), LR +, and LR- of TVUS for USL and TU were 0.895, 96.6%, 82.1%, 85.0%, 95.8%, 5.41, and 0.04 and 0.866, 83.9%, 89.4%, 89.0%, 84.4%, 7.92, and 0.18, respectively, and for PVF were 0.936, 87.0%, 94.6%, 71.4%, 97.9%, 16.20, and 0.14, respectively.

In a prospective study of 120 patients, Goncalves et al. [37] evaluated the value of TVUS with bowel preparation (TVUS-BP) when diagnosing ovarian and DPE locations compared to diagnostic laparoscopy. The results showed that the diagnostic performances were significantly different depending on the disease site. Laparoscopy was not able to diagnose vaginal endometriosis (sensitivity and specificity 0%), whereas TVUS-BP exhibited a respective sensitivity and specificity, of 85.7% and 99.1%, respectively. For rectosigmoid endometriosis, laparoscopy had a poor sensitivity, of 3.7–5.6%, compared to 96.3% for TVUS ($p < 0.001$). However, importantly, the evaluators of the laparoscopic video were blinded to the physical examination.

In a meta-analysis, Zhou et al. [38] evaluated the accuracy of TVUS for USL endometriosis. Among 7562 studies, 11 were included in the meta-analysis. The pooled sensitivity, specificity, positive probability ratio (LR+), and negative probability ratio (LR−) of TVUS in detecting USL endometriosis were 65% (95% CI: 43–83), 92% (95% CI: 84–96), 7.80 (95% CI: 4.7–13.0), and 0.38 (95% CI: 0.22–0.66), respectively. There was significant heterogeneity in sensitivity (I^2: 97.40%; Cochran Q, 385.09; $p < 0.001$) and specificity (I^2, 93.89%; Cochran Q, 163.75; $p < 0.001$).

Another review including 22 articles and focusing on USL endometriosis, Maple et al. [39] underlined that most (20/22) studies described abnormal criteria for USL on TVUS, but only five determined the appearance of normal USL, and only 11 provided the techniques applied. This review underlined the lack of data and consensus on the analysis of USL.

In a meta-analysis, Alcazar et al. [40] reported the diagnostic accuracy of the sliding sign on TVUS in detecting pouch of Douglas obliteration and bowel endometriosis compared to laparoscopy. Among 334 studies, eight were included in the meta-analysis, resulting in 938 and 963 patients available for analysis. The mean prevalence values of pouch of Douglas obliteration and bowel involvement were 37% and 23%, respectively. The pooled estimated sensitivity, specificity, LR+, LR−, and diagnostic odds ratio of the sliding sign on TVS for detecting pouch of Douglas obliteration were 88% (95% CI: 81–93%), 94% (95% CI: 91–96%), 15.3 (95% CI: 10.2–22.9), 0.12 (95% CI: 0.07–0.21), and 123 (95% CI: 62–244), respectively. The heterogeneity was moderate for sensitivity and low for specificity in detecting pouch of Douglas obliteration. The pooled estimated sensitivity, specificity, LR+, LR−, and diagnostic odds ratio on TVUS for detecting bowel involvement were 81% (95% CI: 64–91%), 95% (95% CI: 91–97%), 16.0 (95% CI: 9.0–28.6), 0.20 (95% CI: 0.10–0.40), and 81 (95% CI: 34–191), respectively. The heterogeneity of data on diagnostic accuracy for bowel involvement was high. On the contribution of using the sliding sign to diagnose DPE, this technique raises some concerns on the acceptability of TVUS given the relation between sonographic signs of endometriosis and the occurrence of pain.

In a meta-analysis including 10 prospective studies, Gerges et al. evaluated USL, rectovaginal septum (RVS), and vagina endometriosis via TVUS and MRI compared to surgery [41]. For USL endometriosis, the respective pooled sensitivity and specificity for all TVS and MRI techniques were 60% (95% CI: 32–82%) and 95% (95% CI: 90–98%) for TVS techniques and 81% (95% CI: 66–90%) and 83% (95% CI: 62–94%) for MRI techniques. For RVS endometriosis, the respective pooled sensitivity and specificity for all TVUS techniques were 57% (95% CI: 30–80%) and 100% (95% CI: 92–100%). For vaginal endometriosis, the respective pooled sensitivity and specificity for all TVS and MRI techniques were 52% (95% CI: 29–74%) and 98% (95% CI: 95–99%) for TVS techniques and 64% (95% CI: 40–83%) and 98% (96% CI: 93–99%) for MRI techniques. Pooled analyses were not possible for other imaging modalities. Despite some limits linked to the low quality of evidence, the high risk of bias, and the heterogeneity of the included studies, MRI outperformed TVUS in the diagnosis of USL, RVS, and vaginal endometriosis, with higher sensitivities but similar specificity for both techniques. The results were improved with the addition of bowel preparation or ultrasound gel, although this conclusion is based on individual studies.

More recently, a large international consensus statement [42] related to the use of imaging techniques for the noninvasive diagnosis and classification of DPE focused their analysis on the different sites of DPE and separately analyzed uterosacral ligaments, the vaginal pouch, rectosigmoid locations, perimetrium locations, and bladder locations.

1. *The rectosigmoid*

   They concluded that TVUS demonstrated equal sensitivity (0.89) and equal specificity (0.97) to that of MRI in diagnosing rectosigmoid. Also, they reached a consensus of 86.8% of yes among 51 experts to the following question: “Imaging with TVS can reliably preoperatively predict, and is recommended to detect, the presence of DPE in the rectum but is less accurate in sigmoidal DPE due to limited visibility.”
2. *Uterosacral ligaments, the rectovaginal septum, and the vagina*

   An intersociety consensus statement concludes that in most studies, including the meta-analysis of prospective studies by Gerges et al. [41], TVUS is consistently outperformed by MRI, with sensitivities and specificities for USL of 60%/95% and 81%/83%, respectively, and those for vaginal of 52%/97% and 64%/98%, respectively.
3. *The bladder*

   A few studies exist on the lower frequency of this location. Intersociety consensus reveals the equal poor/high sensitivity of both TVUS and MRI.
4. *The parametrium*

   TVUS is less precise than MRI in assessing this also-infrequent location due to the distance of these locations (lateral as posterior ones) to the probe and their usual poor contrast.

The intersociety consensus paper stated that TVUS performed by adequately trained operators is recommended as first-line imaging tool due to its availability, good test performance, cost-efficiency, and low environmental impact when compared to other imaging methods (level evidence 1a, grade of statement A, consensus 96.2% (49/51)). If TVUS is sensitive enough to diagnose endometrioma and rectal locations, MRI is recommended to exclude other deep pelvic locations, such as USLs and the parametrium.

Some authors have suggested the potential of using contrast-enhanced ultrasonography in the diagnosis of endometriosis, particularly in evaluating vascularity and the inflammation associated with endometriotic lesions.

1.4.3.3 Magnetic Resonance Imaging

MRI is more sensitive than ultrasound in detecting DPE, especially for uterosacral ligaments, the vagina, and the rectovaginal septum, which are the most frequent locations of deep pelvic endometriosis. Several meta-analyses have demonstrated that MRI is recommended as a second-line technique in a symptomatic patient in the context of negative US findings [43, 44]. MRI can provide detailed anatomical information and give functional information relative to the detection of hemorrhagic implants that suggest the presence of active disease that may be sensitive to medical hormonal treatment. Optimally, MRI should be combined with TVUS and a physical examination to improve its specificity. In a recent study, our team demonstrated the value of a model combining a physical examination, TVUS, and MRI to correctly diagnose endometriosis in the uterosacral ligament and in the vagina [32]. This model suggests positivity when two of three modalities are positive. This is a way to solve the lack of specificity of MR imaging in the diagnosis of uterosacral locations. Another way is to use the fusion technique: A fused MR/US examination helps the sonographer to focus on the region of interest and ensure that they are searching for the USL in the right place.

In addition, a third meta-analysis showed that MRI is a useful preoperative test for predicting the diagnosis of multiple sites of DPE [45]. Indeed, MRI provides an exhaustive mapping of all endometriotic locations and assesses the extent of disease involvement, aiding in surgical planning. In this setting, during the development of a classification, such as the deep Pelvic Endometriosis INdex (dPEI) classification [46], that classification must demonstrate its ability to accurately predict the operating duration, hospital stay, and postoperative complications. The major strength of this classification is the correlation of the score with the presence of lateral locations, giving two points when the patient has lateral and posterior parametrial locations. No other techniques, including laparoscopy, can exhaustively describe these lateral locations. This is why MRI is so preoperatively crucial to limit the number of inefficient surgeries that lead to pelvic pain recurrence. This point also underlines the methodological limitations of many studies on TVUS that take laparoscopy as a reference standard.

With a goal to externally validate dPEI scores and the necessity of standardizing the analysis of MR imaging, Rousset et al. elaborated a lexicon of image interpretation and a standardized region-based reporting of DIE with MRI using the RAND-UCLA Appropriateness Method to attain consensus guidelines [47]. A consensus regarding pelvic compartment delineation and DIE reporting was thereby attained. The pelvis was divided into nine compartments and extra-pelvic lesions were assigned to an additional (tenth) compartment. A consensus was also reached for each structure attributed to a compartment and each reporting template item among the experts. No consensus was reached on the normal presentation of uterosacral ligaments, but a consensus was reached on an unequivocal involvement leading to a positive diagnosis and an equivocal involvement leading to an uncertain diagnosis. An external validation of a dPEI score was performed in France in seven endometriotic expert centers and demonstrated a linear correlation between operating time and hospital stay [48]. Moreover, this score defines three levels of the severity of the disease regarding its risk of postoperative complications: a low-risk disease (3%) (score 1–2), a moderate-risk disease (7%) (score 3–4) and a high-risk disease (10%) (score 5 and more).

In the context of presurgical staging, imaging techniques should be combined because MRI will be more accurate or TVUS will be more accurate depending on the surgeon. For example, regarding the digestive tract, multifocality and multicentricity as well as the distance to the anal margin will be better via MRI than TVUS, whereas the length, thickness, and circumference of the nodule in the rectal wall will be better assessed via TVUS than MRI.

1.4.3.4 Rectal Echoendoscopy

Rectal echo endoscopy is not recommended as a simple diagnostic technique. This is a third-line technique that can be useful before planning a surgery. This technique is particularly accurate in evaluating the rectal wall and thus the depth and the length of rectal disease, allowing the discussion of the type of colorectal surgery, including rectal shaving, discoid excision, or segmental resection [49].

1.4.4 Role of Biological Markers

Concerning biological endometriosis diagnosis, a variety of tests utilizing blood markers, eutopic endometrium characteristics, urinary markers, or peritoneal fluid components have been suggested as diagnostic tools of endometriosis. Although large numbers of the reported markers have distinguished women with and without endometriosis in small pilot studies, many have not shown convincing potential as a diagnostic test when evaluated in larger studies by different research groups. The diagnostic value of these tests has been fully evaluated by a Cochrane Review [34], concluding that no simple noninvasive test for the diagnosis of endometriosis is routinely implemented in clinical practice. This explains why 2022 ESHRE recommendations [50] did not recommend the use of a biological test for endometriosis diagnosis. Since the publication of these guidelines, new tools deserve to be underlined. In a study involving 80 patients with endometriosis and 80 controls, Chunli Lin et al. evaluated in serum samples the expression of miR-17-5p, miR-424-5p, VEGFA, IL-4, and IL-6 levels. For endometriosis diagnosis, the AUC of miR-17-5p was 0.865 (a cutoff value of 0.890 with respective sensitivity and specificity values of 91.3% and 85%), the AUC of miR-424-5p was 0.737 (a cutoff value of 0.915 with respective sensitivity and specificity values of 98.8% and 61.2%) [51]. The AUC of the combination of miR-424-5p with miR-17-5p was 0.938 (a cutoff value of 2.205 with respective sensitivity and specificity values of 93.8% and 88.7%). In a retrospective series involving 85 patients with endometriosis and 86 controls, Shan et al. explored the plasma extracellular vesicle–derived lncRNA using qRT-PCR. Among 210 patients with dysregulated lmicroRNA, the expression of LINC01569, RP3-399 L15.2, FAM138B, and CH507-513H4.6 was decreased, whereas the expression of RP11-326 N17.2, KLHL7-AS1, and MIR548XHG was increased in patients with endometriosis. At the cutoff point, the combined expression of RP3-399 L15.2 and CH507-513H4.6 revealed a sensitivity of 80%, a specificity of 85.45%, and an AUC of 0.9045. Moreover, CH507-513H4.6 alone may be useful in detecting early-stage endometriosis lesions. As endometriosis could be considered an autoimmune disorder, in a cross-sectional study, Svensson et al. evaluated the serum levels of TSH receptor antibodies (TRAb), showing that TRAb IgG above ≥0.3 IE/L was observed in 94.5% of patients with endometriosis compared to 7.9% of the controls ($p < 0.001$), but no increase in autoantibodies against FSH, FSH receptor (FSHR), hCG, LH, LH receptor (LHR), or TSH was observed. Thanks to the absence of cross-reactivity with other autoantibodies, TRAb could be used as a diagnostic tool for endometriosis. Moreover, TRAb titers did not correlate with age, disease duration, AXIN1, TSH, thyroid hormones, or gastrointestinal symptoms. In a cross-sectional study of adolescents and young adults (142 with endometriosis at laparoscopy and 74 controls), Sasamoto et al. evaluated 1305 plasma protein levels with the multiplex aptamer–based proteomics discovery platform SOMAscan. They identified 63 proteins associated with endometriosis with an absolute fold change >1.2. Dysregulated proteins were related mainly to angiogenesis and cell migration [52]. Visnic et al.

reported, in a preliminary study evaluating urinary proteins via chromatography and mass spectrometry (LC–MS/MS) in 16 patients with endometriosis and 16 control patients, that 17 proteins were differentially expressed from among the groups. Among these proteins, five are implicated in invasion, migration, and cell proliferation (Lumican, TGF beta receptor type-2, Tetraspanin-1, CD44 antigen, and Tenascin), two in cell proteolysis (Cathepsin G and Cathepsin L), three in immune reactions (inducible T-cell costimulatory ligand, Interleukin-18-binding protein and Annexin A2), six in cell adhesion (Desmoplakin, Thrombospondin 1, Protocadherin 1, Protocadherin gamma-C3, SPARC-like1, and Zinc-alpha-2-glucoprotein), and one in the vascular system (Endoglin) [53]. Jansa et al. evaluated the plasma levels of the cartilage oligomeric matrix protein (COMP) and transforming growth factor-b-induced protein ig-h3 (TGFBI) via the enzyme-linked immuno sorbent assay (ELISA) technique alone or in combination with CA-125 in a discovery phase (32 patients with endometriosis and 24 control patients) and then in a validation phase (166 patients with endometriosis and 71 control patients) [54]. TGFBI exhibited a fair diagnostic potential (AUC = 0.77, sensitivity = 58%, and specificity = 84%). TGFBI and CA-125 had a better relevance (AUC = 0.91, sensitivity = 88%, and specificity = 75%), whereas no difference was observed for COMP. Using the Gene Expression Omnibus (GEO) and Array-Express database, thanks to the development of sequencing technology and a random forest classifier, She et al. identified seven differentially expressed genes (DEGs) (COMT, NAA16, CCDC22, EIF3E, AHI1, DMXL2, and CISD3) in patients with endometriosis. Among them, AHI1, DMXL2, and CISD3 had not been previously reported [55]. The seven DEGs were included in 15 hub genes identified from the constructed protein–protein interaction (PPI) network. The AUC values of the seven DEGs were 0.8226, 0.6623, 0.6836, 0.6625, 0.8367, 0.8471, and 0.8617. In the verification results of the GSE7307 dataset, the AUC values of the seven DEGs were 0.74, 0.64, 0.70, 0.63, 0.90, 0.82, and 0.83. Qin et al. showed that small molecular metabolites derived from gut microbiota, including second bile acid biosynthesis and alpha-linolenic acid (ALA) metabolism, are enriched in endometriosis patients [56]. Huang et al. demonstrated that the predictive value of vaginal microbiota had a lower diagnostic value than gut microbiota. Ruminococcus and pseudomonas have been identified as potential biomarkers in intestinal and peritoneal fluids for diagnosing endometriosis [57].

The most relevant study is the prospective trial using next-generation sequencing (NGS), artificial intelligence (AI) and machine learning (ML) to analyze the human miRNome [58]. These authors developed a blood-based miRNA diagnostic signature for endometriosis. After internal validation, the signature composed of 86 miRNAs was confirmed to provide respective sensitivity, specificity, and AUC values of 96.8%, 100%, and 98.4, which are sufficiently robust and reproducible to replace the gold standard of diagnostic laparoscopy. Subsequently, on the same prospective cohort, the authors developed a salivary miRNA signature of endometriosis composed of 109 miRNAs [58]. The respective sensitivity, specificity, and AUC values for the diagnostic miRNA signature were 96.7%, 100%, and 0,98. Finally, in an interim external validation, the authors confirmed the relevance of the saliva miRNA signature for endometriosis with respective sensitivity, specificity, and AUC values of 96.2%, 95.1%, and 0.96 [33], rendering diagnostic laparoscopy obsolete. Recently, according to the final data of the external multicentric external validation of the saliva miRNA signature (not yet published), the French minister of health has accepted the reimbursement for this noninvasive test from 2025.

Thanks to the development of the saliva miRNA signature, the role of diagnostic laparoscopy is questionable. On one hand, laparoscopy, even less invasive than laparotomy, by nature cannot be transformed into a mini-invasive tool because it would impose surgery with anesthesia and expose patients to some surgical complications. On another hand, in a review on the diagnostic tools available to diagnose endometriosis, the respective sensitivity and specificity values of laparoscopy were 90–94% and 40–79% depending on surgeon experience, so negative laparoscopy did not exclude the diagnosis. Finally, the definition of *noninvasive* varies between medical dictionaries, but a consensus exists on preferring a procedure that does not involve the penetration of skin or physical entrance into the body [59–61]. Some imaging techniques with an intracavitary approach (transvaginal or transrectal sonography) must be qualified as invasive rather than noninvasive or minimally invasive, especially when the goal is to correlate pain with imaging abnormalities.

1.5 Diagnostic and Treatment Strategies

Several scientific societies have proposed different diagnostic algorithms to define the place of clinical, imaging, and biological features in improving diagnostic strategies and in reducing the delay of diagnosis in a context of long delay before applying any diagnostic of endometriotic disease. In 2017, the French college of gynecologists and obstetricians (CNGOF) published an algorithm validated by the High Authority of French Health [62] (Fig. 1.1). According to the strategy proposed, management is divided into three levels. The first level is a screening level with a first-line strategy performed by a family physician, midwife, or gynecologist; a second-line strategy involving an expert gynecologist, radiologist, and sonographer; and a third-line strategy dedicated to preoperative staging if a surgery is selected. In this algorithm are different levels of expertise for transvaginal ultrasonography and a mention of radiological expertise in endometriosis. This algorithm has many similarities with the one proposed in 2022 by the European Society of Reproductive Health Endometriosis (ESHRE) (Fig. 1.2) [50]. Empirical medical treatment has a place in a diagnostic strategy. ESHRE recommendations did not exclude the possibility of diagnostic laparoscopy in the case of a failure of empirical treatment and discordance between clinical symptoms and imaging results. Several authors have demonstrated a strong correlation between the history/number of surgeries for endometriosis and the severity of endometriosis disease [63]. However, iterative surgeries for DPE have been well demonstrated to potentially induce pelvic adhesions that may increase pain symptoms [64].

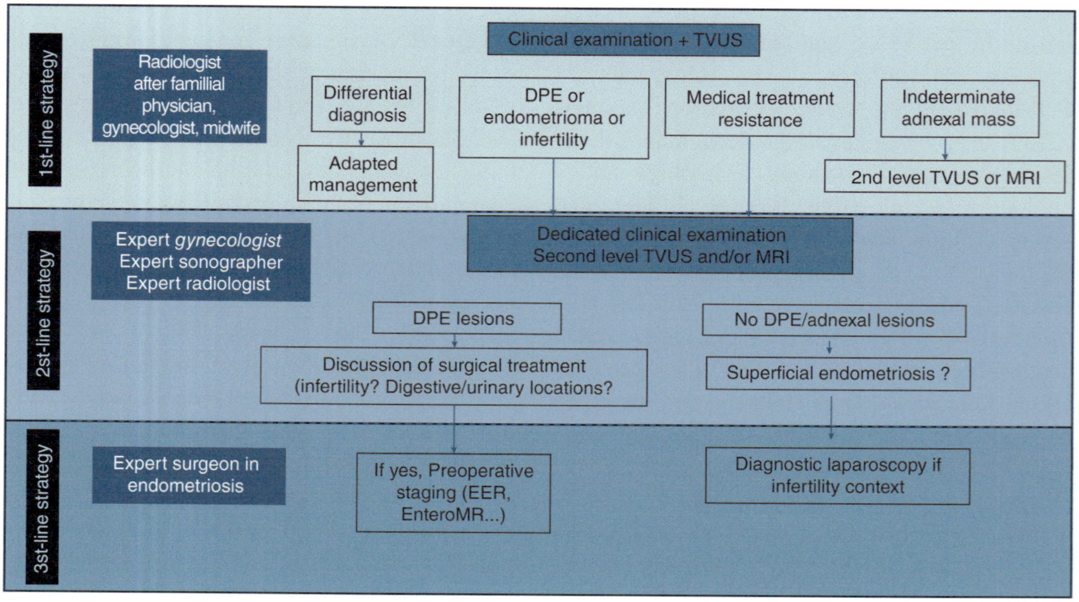

Fig. 1.1 CNGOF-HAS diagnostic strategy algorithm

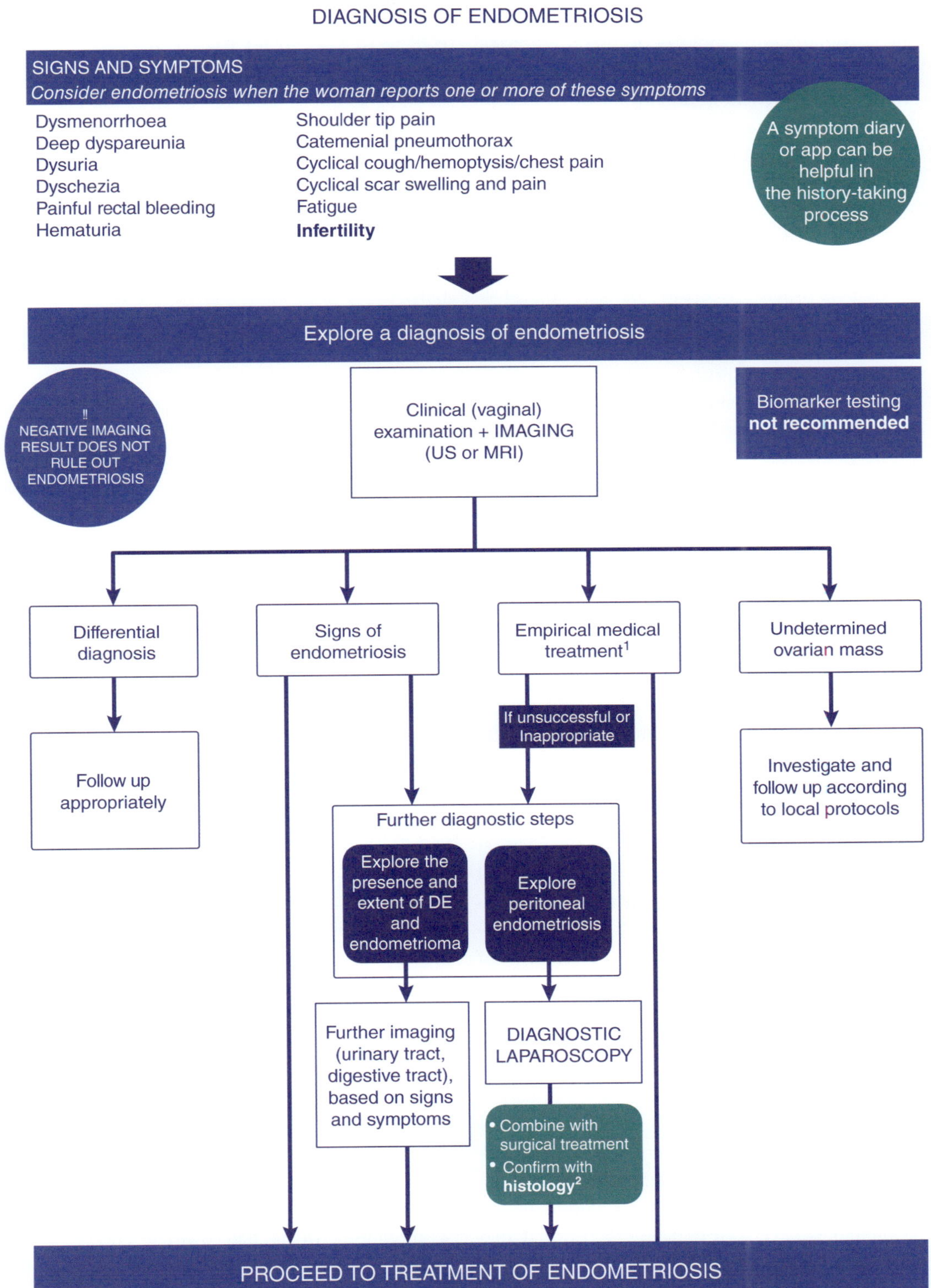

Fig. 1.2 ESHRE diagnostic strategy algorithm

Thus, the main objective of the improvement of a diagnostic strategy would be to avoid empirical therapy that is associated with a high failure rate and high dissatisfaction among patients, to limit the number of unsuccessful surgeries and to reserve surgical indication to resistant pelvic pain and fertility issues with a therapeutic objective. Many authors have demonstrated the role of colorectal surgery for DPE to improve the fertility of patients [65–67], and depending on the age of the patient and the history of infertility, if an assisted reproductive technology (ART) was already begun, a dedicated multidisciplinary team session will indicate a DPE surgery.

ESHRE recommendations specify the absence of a place for biomarker testing in a diagnostic strategy. The development and validation of a saliva-based miRNA diagnostic signature for endometriosis with sensitivity and specificity values >90% [33] may change diagnostic strategies in the next future.

1.5.1 Adolescents

The exact prevalence of endometriosis in adolescents remains unknown, although estimates suggest that about two-thirds of female adolescents with chronic pelvic pain that is nonresponsive to nonsteroidal anti-inflammatory drugs (NSAIDs) or oral contraceptives exhibit endometriosis at laparoscopy [68, 69]. In this review, the largest review, including 880 adolescents with dysmenorrhea or pelvic pain, Janssen E. et al. laparoscopically confirmed the presence of endometriosis in 62% of cases.

Although the relationship between endometriosis and dysmenorrhea in adolescents remains unclear, dysmenorrhea is the most common gynecological symptom in adolescence, with a prevalence of 50% to 90% [2], affecting physical and mental health in the form of school absenteeism, sleep disturbances, anxiety, and depression, representing an important social public health problem [70, 71]. Dai et al. demonstrated that adolescents experiencing dysmenorrhea had an increased risk of developing adult endometriosis (OR = 18.874, 95% CI = 10.309–34.555) compared to patients with occasional dysmenorrhea [72]. The risk of developing endometriosis was higher in adolescents experiencing dysmenorrhea lasting more than 12 months after menarche (OR = 5.257, 95% CI = 3.343–8.266). Adolescents experiencing dysmenorrhea frequently reported gastrointestinal and urinary symptoms, which came with a risk of misdiagnosis and delayed diagnosis. Thus, adolescent endometriosis diagnosis is a crucial challenge. Indeed, Dun et al. [73] reported that teenagers experiencing pain for at least 22.8 months were evaluated by at least three specialists before endometriosis was diagnosed [73].

The evaluation of an adolescent with endometriosis suspicion should include a comprehensive medical, gynecologic, and family history. Age at menarche, the regularity of the menstrual cycle, menstruation duration, the characteristics of menstrual bleeding, and the time interval between menarche and dysmenorrhea onset should be recorded [74]. A pelvic examination should be considered to exclude differential diagnosis, such as a pelvic mass or a reproductive tract abnormality. But gynecological examination is not possible in nonsexually active adolescents, and a digital rectal examination is not always acceptable. In this setting, imaging techniques play a crucial role but also have some limits, especially the feasibility of TVUS in virgin adolescents [75]. Moreover, as aforementioned, both TVUS and MRI can ignore endometriosis. Indeed, in a recent register-based cross-sectional cohort study, Rasp et al. reported that peritoneal endometriosis and ovarian endometriosis were the most common types: 72% and 23%, respectively. The incidence rate of surgically confirmed endometriosis per 100,000 person-years varied from 5.63 (95% CI: 4.24–7.33) to 11.42 (95% CI: 9.64–13.44). These results contrast with those of Millischer et al., who reported that the prevalence of endometriosis at MRI was 39.3% and that 20.7% of adolescents with endometriosis had ovarian endometriosis and 88.4% had DPE. In this paper, the authors demonstrated that severe endometriosis phenotypes (Ovarian endometriosis and/or Deep endometriosis) can be observed in adolescents with intense dysmenorrhea, with a linear increase in prevalence over time that results in a clear predominance after 18 years of age [76].

All these data underline the need for new tools accurately to assess the diagnosis of endometriosis in adolescents who avoid diagnostic laparoscopy. In this setting, thanks to the high accuracy of the saliva miRNA signature of endometriosis in adults, we are expecting the results of the ongoing trial evaluating this biological signature in the adolescent population.

1.5.2 Postoperative Endometriosis

The risk of disease recurrence is influenced by factors such as the disease's location and severity and by the surgeon's expertise and the invasiveness of the surgical procedure [77, 78]. The recurrence of ovarian disease is contingent upon the type of resection performed and can be readily diagnosed by radiologists using transvaginal ultrasonography (TVUS) or magnetic resonance imaging (MRI). Conversely, diagnosing recurrence in patients who have undergone surgery for deep pelvic endometriosis can be challenging because the imaging features of postoperative fibrotic scarring may mimic deep pelvic endometriosis. In such cases, radiologists require precise information on the surgery date, the type, any postoperative complications, and hormonal blockade [79]. Although consensus is lacking on the optimal timing for postsurgical imaging, waiting at least 6 months, at which time surgical tissue repair activity is minimal, is generally recommended [79]. No studies have directly compared the effectiveness of TVUS versus MRI in this context. Both modalities may reveal fibrotic scars as bands, plaques, or linear tracks in dissected peritoneal areas. With TVUS, these scars appear as low-echogenic infiltrations with acoustic shadowing, complicating examination interpretation [80]. Conversely, on MR imaging, these scars typically present with low T2 signal intensity, appearing darker and thinner than fibrotic endometriotic tissue. However, distinguishing these scars from recurrent or residual endometriotic tissue after surgery remains challenging [80]. In our clinical practice, MRI is preferred over TVUS due to its ability to detect hemorrhagic implants, which are specific features of recurrence. Radiologists must carefully evaluate these imaging findings to avoid false positives because misdiagnosis may lead to unnecessary, more-complex surgeries with higher postoperative complication risks compared to the initial procedure. Failure to detect recurrence can have detrimental consequences for the patient.

1.6 Conclusion

Another crucial issue of endometriosis diagnosis algorithms is the obsolescence of medical knowledge. This highlights the need for constantly analyzing and updating medical guidelines. Indeed, as stated by Densen [81], although the evolution of medical knowledge took about 50 years to double in 1950, it took only about 7 years to double in 1980, 3.5 years in 2010, and 73 days in 2020. Therefore, although this current work could be the object of similar criticism, our aim is to evaluate whether currently available medical data provide sufficient evidence for the evolution of the conventional diagnostic algorithm for endometriosis. The choice of imaging modality depends on various factors, including the patient's symptoms, clinical suspicion, the availability of resources, and the expertise of the healthcare provider. Often, a combination of imaging techniques and clinical assessment is necessary for accurate diagnosis and treatment planning in endometriosis. Combining the assessment of women who have potential DPE by using mini-invasive imaging via TVUS and/or MRI by adequately trained clinicians with the planning of surgical and/or conservative management approaches should be the standard of care in healthcare facilities offering endometriosis therapy.

References

1. Giudice LC, Kao LC. Endometriosis. Lancet. 2004;364(9447):1789–99. https://doi.org/10.1016/S0140-6736(04)17403-5.
2. Zondervan KT, Becker CM, Missmer SA. Endometriosis. N Engl J Med. 2020;382(13):1244–56. https://doi.org/10.1056/NEJMra1810764.
3. Le Moal J, Goria S, Chesneau J, et al. Increasing incidence and spatial hotspots of hospitalized endometriosis in France from 2011 to 2017. Sci Rep. 2022;12(1):6966. https://doi.org/10.1038/s41598-022-11017-x.
4. Yamamoto A, Johnstone EB, Bloom MS, Huddleston HG, Fujimoto VY. A higher prevalence of endometriosis among Asian women does not contribute to poorer IVF outcomes. J Assist Reprod Genet. 2017;34(6):765–74. https://doi.org/10.1007/s10815-017-0919-1.
5. Farland LV, Horne AW. Disparity in endometriosis diagnoses between racial/ethnic groups. BJOG. 2019;126(9):1115–6. https://doi.org/10.1111/1471-0528.15805.
6. Koninckx PR, Oosterlynck D, D'Hooghe T, Meuleman C. Deeply infiltrating endometriosis is a disease whereas mild endometriosis could be considered a non-disease. Ann N Y Acad Sci. 1994;734:333–41. https://doi.org/10.1111/j.1749-6632.1994.tb21763.x.
7. Yuan Z, Wang L, Wang Y, et al. Tubal origin of ovarian endometriosis. Mod Pathol. 2014;27(8):1154–62. https://doi.org/10.1038/modpathol.2013.245.
8. Zubrzycka A, Zubrzycki M, Janecka A, Zubrzycka M. New horizons in the etiopathogenesis and non-invasive diagnosis of endometriosis. Curr Mol Med. 2015;15(8):697–713. https://doi.org/10.2174/1566524015666150921105218.
9. Vassilopoulou L, Matalliotakis M, Zervou MI, et al. Defining the genetic profile of endometriosis. Exp Ther Med. 2019;17(5):3267–81. https://doi.org/10.3892/etm.2019.7346.
10. Rahmioglu N, Nyholt DR, Morris AP, Missmer SA, Montgomery GW, Zondervan KT. Genetic variants underlying risk of endometriosis: insights from meta-analysis of eight genome-wide association and replication datasets. Hum Reprod Update. 2014;20(5):702–16. https://doi.org/10.1093/humupd/dmu015.
11. Shao R, Cao S, Wang X, Feng Y, Billig H. The elusive and controversial roles of estrogen and progesterone receptors in human endometriosis. Am J Transl Res. 2014;6(2):104–13.
12. Yilmaz BD, Bulun SE. Endometriosis and nuclear receptors. Hum Reprod Update. 2019;25(4):473–85. https://doi.org/10.1093/humupd/dmz005.
13. Bulun SE, Yilmaz BD, Sison C, et al. Endometriosis. Endocr Rev. 2019;40(4):1048–79. https://doi.org/10.1210/er.2018-00242.
14. Zondervan KT, Rahmioglu N, Morris AP, et al. Beyond endometriosis genome-wide association study: from genomics to phenomics to the patient. Semin Reprod Med. 2016;34(4):242–54. https://doi.org/10.1055/s-0036-1585408.
15. Sapkota Y, Low S-K, Attia J, et al. Association between endometriosis and the interleukin 1A (IL1A) locus. Hum Reprod. 2015;30(1):239–48. https://doi.org/10.1093/humrep/deu267.
16. Rahmioglu N, Mortlock S, Ghiasi M, et al. The genetic basis of endometriosis and comorbidity with other pain and inflammatory conditions. Nat Genet. 2023;55(3):423–36. https://doi.org/10.1038/s41588-023-01323-z.
17. Kashima K, Ishimaru T, Okamura H, et al. Familial risk among Japanese patients with endometriosis. Int J Gynaecol Obstet. 2004;84(1):61–4. https://doi.org/10.1016/s0020-7292(03)00340-0.
18. Nicolaus K, Reckenbeil L, Bräuer D, Sczesny R, Diebolder H, Runnebaum IB. Cycle-related diarrhea and dysmenorrhea are independent predictors of peritoneal endometriosis, cycle-related Dyschezia is an independent predictor of rectal involvement. Geburtshilfe Frauenheilkd. 2020;80(3):307–15. https://doi.org/10.1055/a-1033-9588.
19. Alkatout I, Wedel T, Maass N. [Combined treatment of endometriosis: radical yet gentle]. Aktuelle Urol. 2018;49(1):60–72. https://doi.org/10.1055/s-0043-122175.
20. Freytag D, Peters G, Mettler L, Gitas G, Maass N, Alkatout I. Perioperative considerations in the treatment of endometriosis. J Turk Ger Gynecol Assoc. 2021;22(4):319–25. https://doi.org/10.4274/jtgga.galenos.2021.2021.0017.
21. Spaczynski RZ, Duleba AJ. Diagnosis of endometriosis. Semin Reprod Med. 2003;21(2):193–208. https://doi.org/10.1055/s-2003-41326.
22. Fauconnier A, Chapron C. Endometriosis and pelvic pain: epidemiological evidence of the relationship and implications. Hum Reprod Update. 2005;11(6):595–606. https://doi.org/10.1093/humupd/dmi029.
23. Ballard KD, Seaman HE, de Vries CS, Wright JT. Can symptomatology help in the diagnosis of endometriosis? Findings from a national case-control study—Part 1. BJOG. 2008;115(11):1382–91. https://doi.org/10.1111/j.1471-0528.2008.01878.x.
24. Tempest N, Hill CJ, Whelan A, et al. Symptomatology and serum nuclear magnetic resonance metabolomics; do they predict endometriosis in fertile women undergoing laparoscopic sterilisation? A Prospective Cross-sectional Study. Reprod Sci. 2021;28(12):3480–90. https://doi.org/10.1007/s43032-021-00725-w.
25. Shafrir AL, Wise LA, Palmer JR, et al. Validity of self-reported endometriosis: a comparison across four cohorts. Hum Reprod. 2021;36(5):1268–78. https://doi.org/10.1093/humrep/deab012.
26. Bendifallah S, Puchar A, Suisse S, et al. Machine learning algorithms as new screening approach for

patients with endometriosis. Sci Rep. 2022;12(1):639. https://doi.org/10.1038/s41598-021-04637-2.
27. Chapron C, Lafay-Pillet M-C, Santulli P, et al. A new validated screening method for endometriosis diagnosis based on patient questionnaires. EClinicalMedicine. 2022;44:101263. https://doi.org/10.1016/j.eclinm.2021.101263.
28. Singh B, Berry J, Volovsky M, et al. The utility and impact of the Painful Periods Screening Tool (PPST) to improve healthcare delivery for people with symptoms of pelvic pain. Reprod Sci. 2023;30(5):1676–83. https://doi.org/10.1007/s43032-022-01119-2.
29. Agarwal SK, Antunez-Flores O, Foster WG, et al. Real-world characteristics of women with endometriosis-related pain entering a multidisciplinary endometriosis program. BMC Womens Health. 2021;21(1):19. https://doi.org/10.1186/s12905-020-01139-7.
30. Ling FW. Randomized controlled trial of depot leuprolide in patients with chronic pelvic pain and clinically suspected endometriosis. Pelvic Pain Study Group Obstet Gynecol. 1999;93(1):51–8. https://doi.org/10.1016/s0029-7844(98)00341-x.
31. Eskenazi B, Warner M, Bonsignore L, Olive D, Samuels S, Vercellini P. Validation study of nonsurgical diagnosis of endometriosis. Fertil Steril. 2001;76(5):929–35. https://doi.org/10.1016/s0015-0282(01)02736-4.
32. Roditis A, Florin M, Rousset P, et al. Accuracy of combined physical examination, transvaginal ultrasonography, and magnetic resonance imaging to diagnose deep endometriosis. Fertil Steril. 2023;119(4):634–43. https://doi.org/10.1016/j.fertnstert.2022.12.025.
33. Bendifallah S, Dabi Y, Suisse S, et al. Validation of a salivary miRNA signature of endometriosis – interim data. NEJM Evid. 2023;2(7):EVIDoa2200282. https://doi.org/10.1056/EVIDoa2200282.
34. Nisenblat V, Bossuyt PMM, Farquhar C, Johnson N, Hull ML. Imaging modalities for the noninvasive diagnosis of endometriosis. Cochrane Database Syst Rev. 2016;2:CD009591. https://doi.org/10.1002/14651858.CD009591.pub2.
35. Abrao MS, Andres MP, Gingold JA, et al. Preoperative ultrasound scoring of endometriosis by AAGL 2021 endometriosis classification is concordant with laparoscopic surgical findings and distinguishes early from advanced stages. J Minim Invasive Gynecol. 2023;30(5):363–73. https://doi.org/10.1016/j.jmig.2022.11.003.
36. Ros C, de Guirior C, Mension E, et al. Transvaginal ultrasound for diagnosis of deep endometriosis involving uterosacral ligaments, torus uterinus and posterior vaginal fornix: prospective study. Ultrasound Obstet Gynecol. 2021;58(6):926–32. https://doi.org/10.1002/uog.23696.
37. Goncalves MO, Siufi Neto J, Andres MP, Siufi D, de Mattos LA, Abrao MS. Systematic evaluation of endometriosis by transvaginal ultrasound can accurately replace diagnostic laparoscopy, mainly for deep and ovarian endometriosis. Hum Reprod. 2021;36(6):1492–500. https://doi.org/10.1093/humrep/deab085.
38. Zhou Y, Su Y, Liu H, Wu H, Xu J, Dong F. Accuracy of transvaginal ultrasound for diagnosis of deep infiltrating endometriosis in the uterosacral ligaments: systematic review and meta-analysis. J Gynecol Obstet Hum Reprod. 2021;50(3):101953. https://doi.org/10.1016/j.jogoh.2020.101953.
39. Maple S, Chalmers KJ, Bezak E, Henry K, Parange N. Ultrasound characteristics and scanning techniques of uterosacral ligaments for the diagnosis of endometriosis: a systematic review. J Ultrasound Med. 2023;42(6):1193–209. https://doi.org/10.1002/jum.16129.
40. Alcázar JL, Eguez PM, Forcada P, et al. Diagnostic accuracy of sliding sign for detecting pouch of Douglas obliteration and bowel involvement in women with suspected endometriosis: systematic review and meta-analysis. Ultrasound Obstet Gynecol. 2022;60(4):477–86. https://doi.org/10.1002/uog.24900.
41. Gerges B, Li W, Leonardi M, Mol BW, Condous G. Meta-analysis and systematic review to determine the optimal imaging modality for the detection of uterosacral ligaments/torus uterinus, rectovaginal septum and vaginal deep endometriosis. Hum Reprod Open. 2021;2021(4):hoab041. https://doi.org/10.1093/hropen/hoab041.
42. Condous G, Gerges B, Thomassin-Naggara I, et al. Non-invasive imaging techniques for diagnosis of pelvic deep endometriosis and endometriosis classification systems: an International Consensus Statement. Eur J Radiol. 2024;176:111450. https://doi.org/10.1016/j.ejrad.2024.111450.
43. Guerriero S, Ajossa S, Orozco R, et al. Accuracy of transvaginal ultrasound for diagnosis of deep endometriosis in the rectosigmoid: systematic review and meta-analysis. Ultrasound Obstet Gynecol. 2016;47(3):281–9. https://doi.org/10.1002/uog.15662.
44. Guerriero S, Saba L, Pascual MA, et al. Transvaginal ultrasound vs magnetic resonance imaging for diagnosing deep infiltrating endometriosis: systematic review and meta-analysis. Ultrasound Obstet Gynecol. 2018;51(5):586–95. https://doi.org/10.1002/uog.18961.
45. Medeiros LR, Duarte CS, Rosa DD, et al. Accuracy of magnetic resonance in suspicious breast lesions: a systematic quantitative review and meta-analysis. Breast Cancer Res Treat. 2011;126(2):273–85. https://doi.org/10.1007/s10549-010-1326-9.
46. Thomassin-Naggara I, Lamrabet S, Crestani A, et al. Magnetic resonance imaging classification of deep pelvic endometriosis: description and impact on surgical management. Hum Reprod. 2020;35(7):1589–600. https://doi.org/10.1093/humrep/deaa103.
47. Rousset P, Florin M, Bharwani N, et al. Deep Pelvic infiltrating endometriosis: MRI consensus lexicon and compartment-based approach from

the ENDOVALIRM group. Diagn Interv Imaging. 2023;104(3):95-112. https://doi.org/10.1016/j.diii.2022.09.004.
48. Thomassin-Naggara I, Monroc M, Chauveau B, et al. Multicenter external validation of the deep pelvic endometriosis index magnetic resonance imaging score. JAMA Netw Open. 2023;6(5):e2311686. https://doi.org/10.1001/jamanetworkopen.2023.11686.
49. Bazot M, Lafont C, Rouzier R, Roseau G, Thomassin-Naggara I, Daraï E. Diagnostic accuracy of physical examination, transvaginal sonography, rectal endoscopic sonography, and magnetic resonance imaging to diagnose deep infiltrating endometriosis. Fertil Steril. 2009;92(6):1825–33. https://doi.org/10.1016/j.fertnstert.2008.09.005.
50. Becker CM, Bokor A, Heikinheimo O, et al. ESHRE guideline: endometriosis. Hum Reprod Open. 2022;2022(2):hoac009. https://doi.org/10.1093/hropen/hoac009.
51. Lin C, Zeng S, Li M. miR-424-5p combined with miR-17-5p has high diagnostic efficacy for endometriosis. Arch Gynecol Obstet. 2023;307(1):169–77. https://doi.org/10.1007/s00404-022-06492-6.
52. Sasamoto N, Ngo L, Vitonis AF, et al. Circulating proteomic profiles associated with endometriosis in adolescents and young adults. Hum Reprod. 2022;37(9):2042–53. https://doi.org/10.1093/humrep/deac146.
53. Višnić A, Čanadi Jurešić G, Domitrović R, Klarić M, Šepić TS, Barišić D. Proteins in urine – possible biomarkers of endometriosis. J Reprod Immunol. 2023;157:103941. https://doi.org/10.1016/j.jri.2023.103941.
54. Janša V, Pušić Novak M, Ban Frangež H, Rižner TL. TGFBI as a candidate biomarker for non-invasive diagnosis of early-stage endometriosis. Hum Reprod. 2023;38(7):1284–96. https://doi.org/10.1093/humrep/dead091.
55. She J, Su D, Diao R, Wang L. A joint model of random forest and artificial neural network for the diagnosis of endometriosis. Front Genet. 2022;13:848116. https://doi.org/10.3389/fgene.2022.848116.
56. Qin R, Tian G, Liu J, Cao L. The gut microbiota and endometriosis: from pathogenesis to diagnosis and treatment. Front Cell Infect Microbiol. 2022;12:1069557. https://doi.org/10.3389/fcimb.2022.1069557.
57. Huang L, Liu B, Liu Z, et al. Gut microbiota exceeds cervical microbiota for early diagnosis of endometriosis. Front Cell Infect Microbiol. 2021;11:788836. https://doi.org/10.3389/fcimb.2021.788836.
58. Bendifallah S, Suisse S, Puchar A, et al. Salivary MicroRNA signature for diagnosis of endometriosis. J Clin Med. 2022;11(3):612. https://doi.org/10.3390/jcm11030612.
59. McGraw-Hill Medical Dictionary for A…, Seeman, Robert 9780073510965. eBay. https://www.ebay.com/itm/315172462207. Accessed 18 Mar 2024.
60. Encyclopedia of Medicine | Gale eBooks. https://www.gale.com/ebooks/encyclopedia-of-medicine. Accessed 18 Mar 2024.
61. Dictionnaire médical de l'Académie de Médecine. https://www.academie-medecine.fr/le-dictionnaire/index.php?q=CD. Accessed 18 Mar 2024.
62. Fauconnier A, Borghese B, Huchon C, et al. [Epidemiology and diagnosis strategy: CNGOF-HAS Endometriosis Guidelines]. Gynecol Obstet Fertil Senol. 2018;46(3):223–230. https://doi.org/10.1016/j.gofs.2018.02.012.
63. Sibiude J, Santulli P, Marcellin L, Borghese B, Dousset B, Chapron C. Association of history of surgery for endometriosis with severity of deeply infiltrating endometriosis. Obstet Gynecol. 2014;124(4):709–17. https://doi.org/10.1097/AOG.0000000000000464.
64. Tummers FHMP, Peltenburg SI, Metzemaekers J, Jansen FW, Blikkendaal MD. Evaluation of the effect of previous endometriosis surgery on clinical and surgical outcomes of subsequent endometriosis surgery. Arch Gynecol Obstet. 2023;308(5):1531–41. https://doi.org/10.1007/s00404-023-07193-4.
65. Daraï E, Marpeau O, Thomassin I, Dubernard G, Barranger E, Bazot M. Fertility after laparoscopic colorectal resection for endometriosis: preliminary results. Fertil Steril. 2005;84(4):945–50. https://doi.org/10.1016/j.fertnstert.2005.04.037.
66. Ferrier C, Roman H, Alzahrani Y, et al. Fertility outcomes in women experiencing severe complications after surgery for colorectal endometriosis. Hum Reprod. 2018;33(3):411–5. https://doi.org/10.1093/humrep/dex375.
67. Ferrier C, Le Gac M, Kolanska K, et al. Comparison of robot-assisted and conventional laparoscopy for colorectal surgery for endometriosis: a prospective cohort study. Int J Med Robot. 2022;18(3):e2382. https://doi.org/10.1002/rcs.2382.
68. Janssen EB, Rijkers ACM, Hoppenbrouwers K, Meuleman C, D'Hooghe TM. Prevalence of endometriosis diagnosed by laparoscopy in adolescents with dysmenorrhea or chronic pelvic pain: a systematic review. Hum Reprod Update. 2013;19(5):570–82. https://doi.org/10.1093/humupd/dmt016.
69. Eisenberg VH, Decter DH, Chodick G, Shalev V, Weil C. Burden of endometriosis: infertility, comorbidities, and healthcare resource utilization. J Clin Med. 2022;11(4):1133. https://doi.org/10.3390/jcm11041133.
70. Uçar T, Timur Taşhan S, Aksoy Derya Y, Nacar G. An analysis of dysmenorrhoea and depressive symptoms in university students: a case-control study. Int J Nurs Pract. 2018;24(5):e12678. https://doi.org/10.1111/ijn.12678.
71. Ishikura IA, Hachul H, Pires GN, Tufik S, Andersen ML. The impact of primary dysmenorrhea on sleep and the consequences for adolescent academic performance. J Clin Sleep Med. 2020;16(3):467–8. https://doi.org/10.5664/jcsm.8238.

72. Dai Y, Luo H, Zhu L, et al. Dysmenorrhea pattern in adolescences informing adult endometriosis. BMC Public Health. 2024;24(1):373. https://doi.org/10.1186/s12889-024-17825-2.
73. Dun EC, Kho KA, Morozov VV, Kearney S, Zurawin JL, Nezhat CH. Endometriosis in adolescents. JSLS. 2015;19(2):e2015.00019. https://doi.org/10.4293/JSLS.2015.00019.
74. Laufer MR, Sanfilippo J, Rose G. Adolescent endometriosis: diagnosis and treatment approaches. J Pediatr Adolesc Gynecol. 2003;16(3 Suppl):S3–11. https://doi.org/10.1016/s1083-3188(03)00066-4.
75. Exacoustos C, Zupi E, Piccione E. Ultrasound imaging for ovarian and deep infiltrating endometriosis. Semin Reprod Med. 2017;35(1):5–24. https://doi.org/10.1055/s-0036-1597127.
76. Millischer A-E, Santulli P, Da Costa S, et al. Adolescent endometriosis: prevalence increases with age on magnetic resonance imaging scan. Fertil Steril. 2023;119(4):626–33. https://doi.org/10.1016/j.fertnstert.2022.12.039.
77. Vignali M, Bianchi S, Candiani M, Spadaccini G, Oggioni G, Busacca M. Surgical treatment of deep endometriosis and risk of recurrence. J Minim Invasive Gynecol. 2005;12(6):508–13. https://doi.org/10.1016/j.jmig.2005.06.016.
78. Neme GL, Guimarães CTS, Dantas PP, et al. Postoperative imaging of endometriosis. Radiographics. 2024;44(4):e230159. https://doi.org/10.1148/rg.230159.
79. Chamié LP, Ribeiro DMFR, Ribeiro GMPAR, Serafini PC. Postoperative imaging findings after laparoscopic surgery for deeply infiltrating endometriosis. Abdom Radiol (NY). 2020;45(6):1847–65. https://doi.org/10.1007/s00261-020-02434-5.
80. Guerra A, Daraï E, Osório F, et al. Imaging of postoperative endometriosis. Diagn Interv Imaging. 2019;100(10):607–18. https://doi.org/10.1016/j.diii.2018.11.003.
81. Densen P. Challenges and opportunities facing medical education. Trans Am Clin Climatol Assoc. 2011;122:48–58.

Part II

Description of the Disease (US/MR/Surgical Correlation) (Radiologist/Surgeon)

Peritoneal Endometriosis

2

Elise Zareski, Aygline Paternostre, and Arnaud Fauconnier

2.1 Introduction

Endometriosis is a chronic inflammatory gynaecological disorder. Pelvic endometriosis can be schematically subdivided into three entities [1, 2]: superficial peritoneal and superficial ovarian endometriosis, cystic ovarian endometriosis, and deeply infiltrating endometriosis (DIE). What they have in common is the presence of the typical histological lesion of endometrial glands and stroma. Endometriosis presents significant challenges to both diagnosis and management, especially in its superficial form.

Historically, laparoscopy with a macroscopic evaluation of the pelvic peritoneum and adjacent organs has long been the gold standard for diagnosis, confirmed via a histological analysis of the lesions removed. Laparoscopies were most often performed for the diagnosis of chronic pelvic pain, including severe dysmenorrhoea, nonmenstrual or noncyclic pelvic pain, and provoked pelvic pain, such as deep dyspareunia.

The prevalence of endometriosis in young women under 25 years of age with chronic pelvic pain (CPP) is reported to be 25%–73%. CPP accounts for 10% of gynaecological visits and 50% of all diagnostic laparoscopies. When gynaecologists used laparoscopy liberally as the gold standard in the assessment of women with CPP, the most common findings at laparoscopy were pelvic endometriosis and adhesions. However, in up to 40% of women with CPP, laparoscopy failed to identify any obvious cause of the pain [3].

Reference imaging, transvaginal ultrasound, and magnetic resonance imaging (MRI) have together taken a prominent place over the past 2 decades and become the standard for endometriosis diagnosis, moving away from the dogma that laparoscopy is the gold standard [4].

Although an accurate diagnosis of deeply infiltrating endometriosis with imaging has been recognised, only a small body of work has looked at the imaging diagnosis of superficial endometriosis. It's a real challenge. Recently, Martire et al. observed at least one ultrasound (US) feature of endometriosis in 13.3% of adolescent girls aged 12–20 years who underwent a transvaginal sonography (TVS) or transrectal sonography (TRS) evaluation for different indications. In adolescents with dysmenorrhoea, the percent-

E. Zareski (✉)
Department of Radiology, Poissy Saint-Germain Hospital, Paris-Saclay University (UVSQ), Poissy, France

Department of Radiology, Gustave Roussy, Villejuif, France
e-mail: elise.zareski@ght-yvelinesnord.fr

A. Paternostre · A. Fauconnier
Department of Gynaecology and Obstetrics, Poissy Saint-Germain Hospital, Paris-Saclay University (UVSQ), Poissy, France
e-mail: arnaud.fauconnier@ght-yvelinesnord.fr

I. Thomassin-Naggara (ed.), *Imaging of Endometriosis: A Comparative Guide of US, MRI and Surgery*, https://doi.org/10.1007/978-3-031-82750-1_2

age of endometriosis detected via an US scan increased to 21% [5].

The diagnostic management of superficial endometriosis poses more challenges than do other types, which are crucial to understanding the diagnostic approach. The first challenge is determining the exact prevalence of this condition, which is often considered as 'invisible' on imaging—raising the question whether peritoneal endometriosis can be diagnosed through imaging at all. The second challenge is understanding whether superficial endometriosis is actually responsible for painful symptoms or infertility. Lastly, the question of the morphological definition of this presumed superficial disease on imaging and the question of how well it correlates with the surgical diagnosis remain.

2.2 Definition of Superficial Endometriosis

The definition of *superficial endometriosis* or *peritoneal endometriosis* is anatomopathological. Superficial or peritoneal endometriosis is characterised by functional ectopic endometrium-like tissue consisting of endometrial glands and stroma residing outside of the uterine cavity, extending up to 5 mm under the peritoneal pelvic surface and/or the serosa of pelvic viscera. The most common peritoneal sites of involvement (in decreasing order of frequency) are the ovaries, uterosacral ligaments, pouch of Douglas and pelvic peritoneum reflected over the uterus, fallopian tubes, rectosigmoid, and bladder. Rare extraperitoneal sites include the lungs and the central nervous system [6].

Lesions are present on the surface of the pelvic peritoneum and serosa of the pelvic organs (the uterus, vagina, rectum, sigmoid, and fallopian tubes). Ovarian lesions, on the other hand, are located directly on the cortex, due to the absence of serosa in this organ. Superficial lesions may penetrate more or less deeply beneath the peritoneal surface in the form of small finger-like invaginations of endometrial tissue [7]. Some lesions have a characteristic macroscopic appearance, which is why they are referred to as 'typical' lesions. These are pigmented lesions in the form of small millimetric granulations or patches of blue, brown, or black. These lesions are often associated with small white fibrous plaques of varying degrees of retractility. This appearance has long been recognised as specific to endometriosis [8].

The existence of so-called atypical lesions was recognised in the 1980s. These nonpigmented lesions are in fact more common than the 'typical' ones [9], but their appearance is heterogeneous and much less characteristic. Macroscopically, these lesions present as raised, papular, vesicular, or polypoid lesions, which have a soft consistency and are lightweight and raspberry, red, or burgundy in colour. They may also present as inflammatory, petechial lesions surrounded by intense visible vascularisation [10]. Other atypical lesions have been described [9], including isolated white patches, peritoneal pockets, and yellow-brown spots. The possibility of microscopic lesions without macroscopic translation visible at laparoscopy has also been well documented [11, 12].

The natural history of these lesions is complex and hypothetical. Microscopic, clear or red lesions must be considered as early and active lesions as opposed to pigmented and fibrous lesions, which are older and would constitute a scarring form of the disease. In contrast to the latter lesions, the former show a cyclical activity similar to that of the normal endometrium, are located more on the surface of the peritoneum [13], show greater neoangiogenesis [14] and inflammatory phenomena [10], and have higher mitotic activity [14]. The transition from clear or red lesions to pigmented or white lesions was recognised via follow-up laparoscopy 6 to 12 months later [9]. This transformation would take place through the appearance of fibrosis (in the form of white patches), which would progressively replace the inflammatory lesions and neovessels [13]. Glandular lesions would then become few in number, lose their cyclicity, and take on a pigmented appearance or disappear altogether [13]. As we shall see, this model is largely invalidated by the existence of deep endometriosis lesions.

A recent consensus piece on the terminology of endometriosis refined the subtype definitions of endometriosis. *Superficial endometriosis* is now defined as an endometriosis lesion involving the peritoneal surface, whereas deep endometriosis lesions extend beneath the peritoneal surface or invade adjacent structures such as the bowel, bladder, and/or ureters [15]. The concept of a deeply infiltrating disease has been abandoned, and these updated definitions suggest that endometriosis that is not on the surface of the peritoneum should be classified as deep endometriosis [16].

Superficial endometriosis is the most frequently observed form of endometriosis, because when carefully investigated, it can be found in all three forms in up to 50% of fertile asymptomatic women [12, 17]. This frequency raises the question whether the lesions are pathological [2]. Indeed, microscopic, or red, lesions can likely appear in anyone [12, 13]. These lesions may then regress or develop into more-advanced lesions.

2.3 Transvaginal Sonography

Transvaginal sonography (TVS) is the primary imaging technique for evaluating and diagnosing suspected endometriosis [18]. However, its use may be limited in virgin patients. In such cases, a transrectal sonography probe can be utilised to assess the pelvic organs with comparable accuracy to that of TVS [5]. In practice, endorectal ultrasound is *never* performed on virgin patients (the patient is also an anal virgin).

2.3.1 Technical Aspects

Evaluation is typically performed on patients with an empty bladder and without bowel preparation. If bladder endometriosis is suspected on the basis of symptoms, patients should be asked to not completely empty their bladder before the ultrasound examination: A slightly filled bladder facilitates the evaluation of the walls of the bladder and the detection of endometriotic nodules.

TVS, with or without bowel preparation, was shown in a meta-analysis to accurately predict rectosigmoid deeply infiltrating endometriosis [19]. Some practitioners introduce sterile ultrasound gel into the posterior fornix of the vagina by using a plastic syringe to create an acoustic window or 'standoff' effect between the TVS probe and the surrounding structures, enhancing the visualisation of the pelvic compartment structures [20].

Several studies have sought to systematise the ultrasound evaluation of the pelvis in patients with suspected endometriosis. In 2016, Menakaya et al. created the ultrasound-based endometriosis staging system (UBESS) for predicting the level of complexity in laparoscopic surgery for endometriosis and guiding patients towards appropriate management. The classification involves a systematised and dynamic ultrasound approach based on five domains for pelvis evaluation in endometriosis: the uterus and adnexa, site-specific tenderness (SST), organ mobility, non-bowel DIE, and bowel DIE. This classification takes into account soft markers such as adhesions and site-specific tenderness, which may reflect underlying superficial endometriosis [20].

The International Deep Endometriosis Analysis (IDEA) consensus has also developed a systematic and structured sonographic approach to enhance the detection of endometriosis at pelvic ultrasound [18]. This approach evaluates four components via dynamic ultrasonography: the uterus and adnexa, soft markers, sliding signs, and deeply infiltrating endometriosis (DIE).

2.3.2 Soft Markers

Evaluating transvaginal sonographic 'soft markers', such as site-specific tenderness and fixed ovaries, is essential for assessing the presence of pelvic pathology [3]. The presence of soft markers increases the likelihood of superficial endometriosis and adhesions [18]. Ultrasound manoeuvres must be gentle and it is recommended to avoid pain, in which case the manoeuvres must be stopped. These indirect signs must also be interpreted with caution to avoid false positives.

2.3.2.1 Adhesions

The search for adhesions requires studying organ mobility—hence the importance of a dynamic examination, which is the strength of ultrasound. If pelvic fluid is present, fine strands of tissue (adhesions) may be seen between the ovary (with or without endometrioma) and the uterus or the peritoneum of the pouch of Douglas (POD). Ovarian mobility is routinely assessed in three planes on TVS to evaluate the fixation or adhesions [21]. By applying pressure between the uterus and the ovary, one can assess whether the ovary is fixed to the uterus medially, to the pelvic side wall laterally, or to the uterosacral ligament (USLs). Adhesions may also be suspected if the ovaries or uterus feel fixed to any adjacent structures (the broad ligament, POD, bladder, rectum, or parietal peritoneum) during palpation with the probe, and/or abdominal palpation with one's free hand.

Additionally, the presence of hydrosalpinx/hematosalpinx and peritoneal cysts should be investigated and reported because adhesions may distort the normal course of the fallopian tubes and because occlusion may occur due to endometriotic foci or distal tubular adhesions [18]. The detection of thickened pericolic fat has been associated with mild-to-moderate endometriosis [22].

Studies have shown that ovarian immobility on ultrasound has high specificity and negative predictive value but poor sensitivity and positive predictive value for disease location in isolated superficial endometriosis—suggesting that visualising a mobile ovary indicates a low probability of the presence of pelvic sidewall superficial endometriosis. Additionally, ipsilateral ovarian immobility is associated with an increased risk of uterosacral ligament and pelvic sidewall endometriosis [23].

2.3.2.2 Sliding Sign

Organ mobility is tested by looking for a slippage zone between the organ and its surroundings by using an abdominal hand opposite the organ to be mobilised and the tip of the probe that mobilises the organ. The sliding-sign technique is used to assess the status of the pouch of Douglas (POD) obliteration. In patients with an anteverted uterus, gentle pressure is placed against the cervix by using the tip of the transvaginal probe to establish whether the anterior rectum glides freely across the posterior aspect of the cervix and posterior vaginal wall. The examiner places their nonscanning hand over the woman's lower anterior abdominal wall to mobilize the uterus between the palpating hand and the transvaginal probe to assess whether the anterior bowel glides freely over the posterior aspect of the upper uterus/fundus. For patients with a retroverted uterus, gentle pressure is applied against the posterior upper uterine fundus with the transvaginal probe to establish whether the anterior rectum glides freely across the posterior upper uterine fundus. Place the nonscanning hand over the woman's lower anterior abdominal wall to support the uterus while assessing whether the anterior sigmoid glides freely over the anterior lower uterine segment [18] (Fig. 2.1). Operators evaluate the posterior sliding of the posterior uterine and retrocervix serosa against the contents (anterior rectal wall or anterior sigmoid wall). A positive sliding sign indicates the sliding of the contents, whereas a negative sliding sign indicates the absence of sliding [21], because of which the POD is recorded as obliterated. However, the sliding test should be interpreted cautiously because a negative sliding sign may be caused by inflammatory changes and postoperative adhesions, such as those resulting from pelvic surgery or pelvic inflammatory disease [24]. If a negative TVS sliding sign, suggesting POD obliteration, is observed during the initial scan, these patients should be referred to an advanced gynaecological ultrasound unit for further preoperative imaging to assess the presence, location, and extent of DIE lesions [25]. The posterior sliding-sign technique can be transposed to the anterior compartment by looking for a sliding zone between the posterior surface of the bladder and the anterior uterine serosa, which would be carried out to detect adhesions linked to the possible superficial endometriosis of the vesicouterine cul-de-sac.

2.3.2.3 Site-Specific Tenderness (SST)

Given that tenderness in specific structures (e.g. uterosacral ligament) may be associated with

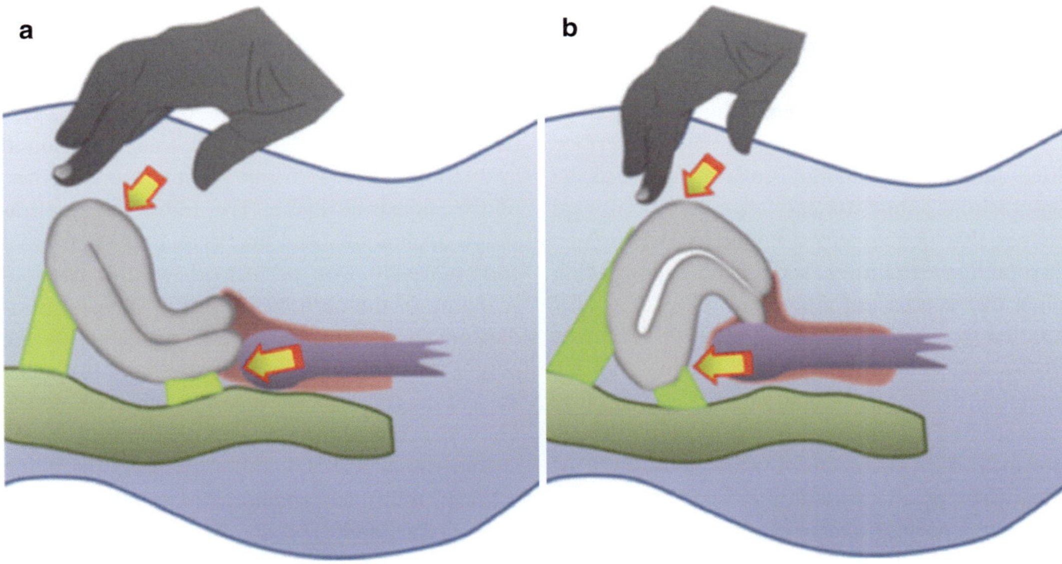

Fig. 2.1 Schematic drawings demonstrating how to elicit the 'sliding sign' in (**a**) an anteverted uterus and (**b**) a retroverted uterus. Reproduced with permission from [18]

underlying endometriosis, site-specific tenderness can be assessed in different pelvic anatomical locations using the TVS probe and the Visual Analogue Scale for pain (VAS range: 0–10), such as in the UBESS approach. Locations include the POD, the left and right USL, the corpus uteri, and the left and right ovaries. The presence of elective pain should prompt a more thorough search for signs of endometriosis, especially if the pain is in the posterior compartment [20].

Another approach to tenderness-guided ultrasound examination includes patient involvement in indicating sites of tenderness experienced during the exam. However, tenderness elicited during physical and TVS examinations has a high false-positive rate and may not be useful in locating superficial endometriosis [26]. Indeed, pain feeling is highly subjective and personal in terms of intensity, and it yields many false positives. For example, patients with irritable bowel may have pain along the rectosigmoid digestive tract, especially in the left periovarian towards the left iliac fossa, and enlarged micropolycystic ovaries are painful to mobilise. Additional large-scale studies are needed to evaluate the usefulness of soft markers for localising isolated superficial endometriosis. Inversely, the absence of pain on tensioning the uterosacral ligaments is much more interesting because it often rules out the presence of endometriosis.

2.3.3 Visible Sonographic Markers of Superficial Endometriosis

The direct visibility of superficial endometriosis at transvaginal sonography (TVS) is debated. Detecting superficial endometriosis requires the meticulous study of the peritoneal and ovarian surfaces with a systematic scanning of each compartment from right to left in search of differences in echogenicity or surface irregularities. Operators should be experienced and look for signs of certainty to avoid false positives. The probe should be positioned as close as possible to the structures: a probe in the anterior cul-de-sac when studying the vesicouterine space, a probe in the posterior vaginal cul-de-sac when studying the POD peritoneum, and a probe as close as possible to the uterosacral ligaments.

Bailey et al. demonstrated that the detection of superficial endometriosis in the POD is possible with high specificity by using routine TVS. A detailed assessment of the peritoneum of the

POD was performed by positioning the TVS probe in the posterior fornix of the vagina behind the cervix in the longitudinal plane and then tracking left and right to view the whole peritoneum at the back of the vagina. They described three landmarks: vaginal muscle, hypoechoic/hyperechoic subperitoneal fat, and a peritoneal surface that demarcates a boundary over which surrounding structures should be seen sliding when probe pressure is applied (Fig. 2.3). This detailed scanning had a high specificity rate (96%) and a low false-positive rate, and the detection of superficial endometriosis was more accurate in the POD than in the bladder surface. However, they observed low sensitivity (50% of those with superficial endometriosis on laparoscopy had a normal scan) [16].

To enhance diagnostic accuracy, a novel transvaginal ultrasonography (TVUS) procedure called saline-infusion sonoPODography has been proposed [21]. This involves instilling saline into the pouch of Douglas via an intrauterine balloon catheter to create an acoustic window between the ultrasound probe and its surrounding structures, allowing a direct visualisation of superficial endometriosis. Superficial endometriosis may appear as hyperechoic projections, hypoechoic areas, filmy adhesions, cystic areas, or peritoneal pockets (as demonstrated via incomplete septations and 'entrapped fluid'). The peritoneum of the pouch of Douglas is commonly affected. The overall diagnostic performance of sonoPODography was found to be 69% accurate, with a sensitivity of 65% and specificity of 100%. In cases without deep endometriosis, endometriomas, or the obliteration of the pouch of Douglas, the diagnostic accuracy was 80%, with a sensitivity of 78% and specificity of 100% [21]. Leonardi et al. described a TVUS diagnosis of superficial endometriosis that used a technique that required minimal invasion and allowed for a better visualisation of the lesions in the peritoneum of the pouch of Douglas, the utero sacral ligaments, the posterior pelvis sidewall, and the rectosigmoid.

A classification of the ultrasound features of superficial endometriosis lesions based on laparoscopic and/or histologic correlations with a precise description of semiology that had never been as detailed before was recently published [27]. To take advantage of the presence of pelvic free fluid after ovulation, all their ultrasound evaluations were performed in the second phase of the menstrual cycle. The transvaginal ultrasound technique used for detecting superficial endometriosis was performed with a detailed scanning of the peritoneum in the anterior, middle, posterior, and lateral compartments of the pelvis. The surface of the ovaries and serosa of the rectosigmoid were also evaluated in detail. They described various presentations of cystic lesions in superficial endometriosis, including solitary, multiple separate, linear clusters, and honeycomb appearances. These lesions often contain hyperechogenic foci, possibly due to hemosiderin deposits or calcifications. However, small cystic lesions may exhibit specular artefacts, simulating hyperechogenic foci. Solitary lesions typically range in diameter from 1 to 5 mm and may appear convex or concave, the latter because peritoneal retraction forms a pocket. Hypoechogenic tissue, indicative of stromal reaction or fibrosis, is commonly associated with cystic lesions. On the basis of these observations, they proposed three main categories of superficial endometriotic lesions: solitary lesions, multiple separate lesions, and cluster lesions. Each lesion may display specific ultrasound features: hypoechogenic associated tissue forming a 'hat', convex 'bulging', concave 'pockets', hyperechoic foci called 'pearls', and filmy adhesions called 'veils' [27] (Fig. 2.2). Examples of the different aspects of superficial endometriotic lesions are illustrated in Figs. 2.3, 2.4, 2.5, 2.6, 2.7, 2.8, 2.9, 2.10, 2.11, 2.12, 2.13, and 2.14.

Taking advantage of the presence of liquid in the pouch of Douglas after ovulation or during the menstrual period for patients on oral contraceptives reproduces, like serum instillation, an acoustic window that highlights the contours of the organs and peritoneum. However, the menstrual period can create false images of superficial endometriosis. Indeed, menstrual reflux is

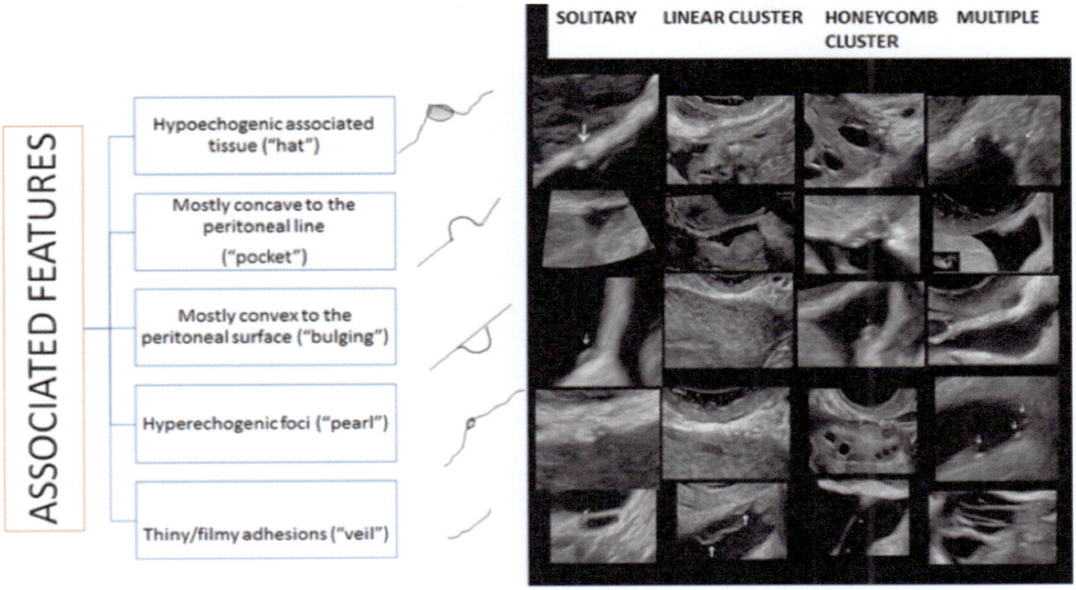

Fig. 2.2 Schematic representation of superficial endometriotic lesions—lesions marked by arrows. Reproduced from Pedrassani 2023. Published in Open Access by MDPI https://www.mdpi.com/2075-4418/13/11/1876, licensed under CC-BY 4.0

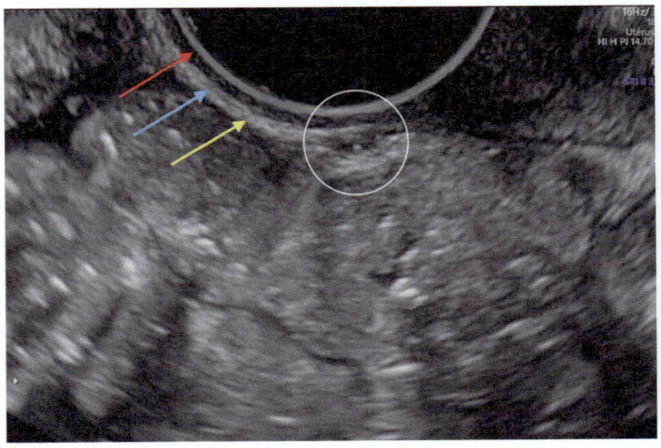

Fig. 2.3 Example of superficial endometriotic lesions in cluster with honeycomb appearance convex to the peritoneum surface (bulging) (white circle). Red arrow: vaginal muscle hypochoic. Blue arrow: subperitneal fat hyperechoic. Yellow arrow: peritoneal surface

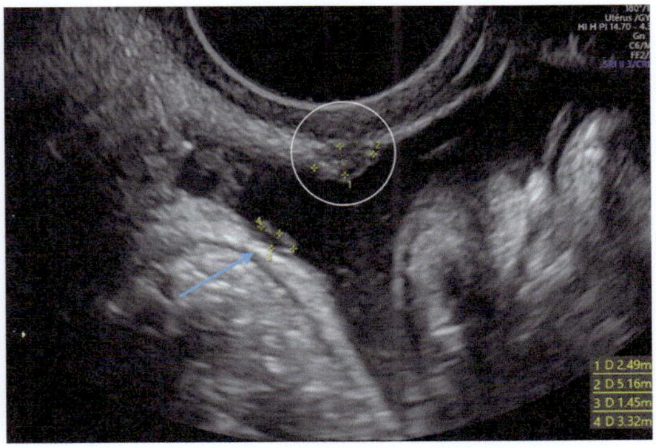

Fig. 2.4 Multiple separate bulging superficial endometriotic lesions with fluid in the pouch of Douglas (POD): one (white circle) convex on the peritoneal surface with honeycomb appearance and the other (blue arrow) a cystic lesion on the serosa of the rectosigmoid like a vesicle aspect

physiologically present in 90% of women, and most of them eliminate endometrial residuals through a process of peritoneal degradation. These hyperechogenic foci are similar to endometriotic implants but may correspond to transient haemorrhagic spots of hyperechogenic blood deposited on the surface of the ovaries and in the peritoneum of the pouch of Douglas. Ultrasound examinations during menstruation can therefore lead to false positives: false images of superficial endometriosis. The persistence of these images outside the menstrual period points

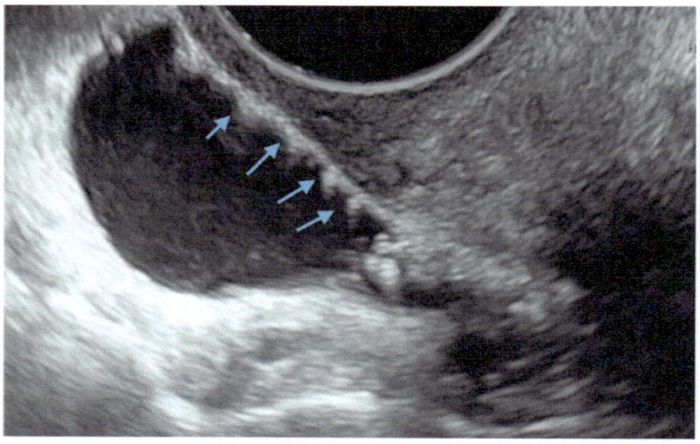

Fig. 2.5 Superficial endometriosis lesions disposed on a linear cluster with hyperechoic foci or hyperechoic spots (pearls) (blue arrows), highlighted by serohematic fluid in the POD

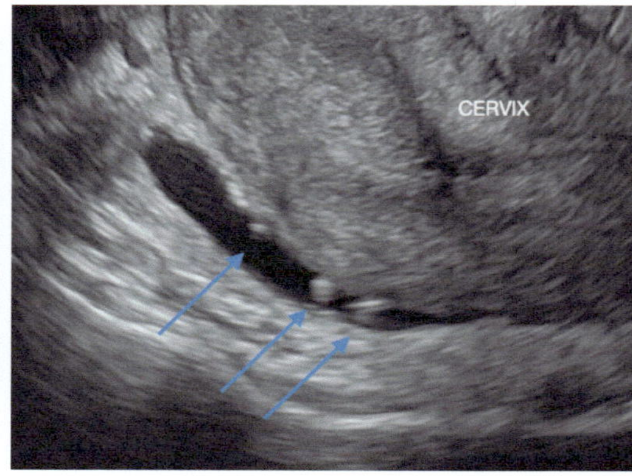

Fig. 2.7 Hyperechoic spots on the back of the cervix (arrows): positioning the TVS probe in the posterior vaginal fornix behind the cervix is essential to better analyse the pouch of Douglas at the back of the vagina

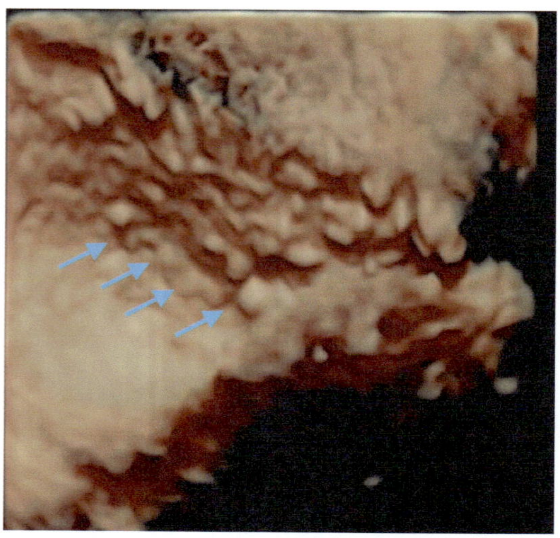

Fig. 2.6 3D view of Fig. 2.5: the hyperechoic foci form a 'pearl mat' on the peritoneal surface (blue arrows)

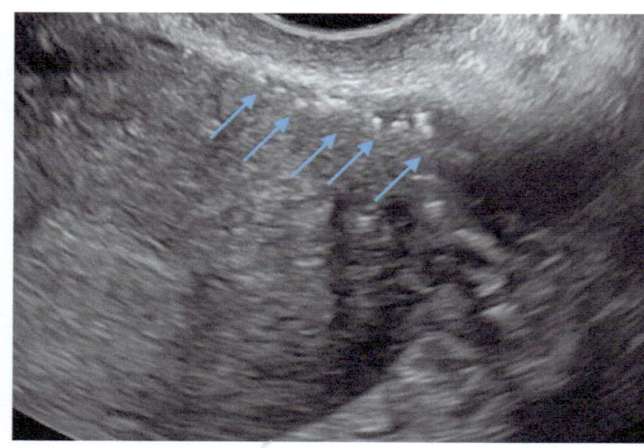

Fig. 2.8 Bulging superficial endometriotic lesions with hyperechoic foci (pearls) forming a 'pearl mat' on the peritoneal surface of the vesicouterine pouch; on an axial plane—hyperechoic foci disposed on a linear cluster on the anterior uterine serosa (blue arrows)

towards endometriotic implants. The same applies to ultrasound images taken just after ovulation: If ovulation is haemorrhagic, this pattern of haemorrhagic spots on the cortex and POD effusion may mimic superficial endometriosis (Fig. 2.12). Care must therefore be taken when interpreting images, depending on the phase of the cycle, and look for more-specific ultrasound signs of superficial endometriosis.

2.3.4 From Superficial to Deep Endometriosis: A Continuum?

Chowdary demonstrated a statistically significant association between uterosacral ligament thickening at TVS (> 3 mm) and the operative finding of superficial endometriosis (sensitivity of 62% and specificity of 73%). For him, this thickening is a marker of inflammation. However, some

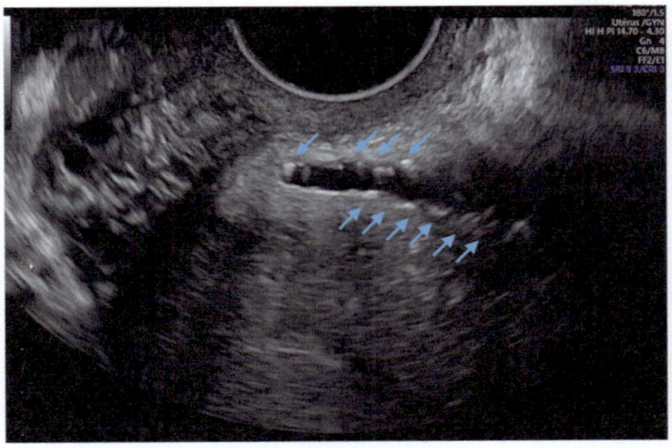

Fig. 2.9 On a longitudinal plane—releasing the pressure on the vaginal probe allows the creation of an acoustic window to better see the hyperechoic foci as they form a mat on the peritoneal surface of the vesiocuterine pouch

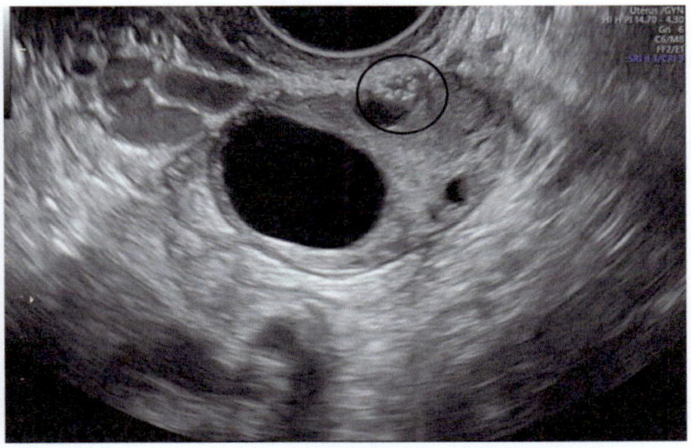

Fig. 2.11 Superficial endometriotic bulging lesions with hyperechoic foci (pearl) disposed on a nonlinear cluster (black circle)

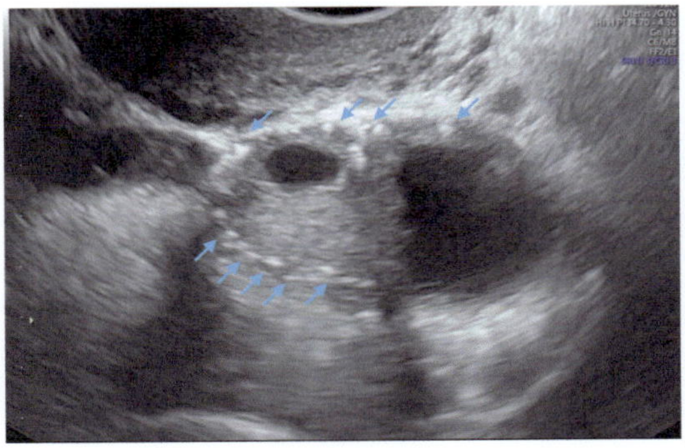

Fig. 2.10 Superficial endometriotic bulging lesions with hyperechoic foci (pearl) disposed on a linear cluster on the ovarian surface; tracking the probe left and right is essential to get a view of the whole cortical surface of the ovarian, where hyperechoic foci form a 'pearl mat' that completely covers the ovarian surface

argue that ligament thickening may actually diagnose deeply infiltrating disease rather than superficial endometriosis. They maintain that the definition of deep disease is endometriosis invading at a depth of ≥5 mm and that a ligament thickening of >3 mm may not be representative of deep disease [22].

This new terminology seems better suited to practice. The average thickness of a nonthickened uterosacral ligament varies between 1.5 and 2.5 mm, with a hyperechoic appearance and regular smooth edges. Superficial endometriosis of the uterosacral ligaments can be seen by finding deposits of hyperechoic foci on its surface and along its course, but its thickness remains normal. On the other hand, when a change in the appearance of the uterosacral ligaments occurs, the involvement becomes subperitoneal and can be described as deep, infiltrating the uterosacral ligament with a heterogeneous hypoechoic thickening with less regular margins: Its thickening is generally >3 mm and indurated, with a surgical correspondence with deep involvement to be excised. Nodular infiltration probably corresponds to the evolution of the infiltration towards retractile fibrosis with the formation of a spiculated nodule in the uterosacral ligament.

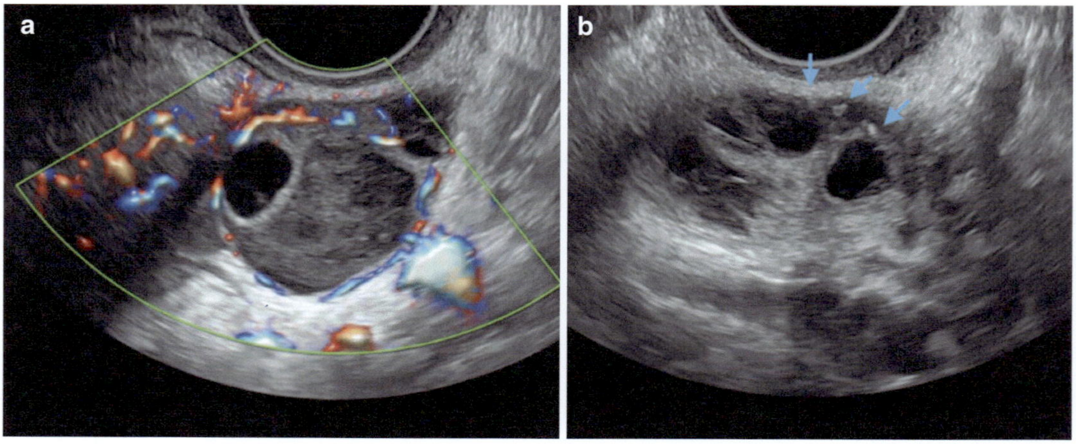

Fig. 2.12 False positive: (**b**) hyperechoic foci on the ovarian surface (blue arrow) contemporary of (**a**) a haemorrhagic cyst of the corpus luteum, and fluid was in the POD

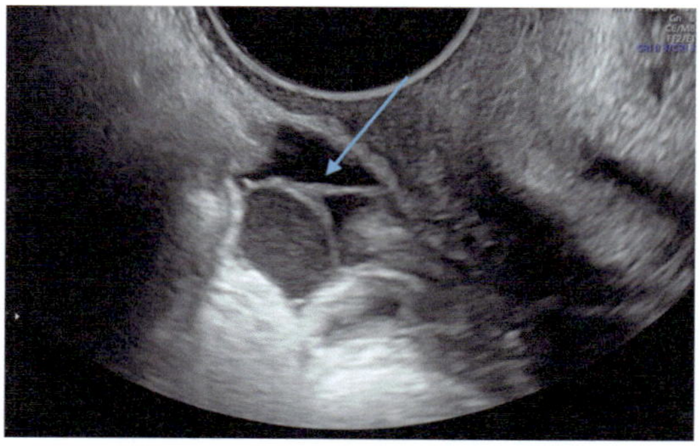

Fig. 2.13 Superficial endometriotic lesions with velamentous adhesions (veils) trapped in serohematic fluid in the POD

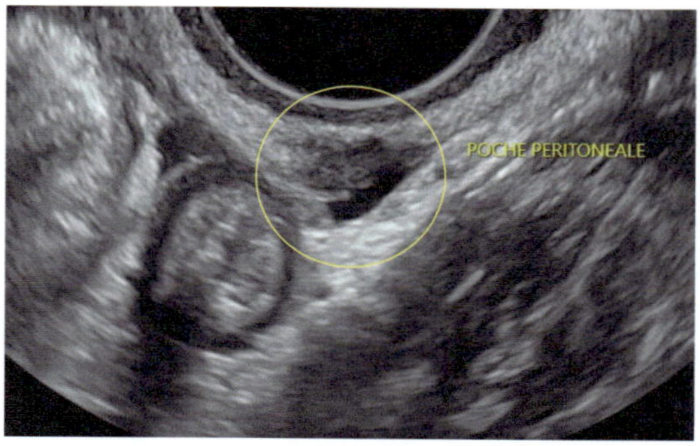

Fig. 2.14 Peritoneal pocket: superficial endometriotic lesions in a cluster with a honeycomb appearance, concave to the peritoneal surface (pocket) (yellow circle)

2.4 MRI

MRI should be considered as a second-line examination technique after ultrasound in the evaluation of pelvic endometriosis [4, 28], particularly for patients with a high clinical suspicion and negative ultrasound findings or before surgery for optimal preoperative staging.

2.4.1 Technical Aspects

The European Society of Urogenital Radiology (ESUR) has published specific guidelines for optimal MRI sequences in the evaluation of endometriosis. Although no specific recommendation exists for the timing of MRI in relation to the menstrual cycle, the presence of pelvic free fluid, such as during menstruation or the postovulatory phase, can sometimes aid in image interpretation.

Both 1.5 T and 3.0 T MRI machines are valuable, utilising pelvic phased array coils and abdominal strapping in the supine position. The prone position can be an option for patients with claustrophobia. Also, administering antiperistaltic agents (intramuscularly or intravenously) when not contraindicated is strongly advised to improve image quality. The bladder should be moderately filled, and vaginal and/or rectal opacification is optional. In practice, the patient is asked to empty their bladder just before the examination. Bowel preparation should be prioritised over rectal or vaginal opacification in MRI protocols [29]. T2-weighted and T1-weighted images with and without fat suppression (or the Dixon technique) are utilised, and where three-dimensional (3D) T2-weighted imaging was once an option, it is now used routinely. There is no place for diffusion-weighted, susceptibility-weighted magnetic resonance (MR) or gadolinium injection in the evaluation of endometriosis via MRI.

MRI offers better than TVS contrast resolution and the ability to detect blood by using T1 hyperintensity in fat saturation, making it valuable for assessing pelvic endometriosis, particularly in case of active peritoneal lesions. However, the diagnosis on MRI depends on the stage of the evolution of endometriosis and also the hormonal environment. Implants can present varied appearances depending on their age, ranging from highly vascular lesions to raised nodular lesions due to fibrosis and hemosiderin deposition [6].

2.4.2 Typical MRI Images of Superficial Endometriosis

The appearance of ectopic endometrial glands on T1- and T2-weighted images varies depending on the age of the haemorrhage. Cases of subacute bleeding typically have a high signal intensity on T1-weighted images with fat suppression that is characteristic of superficial endometriosis (Fig. 2.15), better seen in areas of stasis and slope in the pelvic peritoneal cavity. Chronic endometriosis (Fig. 2.16), on the other hand, can cause reactive fibrosis, leading to lesions with irregular contours and low signal intensity on both T1-weighted images and T2-weighted images [30]. We should therefore focus on identifying T1 FS hyperintense foci to confirm intraperitoneal endometriosis given that a definitive diagnosis is more challenging in the absence of this hyperintensity on T1.

Even though ectopic endometrial glands are hormonal dependent, no significant difference in lesion size may exist between the early and mid-menstrual periods for abdominal wall endometriosis [31]. Women commonly have symptoms of endometriosis, but only minor MRI findings [32].

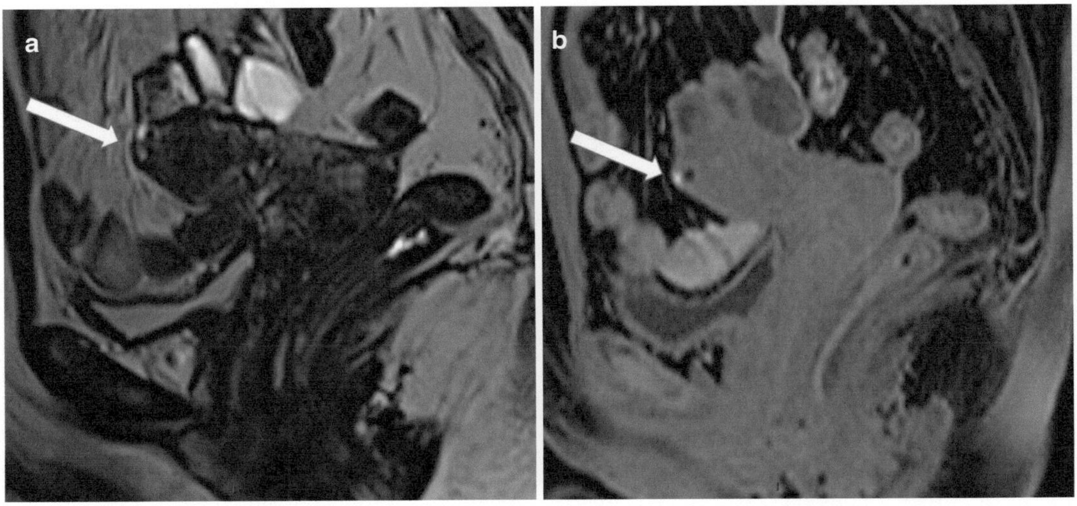

Fig. 2.15 Punctiform T2 hyperintensity of the uterine serosa (**a**) with a slight peripheral T2 hypointense halo, and clear T1 FS hyperintensity (**b**), indicating a haemorrhagic implant of peritoneal endometriosis at the surface of the uterus; the punctiform T2 hyperintensity of the bladder dome, without T1 hyperintensity, could also suggest an implant that would not have been confirmed if it had been seen in isolation

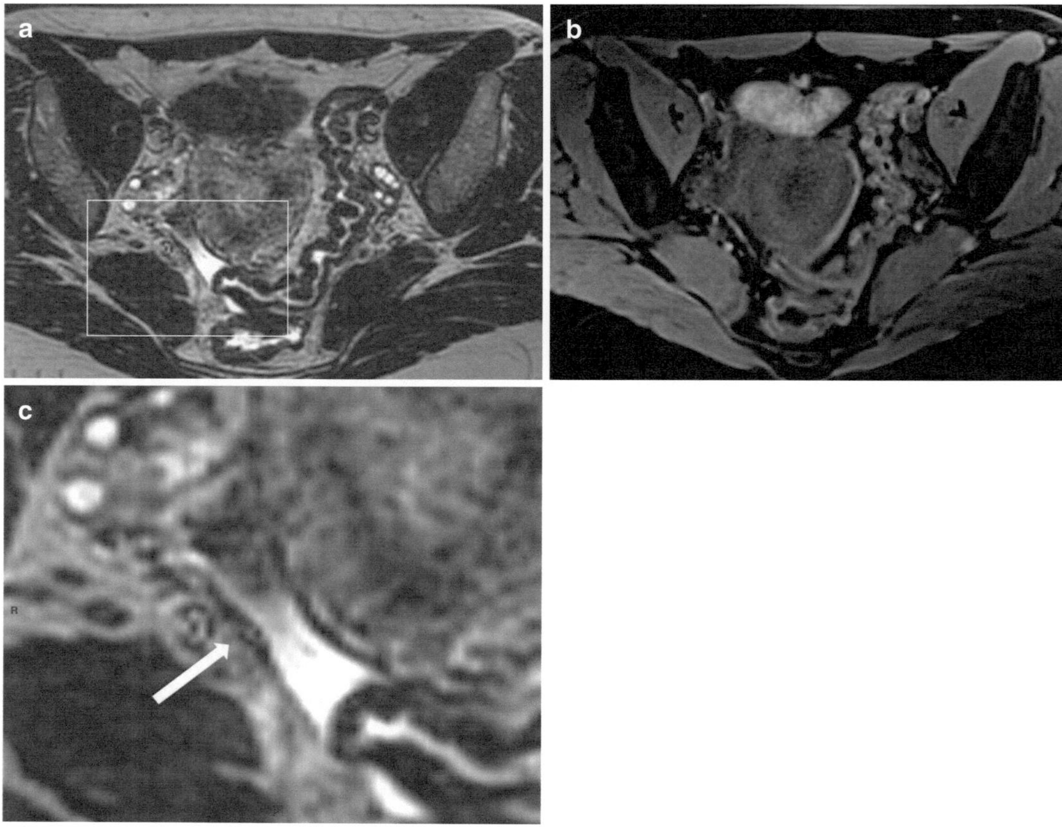

Fig. 2.16 (**a**) Focal thickening of the peritoneum with T2 hypointensity. (**b**) No T1 FS hyperintensity is evident either at the site of this thickening or in any other pelvic location. (**c**) Enlarged image of this pelvic thickening shows a T2 hyperintense spot at the limit of visibility without T1 FS correlation (arrow), so the appearance is ambiguous, preventing a definitive diagnosis of endometriosis, unlike the other presented imaging findings

Thomeer et al. confirmed, despite a small sample size, consisting of 40 patients, that an optimised protocol on a 3.0 T MRI enables the detection of patients with endometriosis more advanced than stage I (according to the r-AFS). Among the 40 patients, seven had false-negative findings on MRI, all of whom were diagnosed with stage I endometriosis on the basis of laparoscopic findings. These seven patients had only small spots of superficial endometriosis visible via laparoscopy. Additionally, they noted that their patient group was limited to those without hormonal suppression, aiming to enhance the visibility of active lesions on T1-weighted images [33]. To our knowledge, no study has evaluated the impact of hormonal treatment, particularly progestin, on the reduced sensitivity of detecting implants on MRI due to endometrial atrophy.

2.4.3 A Sliding Sign in MRI?

Fan et al. evaluated the effectiveness of a single sagittal T2-weighted MRI motion sequence in the preoperative assessment of pelvic mobility for endometriosis patients. Their findings indicate that this MRI sequence can identify pelvic adhesions and immobility, providing valuable insights for surgical planning when TVUS results are inconclusive or not feasible.

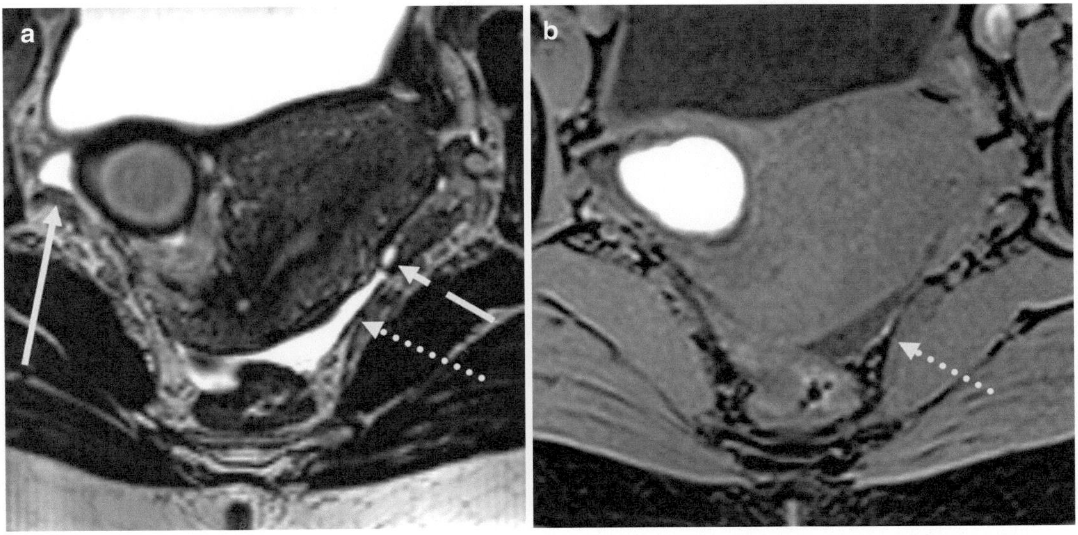

Fig. 2.17 (**a**) Peritoneal fluid outlining the right ovary, which also contains an endometrioma. Because the patient was lying on her back during the MRI, the peritoneal fluid would be expected to accumulate in the Douglas pouch due to gravity. The visualisation of this fluid in the right ovarian fossa is an indirect sign of pelvic adhesions. Additionally, some adhesions have a fibrous signal in T2 hypointensity, partitioning the Douglas pouch on the left. (**b**) Peritoneal thickening is present with T2 hypointensity in the left Douglas pouch, with a punctiform haemorrhagic implant showing T1 FS hyperintensity. Thus, in this patient, the presence of ovarian and intraperitoneal endometriosis can be confirmed

The absence of an MRI sliding sign showed high sensitivity (90%) in diagnosing the absence of a reported TVUS sliding sign. Additionally, the sensitivity in labelling the motion sequence as indicating pelvic bowel adhesions (superficial endometriosis) was very high, at 97% (95% CI: 82–100%), compared to an absent TVUS sliding-sign reference standard. This heightened sensitivity is clinically beneficial, providing increased confidence in assessing a mobile uterus, the absence of rectouterine adhesions, and the potential for less-complicated surgery. The high interobserver agreement in identifying the absence of MRI sliding further supports the reproducibility of this finding [34].

2.4.4 Equivocal Images on MRI

2.4.4.1 Adhesions

In MRI, as in ultrasound, attention should be paid to searching for direct signs through the visualisation of fine strands of tissue, particularly in the ovarian fossa or the Douglas pouch (Fig. 2.17). Unlike ultrasound, no bimanual palpation is available to study the sliding of organs relative to one another. However, an adhesive pelvis can be suggested by the presence of peritoneal trapping. Because MRI is performed with the patient lying on their back, the peritoneal fluid should, due to gravity, position itself in the Douglas pouch. The presence of suspended peritoneal fluid in the ovarian fossae, between intestinal loops (Fig. 2.18), or in the vesicouterine space is an indirect sign of an adhesive pelvis. Of course, this is nonspecific and may be secondary to postsurgical, inflammatory, infectious, or postradiation changes.

The other MRI findings that have been described, particularly in Khashchenko's study on a cohort of 134 adolescent girls, include the tissue heterogeneity of parametric, para-ovarian, and paracervical tissues, which are subjective signs, hypointense foci, and structural abnormalities of ligaments and the peritoneum and the thickening of the tissue of the Douglas pouch

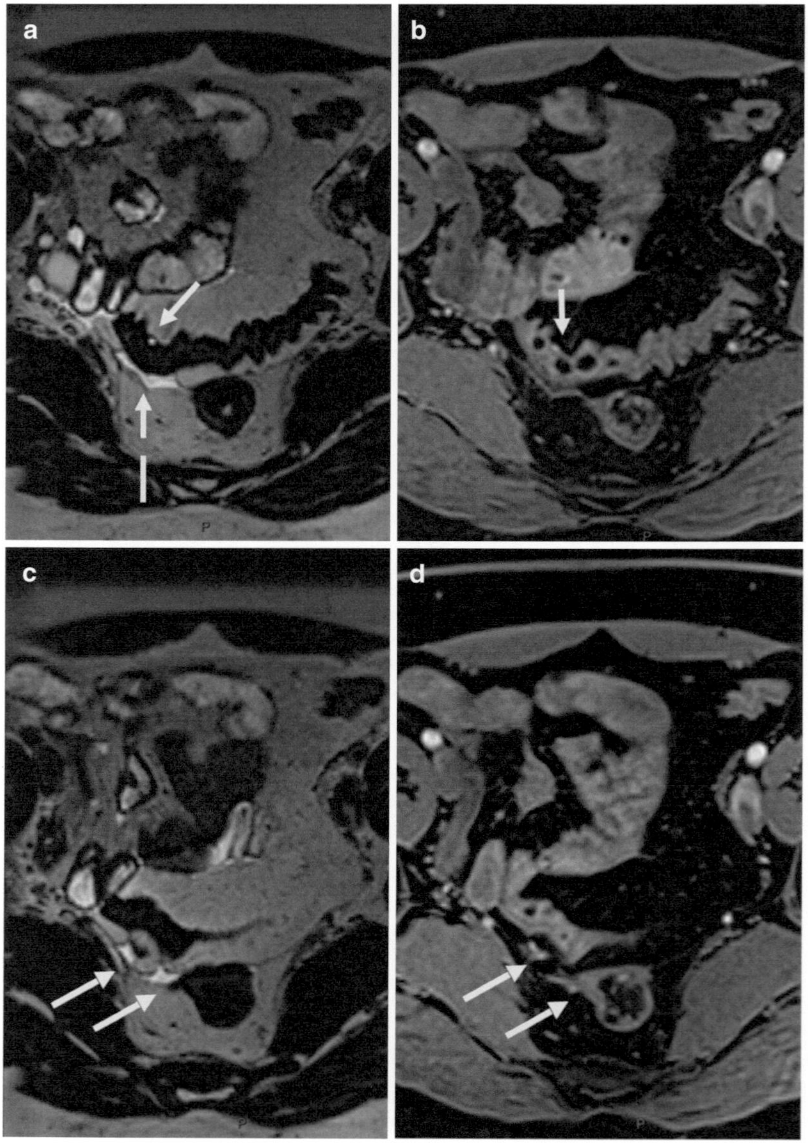

Fig. 2.18 (**a**) **Compartmentalisation of peritoneal fluid** is observed, an indirect sign of adhesions in this patient, accompanied by the fibrous thickening of the peritoneum, displaying T2 hypointensity, and by a hyperintense T2 implant on the sigmoid serosa. (**b**) **A detailed analysis of T1 FS sequences** reveals this implant on the sigmoid serosa with T1 hyperintensity, supporting an endometriotic origin of these adhesive lesions. (**c**) **Other implants** present with a T2 hypointense signal. (**d**) **Varying T1/T2 hyperintensity** may be observed, depending on the age of these implants. Pelvic adhesions, the fibrous thickening of the serosa, or peritoneum can be sequelae from conditions such as pelvic peritonitis, postsurgical changes, or postradiation therapy. The presence of a haemorrhagic implant with T1 hyperintensity, in a suggestive clinical context, supports the diagnosis of intraperitoneal endometriosis

space, of the fallopian tubes, of the capsule of the ovary, and of the serous cover of the uterus [35].

As explained for TVUS, the MRI diagnosis of peritoneal lesions matches the diagnosis of mild forms of subperitoneal disease of the posterior area of the pelvis. Lesions with the millimetric infiltration of the USL or posterior surface of the uterine isthmus (torus uterinum) may have discrete MRI aspects that lead to uncertain diagnoses [36].

An interesting study is the one by Stoppa, which focused solely on the performance of MRI in mild USL endometriosis. This study specifically addressed the issue of cases that radiologists are likely to misidentify as endometriosis. Six criteria were listed with their values for detecting the presence of endometriosis. It concludes that none of the reported criteria have sufficient diagnostic performance to be used alone, and when considered together, they lose all specificity. Asymmetry and thickening (0.69 [95% CI: 0.54–0.80] and 0.51 [95% CI: 0.40–0.63], respectively) were the most sensitive morphological criteria but were associated with moderate specificities (0.52 [95% CI: 0.31–0.73] and 0.62 [95% CI: 0.50–0.72], respectively), whereas the presence of irregularity, a nodule, or a T1 hypersignal spot or the irregular appearance of the USL appeared to have good specificities (0.81 [95% CI: 0.70–0.89], 0.96 [95% CI: 0.89–0.99], 0.95 [95% CI: 0.87–0.99], and 0.99 [95% CI: 0.93–1.00], respectively) but low sensitivities in this population (0.22 [95% CI: 0.14–0.33], 0.12 [95% CI: 0.06–0.21], 0.08 [95% CI: 0.03–0.16], and 0.08 [95% CI: 0.03–0.16], respectively). The best cut-off value for the prediction of endometriosis was found at a diameter of 3.85 mm [37].

2.5 Diagnosing Peritoneal Endometriosis in Adolescents

Focusing specifically on diagnosing peritoneal endometriosis in adolescents is crucial for several reasons. The first one is the high prevalence of primary dysmenorrhoea. Primary dysmenorrhoea is common among young women, affecting between 45% and 95% of menstruating women. It is characterised by painful menstruation in the absence of pelvic pathology [38]. Moreover, even in adolescents with intraperitoneal endometriosis, symptoms are often nonspecific. Khashchenko's study [35] on the early diagnosis of endometriosis in a cohort of 134 patients found that cyclic pain was present in only 9.4% of cases, whereas chronic pelvic pain was a common complaint that often resisted treatment with nonsteroidal anti-inflammatory drugs (NSAIDs) or combined oral contraceptives (COCs). Adolescents with peritoneal endometriosis (PE) typically present with hereditary predisposition, persistent dysmenorrhoea, reduced daily activity, and gastrointestinal symptoms.

The second reason is the nonspecific imaging findings and the lack of clear data on endometriosis imaging description among adolescents. Imaging results are often nonspecific due to the prevalence of subtle intraperitoneal endometriosis in this population (early stages according to the r-ASRM classification). Additionally, the detection of pathological lesions is challenging due to their small size (superficial lesions smaller than 2–3 mm) and their fibrous nature, which appears as a hypointense signal on T2-weighted images, along with the absence of a specific T1 hyperintense signal.

The mild, isolated involvement of the uterosacral ligament may represent the majority of endometriosis cases diagnosed among adolescents [39]. As previously discussed, even for highly experienced radiologists, the specificity of MRI for detecting mild uterosacral ligament involvement can dramatically decrease to 33% [40]. This could lead to a potentially high false-positive rate, especially given the physiological changes occurring during puberty [41]. Therefore, the liberal or restrictive use of MRI in the population of young adolescent women is a significant concern.

When suggestive symptoms such as severe dysmenorrhoea are present, the first aim of imaging should be to rule out an obstructive congenital anomaly in the reproductive tract. These anomalies could include a unicornuate uterus with an unattached rudimentary blind horn, **OR AN** unilateral or bilateral vaginal obstruction, **OR** a vaginal septum, **OR** an imperforate hymen. The second aim is to detect a potential endometriotic cyst. This can be achieved by using a suprapubic abdominal ultrasound.

2.5.1 Use of MRI for Diagnosing Endometriosis in Adolescents with Pelvic Pain: Considerations and Cautions

MRI should be used cautiously in adolescents with pelvic pain, as noted previously [41]. Given the frequent inability to perform transvaginal sonography in this population, MRI is often considered the first-line imaging technique.

Indeed, in an observational study that employed systematic MRI for adolescent women referred for 'severe dysmenorrhoea resistant to nonsteroidal anti-inflammatory treatment', investigators estimated the prevalence of endometriosis to be 39% [39]. However, this result appears to be overestimated compared to the less than 1% prevalence estimated in the general population of young women. This discrepancy likely suggests that the study sample was not representative of the broader adolescent population, probably due to a major referral bias [41].

Increasing the use of MRI in routine practice among adolescents could result in an unacceptable false-positive rate, with potential risks for these young women, including unnecessary laparoscopies. Priority should be given to first-line radiologic examinations, such as pelvic ultrasound—which is sufficient to detect endometrioma—and medical treatment for pelvic pain symptoms. A 'treat first' approach should be prioritised in this population.

Few studies have specifically focused on superficial endometriosis among adolescent, but consensus among all studies has been reached on the low sensitivity of imaging, even among specialised radiology teams. Thus, the challenge of early diagnosis for endometriosis, particularly in the absence of specific implants, necessitates a discussion about increasing sensitivity at the expense of specificity, which could lead to a significant rise in false positives. In Khashchenko's study [35], MRI has a higher sensitivity in detecting peritoneal endometriosis than that of ultrasound. Whereas ultrasound detects peritoneal endometriosis in only 3.3% of cases, MRI identifies it in 78.9%. Persistent dysmenorrhoea and detected MRI parameters predict the laparoscopic confirmation of initial superficial endometriosis in adolescents 84.3% of the time. Therefore, that MRI may yield a large number is not surprising. Carefully interpreting the MRI findings is necessary to avoid misdiagnosis.

The decision to use imaging to detect endometriosis in adolescents should first be based on a thorough medical history and a proper clinical examination, including abdominal palpation and visual inspections of the vulva and hymen. The decision to proceed with an MRI should be guided by three factors: the prevalence of mild endometriosis among adolescents, the risk of falsely labelling a young woman with a chronic disease, and the impact on the management plan.

Not overdiagnosing intraperitoneal endometriosis in adolescents is crucial. In cases featuring uncertainty (e.g. confined ovarian fossae or peritoneal thickening without T1 FS hyperintensity), a follow-up MRI may be proposed to assess progression and to determine whether more-specific signs appear. These young women and those accompanying them should be given thorough information to avoid misunderstanding what diagnostic uncertainty means.

2.6 Conclusions

Contrary to commonly held beliefs and recommendations regarding the imaging of endometriosis, superficial endometriosis is eligible for reference imaging, both TVUS and MRI. Physicians need to know the precise description of the semiology and the practice of a technically relevant examination procedure such as UBESS for ultrasound and the standardised protocol of the European Society of Urogenital Radiology (ESUR) for MRI. These examinations can often guide the diagnosis by looking for signs that are sometimes direct, but often indirect, but if they are part of a suggestive clinical context, they can contribute to a definitive diagnosis. Diagnostic classification using nonbinary criteria could be useful, taking into account the possibility of uncertain cases that may require further investigation or repeat imaging over time.

The central questions are as follows:

1. Is making an early imaging diagnosis of intraperitoneal endometriosis clinically beneficial? Does underdiagnosing superficial endometriosis deprive patients of an opportunity? On the other hand, falsely diagnosing endometriosis may be dangerous; this can lead to unnecessary therapies or interventions and increase patient anxiety, thus contributing to medical errancy. To promote an early imaging diagnosis of superficial endometriosis, we must

better understand the natural history of the disease. Is superficial endometriosis a progressive disease, and in what cases could early detection prevent the later onset of a more severe disease? We currently have no answers to these questions.

2. Will the diagnosis of superficial endometriosis add value to the management and recovery of patients? The recognition of endometriosis disease, even in its minimal or mild forms, is considered beneficial for patients because they feel recognised [42]. Conversely, in the 'treat first' option, the diagnosis of endometriosis does not always lead to new therapeutic solutions. In our practice, as in others, we use the visualisation of target lesions documented via imaging as a marker of surgical efficacy. In the absence of such clearly visible and well-documented lesions, the question of probabilistic treatment, such as hormone therapy or diagnostic surgery, arises. In this context, the contribution of biomarkers currently under development could provide further answers.

References

1. Nisolle M, Donnez J. Peritoneal endometriosis, ovarian endometriosis, and adenomyotic nodules of the rectovaginal septum are three different entities. Fertil Steril. 1997;68(4):585–96.
2. Koninckx PR, Oosterlynck D, D'Hooghe T, Meuleman C. Deeply infiltrating endometriosis is a disease whereas mild endometriosis could be considered a non-disease. Ann N Y Acad Sci. 1994;734:333–41.
3. Okaro E, Condous G, Khalid A, Timmerman D, Ameye L, Huffel SV, et al. The use of ultrasound-based 'soft markers' for the prediction of pelvic pathology in women with chronic pelvic pain—can we reduce the need for laparoscopy? BJOG. 2006;113(3):251–6. Epub 2006/02/21.
4. Dunselman GA, Vermeulen N, Becker C, Calhaz-Jorge C, D'Hooghe T, De Bie B, et al. ESHRE guideline: management of women with endometriosis. Hum Reprod. 2014;29(3):400–12. Epub 2014/01/18.
5. Martire FG, Russo C, Selntigia A, Nocita E, Soreca G, Lazzeri L, et al. Early noninvasive diagnosis of endometriosis: dysmenorrhea and specific ultrasound findings are important indicators in young women. Fertil Steril. 2023;119(3):455–64. Epub 2022/12/10.
6. Gougoutas CA, Siegelman ES, Hunt J, Outwater EK. Pelvic endometriosis: various manifestations and MR imaging findings. AJR Am J Roentgenol. 2000;175(2):353–8. Epub 2000/08/01.
7. Donnez J, Nisolle M, Casanas-Roux F. Three-dimensional architectures of peritoneal endometriosis. Fertil Steril. 1992;57(5):980–3.
8. Sampson J. Peritoneal endometriosis is due to the menstrual dissemination of endometrial tissue into the peritoneal cavity. Am J Obstet Gynecol. 1927;14:422–69.
9. Jansen RP, Russell P. Nonpigmented endometriosis: clinical, laparoscopic, and pathologic definition. Am J Obstet Gynecol. 1986;155(6):1154–9.
10. Brosens IA, Vasquez G, Deprest J, Puttemans P. Pathogenesis of endometriosis. In: Nezhat CR, Berger GS, Nezhat FR, Buttram VC, Nezhat CH, editors. Endometriosis: advanced management and surgical techniques. New York: Springer-Verlag; 1995. p. 9–17.
11. Nisolle M, Paindaveine B, Bourdon A, Berliere M, Casanas-Roux F, Donnez J. Histologic study of peritoneal endometriosis in infertile women. Fertil Steril. 1990;53(6):984–8.
12. Balasch J, Creus M, Fabregues F, Carmona F, Ordi J, Martinez-Roman S, et al. Visible and non-visible endometriosis at laparoscopy in fertile and infertile women and in patients with chronic pelvic pain: a prospective study. Hum Reprod. 1996;11(2):387–91.
13. Brosens IA, Puttemans P, Deprest J, Rombauts L. The endometriosis cycle and its derailments. Hum Reprod. 1994;9(5):770–1.
14. Nisolle M, Casanas-Roux F, Anaf V, Mine JM, Donnez J. Morphometric study of the stromal vascularization in peritoneal endometriosis. Fertil Steril. 1993;59(3):681–4.
15. Tomassetti C, Johnson NP, Petrozza J, Abrao MS, Einarsson JI, Horne AW, et al. An international terminology for endometriosis, 2021. Facts Views Vis Obgyn. 2021;13(4):295–304. Epub 2021/10/22.
16. Bailey F, Gaughran J, Mitchell S, Ovadia C, Holland TK. Diagnosis of superficial endometriosis on transvaginal ultrasound by visualization of peritoneum of pouch of Douglas. Ultrasound Obstet Gynecol. 2024;63(1):105–12. Epub 2023/11/06.
17. Rawson JM. Prevalence of endometriosis in infertile women. J Reprod Med. 1991;36:513–5.
18. Guerriero S, Condous G, van den Bosch T, Valentin L, Leone FP, Van Schoubroeck D, et al. Systematic approach to sonographic evaluation of the pelvis in women with suspected endometriosis, including terms, definitions and measurements: a consensus opinion from the International Deep Endometriosis Analysis (IDEA) group. Ultrasound Obstet Gynecol. 2016;48(3):318–32. Epub 2016/06/29.
19. Hudelist G, English J, Thomas AE, Tinelli A, Singer CF, Keckstein J. Diagnostic accuracy of transvaginal ultrasound for non-invasive diagnosis of bowel endometriosis: systematic review and meta-analysis. Ultrasound Obstet Gynecol. 2011;37(3):257–63. Epub 2010/10/19.

20. Menakaya U, Reid S, Lu C, Gerges B, Infante F, Condous G. Performance of ultrasound-based endometriosis staging system (UBESS) for predicting level of complexity of laparoscopic surgery for endometriosis. Ultrasound Obstet Gynecol. 2016;48(6):786–95. Epub 2016/01/15.
21. Leonardi M, Robledo KP, Espada M, Vanza K, Condous G. SonoPODography: A new diagnostic technique for visualizing superficial endometriosis. Eur J Obstet Gynecol Reprod Biol. 2020;254:124–31. Epub 2020/09/23.
22. Chowdary P, Stone K, Ma T, Readman E, McIlwaine K, Druitt M, et al. Multicentre retrospective study to assess diagnostic accuracy of ultrasound for superficial endometriosis-are we any closer? Aust N Z J Obstet Gynaecol. 2019;59(2):279–84. Epub 2018/11/10.
23. Reid S, Leonardi M, Lu C, Condous G. The association between ultrasound-based 'soft markers' and endometriosis type/location: a prospective observational study. Eur J Obstet Gynecol Reprod Biol. 2019;234:171–8. Epub 2019/02/02.
24. Alcazar JL, Eguez PM, Forcada P, Ternero E, Martinez C, Pascual MA, et al. Diagnostic accuracy of sliding sign for detecting pouch of Douglas obliteration and bowel involvement in women with suspected endometriosis: systematic review and meta-analysis. Ultrasound Obstet Gynecol. 2022;60(4):477–86. Epub 2022/03/16.
25. Reid S, Condous G. Transvaginal sonographic sliding sign: accurate prediction of pouch of Douglas obliteration. Ultrasound Obstet Gynecol. 2013;41(6):605–7. Epub 2013/05/29.
26. Yong PJ, Sutton C, Suen M, Williams C. Endovaginal ultrasound-assisted pain mapping in endometriosis and chronic pelvic pain. J Obstet Gynaecol. 2013;33(7):715–9. Epub 2013/10/17.
27. Pedrassani M, Guerriero S, Pascual MA, Ajossa S, Graupera B, Pagliuca M, et al. Superficial endometriosis at ultrasound examination—a diagnostic criteria proposal. Diagnostics (Basel). 2023;13(11):1876. Epub 2023/06/10.
28. HAS C. Prise en charge de l'endométriose. [pdf]: Haute Autorité de Santé; 2018 [updated 6 Décembre 2018].
29. Thomassin-Naggara I, Zoua CS, Bazot M, Monroc M, Roman H, Razakamantsoa L, et al. Diagnostic MRI for deep pelvic endometriosis: towards a standardized protocol? Eur Radiol. 2024;34(12):7705–15. Epub 2024/07/03
30. Bourgioti C, Preza O, Panourgias E, Chatoupis K, Antoniou A, Nikolaidou ME, et al. MR imaging of endometriosis: Spectrum of disease. Diagn Interv Imaging. 2017;98(11):751–67. Epub 2017/06/28.
31. Solak A, Sahin N, Genc B, Sever AR, Genc M, Sivrikoz ON. Diagnostic value of susceptibility-weighted imaging of abdominal wall endometriomas during the cyclic menstrual changes: a preliminary study. Eur J Radiol. 2013;82(9):e411–6. Epub 2013/06/15.
32. Le Moal J, Goria S, Chesneau J, Fauconnier A, Kvaskoff M, De Crouy-Chanel P, et al. Increasing incidence and spatial hotspots of hospitalized endometriosis in France from 2011 to 2017. Sci Rep. 2022;12(1):6966. Epub 2022/04/29.
33. Thomeer MG, Steensma AB, van Santbrink EJ, Willemssen FE, Wielopolski PA, Hunink MG, et al. Can magnetic resonance imaging at 3.0-Tesla reliably detect patients with endometriosis? Initial results. J Obstet Gynaecol Res. 2014;40(4):1051–8. Epub 2014/01/17.
34. Fan J, McDonnell R, Jacques A, Fender L, Lo G. MRI sliding sign: using MRI to assess rectouterine mobility in pelvic endometriosis. J Med Imaging Radiat Oncol. 2022;66(1):54–9. Epub 2021/07/10.
35. Khashchenko EP, Uvarova EV, Fatkhudinov TK, Chuprynin VD, Asaturova AV, Kulabukhova EA, et al. Endometriosis in adolescents: diagnostics, clinical and Laparoscopic features. J Clin Med. 2023;12(4):1678. Epub 2023/02/26.
36. Thomassin-Naggara I, Lamrabet S, Crestani A, Bekhouche A, Wahab CA, Kermarrec E, et al. Magnetic resonance imaging classification of deep pelvic endometriosis: description and impact on surgical management. Hum Reprod. 2020;35(7):1589–600. Epub 2020/07/04.
37. Stoppa M, Agostini A, Pivano A, Siles P, Calderon L, Netter A. Mild endometriosis of the uterosacral ligaments: a retrospective study of magnetic resonance imaging performance for diagnosis. Reprod Biomed Online. 2023;46(6):947–55. Epub 2023/04/18.
38. Iacovides S, Avidon I, Baker FC. What we know about primary dysmenorrhea today: a critical review. Hum Reprod Update. 2015;21(6):762–78. Epub 2015/09/09.
39. Millischer AE, Santulli P, Da Costa S, Bordonne C, Cazaubon E, Marcellin L, et al. Adolescent endometriosis: prevalence increases with age on magnetic resonance imaging scan. Fertil Steril. 2023;119(4):626–33. Epub 2023/01/03.
40. Nisenblat V, Bossuyt PM, Farquhar C, Johnson N, Hull ML. Imaging modalities for the non-invasive diagnosis of endometriosis. Cochrane Database Syst Rev. 2016;2:CD009591. Epub 2016/02/27.
41. Margueritte F, Fauconnier A. Adolescent endometriosis: Should we really use magnetic resonance imaging scans in this population? Fertil Steril. 2023;120(3 Pt 2):706. Epub 2023/05/25.
42. Wang CY. Coping with endometriosis. Lancet. 2004;364(9447):1800. Epub 2004/11/16.

Adnexal Endometriosis. Typical Benign Endometriosis

3

Sanja Stojanović, Vesna Kopitović, Luka Anđelić, Stevan Milatović, and Una Molnar

3.1 Introduction

Endometriosis is one of the most enigmatic diseases affecting women of reproductive age. It is defined as the presence of endometria-like tissue (glands and stroma) outside the uterus, which induces a chronic inflammatory reaction, scar tissue, and adhesions that may distort a woman's pelvic anatomy [1]. The most common sites are ovaries. Ovaries are parts of the adnexal structures, which include the ovaries, fallopian tubes, and surrounding ligaments. The healthy appearance of ovaries is a paired structure, usually 3–5 cm across their longest diameter, located on each side of the uterus at the ovarian fossa, close to the pelvic wall. In premenopausal women, ovaries are easily recognized as multiple small cysts, which are follicles in different phases of maturation. Fallopian tubes are a part of the adnexal structures situated on both sides of the uterus, extending to the ovaries, which are housed at the the end of tubes that have fingerlike extensions called fimbriae. Fallopian tubes pass through the layers of a broad ligament, its proximal part. Suspensory ligaments maintain the position of the ovaries connected to uterus. All these adnexal structures could be affected by endometriosis [1].

Surgical treatment was for years considered the gold standard in the treatment of endometriosis, and in certain cases, it still is. Unfortunately, a lack of consensus persists on numerous questions, like when to operate, how radical the operation should be, whether it should be operated on at all, how to treat recurrent endometriosis, and more.

Although ovarian endometriosis is the most common site of the disease and usually the first place where it can be discovered, different perspectives abound about whether to operate. For years, ultrasonography and laparoscopy were regarded as the gold standard, even for the diagnosis of the extent of adnexal endometriosis.

S. Stojanović (✉)
Faculty of Medicine, University of Novi Sad, Novi Sad, Serbia

Center for Radiology, University Clinical Center of Vojvodina, Novi Sad, Serbia
e-mail: sanja.stojanovic@mf.uns.ac.rs

V. Kopitović
Ferona Fertility Clinic, Novi Sad, Serbia

L. Anđelić
General Hospital New Hospital, Novi Sad, Serbia

S. Milatović
Faculty of Medicine, University of Novi Sad, Novi Sad, Serbia

Clinic for Gynecology and Obstetrics, University Clinical Center of Vojvodina, Novi Sad, Serbia
e-mail: stevan.milatovic@mf.uns.ac.rs

U. Molnar
Center for Radiology, University Clinical Center of Vojvodina, Novi Sad, Serbia

Faculty of Sciences, University of Novi Sad, Novi Sad, Serbia
e-mail: una.molnar@df.uns.ac.rs

I. Thomassin-Naggara (ed.), *Imaging of Endometriosis: A Comparative Guide of US, MRI and Surgery*, https://doi.org/10.1007/978-3-031-82750-1_3

3.2 Appearance of Endometriosis on Imaging

Ovaries are the most common sites of endometriosis (20–40% of cases) [2], which may show the following patterns [3]:

- Superficial implants associated with fibrous adhesions (often underdiagnosed at imaging due to their small size (<5 mm)) [3]
- Microintraovarian endometriomas (small (<1 cm) implants inside the ovaries)
- Deep implants with repeated cyclic hemorrhage resulting in endometriotic cysts—endometriomas (pseudocyst with hemorrhagic content, formed by the invagination of endometriosis within the ovarian cortex [4]—frequently multiple and bilateral (50% of cases)), where confirmation that the cyst belongs to an ovary is finding a crescent sign present on MRI and ultrasound imaging (Figs. 3.1 and 3.2)

Hydrosalpinx, Hematosalpinx

In certain cases, the only sign of endometriosis is hydro- or hematosalpinx. Hydrosalpinx develops as a result of adhesions and scarring, and it may appear as a dilated fallopian tube folding on itself, forming a sausage-like C- or S-shaped cystic mass [5]. The signal intensity of the fluid in the fallopian tube depends on the cause of the blockage [6] and the type of the fluid, so it could be hydrosalpinx when no trace of blood products can be found or hematosalpinx when such a trace can be found. When adhesions cause the ovaries to be repositioned to within proximity to each other, this results in the appearance of kissing ovaries on imaging (usually related to superficial endometriosis in the ovarian fossae).

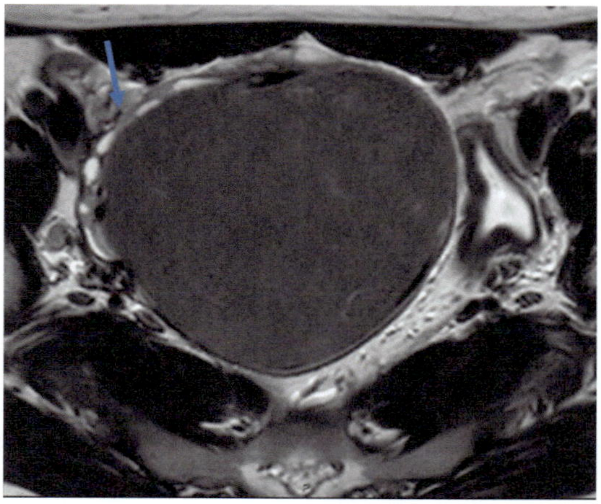

Fig. 3.1 T2W image of endometrial cyst originating from right ovary: semilunar rim of healthy ovarian tissue (crescent sign) (arrow)

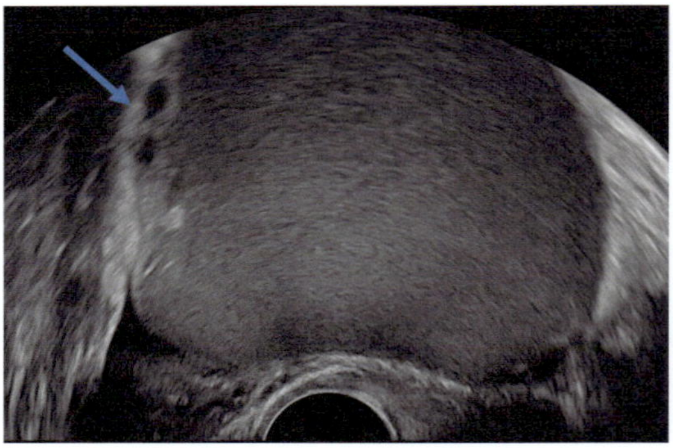

Fig. 3.2 Ultrasound image ofan endometrial cyst, which correlates with MR image: semilunar rim of healthy ovarian tissue (crescent sign) (arrow)

Even though in the differential diagnosis of ovarian endometriosis, transvaginal US is highly sensitive and specific, MR imaging is considered by some authors as the best imaging modality for diagnosing endometriomas due to its high sensitivity and specificity, of 95% and 91%, respectively [7]. According to the Cochrane systematic review, transvaginal ultrasonography (TVUS) and MRI have the same accuracy as that of laparoscopy when diagnosing endometriomas [7]. The added value of MR imaging is to not only allow the diagnosis of benign ovarian cyst, deep pelvic endometriosis, and associated malignancy but also gain insights into the loco-regional extension of the disease. It is also useful in detecting recurrences after medical or surgical treatment.

The overall sensitivity of MRI in diagnosing endometriosis is estimated to be 94% [8]; however, the specificity is slightly lower, leading to a 10% false-positive rate [9]. Computed tomography (CT) is not the modality of choice because patients could come to CT only because of other, usually emergency, reasons. All endometrial cysts on CT look the same as any other cysts; the differentiation is possible only for dermoid cysts because fatty content has a specific appearance.

The image of ovarian endometriosis on ultrasound is quite typical: an ovoid, well-circumscribed cystic mass rising from the ovary and filled with echoic reflections (Figs. 3.3 and 3.4). If it is under acute inflammation, the wall might be thickened. Sometimes endometriomas exhibit septation or multiple septations. Among the most important ultrasound findings are hyperechoic foci seen in the wall, which should not be missed during an initial diagnosis. They are usually smaller and more echogenic than mural nodules are. Endometriomas do not have color Doppler signals.

Improving technology for and the education of dedicated radiologists as they apply to imaging female patients has improved the diagnosis of endometriosis as well.

The typical features of endometriomas at MR imaging are as follows:

- The shading sign can be seen on T2-weighted images as decreased signal intensity (SI), and it results from cyclic bleeding over time. Magnetism-susceptible inhomogeneity based

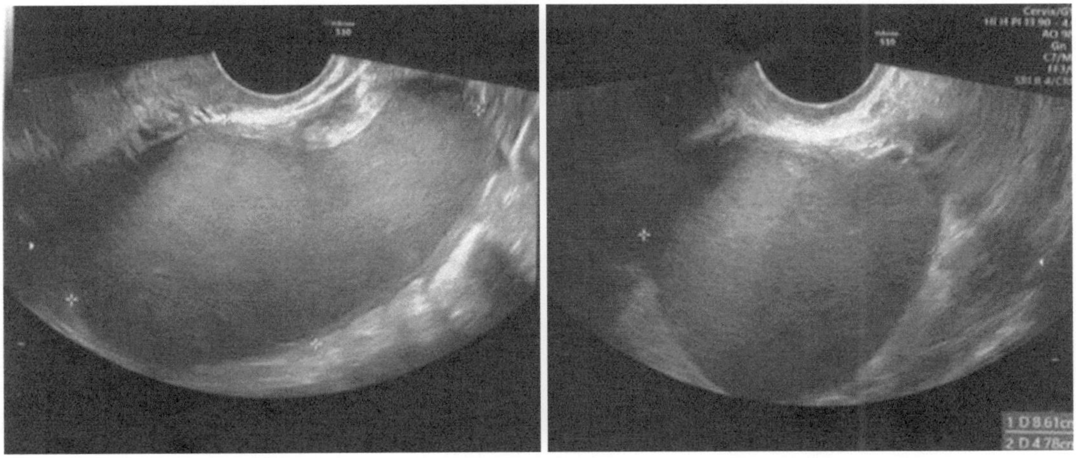

Fig. 3.3 Ultrasound images of a left ovary: unilocular, avascular cyst with ground-glass appearance on internal echo

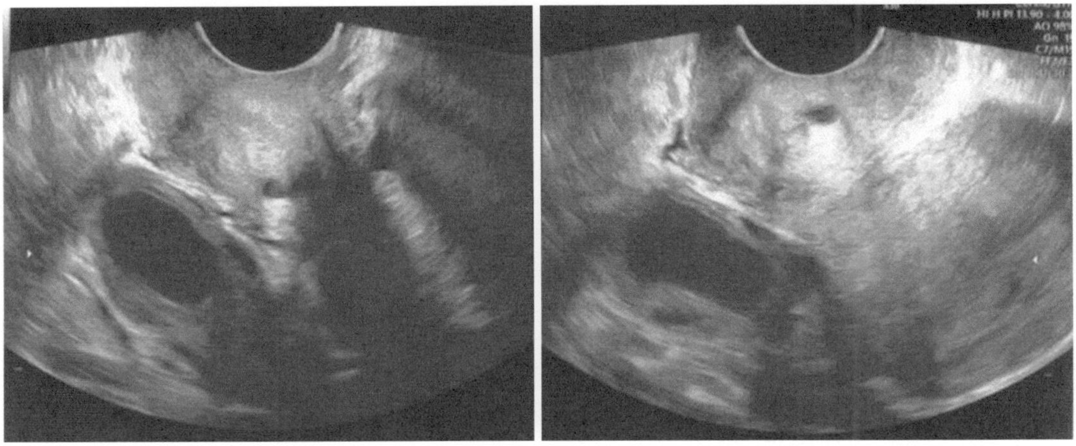

Fig. 3.4 Ultrasound images of a healthy right ovary

on iron concentration and blood viscosity determines a decrease in T2 relaxation time and can be seen in variations from faint, layered signal loss to complete signal loss within a cyst. Therefore, on T2-weighted images, endometriomas will show a gradual loss of signal within the lesion, accompanied by low signal intensity until the entire signal is absent in the declivous portion ("shading"). The presence of "shading" is useful in detecting endometriotic cysts because of its high sensitivity [9]. In patients with a history of endometriosis, endometriomas increasing in size or a loss of shading on T2-weighted images [10, 11] should raise concerns over a potential malignant transformation. The loss of shading on T2 images is thought to be due to fluid secretions by malignant components, diluting the chronic hemorrhagic content.

- T2 dark spot signs—discrete, well-defined, and markedly hypointense foci within a cyst on T2-weighted images, which are often linear, punctate, or oval in shape (Fig. 3.5). According to some speculation, this sign represents the presence of chronic retracted blood clots with high concentrations of protein and hemosiderin [9]. The specificity of this sign was thought to be very high, >90% [12], but in recent papers, the specificity has been shown to be lower given that T2 dark spot signs can sometimes be seen in hemorrhagic cysts as well.
- The rim sign—a curve line around a cystic mass—could appear on T1-weighted images and especially on T2-weighted sequences. It presents as a hypointense line that could be complete (the whole circle) or incomplete and is also regarded as one of the signs of endometriosis (Figs. 3.6 and 3.7).
- T1 high-signal multiplicity—multiple high-signal cysts on T1-weighted images that result from repeated bleeding and the formation of new blood locules—is a characteristic finding [13] (Fig. 3.8).

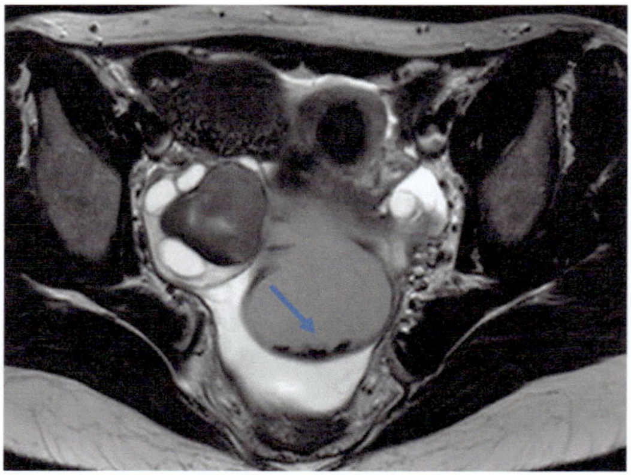

Fig. 3.5 Axial T2W MR image of T2 dark spot sign (arrow)

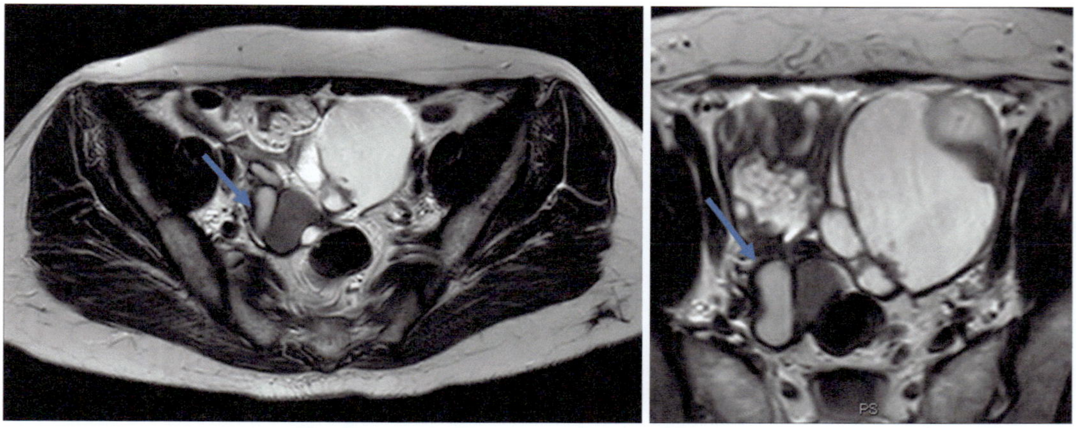

Fig. 3.6 Axial T2W image of incomplete hypointense rim sign (arrow)

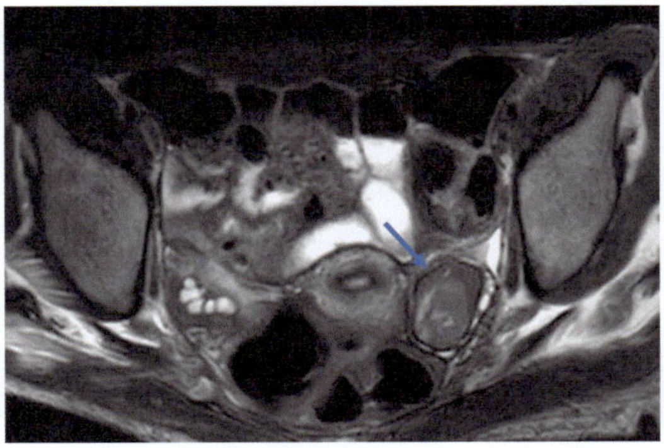

Fig. 3.7 Axial T2W image of complete hypointense rim sign (arrow)

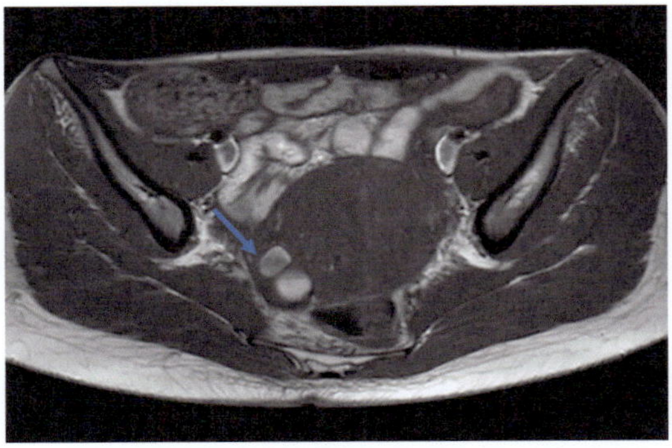

Fig. 3.8 Axial T1W image showing T1 hyperintense signal multiplicity (arrow)

In rare cases (<5%), which depend on the protein and hemosiderin concentrations and on the patient's age, endometriomas may appear as T2-hyperintense [14].

The recommended protocol to explore pelvic endometriosis was updated in 2017 by the European Society of Urogenital Radiology [15], which includes T2-weighted images without fat suppression in all three orthogonal planes and T1-weighted sequences with and without fat suppression. Roles of different MR sequences has now been numbered so readers can better parse following paragraphs.

I T2-weighted sequences without fat suppression are the best sequences for detecting pelvic endometriosis [12], in particular for the evaluation of fibrotic lesions [2]. Ovarian endometriosis varies in its appearance depending on the cyst content, so it could present as different degrees of high SI to even hypo. The most common finding is a different level of a less-intense signal, partial or complete, defined as shading. The most important is the dropping of signal intensity on T2-weighted, compared to T1-weighted, signal intensity, although no quantitative feature has been established for determining the exact degree.

II The fat-suppressed T1-weighted three-dimensional (3D)-gradient echo sequence improves the sensitivity of MR imaging in the detection of small lesions. It is the most sensitive for the detection of bloody foci and peritoneal endometriosis because fat suppression narrows the dynamic signal range, thus accentuating the differences in tissue signal. It also increases MRI specificity because fat-containing lesions such as dermoids are ruled out from the differential diagnosis of endometriomas [16].

The intravenous injection of gadolinium is not mandatory in the setting of typical endometriosis, but it should be performed in the presence of a solid component within an endometrioma to better characterize the lesion [17, 18]. Thus, for the exploration of a complex ovarian mass, adding the following sequences is recommended [19, 20].

III The contrast-enhanced fat-suppressed T1-weighted 3D-gradient echo sequence is useful in specific cases, namely where US or T2-weighted MR sequences suggest potential malignancy, for the detection of enhancing mural nodules within adnexal masses [12]. It also has a significant role in ureter visualization for assessing the anatomical relationship between the ureters and endometrial cysts or implants before surgery, which helps to avoid any possible detachment of ligation during the procedure. Contrast-enhanced dynamic subtraction images are obtained by using a gradient echo sequence [20] and subtractions between enhanced and unenhanced fat-saturated T1-weighted images. They are helpful for distinguishing the true enhancement of solid nodules that may be hard to depict within the already-hyperintense hemorrhagic cystic fluid of endometriomas on T1-weighted sequences [21].

IV T2-weighted sequences* depict magnetic susceptibility effects as signal voids [22].

This pulse sequence is useful in the detection of old hemorrhagic content in endometriomas and endometriotic implants because of its sensitivity to hemosiderin. Nevertheless, because of the susceptibility artifacts caused by intestinal gas, it is not routinely used in the standard MR protocol and represents an optional sequence.

V Diffusion-weighted imaging (DWI) sequences do not possess high specificity in ovarian endometriomas, because both endometriomas, as well as other ovarian lesions can be presented with similar characteristics on DWI. Solid, cellular portions display high signal intensity with an associated low signal on the apparent diffusion coefficient (ADC) map, whereas others can show no signs of diffusion restriction at all. Sometimes, diffusion-weighted sequences are useful to distinguish luteal cysts and endometriomas. Luteal cysts typically display a high-signal rim intensity in contrast with that of endometriomas.

Several authors have suggested that endometriomas are characterized by having lower ADC values than those of other cystic lesions. However, its role in differentiating endometriomas from functional hemorrhagic ovarian cysts is still debated. The recommendations for imaging reporting to improve the ability to predict the success of a fertility procedure are to report on the following: the size and number of endometriomas, uni/bilaterality, any associated dilated tubes, a residual ovarian parenchyma, and a contralateral ovary (its size and number follicles).

3.3 Differential Diagnosis

The differential diagnosis of endometriomas includes lesions with high signal intensity on T1-weighted images: dermoids, mucinous cystic neoplasms, and hemorrhagic masses. The combination of T2-weighted images, DWI signals, and ADC analysis helps to characterize the different types of liquids.

	T1	T1 FS	T2	DW	ADC
Endometriotic	++++	++++	–	+++	–
Fatty	+++	–	+	++	–
Proteinaceous	++	+++	+	+	+
Colloid	++	++	–	–	–
Melanin, Manganese	++	++	+	–	
Methemoglobin	Variable	Unchanged	Variable	Variable	Variable

Note: T1 = T1 - weighted image; T1 FS = fat-suppressed T1 -weighted image; T2 = T2 - weighted image X; DWI = diffusion - weighted image; and ADC = apparent diffusion coefficient

Endometriomas vs. Mucinous Lesions
Mucinous lesions may show high T1-weighted signals but appear in high or intermediate T2-weighted signals without clots, usually displaying thin septations, and when a borderline degeneration occurs, the cyst contains very small papillary projections visible as irregular septa.

Endometriomas vs. Hemorrhagic Masses
Hemorrhagic follicular cysts and hemorrhagic corpus luteum cysts are functional hemorrhagic cysts, which are usually unilocular and unilateral and mostly disappear on follow-up examinations (generally in 4–6 weeks) [16]. They are temporary conditions without any influence on the health status of women and should be solved without surgery. On the other hand, endometrioma is sometimes a sign of a serious health disorder. For several decades, many believed that seeing the shading sign was proof of endometriotic cysts. Unfortunately, the everyday practice denied it, and the "T2 shading sign" can in some cases be found in hemorrhagic cysts as well. In recent papers, the authors have tried to define specific signs, and the T2 dark spot sign showed high specificity and low sensitivity. The rim sign could also be present in certain percentages in both conditions (an incomplete rim sign appears more often in an endometriotic cyst, whereas a complete rim sign appears more often in a hem-

orrhagic cyst) [23]. That raised the idea of trying a texture analysis of the endometriotic and hemorrhagic cystic wall because they show different characteristics. Improving technologies and engaging in further investigation are important to increasing certainty in differentiating those entities. The other useful features that distinguish endometriomas from hemorrhagic cysts are wall thickness (thick for hemorrhagic cyst and thin for endometrioma) and wall enhancement (intense for hemorrhagic cysts). Finally, endometriomas display a homogeneous, internally high DW signal intensity, whereas hemorrhagic cysts show only a high DW signal intensity from the wall.

Endometriomas vs. Dermoids

A dermoid may mimic an endometrioma on TVUS given that both can display a ground-glass high echoic signal with high echoic condensation due to clots or phaneres.

Because different MR sequences are available, the differentiation of dermoid cysts is much easier and more specific (Figs. 3.9 and 3.10). Fat-saturated T1-weighted sequences are helpful to rule out a fat-containing lesion (such as dermoids) because they can show a drop in the SI or can remain hyperintense, the latter confirming the presence of blood [24].

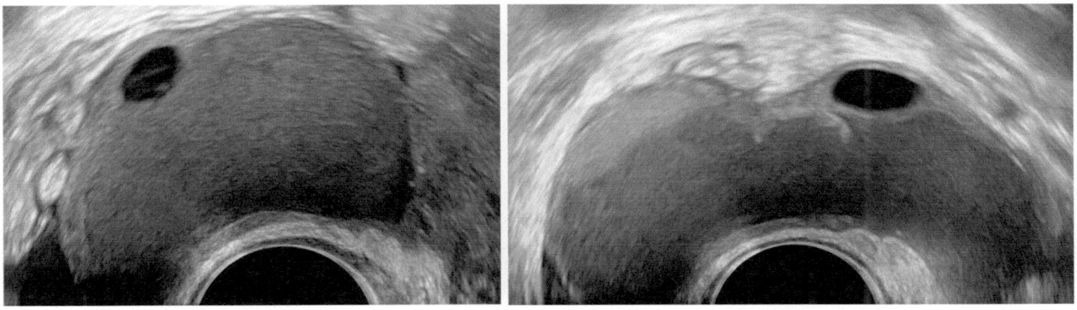

Fig. 3.9 Ultrasound images of the left ovary: unilocular, avascular cyst with ground-glass appearance on internal echo

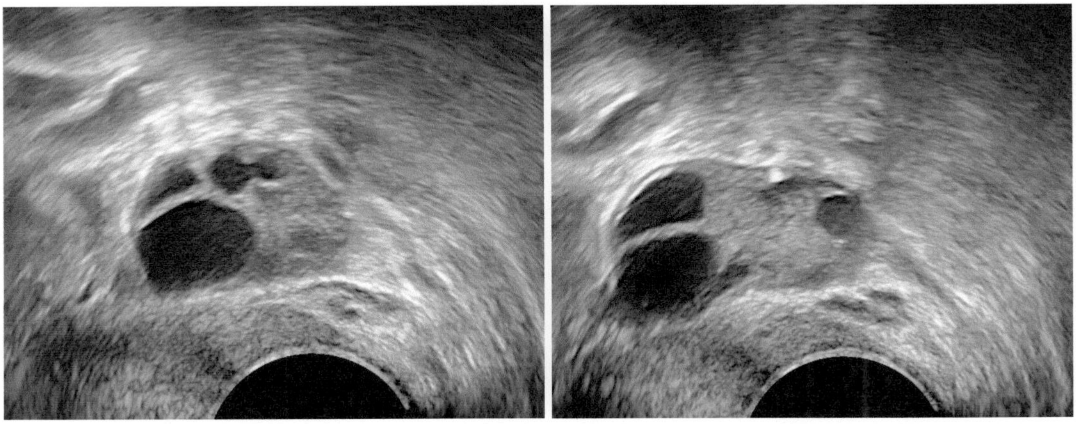

Fig. 3.10 Ultrasound images of the healthy right ovary

3.4 Endometriosis and IVF

Endometriosis is often the cause of infertility in women. In the case of benign ovarian endometriosis, medical strategies have overcome surgical strategies, which are discussed only in cases of medical treatment failure. However, a variety of studies have been carried out to evaluate the impact of surgery for ovarian endometriomas on IVF outcomes.

The main questions are, could the ovarian reserve be significantly reduced after surgery, and will surgery help to yield further IVF results or will it be harmful? Laparoscopic surgery is still a common practice in the treatment of endometriomas in cases of infertility. Many studies have shown a reduced ovarian reserve in affected ovaries, regardless of the operation.

In recent years, patient-tailored therapy has been the usual choice for surgery. Otherwise, conservative therapy is chosen on the basis of several clinical parameters: The size of the endometrioma, the age of the patient, the number of previous fertility attempts, and the results of a sperm analysis are among them. The size of the endometrioma itself could indicate the aggressiveness of the disease: The larger the endometrioma, the less space left for the follicles in the ovary. Both the presence of an endometrioma reducing the functional volume of ovaries and surgery-induced damage could be unfavorable for fertility.

According to the 2014 European Society of Human Reproduction and Embryology guidelines, for patients with endometrioma measuring ≥3 cm, laparoscopic ovarian cystectomy is recommended before IVF either to reduce the risk of infection during oocyte retrieval and facilitate access to the follicles or to improve the ovarian response to controlled ovarian stimulation [25]. Different clinical cases have demonstrated a correlation between MR findings and surgical findings (Cases 3.1, 3.2, 3.3, 3.4, 3.5, 3.6, and 3.7). In Case 3.3, a patient with endometriomas who developed hyperstimulation during IVF is presented. In cases of hyperstimulation, the insemination process must be postponed.

3.5 Ovarian Surgery for Endometriomas Prior to IVF

The association between endometriosis and infertility is still not entirely clear. Among infertile women, the prevalence is estimated to range between 30% and 50% [26]. Although assisted reproductive technology (ART) procedures have been successful in infertile women with endometriosis [27], worse results are still expected for women with the disease, mostly due to reduced ovarian reserve [28]. Numerous medical options are available to treat endometriosis, and they should be regarded as complementary, not competitive, modalities.

Various studies have been carried out to evaluate the impact of surgery for ovarian endometriomas on IVF outcomes, with conflicting results [29]. The main dilemma in this field is whether damage to ovarian reserve is a consequence of endometriosis per se, a result of surgery, or—most likely—a combination of these two factors. Numerous studies have shown reduced ovarian reserve in affected ovaries, regardless of surgery [30, 31]. Both endometrioma-related injury and surgery-mediated damage may be detrimental to fertility. The relative importance of these two factors remains to be clarified.

Expectant management minimizes the risk for the following:

- Surgical damage to the ovaries with decreased ovarian reserve
- Operation complications

The best professionals argue that the surgical management of endometriomas has no significant effect on IVF pregnancy rates or on the ovarian response to stimulation compared with no treatment [31, 32]. Thus, if we cannot expect surgery to improve ovarian response, why should we operate on these women and expose them to risk, especially if numerous studies have shown significant damage to ovarian reserve and very few, if any, complications on expectant management? ESHRE guidelines on endometriosis management indicate that laparoscopic ovarian cystectomy in patients with unilateral endometriomas between 3 and 6 cm in diameter before IVF/ICSI can decrease ovarian response without improving IVF cycle outcomes [33].

Finally, a study of Benchop et al. on interventions for women with endometrioma prior to assisted reproductive technology concluded that surgery (aspiration or

cystectomy) in terms of expectant management (EM) showed no evidence of a benefit for clinical pregnancy with either technique. Cystectomy was associated with a decreased ovarian response to controlled ovarian hyperstimulation (COH) (MD: 510.00; 95% CI: 676.62–343.38); no evidence of an effect on the number of mature oocytes retrieved (NMOR) compared to EM was found [34].

Treatment must be maximally individualized for every patient entering IVF with endometriosis and must consider all aspects of the patient's disease, but the latest results indicate that most patients will benefit from avoiding surgery, so they go directly to IVF instead.

3.6 Pregnancy and Endometriosis

Over the past several years, pregnancy, with all its hormonal and metabolic changes, was considered to have a positive effect on endometriosis. It showed a tendency toward reducing the number and scope of all foci in both the ovaries and the peritoneum, followed by pain relief. That is also the goal of therapy, which leads to artificial amenorrhea, and pregnancy is the natural amenorrhea, representing a good therapy for endometriosis. In clinical practice, inflammatory reactions to endometriosis, the bursting of endometriotic cysts, and possible ovarian and adnexa torsion are rarely seen during pregnancy.

Some authors have even described decidualized endometriosis as a pseudotumor mass with complete reduction during postpartum control examinations [35]. However, an analysis of the increased number of pregnant patients with the presence of endometriosis revealed different changes that mimic the malignant transformation of endometriosis. Reaching a diagnosis of endometriosis during pregnancy is challenging, particularly differentiating between reversible and irreversible changes. Decidualization is a process that affects endometrial tissue both inside and outside the uterus, with specific dynamic changes that can be observed in ovarian endometriomas. One of the signs of decidual endometriosis on MR imaging is the appearance of a hyperintense mural nodule. DWI with a quantification of ADC values can be particularly helpful in differentiating endometriosis from its malignant transformation (a decidualized endometrioma is characterized by higher ADC values compared to those of malignant lesions).

In the following part of this chapter, different cases of benign adnexal endometriosis will be presented, including radiological, diagnostic, and operative images of the cases (Figs. 3.11, 3.12, 3.13, 3.14, 3.15, 3.16, 3.17, 3.18, 3.19, 3.20, 3.21, 3.22, 3.23, 3.24, 3.25, 3.26, 3.27, 3.28, 3.29, 3.30, 3.31, 3.32, 3.33, 3.34, 3.35, 3.36, 3.37, 3.38, 3.39, 3.40, 3.41, 3.42, 3.43, 3.44, 3.45, 3.46, 3.47, 3.48, 3.49, 3.50, 3.51, 3.52, 3.53, 3.54, 3.55, 3.56, 3.57, 3.58, 3.59, 3.60, and 3.61).

Case 3.1

A 28-year-old patient with pelvic discomfort and intermittent pain.

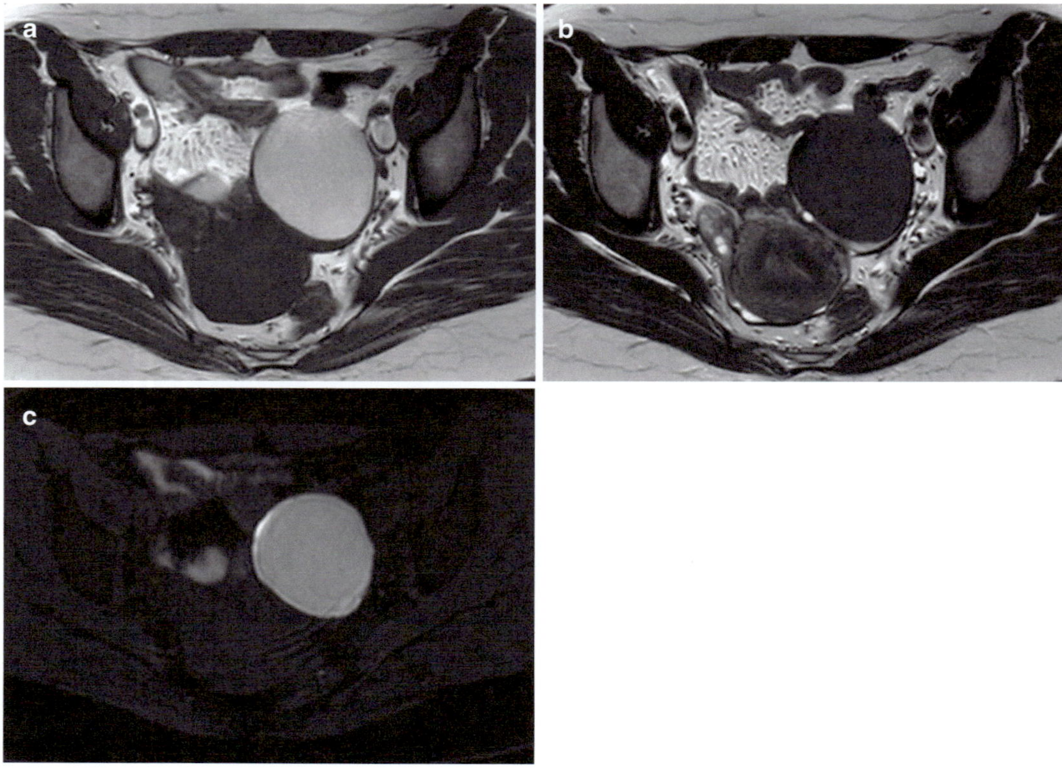

Fig. 3.11 MR images of female pelvis: (**a**) axial T1W, (**b**) T2W, and (**c**) T1W fat-saturated images—with no sign of drop in signal intensity

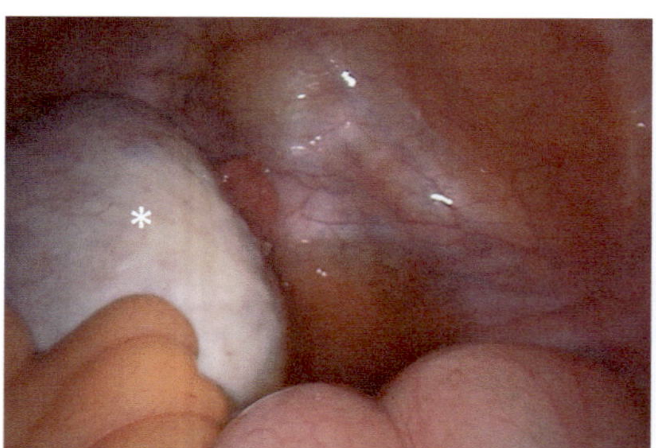

Fig. 3.12 Laparoscopic image of cystic lesion on the left ovary (asterisk) and white smooth capsule with benign characteristics

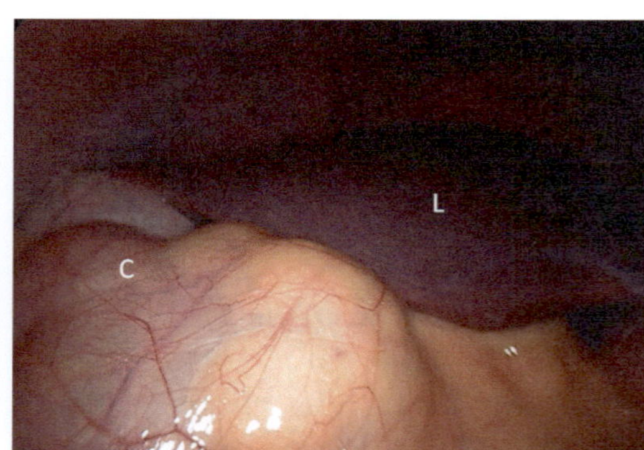

Fig. 3.13 Laparoscopic image of the upper portion of the abdomen, right hemidiaphragm's cupola, (L) liver surface, and (C) part of the colon

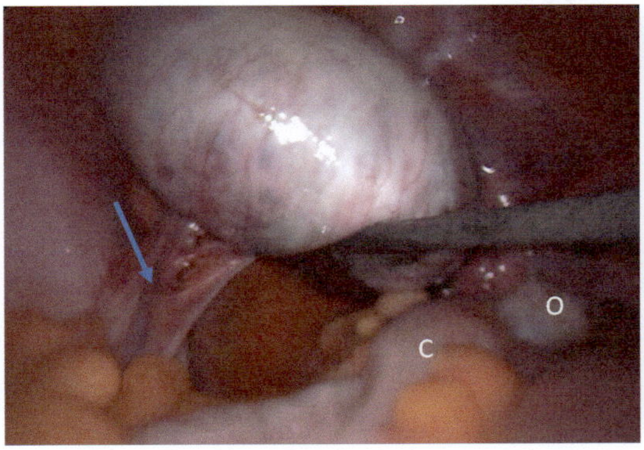

Fig. 3.14 Laparoscopic image of endometriotic cyst released from its adhesions with side pelvic wall (arrow); in the back, sigmoid colon (C) and contours of the right ovary (O)

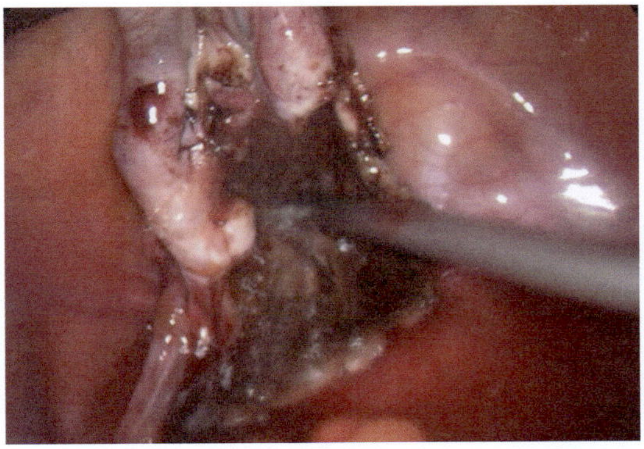

Fig. 3.15 Laparoscopic image of the left ovary's endometriotic cyst opening that is leaking its characteristic "chocolate" content, which represents coagulated blood

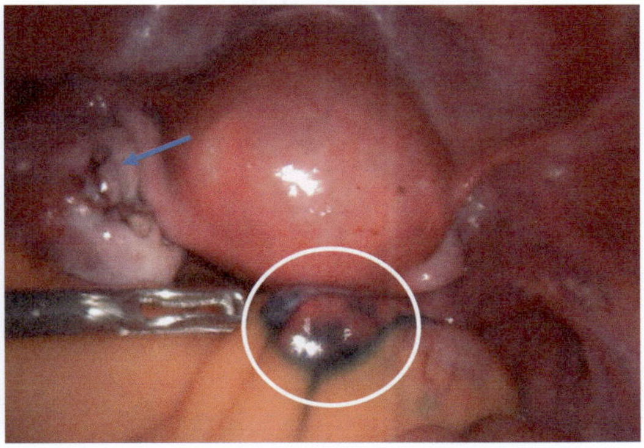

Fig. 3.16 Panoramic laparoscopic view while examining the patency of the ovarian tubes: blue color can be seen in the area of ampullary orifice of the right ovary, which confirms its patency (circled), and on the left side ovary in the area of the removed cyst are laparoscopically inserted stitches (arrow)

Case 3.2

A 32-year-old patient with painful menstrual cycles for years, with increasing pain intensity, multiple cystic formations on both ovaries, and the appearance of kissing ovaries.

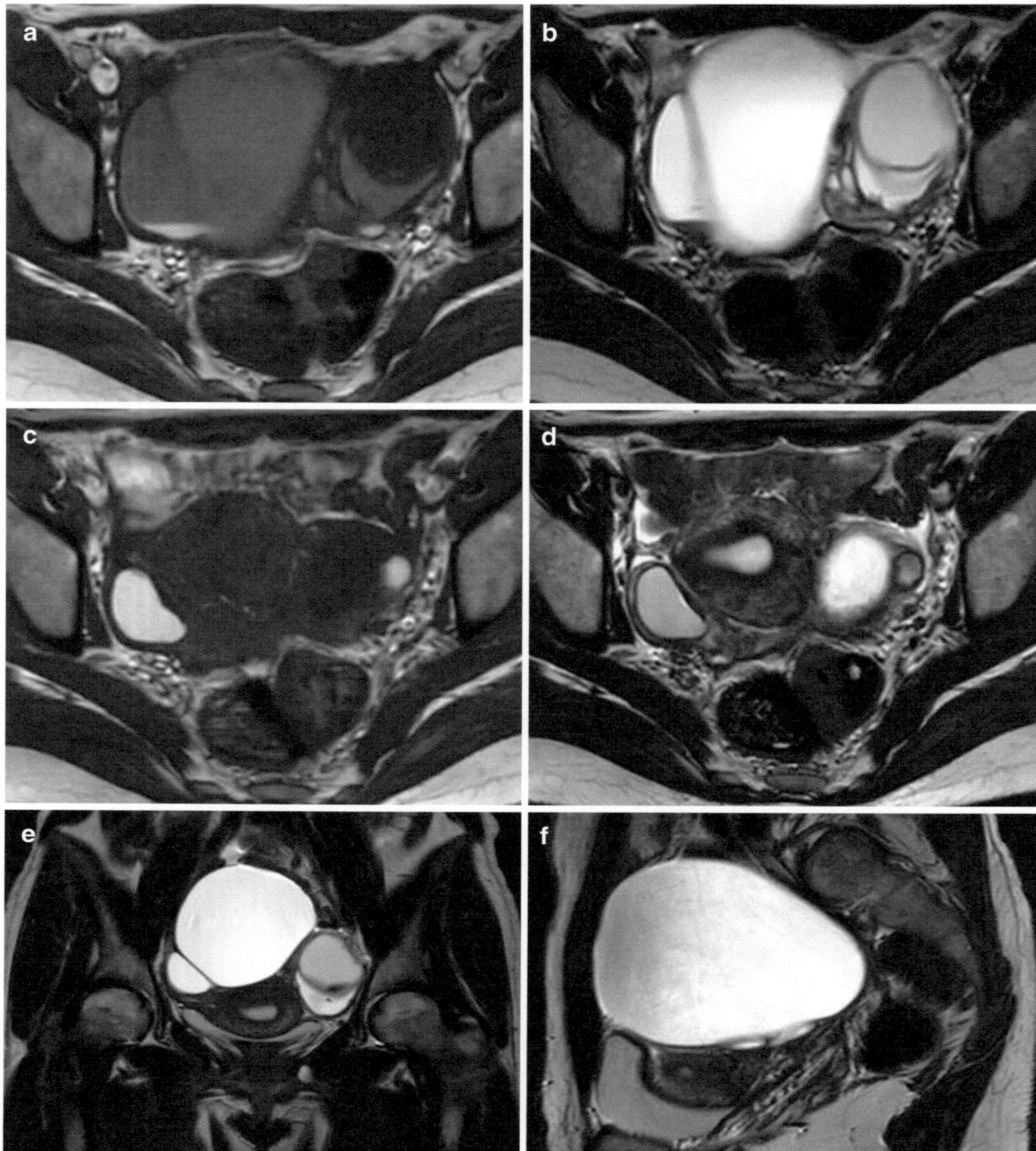

Fig. 3.17 MR images of kissing ovaries with multiple endometriomas: (**a**, **b**) axial T1W images showing level of hyperintensity within cyst of right ovary, (**c**) right fallopian tube, (**b**, **d**) axial T2W images showing discrete shading sign within cystic lesion in left ovary, (**e**, **f**) coronal and sagittal T2W images, and (**g**) axial T1W fat-saturated image

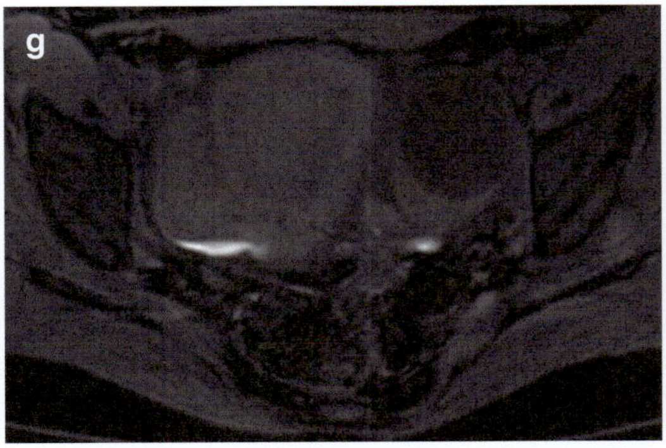

Fig. 3.17 (continued)

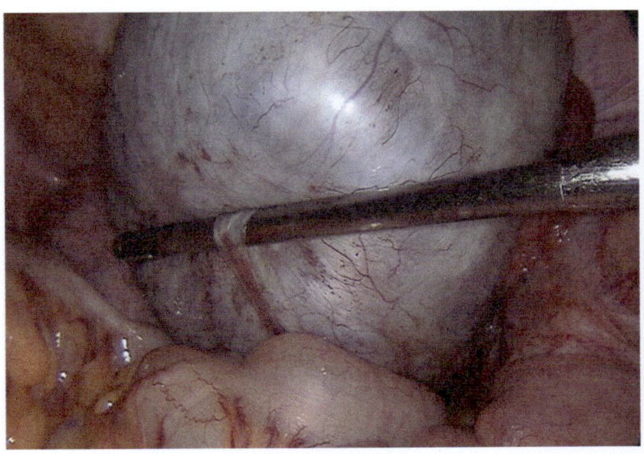

Fig. 3.18 Laparoscopic image of big cystic change in left ovary with benign characteristics, showing endometriosis

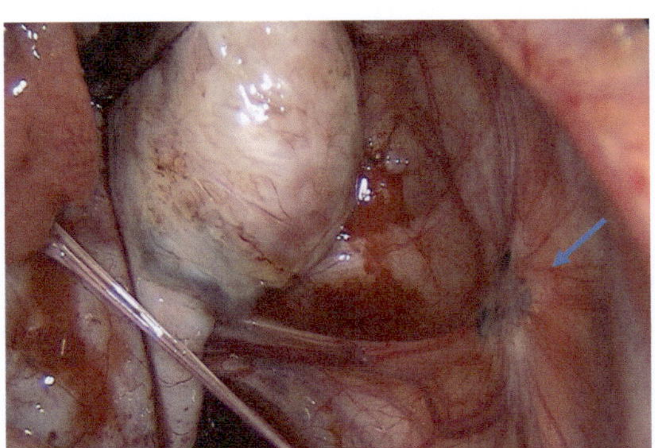

Fig. 3.19 Laparoscopic image of focal endometriosis (arrow) on the peritoneum next to the right ovary

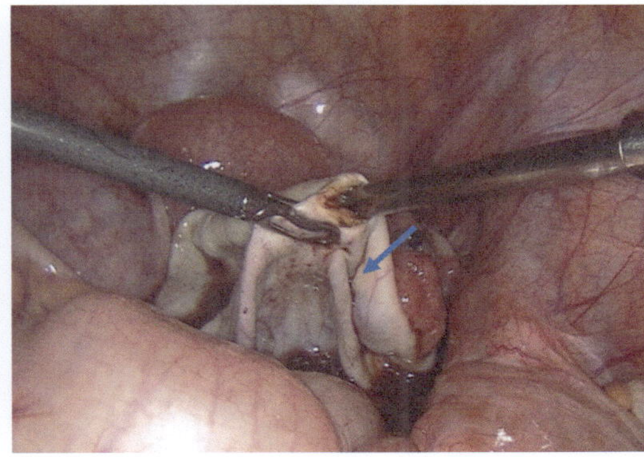

Fig. 3.20 Laparoscopic image of incision and content aspiration of endometriotic cyst and emptied capsule of the cyst (arrow)

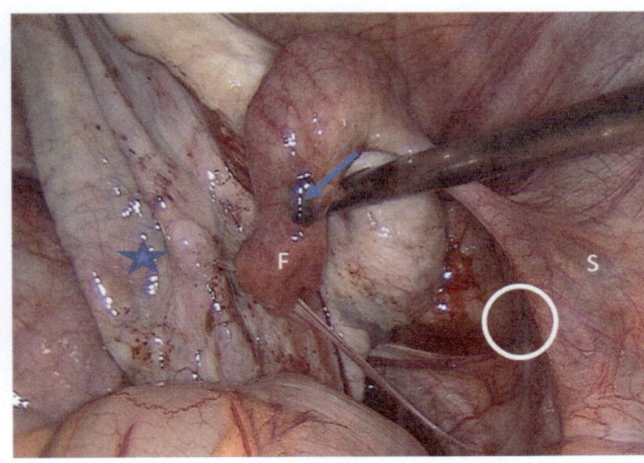

Fig. 3.21 Laparoscopic image of cystectomy of right ovary's big endometriotic cyst with adhesions (asterisk); evaporated endometriosis—fossa ovary (circled); endometriosis (arrow); lig. Suspensorium ovarii (S); and a fallopian tube (F)

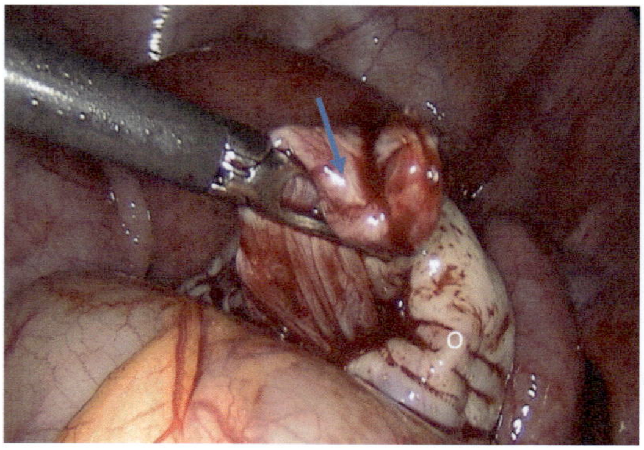

Fig. 3.22 Laparoscopic image of endometriotic cyst capsule (arrow) with remaining tissue of the left ovary (O)

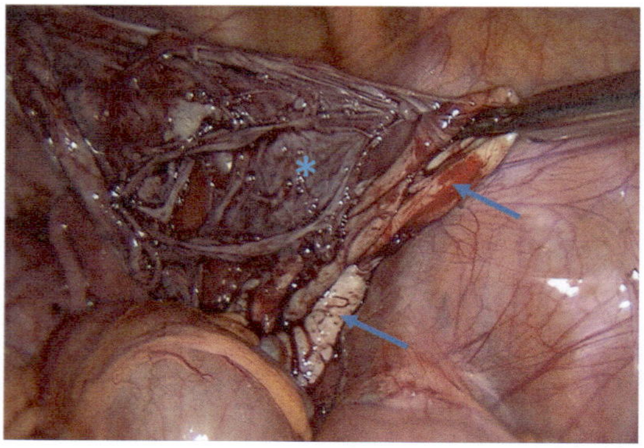

Fig. 3.23 Laparoscopic image of endometriotic cyst capsule (asterisk) with remaining ovary tissue (arrow)

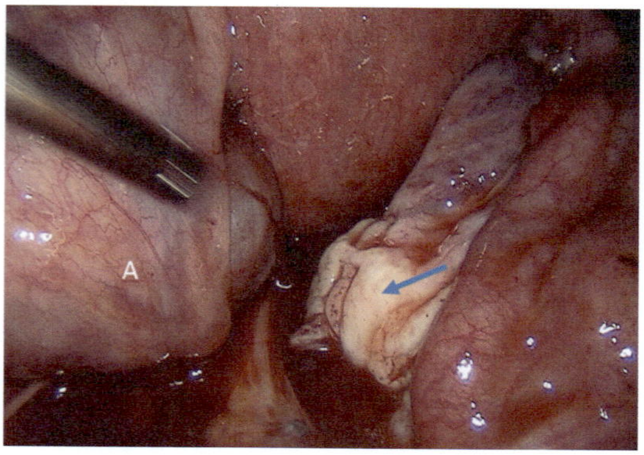

Fig. 3.24 Laparoscopic image of right ovary after cystectomy (in toto) (arrow), with left adnexa in block (A)

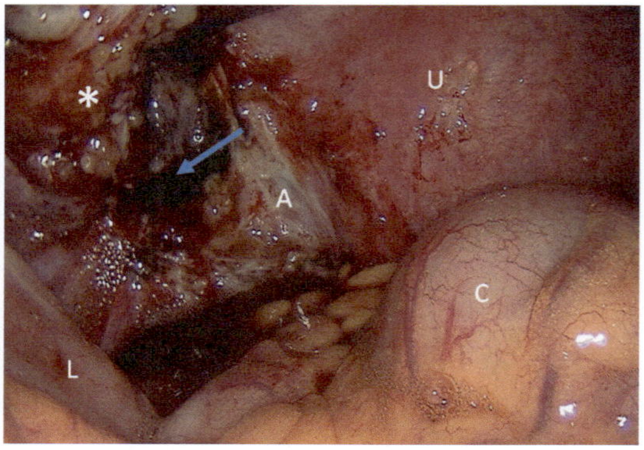

Fig. 3.25 Laparoscopic image of opening left ovary's endometriotic cyst capsule and leaking its content; uterus (U), ligamentum ovarii proprium (L), colon (C), and left adnexa (asterisk); and the detachment place of adhered part of the ovary (arrow)

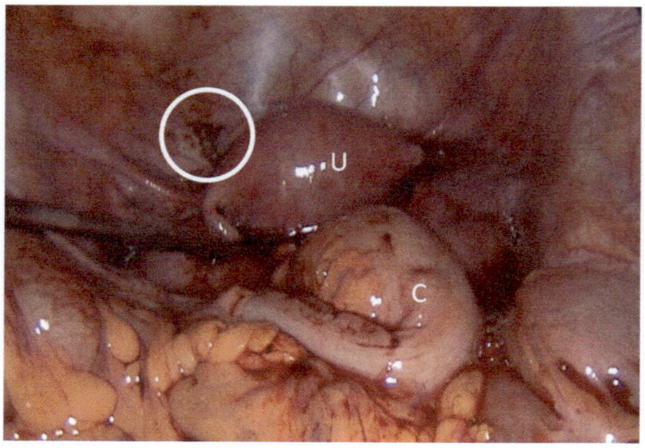

Fig. 3.26 Laparoscopic image after endometriotic cyst removal: uterus (U), colon (C), and focal superficial endometriosis (circled)

Case 3.3

A 32-year-old patient with no previous pregnancies and in a program of in vitro fertilization (second attempt).

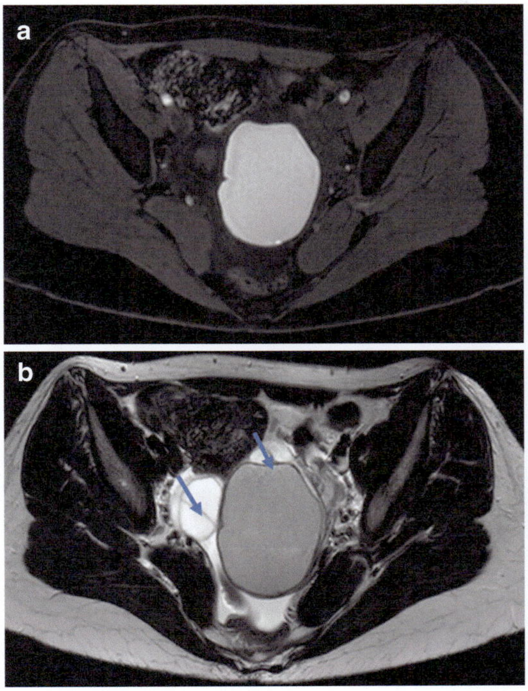

Fig. 3.27 Multiple follicles on both ovaries (hyperstimulation) (arrows) on (**a**) axial T1W fat-saturated image and (**b**) T2W MR image

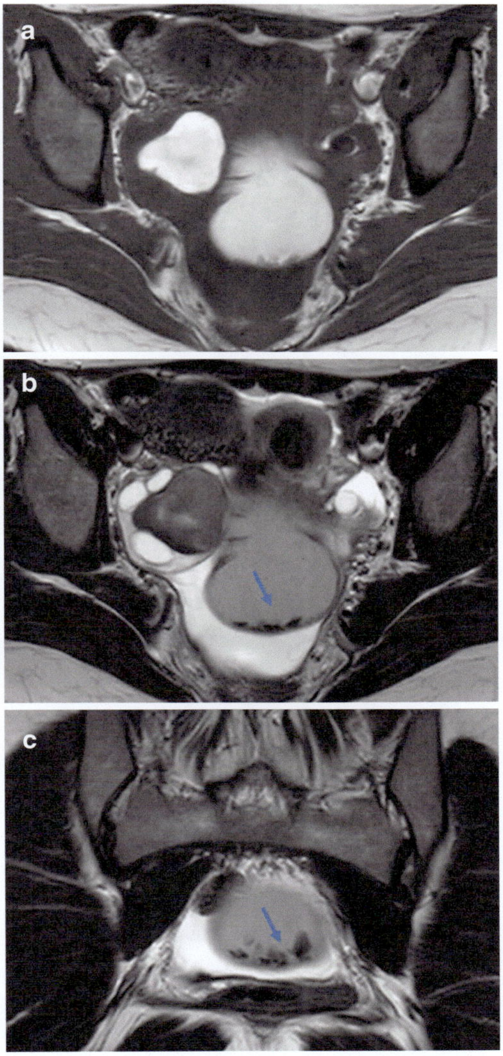

Fig. 3.28 MR images of dark spot sign (arrows) on (**a**) axial T1W image and (**b**) T2W image and (**c**) a coronal T2W image

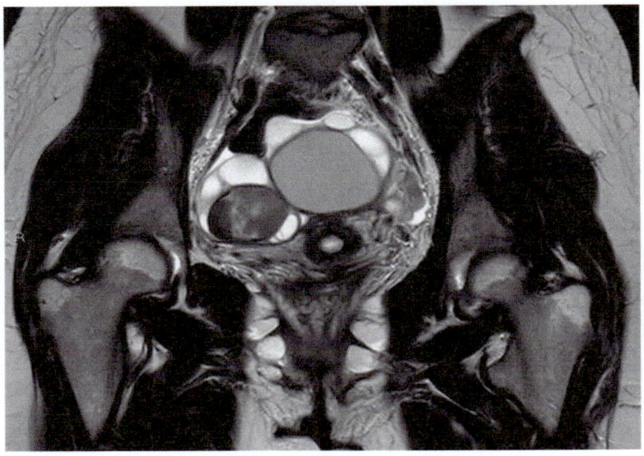

Fig. 3.29 Coronal T2W MR image of multiple follicles on both ovaries

Case 3.4

A 43-year-old patient with infertility.

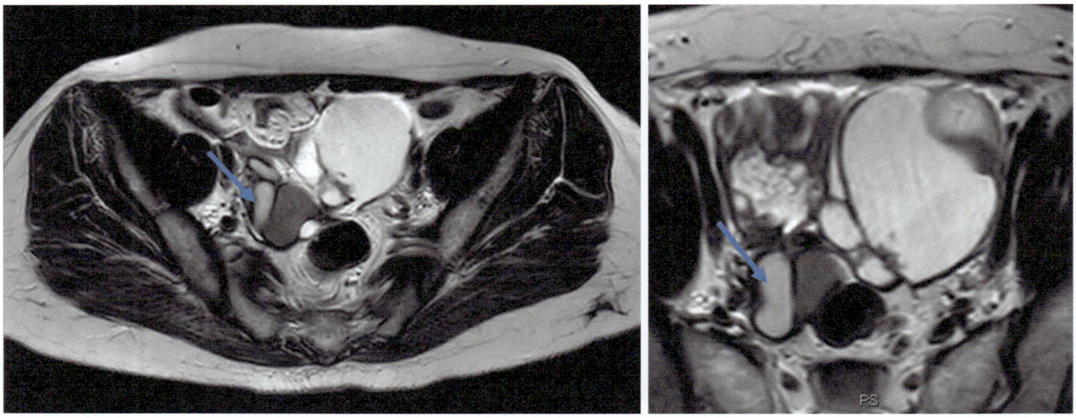

Fig. 3.30 Axial T2W image of hematosalpinx (arrow) with incomplete hypointense rim

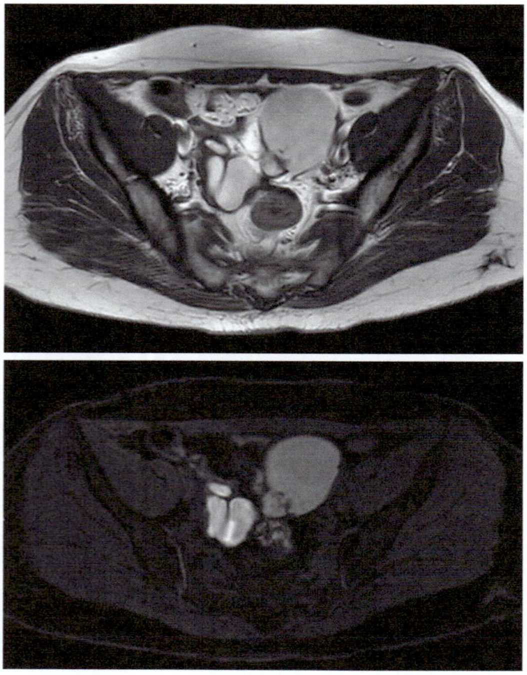

Fig. 3.31 T1W and T1W fat-saturated MR images confirming the presence of blood

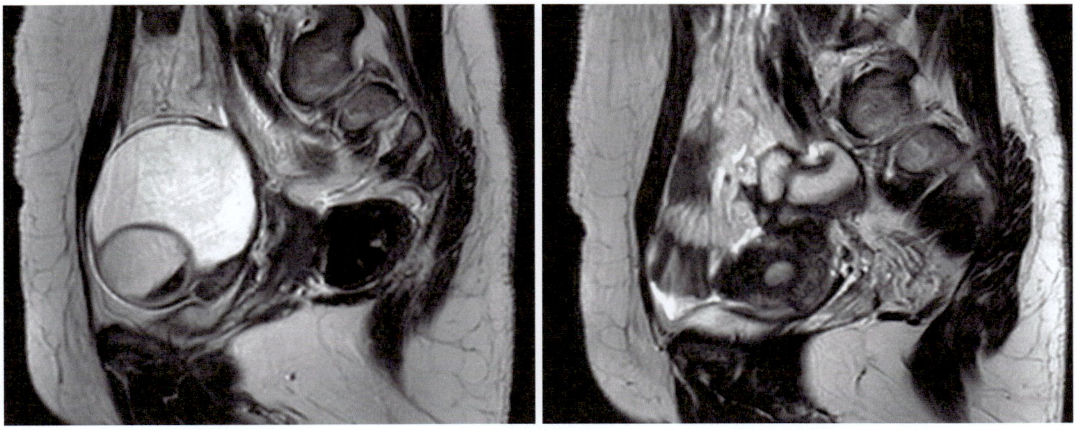

Fig. 3.32 Sagittal T2W MR images of the cyst and hematosalpinx

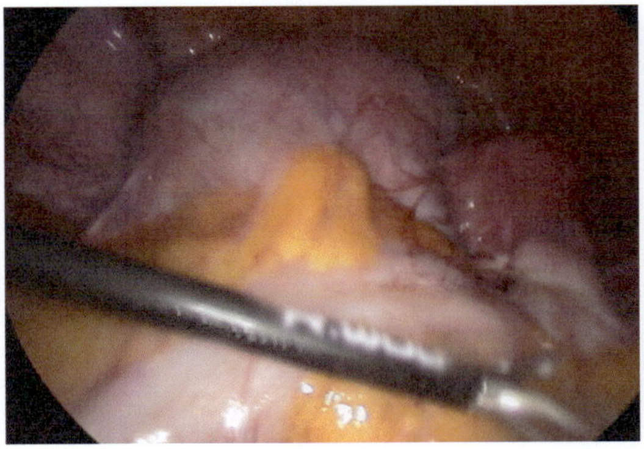

Fig. 3.33 Laparoscopic image of frozen pelvis (multiple perigenital adhesions): extensive adhesions on the intestines and omentum with a back wall in the uterus and the peritoneum of the Douglas pouch

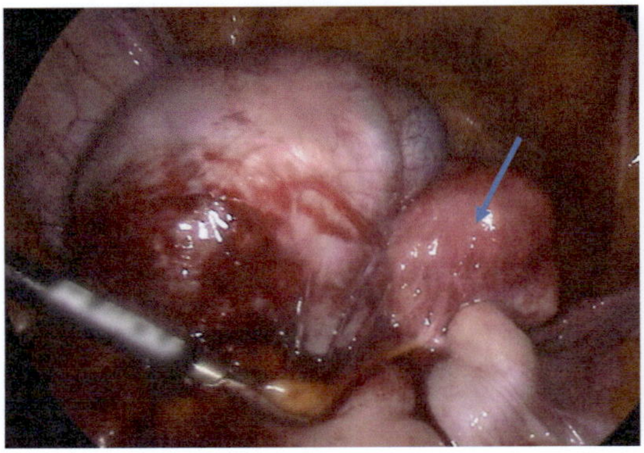

Fig. 3.34 Laparoscopic image of right hydrosalpinx, where the fallopian tube is extended and obstructed by a sack filled with liquid (arrow)

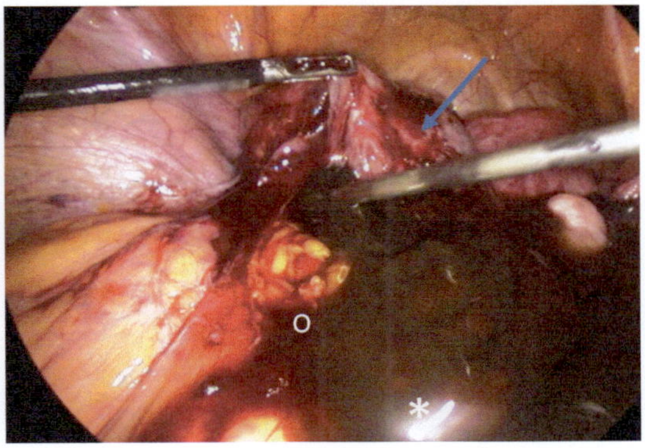

Fig. 3.35 Laparoscopic image of the intraoperative leaking of the characteristic "chocolate" content from left ovary cyst capsule (asterisk): left hydrosalpinx (arrow) and omentum (O)

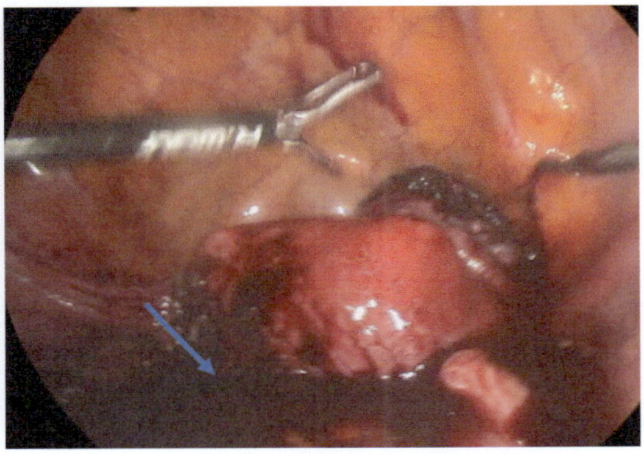

Fig. 3.36 Laparoscopic image of detached left adnexa ready to be removed and coagulated spot of the left adnexa removal (arrow)

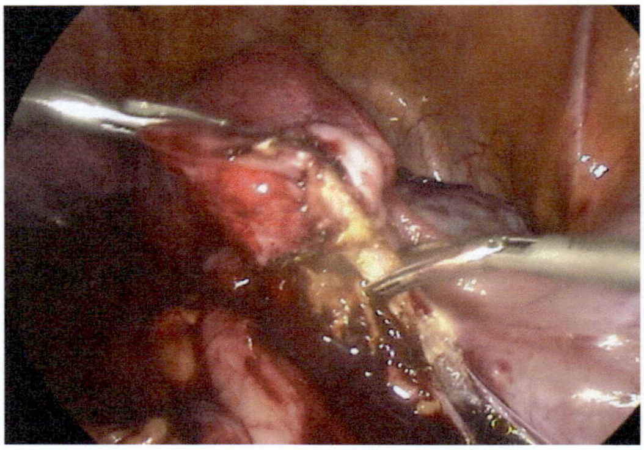

Fig. 3.37 Laparoscopic image of right salpingectomy, showing right fallopian tube removed and hemostatic coagulation

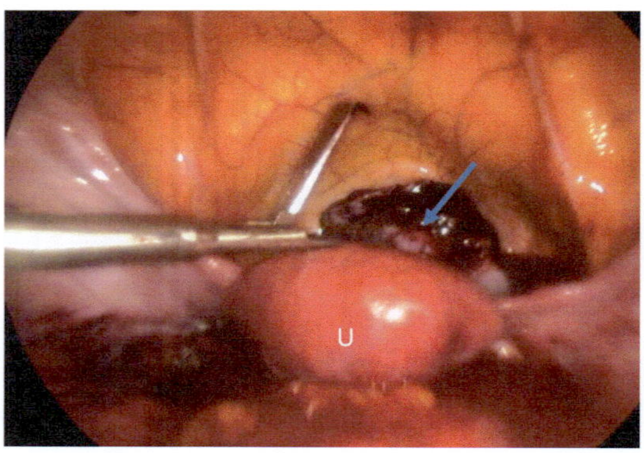

Fig. 3.38 Laparoscopic image of uterus (U) with the left adnexa removed (arrow)

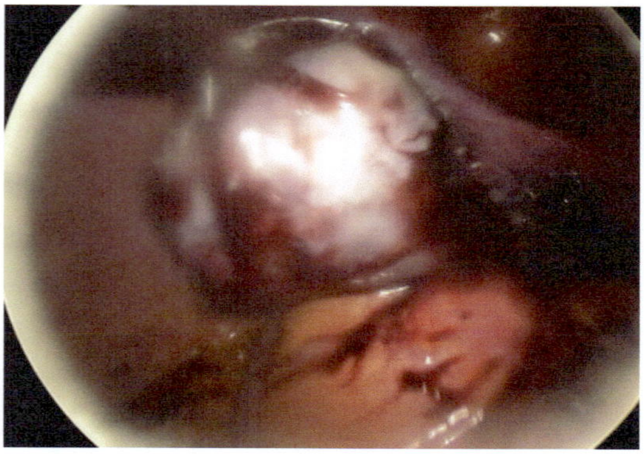

Fig. 3.39 Laparoscopic image of endobag with the removed ovary inside

Case 3.5

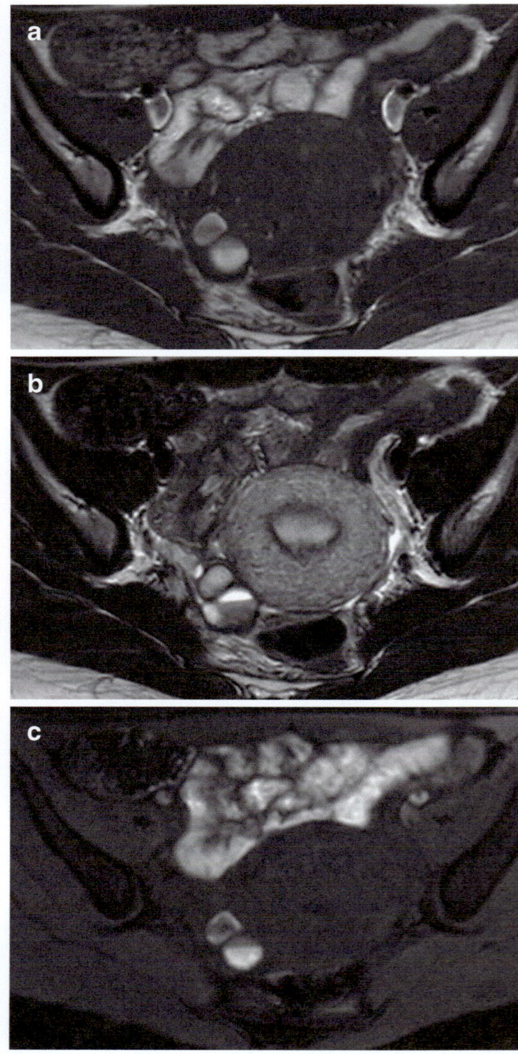

Fig. 3.40 (**a**) Axial T1W, (**b**) T2W, and (**c**) T1 W fat-saturated, showing hyperintense cystic lesions

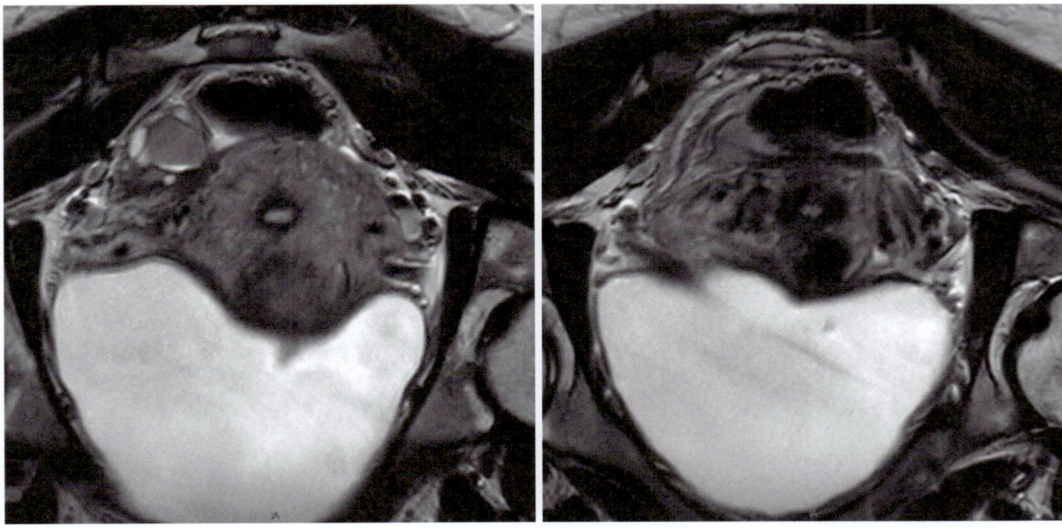

Fig. 3.41 Axial T2W MR image showing T2 shading sign of the right ovarian cyst

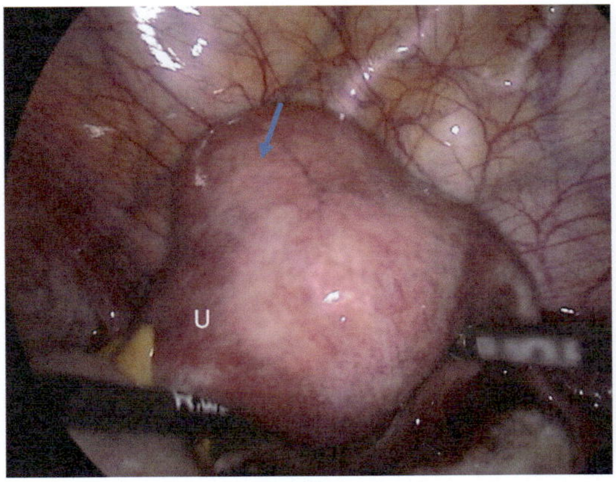

Fig. 3.42 Laparoscopic image of uterus (U) with intramural myoma (arrow)

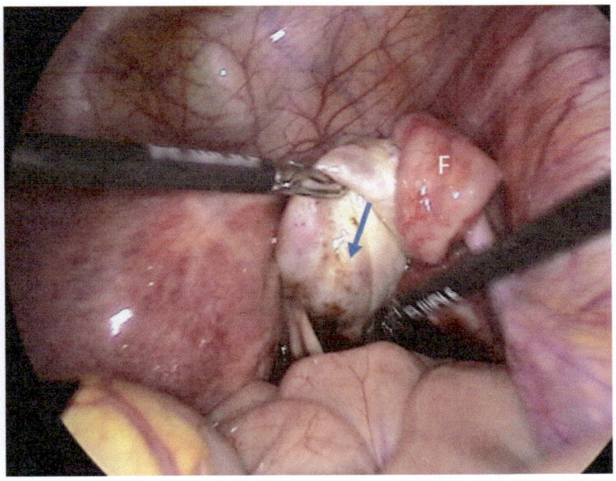

Fig. 3.43 Laparoscopic image of endometriosis with adhesions (arrow) and right fallopian tube (F)

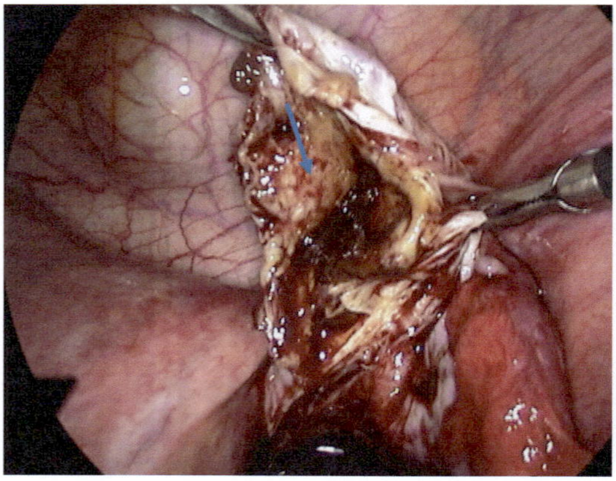

Fig. 3.44 Laparoscopic image of the base of the cyst capsule (arrow) and the characteristic brown content of endometriosis

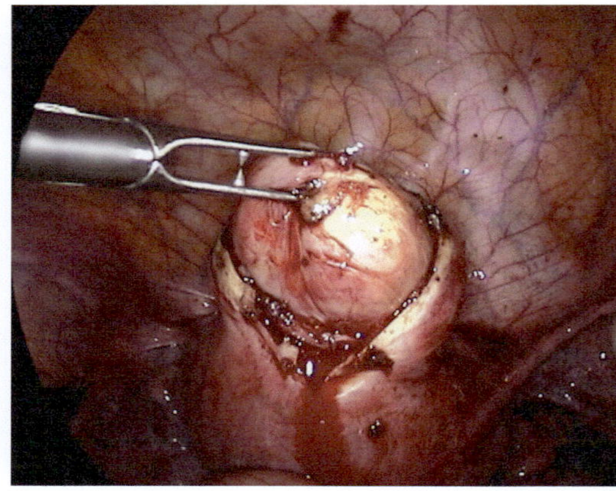

Fig. 3.46 Laparoscopic image of intramural myoma extraction

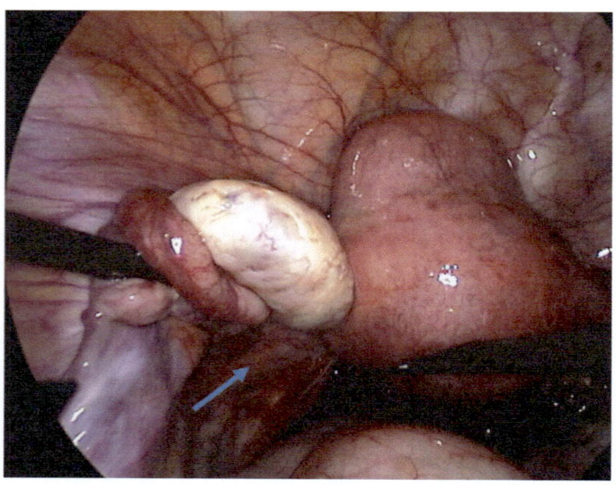

Fig. 3.45 Laparoscopic image of left ovary and fallopian tube and of uterus with myoma, where endometriotic adhesions (arrow) appear on the lower pole of the left ovary

Case 3.6

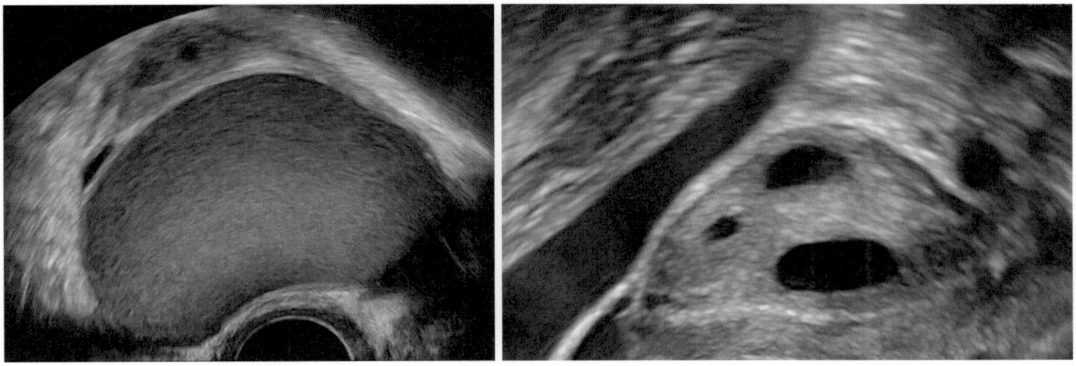

Fig. 3.47 Ultrasound images showing right ovarian cyst (left) and healthy left ovary (right)

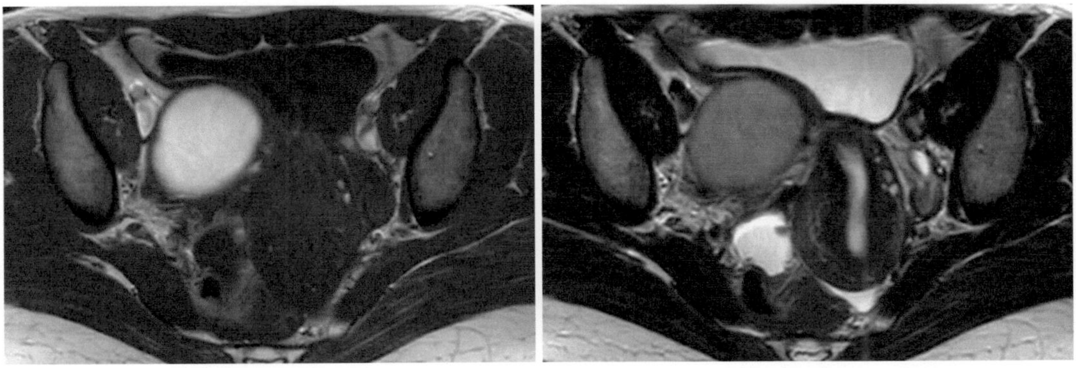

Fig. 3.48 Axial T1W and T2W MR images showing right ovarian cyst and healthy left ovary

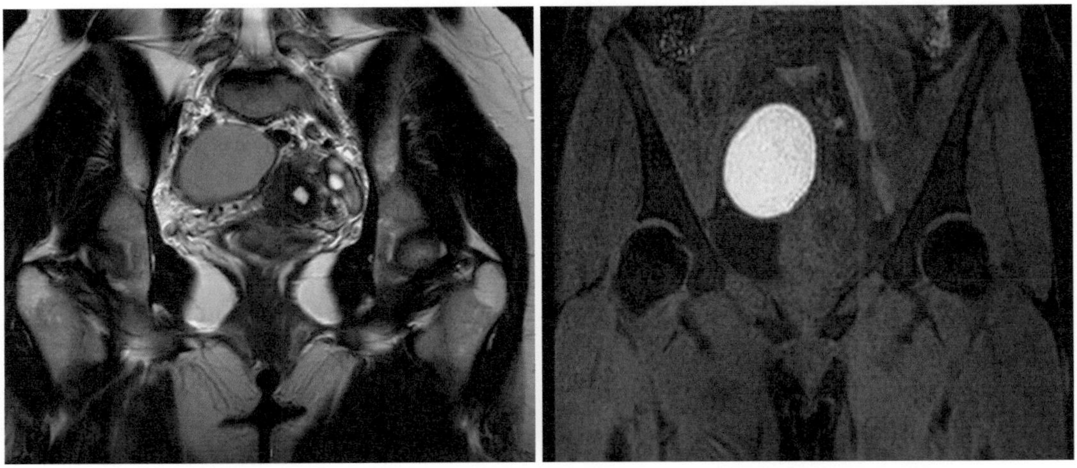

Fig. 3.49 Coronal T2W and T1W fat-saturated MR images showing right ovarian cyst and healthy left ovary

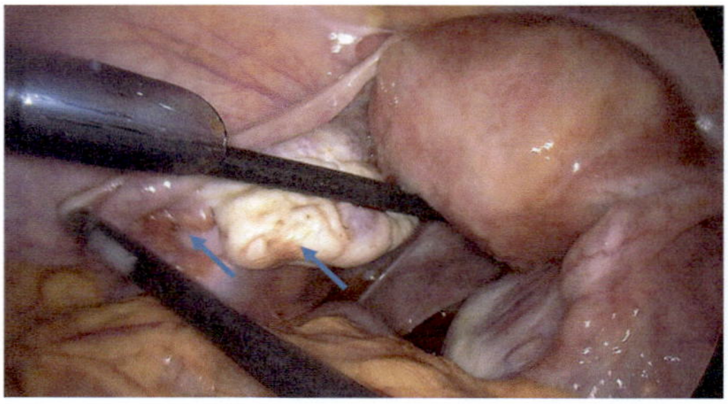

Fig. 3.50 Laparoscopic image of endometriosis on the left ovary and side peritoneum (arrows)

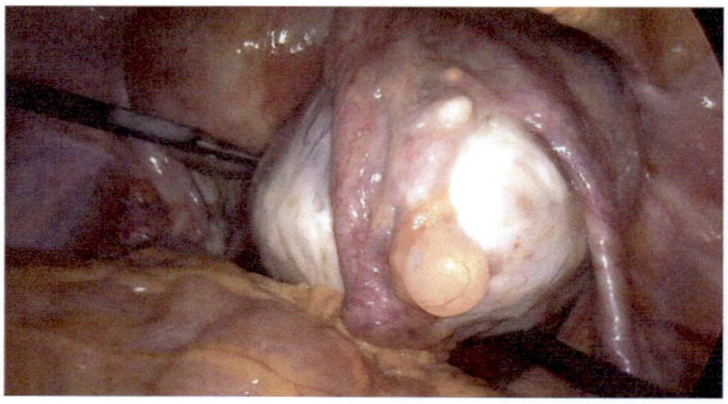

Fig. 3.51 Laparoscopic image of paratubal cyst

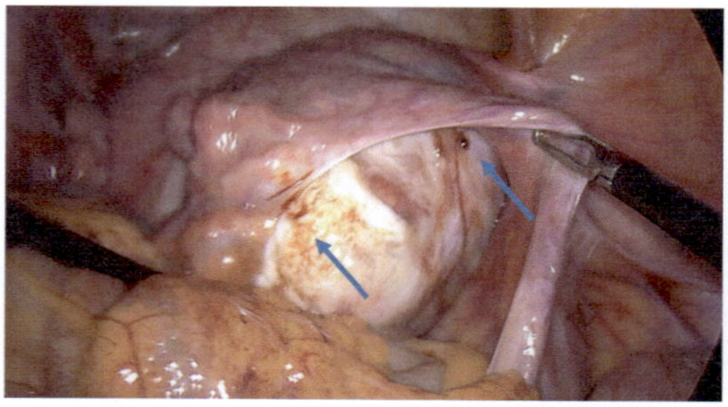

Fig. 3.52 Laparoscopic image of endometriosis adhesions on right ovary (arrow)

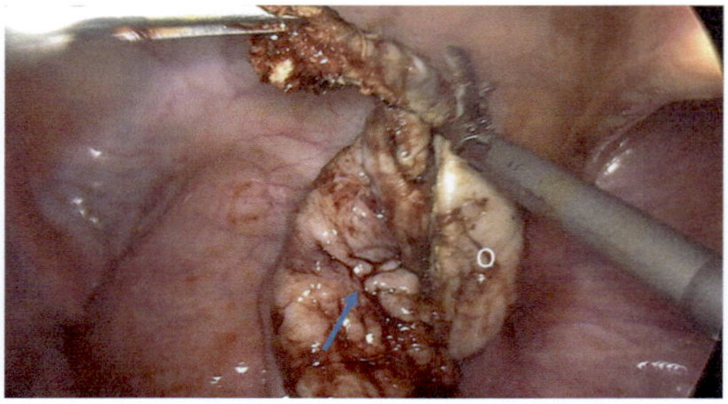

Fig. 3.53 Laparoscopic image of ablation of the right ovarian cyst (extirpation) and of healthy ovary (O) and cyst capsule (arrow)

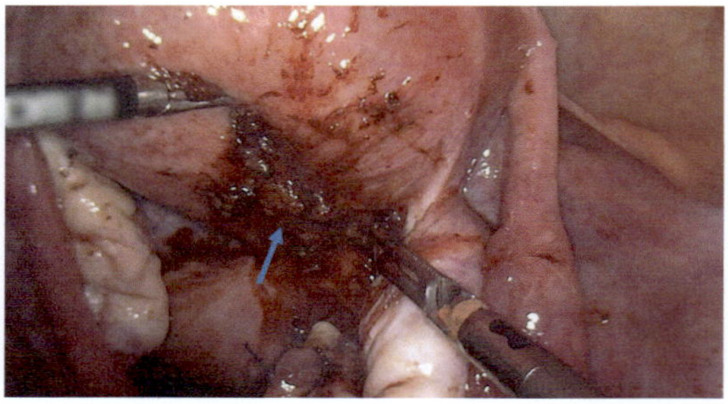

Fig. 3.54 Endometriosis on the back wall of the uterus (arrow)

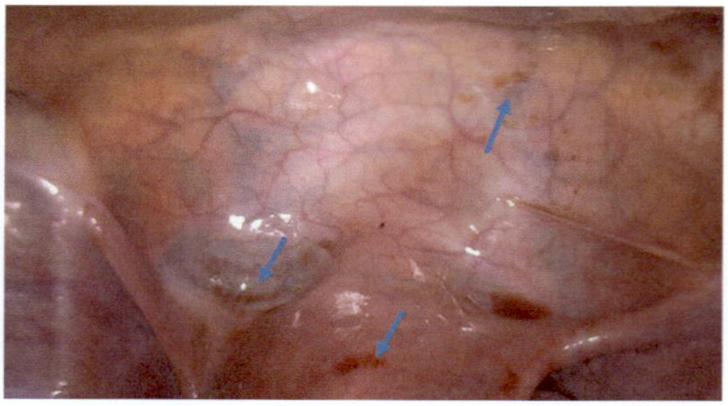

Fig. 3.55 Endometriosis on bladder peritoneum (arrows)

Case 3.7

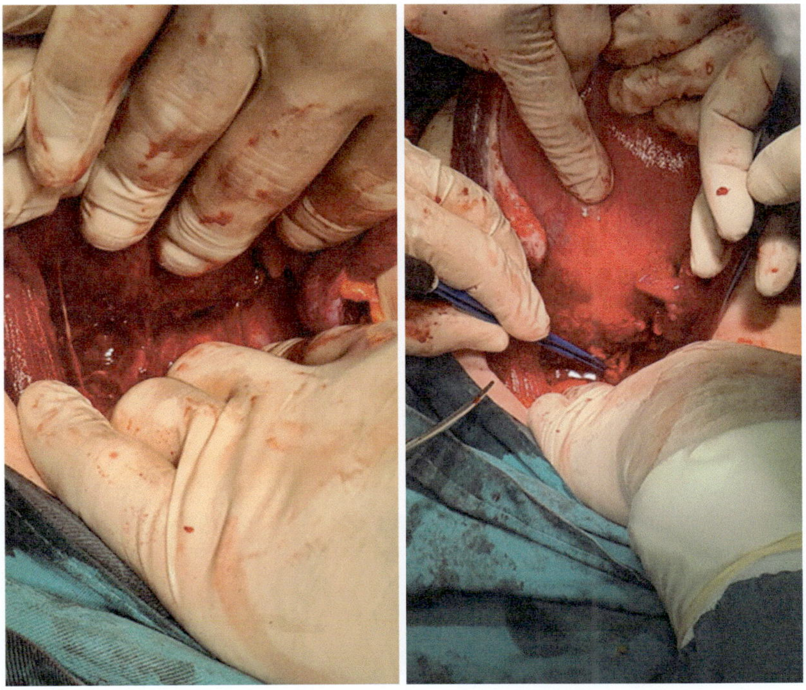

Fig. 3.56 Caesarian section in patient with endometriosis

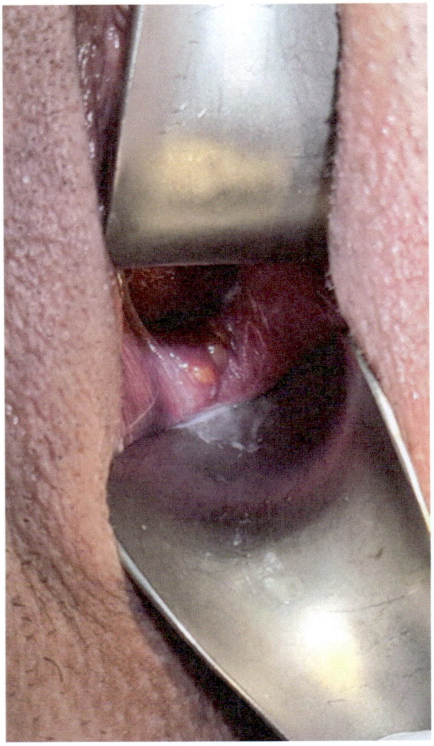

Fig. 3.57 Focal endometriosis in the vagina

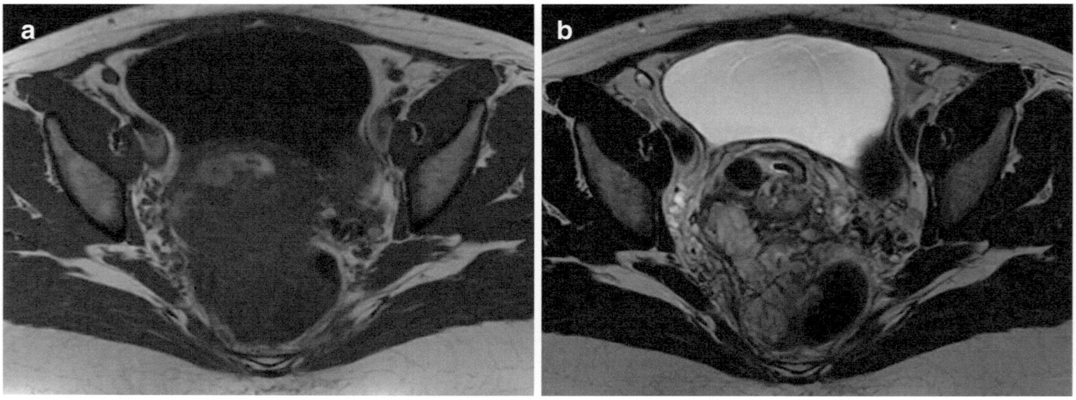

Fig. 3.58 (**a**) T1W and (**b**) T2W MR images of the same patient at 22 weeks of spontaneous pregnancy with bleeding and pelvic pain—diagnosed with deep endometriosis, had previous caesarian section 2 years earlier, and focal endometriosis in vagina

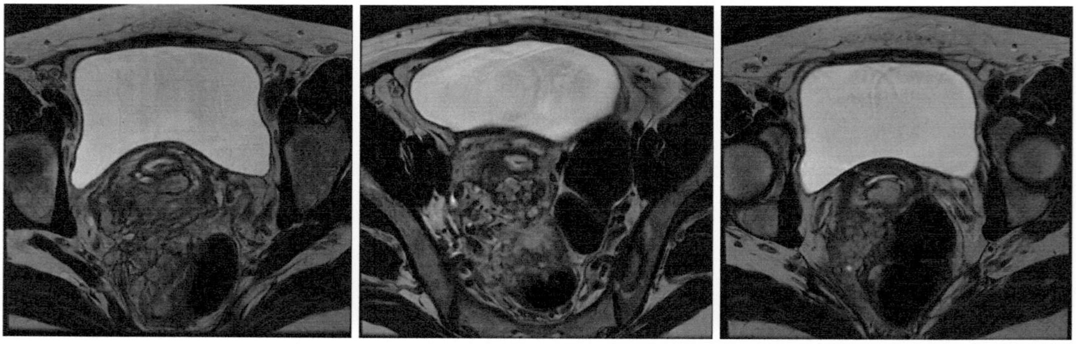

Fig. 3.59 Axial T2W images of huge pelvic mass involving cervical region, rectum, and sacrouterine ligament

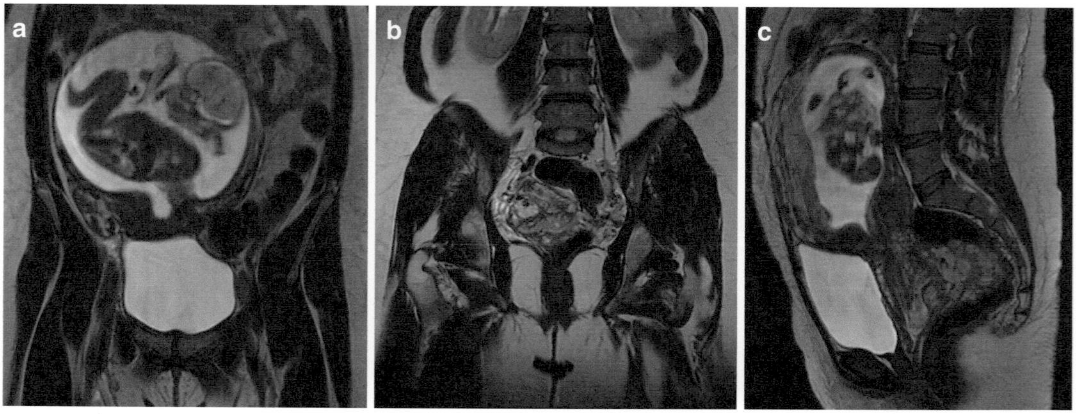

Fig. 3.60 Coronal T2W MR images: (**a**, **b**) graviditas showing periuterine mass and (**c**) sagittal T2W showing the propagation of retrouterine mass

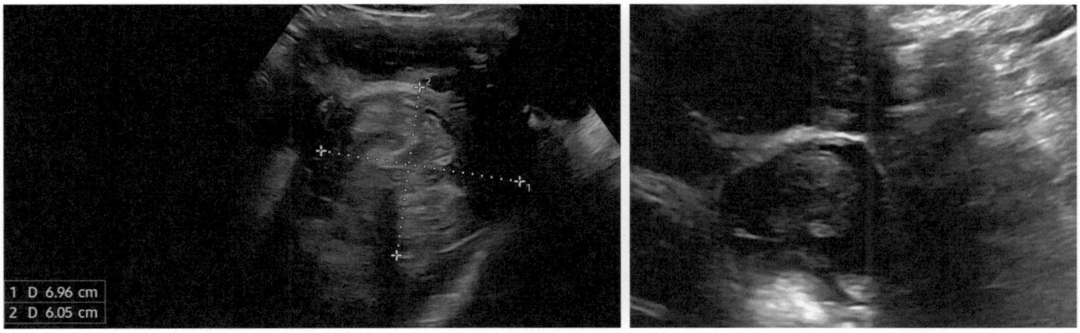

Fig. 3.61 Transabdominal ultrasound images of retrovesical mass in pregnant patients

References

1. Smolarz B, Szyłło K, Romanowicz H. Endometriosis: epidemiology, classification, pathogenesis, treatment and genetics (review of literature). Int J Mol Sci. 2021;22(19):10554. https://doi.org/10.3390/ijms221910554. PMID: 34638893; PMCID: PMC8508982.
2. Chamié LP, Blasbalg R, Pereira RM, Warmbrand G, Serafini PC. Findings of pelvic endometriosis at transvaginal US, MR imaging, and laparoscopy. Radiographics. 2011;31(4):E77–100. https://doi.org/10.1148/rg.314105193.
3. Viala-Trentini M, Maubon A, Filhastre M, Georges P, Rouanet J-P. Imagerie de l'hypofertilité de la femme. EMC Encyclopédie Médico-Chirurgicale (Elsevier SAS, Paris; 2006), Radiodiagnostic—Urologie-Gynécologie, 34–620-E-10.
4. Hsu AL, Khachikyan I, Stratton P. Invasive and non-invasive methods for the diagnosis of endometriosis. Clin Obstet Gynecol. 2010;53(2):413–9. https://doi.org/10.1097/GRF.0b013e3181db7ce8.
5. Outwater EK, Siegelman ES, Chiowanich P, et al. Dilated fallopian tubes: MR imaging characteristics. Radiology. 1998;208:463–9. https://doi.org/10.1148/radiology.208.2.9680577.
6. Foti PV, Ognibene N, Spadola S, et al. Non-neoplastic diseases of the fallopian tube: MR imaging with emphasis on diffusion-weighted imaging. Insights Imaging. 2016;7:311–27. https://doi.org/10.1007/s13244-016-0484-7.
7. Nisenblat V, Bossuyt PM, Farquhar C, Johnson N, Hull ML. Imaging modalities for the non-invasive diagnosis of endometriosis. Cochrane Database Syst Rev. 2016;2:CD009591.
8. Medeiros LR, Rosa MI, Silva BR, et al. Accuracy of magnetic resonance in deeply infiltrating endometriosis: a systematic review and meta-analysis. Arch Gynecol Obstet. 2015;291:611–21. https://doi.org/10.1007/s00404-014-3470-7.
9. Corwin MT, Gerscovich EO, Lamba R, Wilson M, McGahan JP. Differentiation of ovarian endometriomas from hemorrhagic cysts at MR imaging: utility of the T2 dark spot sign. Radiology. 2014;271:126–32.
10. Bazot M, Lafont C, Rouzier R, Roseau G, Thomassin-Naggara I, Daraï E. Diagnostic accuracy of physical examination, transvaginal sonography, rectal endoscopic sonography, and magnetic resonance imaging to diagnose deep infiltrating endometriosis. Fertil Steril. 2009;92:1825–33.
11. Sampson JA. Peritoneal endometriosis due to menstrual dissemination of endometrial tissue into the peritoneal cavity. Am J Obstet Gynecol. 1927;14:422–69.
12. Bazot M, Bharwani N, Huchon C, Kinkel K, Cunha TM, Guerra A, et al. European society of urogenital radiology (ESUR) guidelines: MR imaging of pelvic endometriosis. Eur Radiol. 2017;27:2765–75.
13. Togashi K, Nishimura K, Kimura I, Tsuda Y, Yamashita K, Shibata T, et al. Endometrial cysts: diagnosis with MR imaging. Radiology. 1991;180:73–8.
14. Jeong Y-Y, Outwater EK, Kang HK. Imaging evaluation of ovarian masses. Radiographics. 2000;20:1445–70.https://doi.org/10.1148/radiographics.20.5.g00se101445.
15. Coutinho A Jr, Bittencourt LK, Pires CE, et al. MR imaging in deep pelvic endometriosis: a pictorial essay. Radiographics. 2011;31(2):549–67. https://doi.org/10.1148/rg.312105144.
16. Woodward PJ, Sohaey R, TP M Jr. Endometriosis: radiologic-pathologic correlation. Radiographics. 2001;21(1):193–216. https://doi.org/10.1148/radiographics.21.1.g01ja14193.

17. Redwine DB. Diaphragmatic endometriosis: diagnosis, surgical management, and long-term results of treatment. Fertil Steril. 2002;77:288–96. https://doi.org/10.1016/S0015-0282(01)02998-3.
18. Mannan K, Altaf F, Maniar S, Tirabosco R, Sinisi M, Carlstedt T. Cyclical sciatica: endometriosis of the sciatic nerve. J Bone Joint Surg Br. 2008;90(1):98–101. https://doi.org/10.1302/0301-620X.90B1.19832.
19. Tham WP, Busmanis I, Tan WC, Kwek JW. Polypoid endometriosis of post vaginal fornix: utility of MRI imaging of pelvis with diffusion weighted imaging for diagnosis. Med J Malaysia. 2016;71(3):144–6.
20. Pham M, Sommer C, Wessig C, et al. Magnetic resonance neurography for the diagnosis of extrapelvic sciatic endometriosis. Fertil Steril. 2010;94(1):351.e11–4. https://doi.org/10.1016/j.fertnstert.2009.12.046.
21. Di Paola V, Manfredi R, Castelli F, Negrelli R, Mehrabi S, Pozzi MR. Detection and localization of deep endometriosis by means of MRI and correlation with the ENZIAN score. Eur J Radiol. 2015;84(4):568–74. https://doi.org/10.1016/j.ejrad.2014.12.017.
22. Takeuchi M, Matsuzaki K, Nishitani H. Susceptibility-weighted MRI of endometrioma: preliminary results. AJR Am J Roentgenol. 2008;191(5):1366–70. https://doi.org/10.2214/AJR.07.3974.
23. AbedTwfeq RH, Jawad NS. Differentiation between ovarian endometriotic cysts and functional hemorrhagic cysts on magnetic resonance imaging. Iraqi Postgrad Med J. 2021;20(4):361.
24. Foti PV, Attinà G, Spadola S, et al. MR imaging of ovarian masses: classification and differential diagnosis. Insights Imaging. 2016;7(1):21–41. https://doi.org/10.1007/s13244-015-0455-4.
25. Dunselman GA, Vermeulen N, Becker C, Calhaz-Jorge C, D'Hooghe T, De Bie B, et al. ESHRE guideline: management of women with endometriosis. Hum Reprod. 2014;29:400–12.
26. Practice Committee of the American Society for Reproductive Medicine. Endometriosis and infertility. Fertil Steril. 2004;82:40–5.
27. Nisolle M, Donnez J. Peritoneal endometriosis, ovarian endometriosis, and adenomyotic nodules of the rectovaginal septum are three different entities. Fertil Steril. 1997;68:585–96.
28. Barnhart K, Dunsmoor-Su R, Coutifaris C. Effect of endometriosis on in vitro fertilization. Fertil Steril. 2002;77(6):1148–55.
29. Somigliana E, Benaglia L, Vighi V, Ragni G, Vercellini P, Fedele L. Rate of severe ovarian damage following surgery for endometriomas. Hum Reprod. 2010;25(3):678–82.
30. Benaglia L, Somigliana E, Vercellini P, Abbiati A, Ragni G, Fedele L. Endometriotic ovarian cysts negatively affect the rate of spontaneous ovulation. Hum Reprod. 2009;24(9):2183–6.
31. Bongioanni F, Revelli A, Gennarelli G, Guidetti D, Delle Piane LD, Holte J. Ovarian endometriomas and IVF: a retrospective case-control study. Reprod Biol Endocrinol. 2011;9:81.
32. Vercellini P, Crosignani PG, Abbiati A, Somigliana E, Vigano P, Fedele L. The effect of surgery for symptomatic endometriosis: the other side of the story. Hum Reprod Update. 2009;15(2):177–88.
33. Kennedy S, Bergqvist A, Chapron C, D'Hooghe T, Dunselman G, Saridogan E, et al. ESHRE guideline on the diagnosis and management of endometriosis. Hum Reprod. 2005;20(10):2698–704.
34. Benschop L, Farquhar C, van der Poel N, Heineman MJ. Interventions for women with endometrioma prior to assisted reproductive technology. Cochrane Database Syst Rev. 2010;10(11):CD008571.
35. Charkhchi P, Butcher M, Macura KJ. Vanishing pelvic mass: decidualized endometriosis during pregnancy. Radiol Case Rep. 2024;19(6):2535–9. https://doi.org/10.1016/j.radcr.2024.03.018. PMID: 38585388; PMCID: PMC10997803.

Atypical Endometriosis and Malignant Transformation

4

Helena Paixão and Teresa Margarida Cunha

4.1 Endometriosis and Malignant Transformation

Endometriosis, especially ovarian endometriosis, may increase the risk of developing malignancy [3]. According to studies, women with long-term endometriosis are up to 4.2 times more likely to develop ovarian cancer than the general population [15]. However, the risk of malignant transformation into endometriosis is rare and occurs in approximately 1% of patients with ovarian cancer [17].

The first association between endometriosis and ovarian cancer was described by Sampson in 1925 when reporting the criteria for diagnosing ovarian endometrial carcinoma arising from endometriosis, which were as follows: the coexistence of endometriosis and carcinoma within the same ovary; an identical histological pattern; and the exclusion of a second malignant tumor elsewhere [19].

Later, Scott confirmed these criteria and added a fourth criterion, which resulted in the demonstration of a histology transition from benign endometriosis to malignancy [20]. Since then, a substantial number of studies have indicated an increased risk of epithelial ovarian tumors among women with endometriosis [13, 15].

Two types of endometriosis-associated cancers have been described: endometriosis-associated ovarian cancers and endometriosis-associated extra-ovarian cancers, the first one being the most common and representing almost 75% of these tumors [12].

Endometriosis-associated ovarian cancer is a subtype of ovarian cancer with distinct radiological and histological features. Typically, it presents at a younger age, about 10–20 years earlier than other subtypes of epithelial ovarian neoplasms. It can be detected at lower international federation of gynecology and obstetrics (IFGO) stages and has a better prognosis, although it is less sensitive to chemotherapy. That's why early detection and treatment are imperative [17].

On the other hand, endometriosis-associated extra-ovarian cancer is less known and represents approximately 25% of cases of endometriosis-associated cancers. Its definitive diagnosis requires that concomitant endometriosis be identified at surgery or histological analysis. Regarding the most common histological subtypes, there is some discrepancy relative to endometriosis-associated ovarian cancer given that some researchers have reported a predominance of endometrioid carcinomas and sarcomas, whereas others have described histopathological similarities with endometriosis-associated ovarian cancer [12].

H. Paixão (✉) · T. M. Cunha
Department of Radiology, Instituto Português de Oncologia de Lisboa Francisco Gentil, Lisbon, Portugal
e-mail: paixao@campus.ul.pt

I. Thomassin-Naggara (ed.), *Imaging of Endometriosis: A Comparative Guide of US, MRI and Surgery*, https://doi.org/10.1007/978-3-031-82750-1_4

4.2 Pathogenesis of the Malignant Transformation of Endometriosis

Endometriosis-associated ovarian cancer has been described as an ovarian cancer with one of the following criteria:

1. Having both cancer cells and endometriosis in the same ovary
2. The presence of cancer in one ovary and endometriosis in the second ovary
3. The presence of ovarian cancer and pelvic endometriosis
4. A histopathology demonstrating the transition from benign endometriosis to malignancy [7]

Several histologic subtypes comprise endometriosis-associated neoplasms, including endometrioid carcinoma, clear cell carcinoma, seromucinous borderline tumor (endocervical-like mucinous borderline tumor and Müllerian mucinous borderline tumor), squamous cell carcinoma, Müllerian adenosarcoma, and endometrioid stromal sarcoma, the first two being the most common histologic subtypes [14, 16–18].

Atypical endometriosis has been considered in multiple studies as the direct precursor of endometrioid and clear cell ovarian carcinomas because atypical endometriosis has been identified as contiguous with these histological tumor subtypes [1, 3]. The risk of the malignant transformation of atypical endometriosis is estimated to be about four times greater than in women with no history of endometriosis [7]. Atypical endometriosis includes different histological findings: cellular atypia or cytological atypia and architectural atypia or hyperplasia [3, 14].

The mechanism proposed for malignant transformation in endometriosis has yet to be well defined. However, oxidative stress, cytokines, genetic mutations (including, for example, the activation of oncogenic KRAS and PI3 K pathways and the inactivation of tumor suppressor genes PTEN and ARID1A), and a hyperestrogenic environment (endogenous and exogenous states) may have a role in the carcinogenesis from benign endometriosis to AE and EAOC [17]. Many studies still need to be carried out on the carcinogenetic potential of endometrioma to clarify the pathogenesis of ovarian cancer and to adopt effective preventive strategies.

Increased awareness of the characteristics, namely radiologic, of atypical endometriomas will improve the early diagnosis of patients with endometriosis who are at risk of endometriosis-associated ovarian cancer [7]. Some of these characteristics will be further explored.

4.3 Clinical Presentation and Biomarkers of Endometriosis-Associated Cancer

The clinical presentation of ovarian and extra-ovarian cancer is often nonspecific. It might consist of vague symptoms and also some overlap might exist with symptoms of benign endometriosis, including dysmenorrhea and dyspareunia [17].

Biomarkers are also unreliable, and none of them has evidence to justify their use in clinical practice [3] because, for example, normal CA-125 levels can be seen with endometriosis-associated ovarian cancer and can be elevated in benign endometriosis [17].

4.4 Imaging Endometriosis-Associated Ovarian and Extraovarian Cancers

4.4.1 Ultrasound

Pelvic and gynecologic transvaginal ultrasound (TVUS) are frequently the first imaging techniques recommended by primary care physicians to assess symptoms of pelvic pain or anomalies discovered on physical examination. There are operator-dependent techniques that require years of experience.

Typical endometrioma (Fig. 4.1 is classically, a cystic tumor with homogeneous and hypoechogenic internal echoes and usually uniloculate [8, 16, 17]. In contrast, atypical endometrioma and endometriosis-associated ovarian cancer (Figs. 4.2 and 4.3) tend to present as larger tumors with more-variable internal content that can be anechogenic, hypoechogenic, or mixed; they have solid mural nodules and/or papillary projections with Doppler signals and are often more multiloculated [8, 16, 17]. These characteristics of both tumors are summarized in Table 4.1.

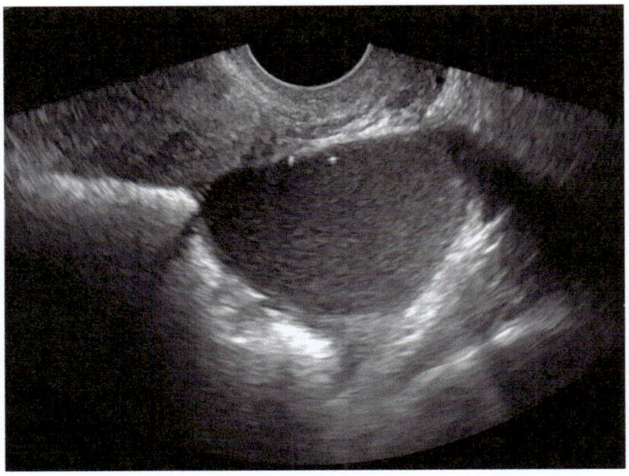

Fig. 4.1 A transvaginal gynecologic ultrasound of a 33-year-old woman shows a classic ultrasound appearance of an endometrioma, an uniloculated cystic tumor of the left ovary, with low-level internal echoes and with small hyperechoic foci in the wall

4.4.2 Computed Tomography (CT)

CT is usually not used to characterize an ovary tumor, but sometimes it is performed for another indication and can identify suspicious ovarian lesions and guide a diagnosis [16]. Its role is essentially in staging, to define difficult-to-resect disease (Fig. 4.4), although the hallmark of ovarian cancer staging remains surgical. In addition, CT is used in unresectable stage IV that has been submitted to neoadjuvant chemotherapy, for evaluating the response to treatment and in the follow-up of patients undergoing surgical resection [17].

As previously mentioned, some findings of ovarian tumors are predictors of malignancy, such as solid mural nodules or papillary projections in a cystic tumor, peritoneal metastases, and ascites (Table 4.2). Large-volume ascites tend to be malignant more frequently than small-volume ascites do [11].

4.4.3 Magnetic Resonance Imaging (MRI)

The use of MRI in evaluating adnexal tumors is becoming increasingly significant due to its ability to offer a more comprehensive and detailed assessment, especially when sonographic findings are inconclusive. Also, it allows the diagnosis of deep pelvic endometriosis and associated malig-

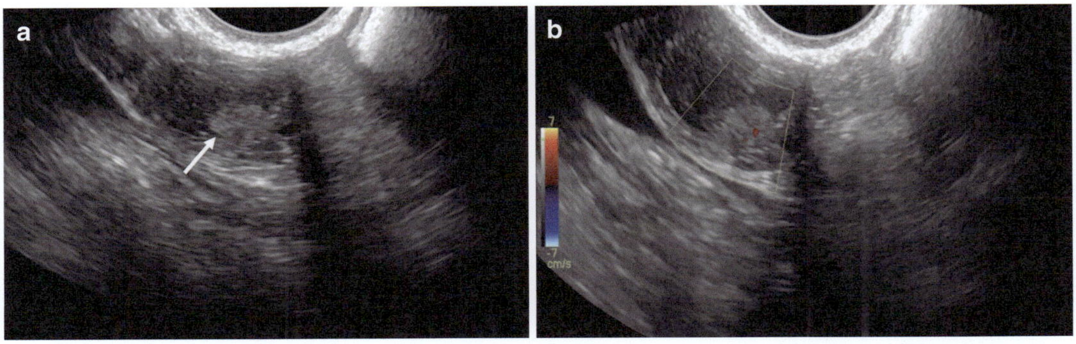

Fig. 4.2 Transvaginal gynecologic ultrasound of a 49-year-old woman with a history of endometriosis: an endometrioma of the right ovary (**a**) with a hyperechogenic nodule (arrow), with Doppler signal (**b**), which turned out to be a 6 mm endometrioid carcinoma arising in an endometrioma

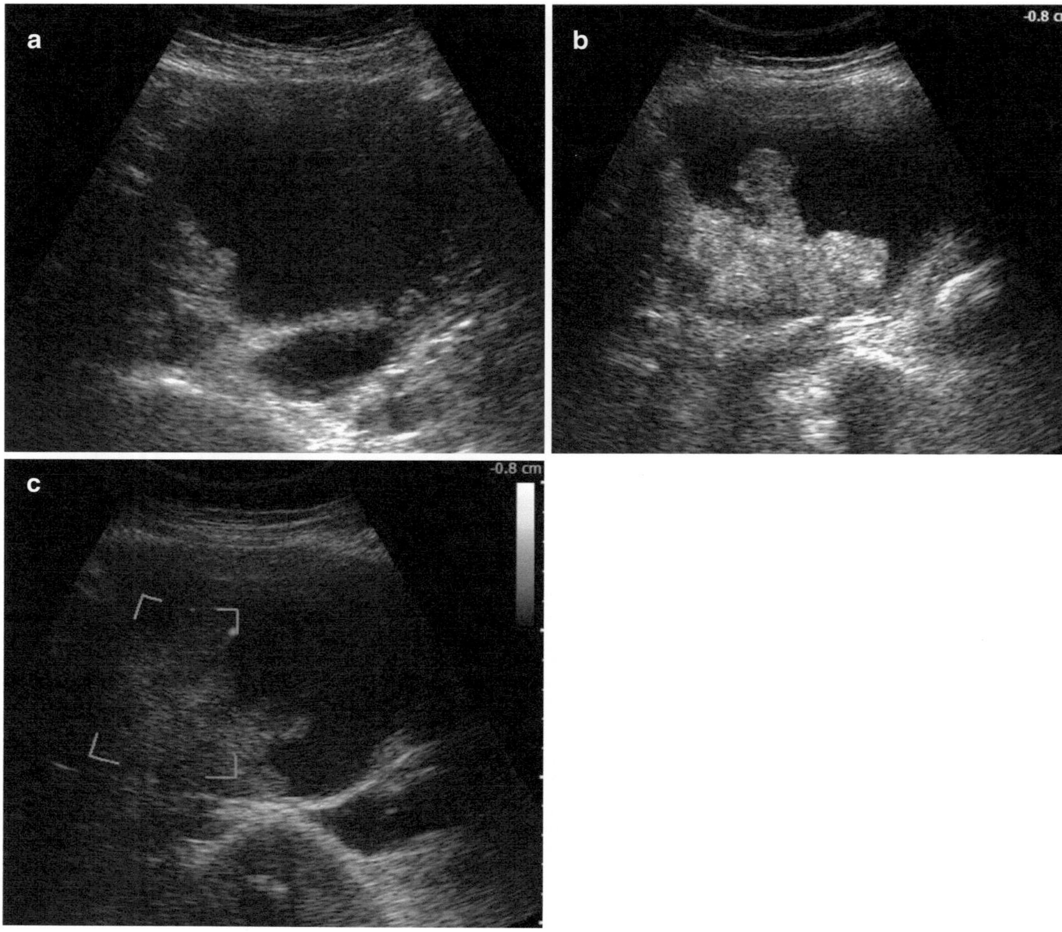

Fig. 4.3 Ultrasound appearance of a malignant endometrioma in a 55-year-old woman: a multiloculated cystic tumor (**a**), with hyperechogenic vegetation (**b**), with Doppler signal (**c**), which turned out to be an endometrioid carcinoma of the right ovary

Table 4.1 Ultrasound characteristics of endometriosis-associated ovarian cancer and endometriosis

Endometriosis-associated ovarian cancer	Endometriosis
Larger tumor	Smaller tumor
Solid mural nodules and/or papillary projections with Doppler signal	Homogeneous, hypoechogenic internal content
More variable internal content: anechogenic, hypoechogenic, mixed internal echogenicity	
Multiloculated	More uniloculated

nancy, the appreciation of the loco-regional extension of the disease, and the detection of recurrences after medical or surgical treatment [16].

By reducing the need for unnecessary surgical interventions and imaging follow-ups, MRI not only contributes to more cost-effective healthcare but also minimizes patient stress and uncertainty [6].

Some MRI characteristics should make us alert and suspect a possible malignant transformation into ovarian endometriosis

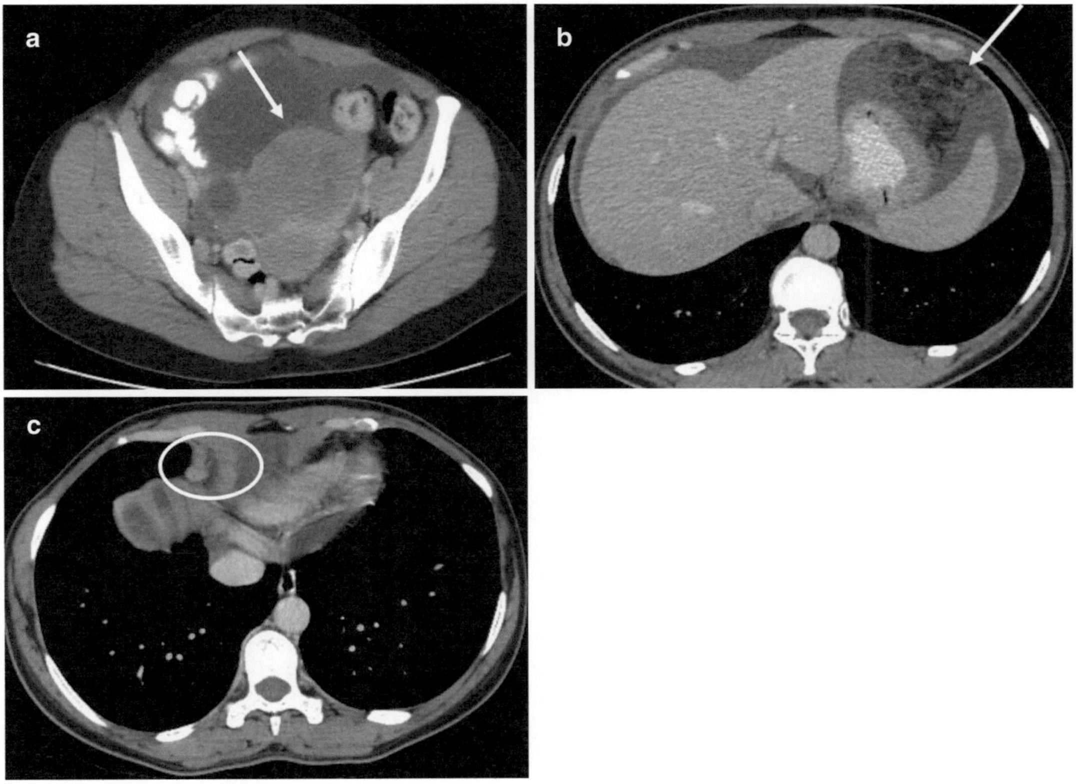

Fig. 4.4 CT staging of a high-grade endometrioid metastatic carcinoma of the left broad ligament (**a**—arrow) best characterized on MRI in Fig. 4.15, showing moderate ascites with peritoneal metastasis on the gastrosplenic ligament (**b**—arrow) and cardiophrenic lymph node metastases (**c**—circle)

Table 4.2 CT features of ovarian tumors predictive of malignancy

CT findings of ovarian tumors predictive of malignancy
Solid mural nodules
Papillary projections in cystic tumor
Peritoneal metastases
Ascites

Table 4.3 MRI findings of endometriosis-associated ovarian cancer

MRI findings of endometriosis-associated ovarian cancer
Solid-enhancing mural nodules
Septations with nodules
Loss of T2 shading
Diffusion restriction of solid-enhancing mural nodules and septations
Endometrioma with increasing size on MRI
Ancillary findings (ascites and peritoneal metastases)

(including solid enhancing mural nodules, septations with nodules, a loss of T2 shading, diffusion restriction, and endometrioma with increasing size on MRI [12]) and in extra-ovarian endometriosis (including the solid tumor in typical extra-ovarian endometriosis localizations, with intermediate signal intensity on T1- and T2-weighted sequences, with restricted diffusion and enhancement on dynamic sequences, the presence of metastatic spread, and the malignant transformation of endometriosis into postoperative scarring in a patient with no history or with evidence of pelvic endometriosis). Each of them will be individually described next and are summarized in Tables 4.3 and 4.4. In addition, a typical endometrioma does not show any wall enhancement. In contrast, if a degeneration occurs, one of the first signs is the appearance of wall enhancement that is not specific (because

Table 4.4 MRI findings of endometriosis-associated extra-ovarian cancer

MRI findings of endometriosis-associated extra-ovarian cancer
Solid tumor in typical extra-ovarian endometriosis localizations (including the pouch of Douglas, pelvic ligaments, vagina or post-hysterectomy vaginal vault, rectum, bladder, or post-cesarean scar)
Tumor with intermediate signal intensity on T1- and T2-weighted sequences, with restricted diffusion and enhancement on dynamic sequences
Metastatic spread
Endometriosis identified at MRI or surgery, or a history of gynecologic surgery in the absence of known endometriosis

Table 4.5 Proposed MRI protocol for diagnosis of endometriosis-associated ovarian cancers

MRI protocol for diagnosis of endometriosis-associated ovarian cancers
T2W sequences
T1 sequences with and without fat suppression
Diffusion study and ADC map
Non-enhanced and dynamic-contrast-enhanced fat-suppressed T1W (including delayed acquisition) images with subtraction

many other phenomena may be responsible for that, such as inflammatory transformation) but that has to alert any radiologist.

Before that, we propose an optimal MRI protocol that considers recommendations from ESUR and is also used at our institution and that should be used to diagnose cases of suspected endometriosis-associated ovarian cancer [4]. Table 4.5 summarizes this protocol. Once again, the subtraction images derived from T1-weighted fat-suppressed images without and after contrast should not be forgotten, because they offer better visibility of enhanced mural nodules against the intrinsically high background signal intensity of endometrioma.

In addition, patient preparation before MRI should be recommended, which includes fasting for 3 to 6 h, bladder emptying 1 h before the examination, and taking an antiperistatical agent to prevent evacuation artefacts, unless contraindicated. Vaginal or rectal opacification with a gel is considered optional [4].

4.4.4 MRI Findings of Endometriosis-Associated Ovarian Cancer

4.4.4.1 Solid-Enhancing Mural Nodules

Studies have shown that the most sensitive MR imaging feature for the diagnosis of malignancy in an endometrioma is the presence of an enhancing mural nodule [12, 17]. Such nodules are frequently iso- to hypointense on T1-weighted precontrast sequences and homogeneously or heterogeneously enhanced on T1-weighted postcontrast sequences. The signal intensity on T2-weighted sequences is variable (Figs. 4.5, 4.6 and 4.7) [12, 17]. Subtraction imaging helps evaluate small nodularities because of the intrinsic high signal intensity of the underlying endometrioma at the T1-weighted sequence (Figs. 4.5, 4.7 and 4.11) [16].

4.4.4.2 Septations with Nodules

Septations within endometriomas occur, and differentiating benign from malignant septations can be challenging. However, some clues can help us in this classification. Benign septations should be smooth even if they are thick. Conversely, irregular or nodular septations with enhancing and restricted diffusion should be considered highly suspicious (Fig. 4.8) [17].

4.4.4.3 Loss of T2 Shading

Endometriomas classically exhibit the MR feature of *T2 shading*. This feature is characterized by ranging from a homogeneous signal void to various gradations of decreased signal intensity seen at T2-weighted sequences in lesions that show signal hyperintensity at T1-weighted sequences [21].

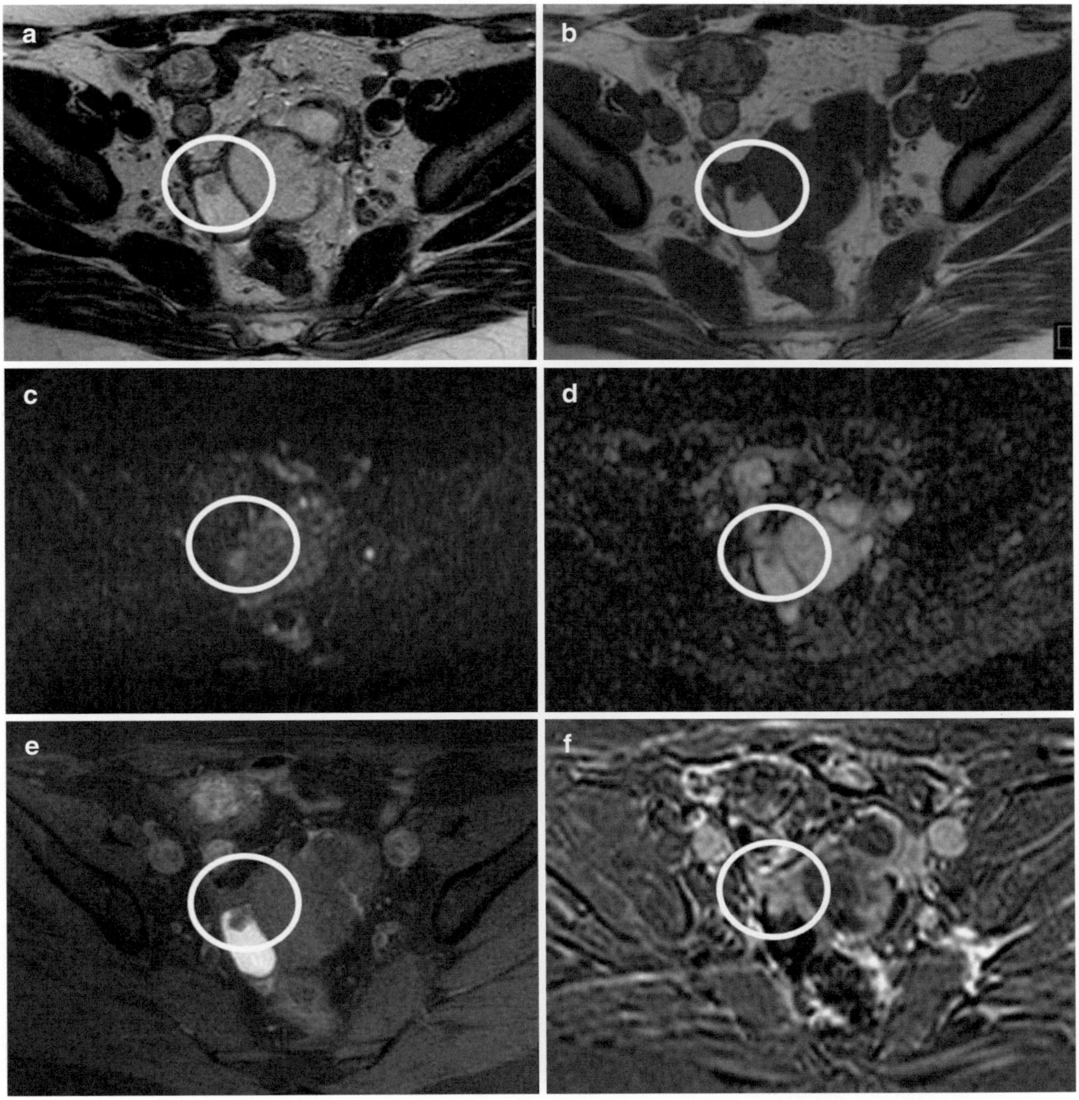

Fig. 4.5 MRI of a borderline serous tumor of the right ovary in a histerectomizated patient with a history of endometriosis: axial images of the pelvis show a small solid nodule in the endometrioma of the right ovary (circle), and the solid nodule is mostly hypointense on T2 (**a**), T1 (**b**), and T1 with fat saturation (**e**), with diffusion restriction (**c**—DWI b-1000, **d**—ADC-map) and enhancement on postcontrast dynamic T1 with fat saturation, best demonstrated in the subtraction (**f**). Image subtraction after contrast administration is essential to evaluate small nodules, namely their enhancement, which can be masked by the hyperintense signal of endometrioma on T1 images

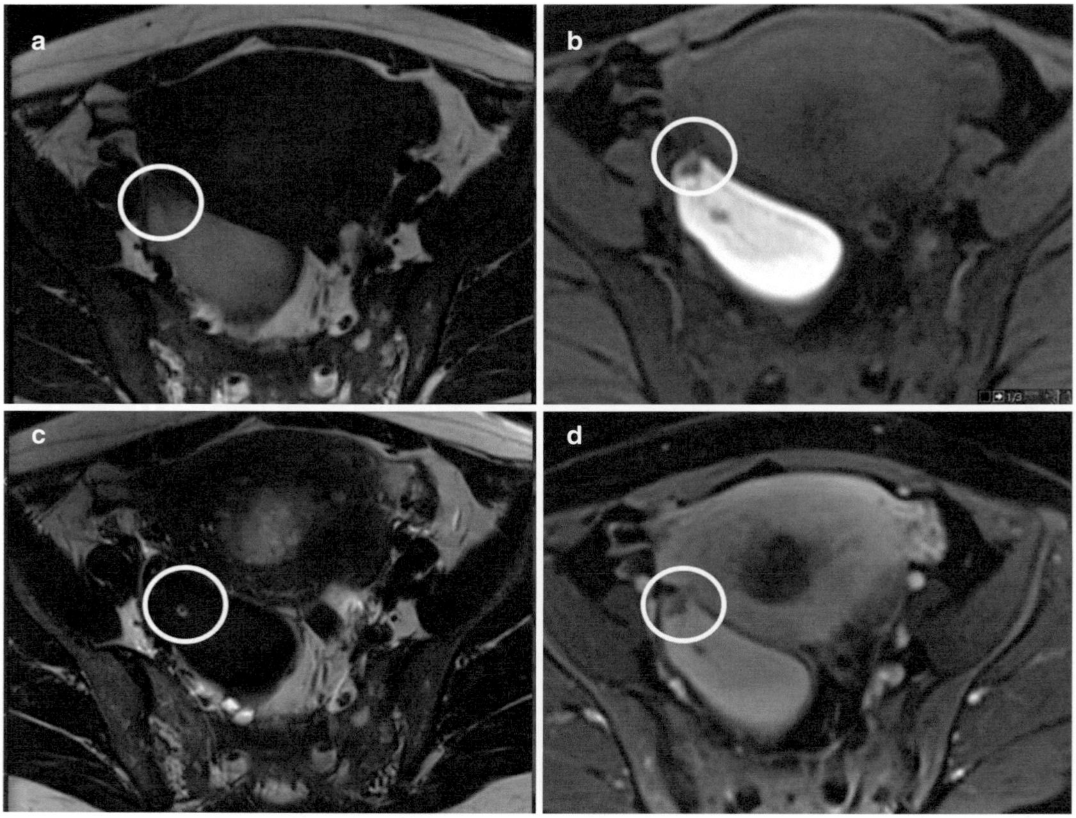

Fig. 4.6 MRI of a borderline intestinal-type mucinous tumor in right ovary endometrioma on MRI: axial images of the pelvis show a small solid nodule in the endometrioma of the right ovary (circle), and the solid nodule is mostly hypointense on T2W (**a**), T1W (**c**), and T1 with fat saturation (**b**), with enhancement after contrast administration (**d**)

Malignant endometriomas can demonstrate the loss or absence of this T2 shading, perhaps due to the dilution of the hemorrhagic contents by the nonhemorrhagic fluid produced by the malignant tumors (Fig. 4.8) [12]. However, this feature alone is nonspecific and can also be seen in benign endometriomas, so it is more helpful when presented in conjunction with other features of malignancy (Fig. 4.9) [5, 17].

4.4.4.4 Diffusion Restriction

Abnormal restricted diffusion occurs in the malignant transformation of endometriomas. Usually, these areas of restricted diffusion and low apparent diffusion coefficient apparent diffusion coefficient (ADC) values should overlap with solid mural nodularities and enhanced nodular septations of the lesion (Figs. 4.5, 4.7, 4.9, 4.10, and 4.11).

Abnormal restricted diffusion in solid tissue is not specific to malignancy. Carefully placing Region-of-Interest (ROI) in solid tissue is crucial because the ADC value in the cystic component is typically low. Thus, a gadolinium injection with subtraction is particularly useful in this setting. It can also be seen in benign lesions such as endometriomas, although in this case, the typical pattern of diffusion restriction is more diffuse in the lesion's cystic portion. Intracystic blood clots may also demonstrate restricted diffusion, mimicking a mural nodule. However, blood clots usually do not enhance after contrast administration [16, 17].

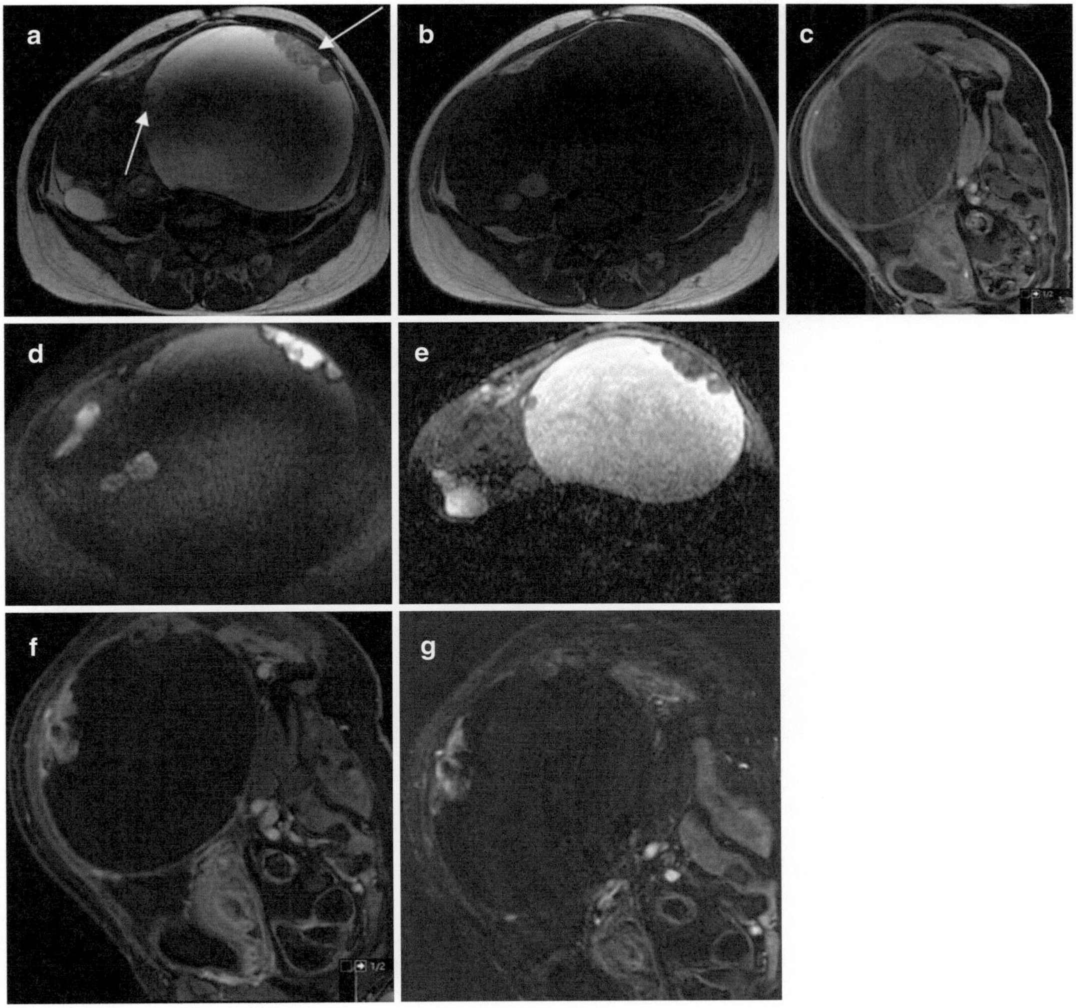

Fig. 4.7 MRI of a clear cell carcinoma in a woman with endometriosis: axial and sagittal images of the pelvis show a cystic tumor with some vegetations (arrows) hypointense on T2W (**a**), T1W (**b**), and T1W with fat saturation (**c**), with restriction on diffusion (**d** and **e**) and with enhancement after contrast on T1 with fat saturation (**f**), which is better demonstrated with subtraction (**g**)

4.4.4.5 Endometrioma with Increasing Size on MRI

Endometrioma growth is another alarming finding for malignant transformation in endometrioma (Fig. 4.11) [9, 12]. An endometriotic cyst diameter of ≥9 cm was an independent predictive factor for the future development of ovarian malignant tumor [10].

4.4.4.6 Ancillary Findings

Ancillary findings suggestive of metastases, including voluminous ascites and peritoneal metastases, are not a great help in this diagnosis, because they are exceedingly rare in patients with a malignant transformation of an endometrioma [12]. However, when they are present, malignancy should be suggested.

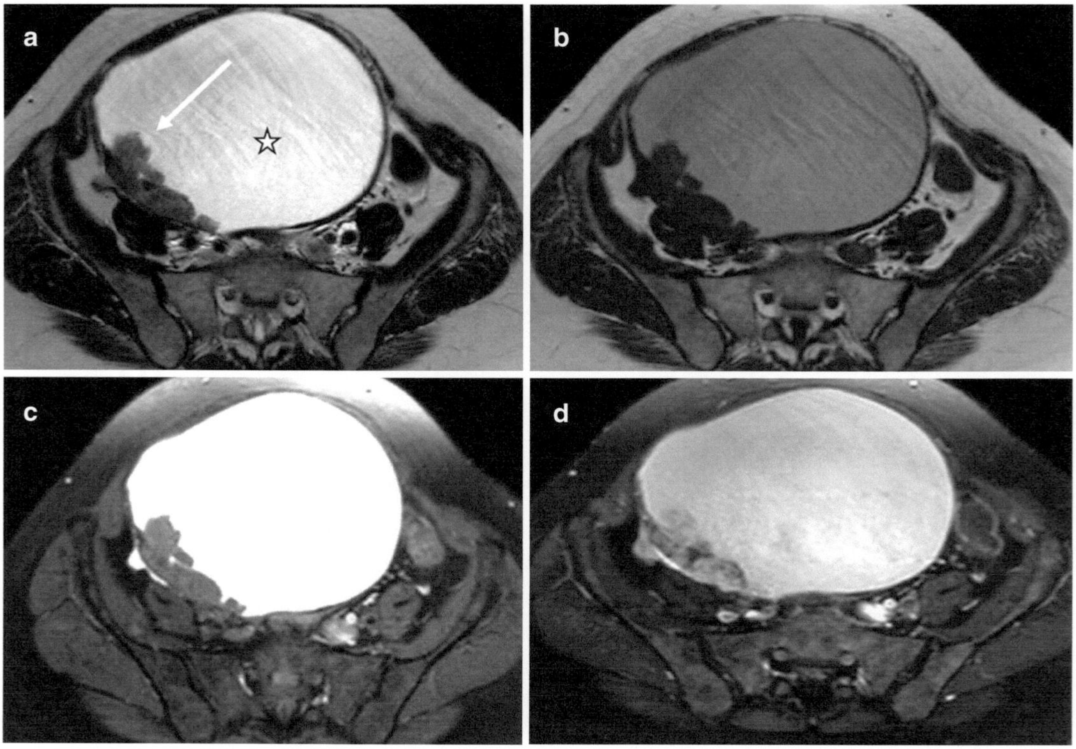

Fig. 4.8 A poorly differentiated endometrioid carcinoma of the right ovary on MRI: axial images show a cystic pelvic lesion containing nodular, irregular, enhancing septations (arrow), and a loss of shading is noticeable in the endometrioma, which is T2 hyperintense (star). **a**—T2W, **b**—T1W, **c**—T1W with fat saturation, and **d**—post-contrast T1W with fat saturation

4.4.5 MRI Findings of Endometriosis-Associated Extra-Ovarian Cancer

A solid tumor in the pouch of Douglas, pelvic ligaments, vagina or post-hysterectomy vaginal vault, rectum, bladder, or post-cesarean scar can be seen on MRI. The distribution of endometriosis-associated extra-ovarian malignancies usually mirrors that of extra-ovarian endometriosis, with a higher prevalence on rectovaginal sites (Fig. 4.12) [12].

4.4.5.1 Tumor with Intermediate Signal Intensity on T1- and T2-Weighted Sequences, with Restricted Diffusion and Enhancement on Dynamic Sequences

Endometriosis-associated extra-ovarian cancers present as predominantly solid-enhancing tumors, with intermediate signal intensity on T1- and T2-weighted sequences and restricted diffusion. These tumors also characteristically enhance after an intravenous administration of gadolinium-based contrast (Figs. 4.12, 4.13, and 4.14) [12].

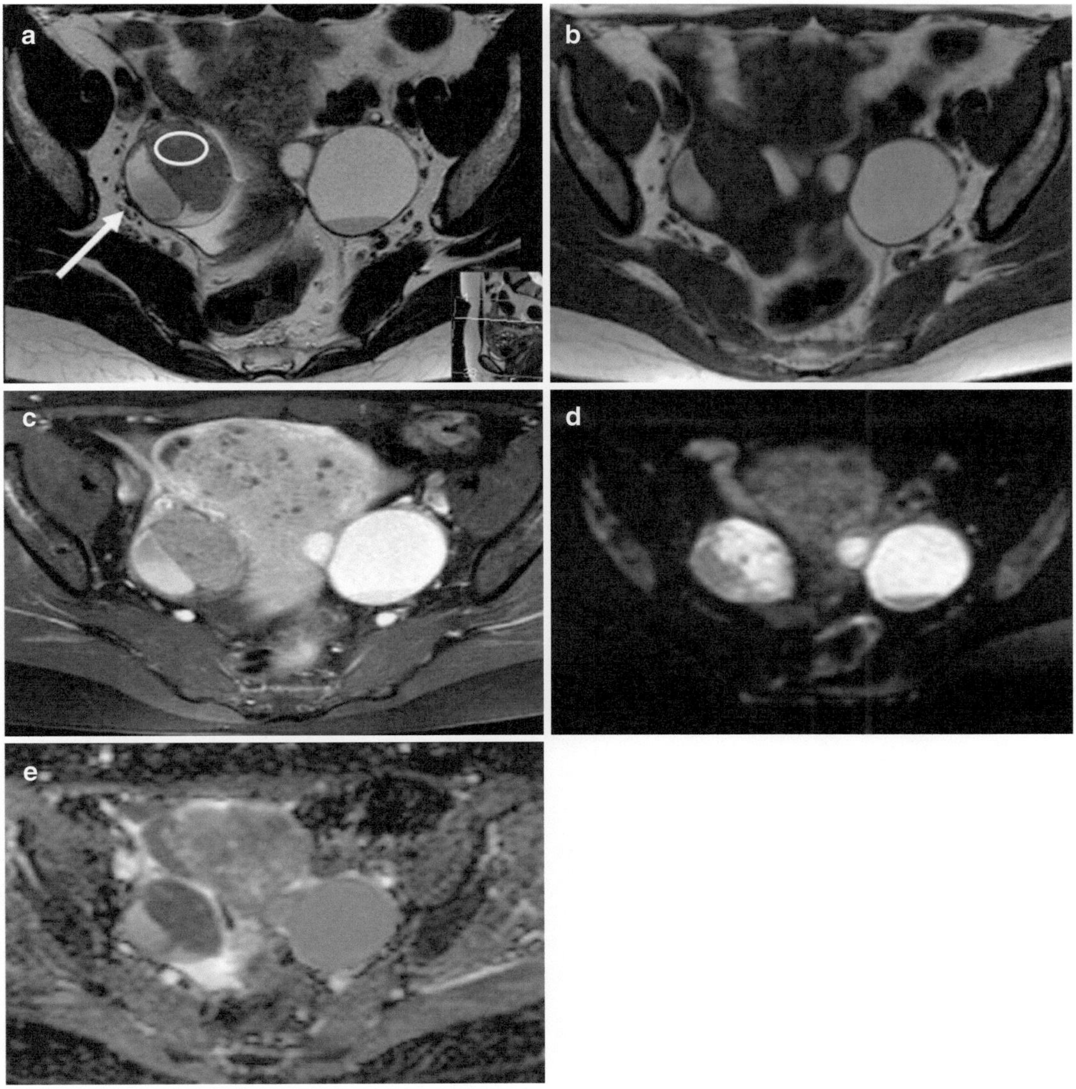

Fig. 4.9 MRI of an endometrioid carcinoma (circle) arising from an endometriotic right ovary cyst that did not lose T2 shading (arrow). **a**—T2W, **b**—T1W, **c**—postcontrast T1W with fat saturation, **d**—DWI *b*-1000, and **e**—ADC-map

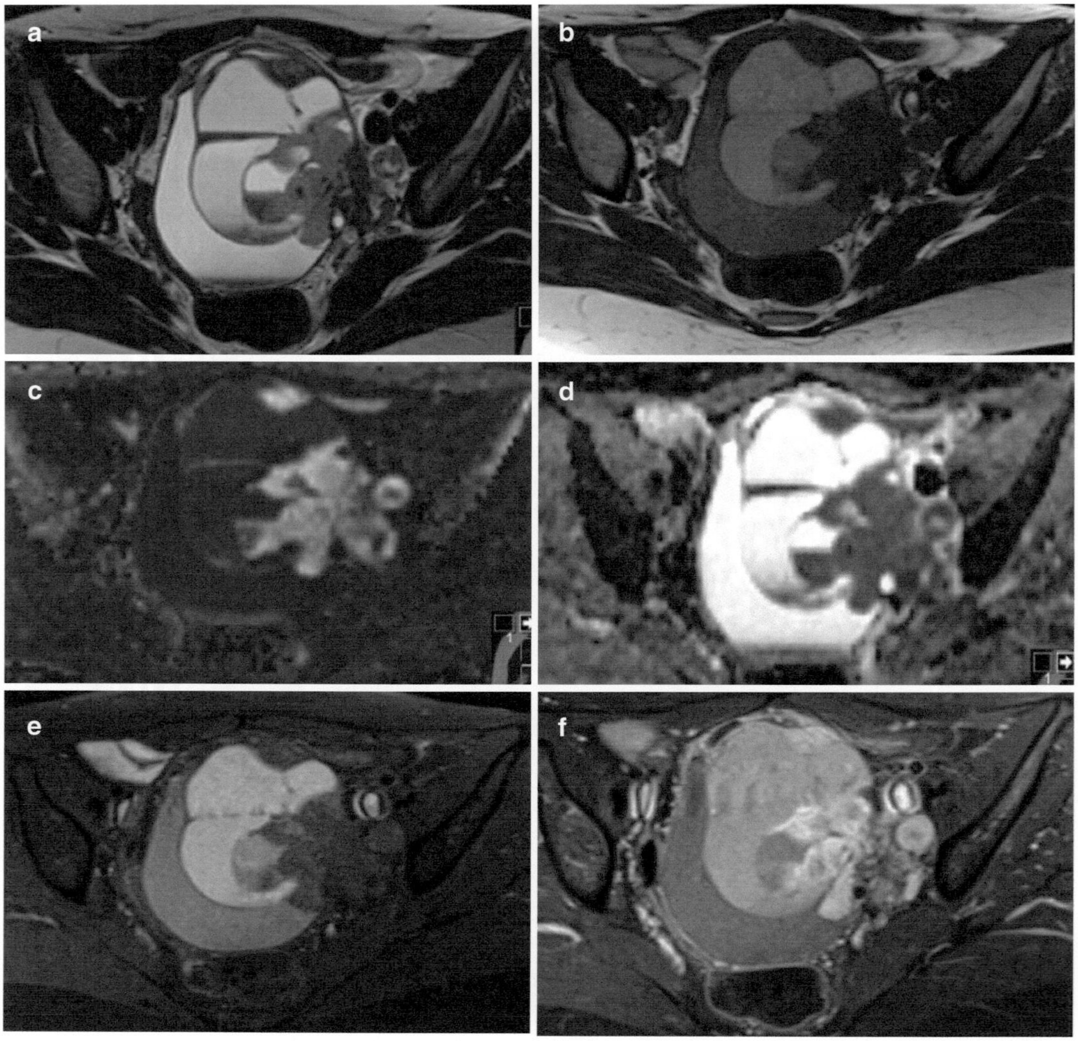

Fig. 4.10 Low-grade endometrial stromal sarcoma within a left ovarian endometrioma in a 42-year-old woman: axial MRI images show a large multiloculated cystic ovarian tumor with nodular septations hypointense on T2W (**a**), T1W (**b**), and T1W with fat saturation (**e**) that restricts in response to diffusion (**c**, **d**) and enhances after contrast administration on T1W with fat saturation (**f**). **c**—DWI *b*-1000, **d**—ADC map, and **f**—postcontrast T1W with fat saturation

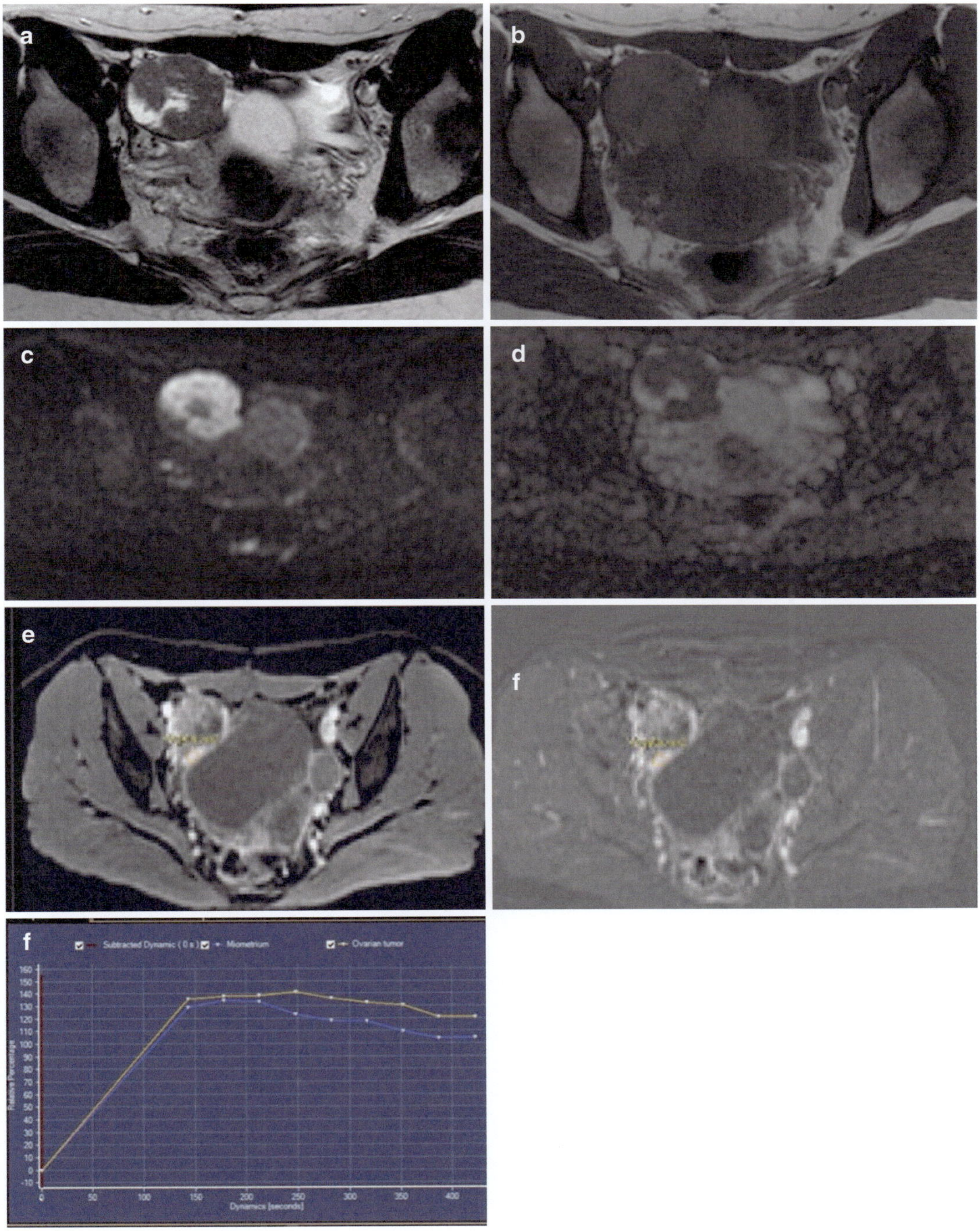

Fig. 4.11 MRI of an endometrioid carcinoma of the right ovary in a 17-year-old girl: axial MRI images show a solid area, hypointense on T2W and T1W (**a** and **b**, respectively), with restricted diffusion (**c** and **d** are DWI *b*-1000 and ADC-map, respectively) and enhancement after contrast on dynamic post-contrast T1W with fat saturation (**e**) and best demonstrated in the subtraction (**f**), within the cystic lesion of the right ovary; the solid component shows a high risk type curve (**g**), the mass was scored O RADS IRM 5; and on the previous MRI (not shown) was a smaller endometrioma without a solid component

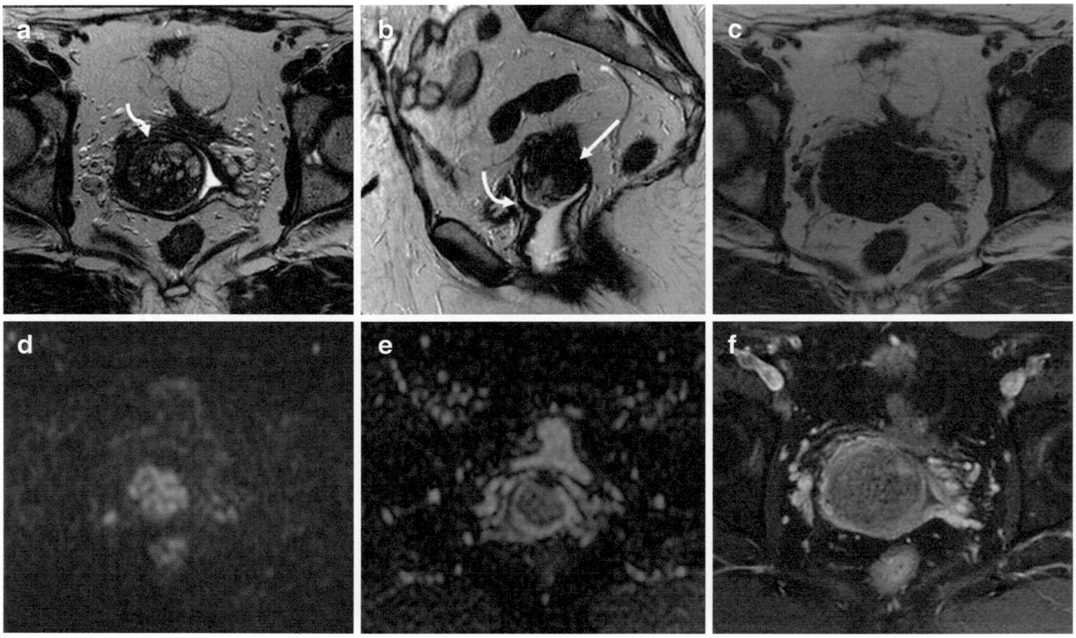

Fig. 4.12 Clear cell carcinoma of the vagina with concomitant endometriosis identified: in the vaginal dome, a solid tumor is observed in the vaginal lumen, heterogeneous, hypointense in its upper half on T2 sagittal (arrow), and without diffusion restriction; in its lower half is hyperintense on T2 (**a** and **b**, curved arrows), hypointense on T1 (**c**), with diffusion restriction (with high signal intensity on the DWI *b*-1000 (**d**) and hyposignal on the ADC map (**e**)) and with enhancement after contrast (**f**) showing suspicious aspects that favor the diagnosis of vaginal endometriosis with malignant transformation in its lower half, which was later histologically confirmed

4.4.5.2 Lymphadenopathy

The metastatic spread of extra-ovarian endometriosis-associated malignancies generally occurs via lymphatic and/or hematogenous routes. Perineural spread has also been observed (Fig. 4.15) [12].

4.4.5.3 Endometriosis Identified at MRI or Surgery in the Absence of Known Endometriosis

The definitive diagnosis of endometriosis-associated extra-ovarian cancer requires that concurrent endometriosis be identified. So, we should remember to consider the diagnosis of endometriosis-related extra-ovarian malignancy when such a lesion is seen in a woman with a history of endometriosis or when a lesion with endometriotic characteristics and another lesion with malignant features are seen simultaneously on MRI.

Sometimes the malignant transformation of an endometriotic lesion into a postoperative scar can be found in a patient with no history or evidence of endometriosis. In these cases, the definitive diagnosis requires a biopsy of the suspicious lesion [12].

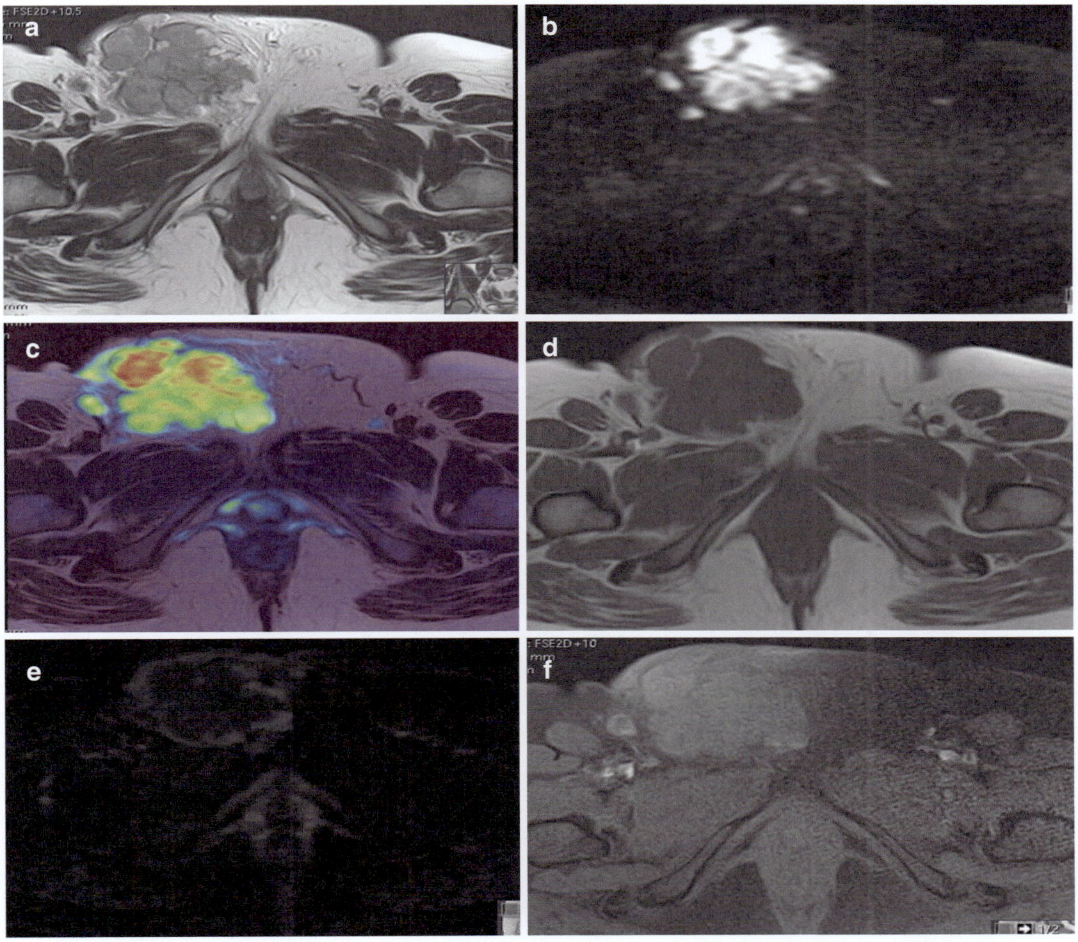

Fig. 4.13 Clear cell carcinoma originating from endometriosis on the right Nuck's canal: axial pelvic MRI shows a multiloculated tumor in the right Nuck's canal, with intermediate signal intensity on T2W (**a**) and T1W (**d**), with diffusion restriction (**b** and **e**) and enhancement after contrast on T1W with fat saturation (**f**). **c**—fusion between T2W and DWI *b*-1000

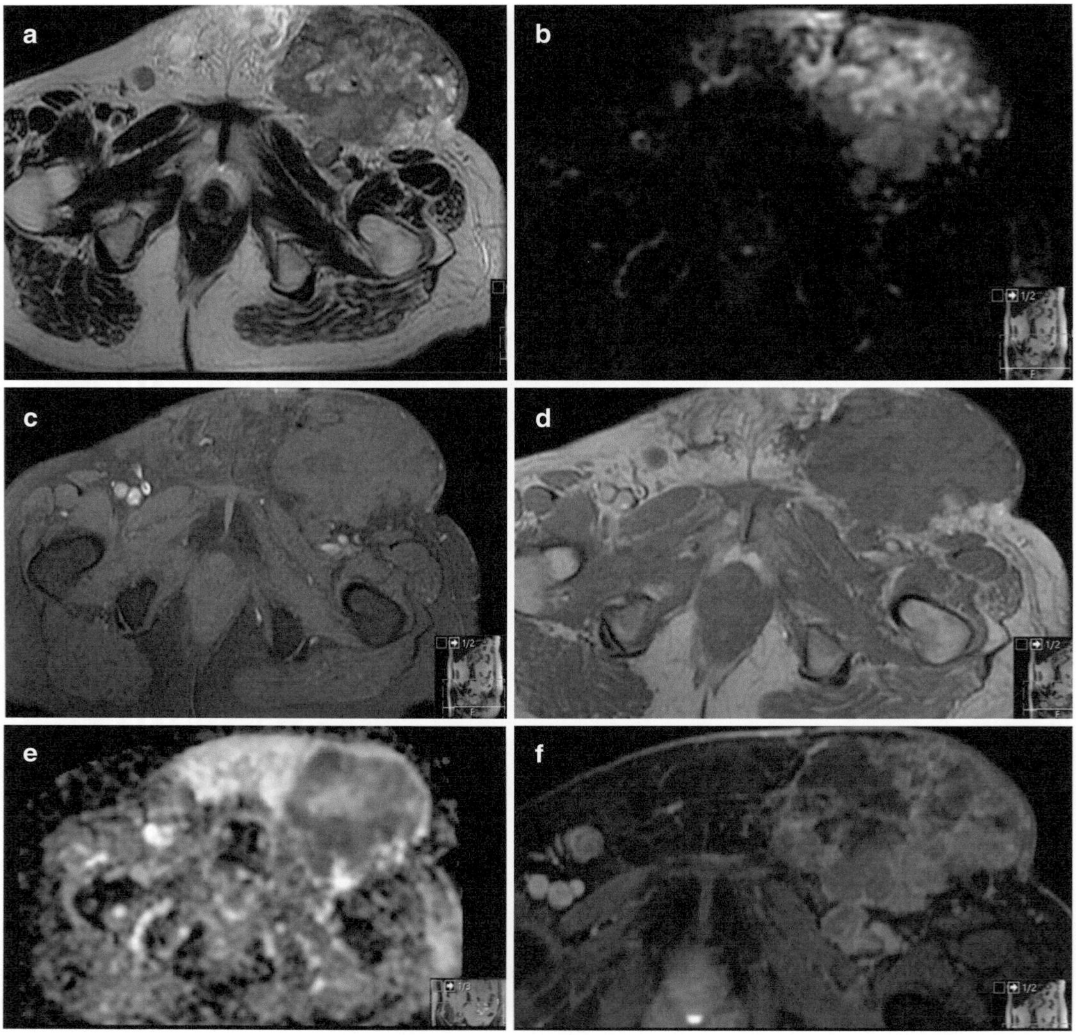

Fig. 4.14 High-grade serous carcinoma originating from endometriosis on the left Nuck's canal: it is a solid tumor with discreet cystic areas, with intermediate signal intensity on T2W (**a**), T1W (**d**), and T1W with fat saturation (**c**) and with diffusion restriction (**b** and **e**) and enhancement after contrast on T1 with fat saturation (**f**)

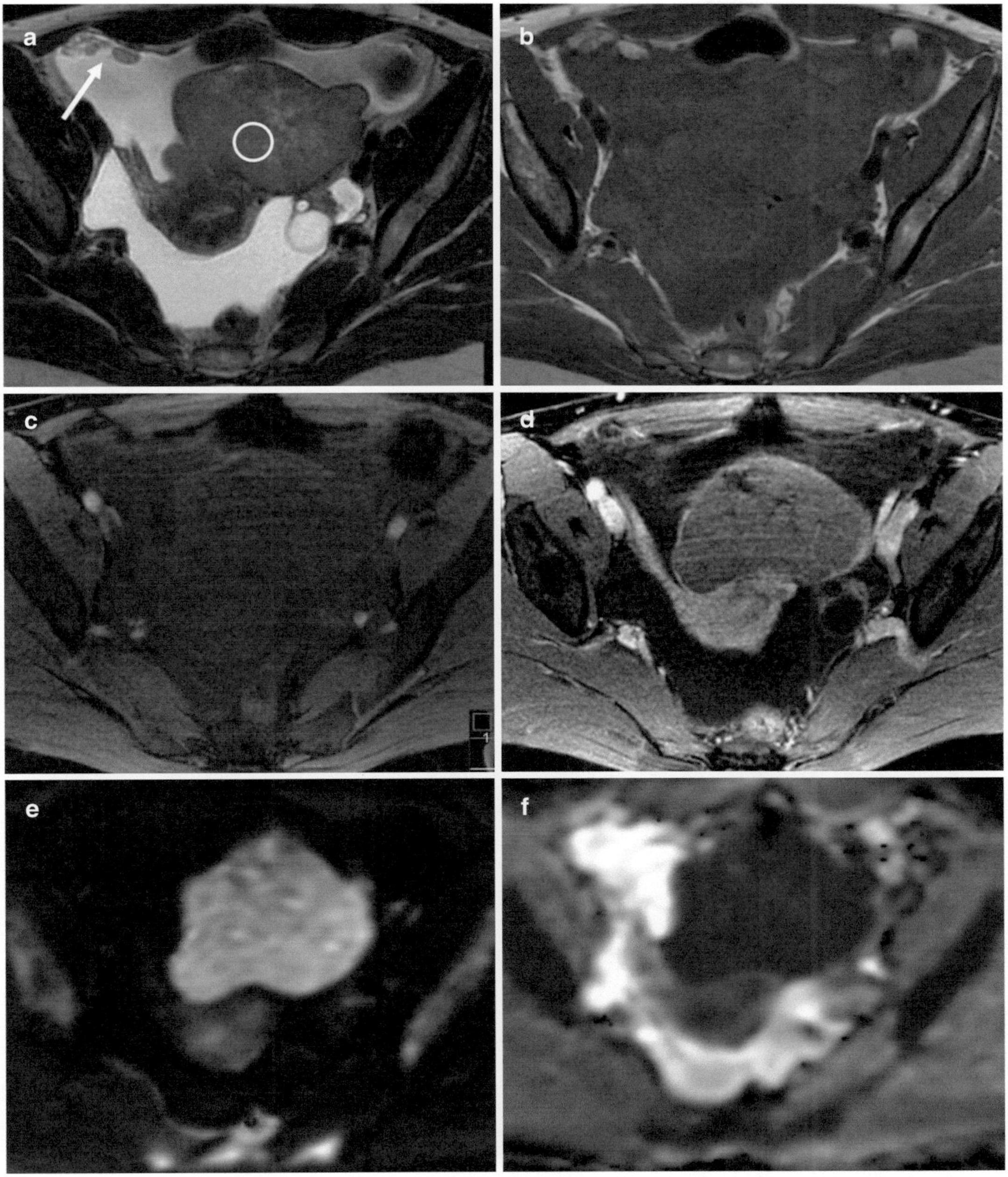

Fig. 4.15 High-grade endometrioid metastatic carcinoma of the left broad ligament on MRI: axial pelvic MRI shows a solid tumor of the left broad ligament (circle), with intermediate signal intensity on T2W (**a**), T1W (**b**), and T1W with fat saturation (**c**) and with enhancement after contrast on T1W with fat saturation (**d**) and with diffusion restriction (**e** and **f**) ascites and peritoneal metastases (arrow) are also shown

4.5 Differential Diagnosis and Pitfalls of MRI

As radiologists, we must be aware of different mimickers of endometriosis-associated ovarian cancer, such as the usual ovarian parenchyma, the decidualization of endometriomas, and polypoid endometriosis (Table 4.6). The usual ovarian parenchyma adjacent to an endometrioma can be mistaken as an enhancing mural solid nodule. However, its crescent shape with follicles that are T2 hyperintense and nonenhancing should differentiate itself from irregular and papillary nodules of endometriosis-associated ovarian cancer [17].

The decidual reaction of endometriomas during pregnancy is rare, but it could mimic endometriosis-associated ovarian cancer. During pregnancy, hormonal changes lead to the hypertrophy of the endometrial stromal cells that line the endometrioma and the gravid uterus, and thus, endometrioma can exhibit solid mural nodules or rapid growth, all features of endometriosis-associated ovarian cancer. However, some of the findings that can point to the decidualization of endometrioma are the maintenance of T2 shading in the endometrioma and the recognition that the solid nodules follow the signal intensity of the decidualized uterine endometrium (which characteristically shows as T2 hyperintense and with T2 shine-through, which means that it has high signal intensity on diffusion weighted imaging (DWI) and ADC maps—as opposed to solid mural nodules from endometriosis-associated ovarian malignancy, which show diffusion restriction). Of course, these lesions should be followed in the postpartum period to ensure that they are benign and disappear [9, 17].

Table 4.6 Differential diagnosis and pitfalls of endometriosis-associated cancers on MRI

Differential diagnosis and pitfalls of MRI
Ovarian parenchyma adjacent to an endometrioma
Decidualization of endometrioma
Polypoid endometriosis

Polypoid endometriosis, a rare form of endometriosis, is associated with exogenous hormone therapy (for example, Tamoxifen) and may also mimic malignant transformation in an endometrioma. As opposed to endometriosis, which classically affects women of reproductive age, polypoid endometriosis affects women over 50 years old. This lesion is characterized by being a polypoid tumor that grows from the serosal surface or mucosa of the bowel (particularly the rectum and sigmoid colon), an endometrioma, or the bladder. On MRI, it typically appears hyperintense with a peripheral hypointense rim on T2, with marked enhancement similar to that of the endometrium and with T2 shine-through (Fig. 4.16) [9, 17].

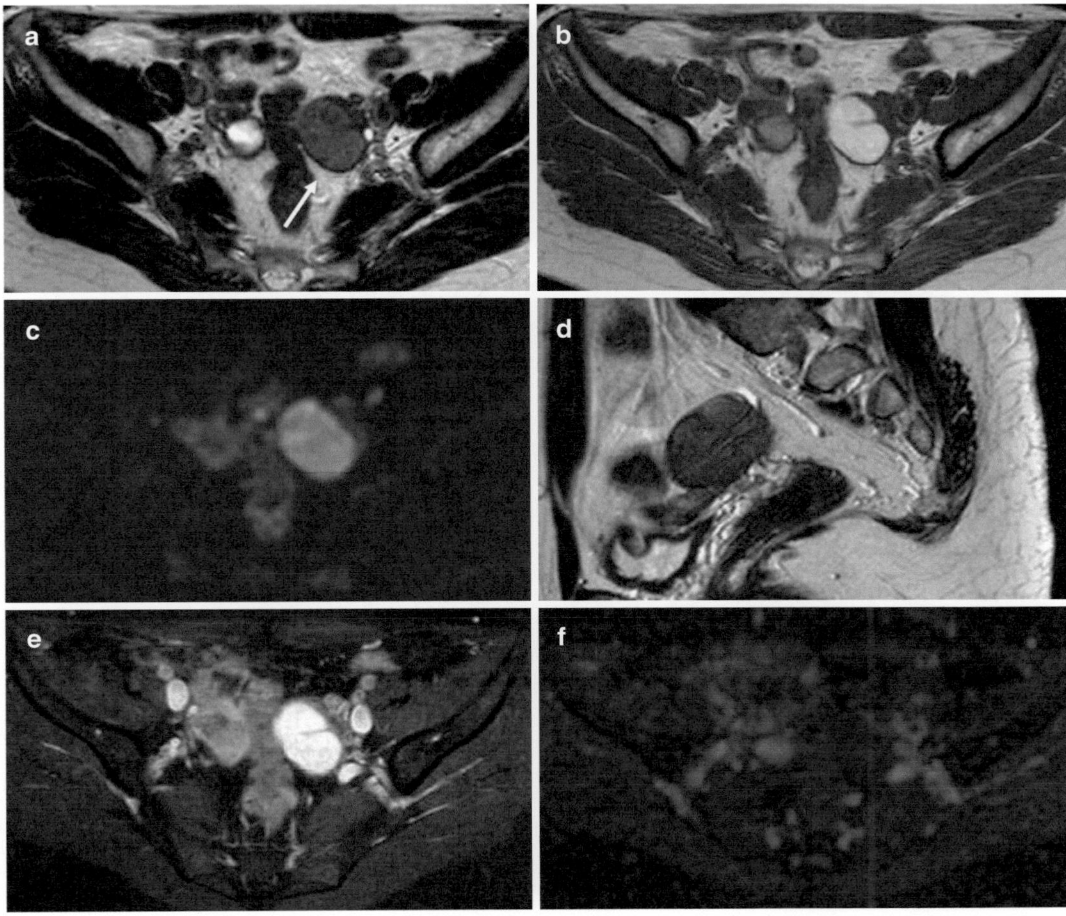

Fig. 4.16 Polypoid endometriosis of the sigmoid colon: axial pelvic MRI shows a solid tumor (arrow) without a cleavage plane with the sigmoid colon, slightly hyperintense with a peripheral hypointense rim on T2W (**a** and **d** are axial and sagittal, respectively), hyperintense on T1W (**b**), with enhancement after contrast on T1W with fat saturation (**e**) and without diffusion restriction (**c** and **f**)

4.6 Conclusion

Ovarian cancer risk is markedly increased in women with ovarian endometrioma or deep pelvic endometriosis according to a recent cohort study on 78,893 women (HR = 966) in both type 1 and type 2 ovarian cancer [2]. Endometriosis-associated cancer is a distinct disease in its clinical presentation, imaging appearance, pathologic characteristics, and prognostic implications. Diagnosing endometriosis-associated cancer may be challenging, but an optimized MR protocol, including dynamic subtraction images, is the key to achieving it. A comprehensive understanding of the imaging features associated with atypical endometriosis and endometriosis-associated cancer is so fundamental because it aids in an early diagnosis and aids clinicians in making informed decisions on treatment strategies, contributing to improved patient outcomes.

References

1. Anglesio MS, Yong P. Endometriosis-associated ovarian cancers. Clin Obstet Gynecol. 2017;60(4):711–27. https://doi.org/10.1097/GRF.0000000000000320.
2. Barnard ME, Farland LV, Yan B, Wang J, Trabert B, Doherty JA, et al. Endometriosis Typology and Ovarian Cancer Risk. JAMA. 2024;332(6):482–9. Published online July 17, 2024.
3. Bartiromo L, Schimberni M, Villanacci R, Mangili G, Ferrari S, Ottolina J, et al. A systematic review of atypical endometriosis-associated biomarkers. Int J Mol Sci. 2022;23(8):4425. https://doi.org/10.3390/ijms23084425.
4. Bazot M, Bharwani N, Huchon C, Kinkel K, Cunha TM, Guerra A, et al. European Society of Urogenital Radiology (ESUR) guidelines: MR imaging of pelvic endometriosis. Eur Radiol. 2017;27(7):2765–75. https://doi.org/10.1007/s00330-016-4673-z.
5. Dias JL, Gomes FV, Lucas R, Cunha TM. The shading sign: is it exclusive of endometriomas? Abdom Imaging. 2015;40(7):2566–72. https://doi.org/10.1007/s00261-015-0465-1.
6. Forstner R, Thomassin-Naggara I, Cunha TM, Kinkel K, Masselli G, Kubik-Huch R, et al. ESUR recommendations for MR imaging of the sonographically indeterminate adnexal mass: an update. Eur Radiol. 2017;27(6):2248–57. https://doi.org/10.1007/s00330-016-4600-3.
7. Grandi G, Toss A, Cortesi L, Botticelli L, Volpe A, Cagnacci A. The association between endometriomas and ovarian cancer: preventive effect of inhibiting ovulation and menstruation during reproductive life. Biomed Res Int. 2015;2015:751571. https://doi.org/10.1155/2015/751571.
8. Huang KJ, Li YX, Wu CJ, Chang WC, Wei LH, Sheu BC. Sonographic features differentiating early-stage ovarian clear cell carcinoma from endometrioma with atypical features. J Ovarian Res. 2022;15(1):84. https://doi.org/10.1186/s13048-022-01019-8.
9. Kido A, Himoto Y, Moribata Y, Kurata Y, Nakamoto Y. MRI in diagnosis of endometriosis and related diseases. Korean J Radiol. 2022;23(4):426–45. https://doi.org/10.3348/kjr.2021.0405.
10. Kobayashi H, Ooi H, Yamada Y, Sakata M, Kawaguchi R, Kanayama S, et al. Serum CA125 level before the development of ovarian cancer. Int J Gynaecol Obstet. 2007;99(2):95–9. https://doi.org/10.1016/j.ijgo.2007.06.003.
11. Li X, Ye Z. Clear cell carcinoma of the ovary: multi-slice computed tomography findings. World J Surg Oncol. 2015;13:133. https://doi.org/10.1186/s12957-015-0546-1.
12. McDermott S, Oei TN, Iyer VR, Lee SI. MR imaging of malignancies arising in endometriomas and extraovarian endometriosis. Radiographics. 2012;32(3):845–63. https://doi.org/10.1148/rg.323115736.
13. Melin A, Sparen P, Persson I, Bergqvist A. Endometriosis and the risk of cancer with special emphasis on ovarian cancer. Hum Reprod. 2006;21(5):1237–42. https://doi.org/10.1093/humrep/dei462.
14. Mikami Y. Endometriosis-related ovarian neoplasms: pathogenesis and histopathologic features. Diagn Histopathol. 2014;20(9):357–63. https://doi.org/10.1016/j.mpdhp.2014.07.002.
15. Nezhat F, Datta MS, Hanson V, Pejovic T, Nezhat C, Nezhat C. The relationship of endometriosis and ovarian malignancy: a review. Fertil Steril. 2008;90(5):1559–70. https://doi.org/10.1016/j.fertnstert.2008.08.007.
16. Radzynski L, Boyer L, Kossai M, Mouraire A, Montoriol PF. Pictorial essay: MRI evaluation of endometriosis-associated neoplasms. Insights Imaging. 2023;14:144. https://doi.org/10.1186/s13244-023-01485-8.
17. Robinson KA, Menias CO, Chen L, Schiappacasse G, Shaaban AM, Caserta MP, et al. Understanding malignant transformation of endometriosis: imaging features with pathologic correlation. Abdom Radiol. 2020 Jun;45(6):1762–75. https://doi.org/10.1007/s00261-019-01914-7.
18. Rodrigues S, Braga M, Félix A, Cunha TM. Clear cell carcinoma of the ovary: clues for radiologists to perform a correct diagnosis. Curr Probl Diagn Radiol. 2023;53(2):271–9. https://doi.org/10.1067/j.cpradiol.2023.10.003.
19. Sampson JA. Endometrial carcinoma of the ovary, arising in endometrial tissue in that organ. Arch Surg. 1925;10(1):1–72. https://doi.org/10.1001/archsurg.1925.01120100007001.
20. Scott RB. Malignant changes in endometriosis. Obstet Gynecol. 1953;2(3):283–9.
21. Tran-Harding K, Nair RT, Dawkins A, Ayoob A, Owen J, Deraney S, et al. Endometriosis revisited: an imaging review of the usual and unusual manifestations with pathological correlation. Clin Imaging. 2018;52:163–71. https://doi.org/10.1016/j.clinimag.2018.07.017.

5 Anterocentral Compartment (Bladder, Round Ligament)

Heng Zhang, Christine O. Menias, and Priyanka Jha

5.1 Introduction

Deep infiltrative endometriosis is determined by the presence of ectopic endometrial glands and stroma outside the endometrial cavity. This condition is commonly associated with chronic pelvic pain and infertility and affects approximately 10% of women of reproductive age. Anterior compartment endometriosis can present with symptoms of dysuria and hematuria when bladder involvement is present. Endometriotic nodules and plaques tend to invade through the peritoneal surface and extend subperitoneally, and they can even invade adjacent organs, eventually causing fibrosis and distorting the patient's anatomy. Like eutopic endometrium, ectopic endometrial glands can also respond to hormonal influences, causing cyclical bleeding and hemorrhage, which provokes scarring and fibrosis. The imaging features of endometriosis reflect these pathologic processes and include the features of hemorrhage in glandular components, endometriomas and endometriosis plaques, and architectural distortion from repeated cycles of hemorrhage and scarring. When analyzing imaging for the presence of endometriosis, a compartmental approach is helpful to allow for an algorithmic and complete assessment of all the potential sites of endometriosis. Several compartment-based approaches have been proposed, including a tricompartmental approach of the anterior, middle, and posterior compartments, as advocated by the Society of Abdominal Radiology (SAR) endometriosis consensus lexicon; a more detailed nine-compartmental approach has also been validated by several ENDOVALRIM publications. The latter approach further divides the anterolateral, anterocentral, posterolateral, and posterocentral compartments.

The anterior compartment is the least common site of deep endometriosis involvement. It is impacted in approximately 6% of patients with endometriosis and commonly coexists with endometriosis elsewhere in the pelvis. Anatomically, the anterior compartment extends posteriorly from the pubic symphysis up to the anterior uterus. Deep endometriosis assessment in the anterocentral compartment includes the assessment of the urinary bladder, the proximal one-third of the intra-pelvic round ligament, and adjacent spaces, such as the prevesical, vesico-

H. Zhang
Department of Radiology, Body Imaging Division, Stanford University, Stanford, CA, USA

Department of Radiology, West China Second University Hospital, Sichuan University, Chengdu, Sichuan, China

C. O. Menias
Mayo Clinic, Phoenix, AZ, USA
e-mail: menias.christine@mayo.edu

P. Jha (✉)
Department of Radiology, Body Imaging Division, Stanford University, Stanford, CA, USA
e-mail: jhap@stanford.edu

I. Thomassin-Naggara (ed.), *Imaging of Endometriosis: A Comparative Guide of US, MRI and Surgery*, https://doi.org/10.1007/978-3-031-82750-1_5

uterine, vesicocervical, and vesicovaginal spaces [1, 2]. The distal two-thirds of the intra-pelvic round ligament is considered a part of the anterolateral compartment, after which point the ligament enters the inguinal canal, forming the extra-pelvic portion of the round ligament [2–4]. For clarity and coherence, this chapter will discuss endometriosis affecting the anterocentral compartment, including the urinary bladder and the proximal part of the round ligament. Given the similarity, we will also discuss the distal part of the round ligament in its intra-pelvic and extra-pelvic parts, which correspond to the anterolateral compartment.

5.2 Bladder Endometriosis

Bladder endometriosis (BE) is present in less than 1% of all patients with endometriosis [5], and its prevalence increases to upward of 14% in patients that have undergone surgery for deep endometriosis [6, 7]. The bladder is the most commonly affected site in urinary tract endometriosis, accounting for 85% of cases of urinary endometriosis [8]. Patients tend to present with dysuria and hematuria, and this can commonly be seen in patients with a history of prior cesarean delivery.

5.2.1 Pathology and Pathogenesis

Bladder endometriosis is defined as the presence of endometrial glands and stroma in the bladder muscularis layer. Endometriotic lesions usually present as an outside-in pattern, starting with disease on the serosal surface of the bladder, with varying depths of detrusor invasion. The implants may extend partially into the detrusor muscle and with increasing disease severity may infiltrate through its full thickness and protrude into the bladder lumen. The mucosal layer of the bladder is rarely infiltrated, and mucosal ulceration is extremely rare. Bladder endometriosis can be multifocal, where the posterior wall, adjacent to the vesicouterine space, is the most frequent site of involvement [9, 10]. Lesions involving only the serosa of the bladder fall into the category of superficial peritoneal endometriosis.

Multiple hypotheses exist for the pathogenesis of bladder endometriosis. The four main etiologic hypotheses are the migratory theory, the iatrogenic theory, the transplantation theory, and the embryonal theory. Among these, the migratory theory is the most widely accepted theory, which postulates that with retrograde menstruation, menstrual endometrium regurgitates through the fallopian tube into the pelvis and then implants on the bladder wall [7, 11]. The implants then cause an inflammatory process in the peritoneum, resulting in adhesions and fibrotic reactions in the vesicouterine space and the vesicovaginal septum. This theory can explain why the central part of the bladder is the most frequent site of disease involvement: Its dependent location is in the vesicouterine space. This theory also explains why BE is seldom seen in retroverted uteruses when the potential dependent space in the vesicouterine pouch is absent [12]. It also explains why bladder endometriosis nearly always coexists with other peritoneal lesions [5, 7]. The iatrogenic theory suggests that bladder lesions may be caused by the intraoperative dissemination of endometrial cells or disruption to the uterine incision [5]. This theory is supported by cases of endometriosis in the surgical scars after cesarean sections and other gynecologic procedures and the increased frequency of bladder endometriosis in patients who have undergone previous gynecologic surgery. The transplantation and embryonal theory proposes that bladder endometriosis might originate from the extension of adenomyotic lesions in the myometrium and the Müllerian remnants. However, as of now, not enough evidence supports these two theories.

5.2.2 Demographics and Clinical Presentation

Bladder endometriosis typically affects women of reproductive age, at an average age of 35 years [8]. It is rarely seen in postmenopausal women. Symptoms of bladder endometriosis can vary and are largely dependent on the location and size of the lesions, the depth of infiltration, and the presence of coexisting lesions at other locations. Approximately 30% of patients are asymptomatic, in which lesions are usually small and superficial [8]. Symptomatic patients can present with dysuria, cramping, painful voiding, urinary frequency, recurrent urinary tract infections, hematuria, and, in rare and severe cases, ureteral stenosis and occlusion. Dysuria is the most frequent symptom in bladder endometriosis (up to 70% of patients), particularly when the detrusor is involved, especially with plaques involving the trigone and dome [8, 13]. The severity of dysuria correlates with the size of the lesions [13]. Hematuria, and less commonly cyclical menouria (hematuria during menstruation), is seen in 20–35% of patients because bladder endometriosis rarely infiltrates and ulcerates the mucosa [8]. The ureter and ureteral orifice are rarely involved in BE; therefore, hydronephrosis is uncommon with isolated bladder endometriosis [12].

5.2.3 Physical Examination and Operative Findings

Bimanual examination is critical and reliable for the diagnosis of BE. A physical exam may identify a focal thickening or a palpable nodule at the vesicovaginal septum region, which may be painful in some patients [14]. Endoscopic visualization with biopsy may confirm the diagnosis. However, the mucosa is only infrequently involved, its typical bluish appearance may not be seen on cystoscopy. Often the endoscopic visualization shows an "extrinsically" appearing mass lesion projecting endoluminally without overlying mucosal abnormalities. With laparoscopic evaluation, the lesions can be identified as endometriosis plaques, commonly causing tethering and fibrosis between the bladder and the anterior uterus. The anterior cul-de-sac may be obliterated with severe disease. Superficial bladder endometriosis can cause punctate powder burn lesions, which have a lesser degree of surrounding fibrosis.

To achieve symptom resolution and improve fertility, the treatment for BE can be expectant, medical, or surgical. When medical treatment is not effective, surgery is usually considered. Surgical planning depends on the depth of the lesions, where partial cystectomy is the most commonly performed procedure for bladder endometriosis.

5.2.4 Imaging of Bladder Endometriosis

The accurate and comprehensive diagnosis of bladder endometriosis and of all the coexisting lesions is essential for management decisions. Therefore, imaging plays an important role in pretreatment diagnosis, disease mapping, and surgical planning. Imaging plays an important role even in patients who may be asymptomatic or present with only nonspecific symptoms.

5.2.4.1 Ultrasonography (US)

Ultrasound is usually the first-line imaging modality for imaging the female pelvis. Due to its widespread availability, low cost, lack of ionizing radiation, and capability for real-time assessment, US remains the first-line imaging modality of choice for the evaluation of any patient presenting with urinary symptoms. Transabdominal ultrasonography, transvaginal ultrasonography, and transrectal ultrasonography have been described for the evaluation of bladder endometriosis, and transvaginal ultrasonography (TVUS) is the most used technique in gynecological practice. TVUS can accurately assess the lesion size as well as detrusor infiltration and its relationship with extravesical lesions. Owing to its higher resolution and increased proximity to sites of interest, TVUS can be very valuable in assessing the depth of detrusor involvement. Compared with TVUS, transrectal ultrasonography does not improve diagnostic accuracy in the evaluation of bladder endometriosis [15]. A recent meta-analysis revealed an overall pooled sensitivity of 72% and a specificity of 99% for the TVUS detection of bladder endometriosis and revealed a sensitivity of 68% and a specificity of 100% for the MRI detection of the same [16], suggesting that both TVUS and MRI performed well on the diagnosis of bladder endometriosis with moderate sensitivity and high specificity. In addition to good diagnostic accuracy, TVUS performed by experienced sonographers is also highly reproducible for bladder endometriosis detection [17]. Three-dimensional TVUS, with its multiplanar acquisition of the sagittal, transversal, and coronal planes, might improve the sensitivity of bladder endometriosis detection compared to conventional two-dimensional TVUS, and it can allow a more detailed investigation of endometriotic nodules as well as a virtual cystoscopy [18]. TVUS can perform a dynamic real-time evaluation, which can help in detecting adhesions between the bladder and the uterus, providing additional input for presurgical planning.

Ultrasound Technique

The evaluation of the urinary bladder is recommended by the Society of Radiologists in Ultrasound (SRU) consensus panel as a part of screening for endometriosis on routine pelvic ultrasound [19]. In the standardized TVUS protocol developed by the International Deep Endometriosis Analysis (IDEA) Consensus Group, performed for the global evaluation and mapping of endometriosis, the evaluation of the bladder is included in the two to four steps, which include a search for bladder lesions and include mobility and tenderness-directed evaluation for endometriosis lesions [20].

Bladder filling and bladder distention are important considerations for a technically adequate evaluation, and a mildly-to-moderately distended bladder is essential for the optimal visualization of the bladder wall musculature and distal ureters. The overdistention of the bladder should be avoided because it may decrease the visibility of the bladder dome and stretch out the endometriosis lesions, limiting their detection. Adequate bladder distention can be achieved via two commonly utilized approaches: Patients can be directed to either empty their bladder and have their bladder examined at the end of the procedure or drink two glasses of water (approximately 300 mL) immediately before the procedure and have their bladder examined first [21, 22]. Imaging with a decompressed bladder is necessary for an adequate assessment of the middle and posterior compartments, and hence, the entire protocol includes imaging with both a distended bladder and a decompressed bladder.

The TVUS probe is placed in the anterior vaginal fornix and tilted anteriorly and superiorly. Sagittal and axial views are obtained through the bladder wall and vesicouterine peritoneum. With a dedicated protocol, evaluating the mobility between the posterior bladder dome and the anterior uterine serosa by applying the sliding sign maneuvers is also important, and this evaluation combines a gentle push of the probe onto the cervix and applying abdominal pressure with a free hand. With a normal sliding sign, free movement is observed between the bladder and uterus. Losing this free movement between the bladder and the uterus constitutes an abnormal sliding sign. The abdominal US assessment of both kidneys to exclude hydronephrosis is also required when bladder endometriosis is noted. The operator also needs to determine whether the patient experiences site-specific pain by applying gentle pressure on the probe.

US Observations of Bladder Endometriosis

On routine pelvic ultrasound, bladder endometriosis nodules can be identified as spiculated hypoechoic nodules, most commonly involving the posterior bladder wall and dome area. Sometimes, internal hyperechoic foci can be seen, which represent the endometrial glands.

The IDEA consensus protocol TVUS evaluation recommends a detailed assessment, which is described in Table 5.1.

Location

According to the IDEA consensus group [20], the urinary bladder is divided into four zones: the trigonal zone, the base, the dome, and the extra-abdominal bladder (Table 5.1). The bladder dome is the most common location for bladder endometriosis.

Table 5.1 Definition of bladder zones based on International Deep Endometriosis Analysis (IDEA) consensus group and frequency of endometriosis involvement

Zone of the bladder	Definition	Frequency of involvement
Trigonal zone	A smooth triangular zone that lies within 3 cm of the urethral opening between the two ureteral orifices and the internal urethral orifice	Rare
Bladder base	Area facing backward and downward adjacent to both the upper vagina and the supravaginal cervix	Common
Bladder dome	The superior and continuous portion of the bladder base, which is intra-abdominal and close to the vesicouterine pouch	Most common
Extra-abdominal bladder	Anterior portion, which is extra-abdominal	Very rare

Size and Morphology

The diameter of endometriotic nodules varies from 1 to 4 cm, which tends to be smaller than that measured at subsequent histological examinations. The detection of bladder endometriosis is strongly related to the lesion size, and smaller lesions may be missed at TVUS. Bladder endometriosis can present as a focal thickening of the bladder wall with irregular, spiculated borders or as a single comma-shaped or spherical nodule [23]. The endometriotic nodule or mass may also be irregular and inseparable from serosal endometriosis in the vesicouterine space and anterior myometrium if present. A large lesion may even extend further out toward the parametrium.

Depth of Infiltration

Bladder endometriosis lesions grow transmurally, invading the bladder wall from the outside serosa and extending into the detrusor muscle. The muscular layer may be partially or completely invaded, and mucosal involvement is rare. Large endometriotic nodules may protrude into the bladder lumen to varying degrees, displaying a "bubble-like," "polyp-like," or "grape-shaped" appearance or presenting as a solid mass that mimics bladder tumors [24–26].

Echogenicity

Endometriotic nodules are usually hypoechoic. Small anechoic cystic areas or hyperechoic foci within the nodule may be seen. A bright hyperechogenic rim is present in half of patients, probably due to the presence of adipose tissue and inflammation around the endometriotic implant [23].

Site-Specific Tenderness and Motility

Patients may experience pain upon the application of pressure with a probe. Due to adhesion, 80% of patients have the vesicouterine pouch obliterated without the sliding of the uterus along the urinary bladder [23]. The uterus may be located in fixed anteversion secondary to adhesions.

Blood Supply and Color Doppler

The color Doppler signal varies depending on the technique and scale settings and usually on the vascularular nature of the lesions. Power Doppler imaging usually reveals the presence of a few blood vessels within the lesion [23].

Distance to the Ureteral Orifice

The distance of the bladder endometriosis plaque from the ureteral orifices needs to be assessed. Although trigone involvement is less frequent, it is also the most serious and the most difficult to treat. Preventive cystoscopic catheterizations of the ureters may be advisable, especially when the distance between the lateral border of the lesion and the interureteric ridge is <2 cm [8]. When ureteral orifice involvement is present, ureteral resection and reimplantation (URR) may become necessary for the complete excision of the lesion. In 75% of cases, the distance between the lesion and the ureteral orifice is usually ≥1 cm [18].

Ureter Involvement and Hydroureteronephrosis

Ureteral involvement is seldom observed in bladder endometriosis [12]. Although BE itself rarely causes hydroureteronephrosis, instances of hydroureteronephrosis can be seen in patients when the ureter is externally compressed by endometriosis lesions from other sites [23, 27].

Malignant Transformation

Currently, there are a few case reports of malignant transformation in bladder endometriosis, and the age of the patients ranges from 35 to 62 [14]. More commonly, bladder endometriosis can mimic a malignancy, particularly when an irregular endometriotic nodule or mass extends through the bladder wall into the perivesical fat. Recognizing the demographics of the patient, typical imaging appearance, and an outside-in pattern of invasion can help suggest the correct diagnosis. Whereas bladder malignancy is more prevalent in postmenopausal women and originates from the urothelium or the mucosal surface of the bladder, bladder endometriosis is common in women of reproductive age and invades the bladder from the external serosa. Moreover, bladder endometriosis may adhere closely to the anterior uterus and may be associated with other pelvic foci of endometriosis, such as external adenomyosis (see Chap. 8).

Surgical Planning and Postoperative Changes

The most common aim of the surgical procedure for symptomatic relief is the complete excision of bladder endometriosis lesions. Incomplete resection is associated with a higher risk of relapse and the incomplete relief of symptoms [24]. Key points for preoperative planning include the precise location of the lesion, the size of the nodule, the depth of infiltration into the detrusor muscle, and the distance from the nodule to the ureteral orifices (Table 5.2).

Table 5.2 Reporting imaging features of bladder endometriosis relevant to surgical planning

Imaging features	Description
Size	Diameters in three orthogonal planes
Location	Dome, base, trigonal zone, extra-abdominal
Depth of infiltration	Partial or full thickness With or without mucosal involvement
Coexisting lesions	Adenomyosis Endometrioma, etc. Deep endometriomas alongside adenomyosis
Ureteral orifices/ureter involvement	Yes/no
Distance to ureteral orifices	Measured in centimeters
Hydroureter and/or hydroureteronephrosis	Yes/no

Postoperative Appearance

Postsurgical appearances for bladder endometriosis include fibrosis, adhesions, and residual lesions [28]. After laparoscopic partial cystectomy, surgical stitches and/or fibrosis of the bladder wall can present hyperechoic fibrotic thickening or irregularities, which are small hypo- or hyperechoic lines or interruptions or are invaginations of the bladder wall. The bladder may be asymmetrical with reduced volume depending on the extent of the resection. Specifically, in the postoperative evaluation, the residual bladder volume is important information to be provided and can be measured immediately at the beginning of TVUS [29]. Adhesions may cause anatomical distortion in the anterocentral compartment, septate and loculated fluid collections, peritoneal inclusion cysts, and a lack of mobility between the uterus and bladder (abnormal sliding sign) [28, 29].

5.2.4.2 Magnetic Resonance Imaging

MRI is a complementary imaging technique for the evaluation of bladder endometriosis after pelvic TVUS and can be considered as second-line imaging modality after transvaginal ultrasonography. Depending on availability and expertise, MRI can be used for diagnosis and presurgical planning for endometriosis. MRI offers notable advantages, including its multiplanar capabilities, excellent soft tissue contrast, lack of operator dependence, and large field view. It is particularly helpful in patients on whom TVUS cannot be performed, such as patients who are not sexually active or experience severe pain during TVUS. MRI has been shown to have good sensitivity (64–68%) and high specificity (98–100%) for the detection of bladder endometriosis [3, 16, 30]. Like TVUS, MRI can evaluate not only the intraluminal lesions but also the invasion of the detrusor muscle and extravesical pelvic involvement. MRI is also recommended as an additional examination in complex cases or prior to surgery, especially when the result of TVUS is equivocal [31].

MRI Magnet Specifications

Both 1.5 T and 3.0 T magnets can be used for the evaluation of endometriosis. A magnet of 3.0 T may improve the signal-to-noise ratio, where T2 sequences result in the acquisition of high-spatial resolution images for the evaluation of the deep endometriosis implants and adhesions. Non-fat-suppressed T2-weighted (T2W) sequences have a higher signal-to-noise ratio, which ensures a better visualization of bladder and bowel surface and uterosacral ligaments. T1 fat-saturation sequences are helpful in identifying intrinsically hyperintense signals in blood products within endometriosis plaques and endometriomas [32]. Pelvic phased-array coils are recommended at both 1.5 T and 3.0 T [31].

Bladder Distension

Similar to ultrasound, adequate bladder filling allows a better visualization of the lesions at the bladder wall, improves the delineation of the vesicouterine pouch by pushing the anteverted uterus backward, and displaces the bowel superiorly, thereby reducing motion artifacts [31]. In the 2016 European Society of Urogenital Radiology (ESUR) guidelines and in the 2020 consensus statement of the Society of Abdominal Radiology on the MRI evaluation of endometriosis, a moderately full bladder is recommended for deep endometriosis evaluation, which can be achieved by asking patients not to empty their bladder for 1 h prior to the examination [31, 33]. A higher bladder distention may ensure a more consistent measurement of the distance from the bladder endometriosis lesions to the ureteral orifices. This is particularly pertinent because the bladder is fully filled during surgical procedures [34]. However, overdistention may limit the detection of the lesions, and hence, a moderately filled bladder is considered a good compromise. Excessive bladder distension can also cause detrusor contractions, resulting in artifacts and the misdiagnosis of small lesions [31].

Protocol

The MRI protocol for evaluating pelvic endometriosis includes a T2W sequence without fat suppression, which should be performed in at least two orthogonal planes, particularly the axial and sagittal planes [31, 33]. A large field-of-view axial or coronal T2W sequence of the upper abdomen can be performed to evaluate the kidneys. T1-weighted (T1W) imaging can be helpful in identifying hemorrhagic bladder endometriosis lesions and should be performed with fat suppression [33]. Although diagnostic accuracy for bladder endometriosis is not increased by using postcontrast T1W imaging [35], it does play a role in the differentiation of endometriosis from neoplasm or infection in case of doubt. Similarly, diffusion-weighted imaging (DWI) helps in the evaluation of malignancy. Susceptibility-weighted imaging (SWI) is sensitive to blood products of all phases of hemorrhage, which may help some authors locate foci that cannot be detected by fat-suppressed T1W imaging [36].

MRI Observations of Bladder Endometriosis

MRI can depict the urinary bladder wall and its relation to perivesical fat and adjacent pelvic structures. On T2W images, the urinary bladder wall is depicted as uniformly low signal intensity due to the detrusor muscle. On T1W images, it appears as intermediate signal intensity. On dynamic T1W contrast-enhanced images, the mucosa exhibits early enhancement, followed by the later enhancement of the detrusor. The urinary bladder wall displays homogeneous enhancement on the delayed postgadolinium images.

Location

More than half of the lesions are at the median of the bladder wall. When the posterior third of the dome is involved, 80% of the cases would extend deep into the bladder base [34].

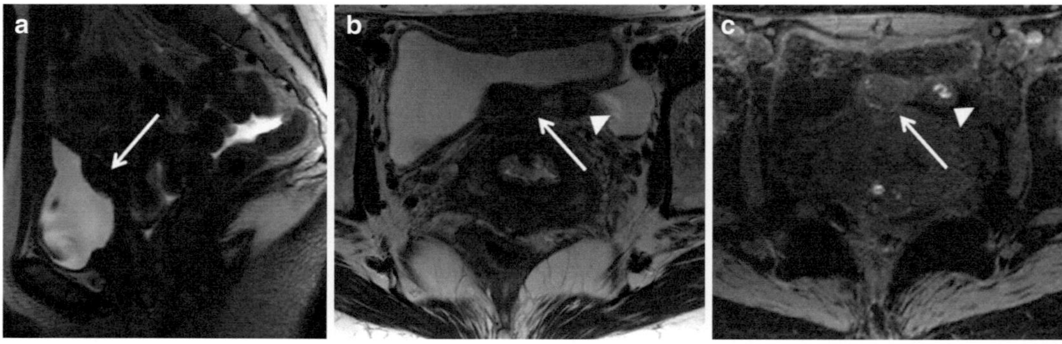

Fig. 5.1 Bladder endometriosis on MRI: 40-year-old patient with prior history of cesarean section delivery presented with cyclical abdominal pain and dysuria, which worsened during menstruation. Sagittal T2W (**a**), axial (**b**) T2W, and axial fat-suppressed T1W (**c**) images show two nodules in the vesicouterine space (arrow and arrow head) with a low signal intensity on T2W, intermediate signal intensity on T1W, and intrinsically hyperintense foci on T1W images. The bigger nodule is located at the median of the bladder wall, involving the posterior third of the dome (arrow)

Size and Morphology

The average size of bladder endometriosis is 3 cm (1 - 4 cm) at MRI. It may manifest as localized or diffuse wall thickening or as a single nodule or mass extending through the bladder wall with the obliteration of the normal muscular layer (Figs. 5.1, 5.2, 5.3, and 5.4). The borders can be regular or irregular. In the majority of cases, a bladder endometriosis lesion is inseparable from the anterior uterine wall, presenting with either a "continuous" pattern or an "hourglass" pattern [10]. Sometimes, the external infiltration of the endometriosis of the anterior uterine wall might extend as deeply as the junctional zone [34].

Depth of Infiltration

MRI without enhancement may be suboptimal in differentiating layers of the bladder wall and in determining the exact infiltration depth, which can be achieved by using intravenous gadolinium-based contrast agent for some authors, which remains an option in certain patients [27, 37]. When the full-thickness infiltration of the detrusor muscle is present, the lesion may project into the bladder lumen and may even resemble bladder cancer [1].

MR Signal Characteristics

Bladder endometriosis nodules frequently exhibit low signal intensity on T2W images and intermediate signal intensity on T1W images. Like deep endometriosis plaques at other sites, they may have internal T1W and T2W hyperintense foci within these nodules due to the presence of cystic and hemorrhagic ectopic endometrial glands (Fig. 5.2). About 70% of patients may have T1W hyperintense foci on fat-suppressed T1W images, indicating an acute or subacute hemorrhage [11, 27]. Stromal decidualization may be induced in bladder endometriosis during pregnancy or under hormonal treatment, which might alter the typical signal characteristics, with implants appearing as relatively more T2W hyperintense [38].

Enhancement

As with endometriosis elsewhere, bladder endometriosis lesions demonstrate delayed enhancement on postcontrast images compared to a healthy bladder detrusor [1] (Figs. 5.2, 5.3 and 5.4).

Distance to the Ureteral Orifice

The distance of the bladder endometriosis lesions to the ureteral orifices should be measured when the bladder is maximally distended. With under-distention, proximity to the ureteral orifices may be overestimated [34].

Associated Lesions

Bladder endometriosis is rarely an isolated disease. Endometriosis of other sites is common, including the involvement of the uterus (external adenomyosis), uterosacral ligaments, ovaries,

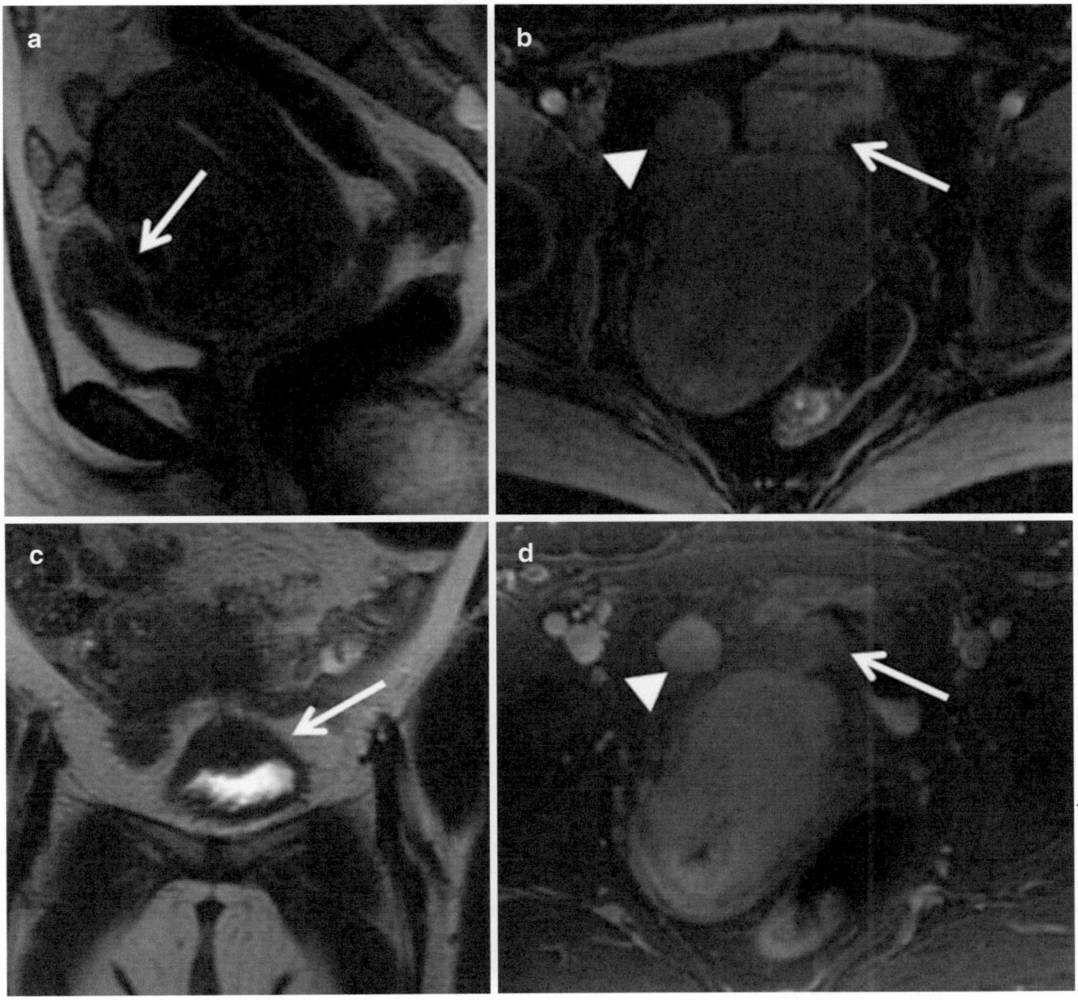

Fig. 5.2 Bladder endometriosis on MRI: 41-year-old patient with dysuria that worsens around the menstrual cycle. Sagittal T2W (**a**), axial fat-suppressed T1W (**b**), coronal T2W (**c**), and axial postcontrast fat-suppressed T1W (**d**) images demonstrate the thickening of the bladder dome wall (arrow), which appears hypointense on T2W images and isointense on T1W images with scattered internal T1 and T2 hyperintense foci, and it displays heterogeneous enhancement. Also, a right ovarian endometrioma appears (arrowhead). In a patient with endometriosis, such a bladder nodule is likely to represent bladder endometriosis with these characteristic imaging features. Urothelial malignancy is considered unlikely with this typical outside-in pattern of invasion

intestine, vagina, rectovaginal septum, round ligament, abdominal wall, etc. Due to the involvement of the anterior uterine wall and adhesions, the uterus is usually anteflexed.

Postoperative Appearance

On MRI, postoperative adhesions and fibrosis might be seen directly as hypointense linear bands on T2W images or indirectly as distortion or even the obliteration of the vesicouterine pouch [39]. The bladder wall may appear asymmetrical and irregular. Hypointense and thickened fibrotic bands may be found on T2W images. After partial cystectomy, the bladder volume might be reduced.

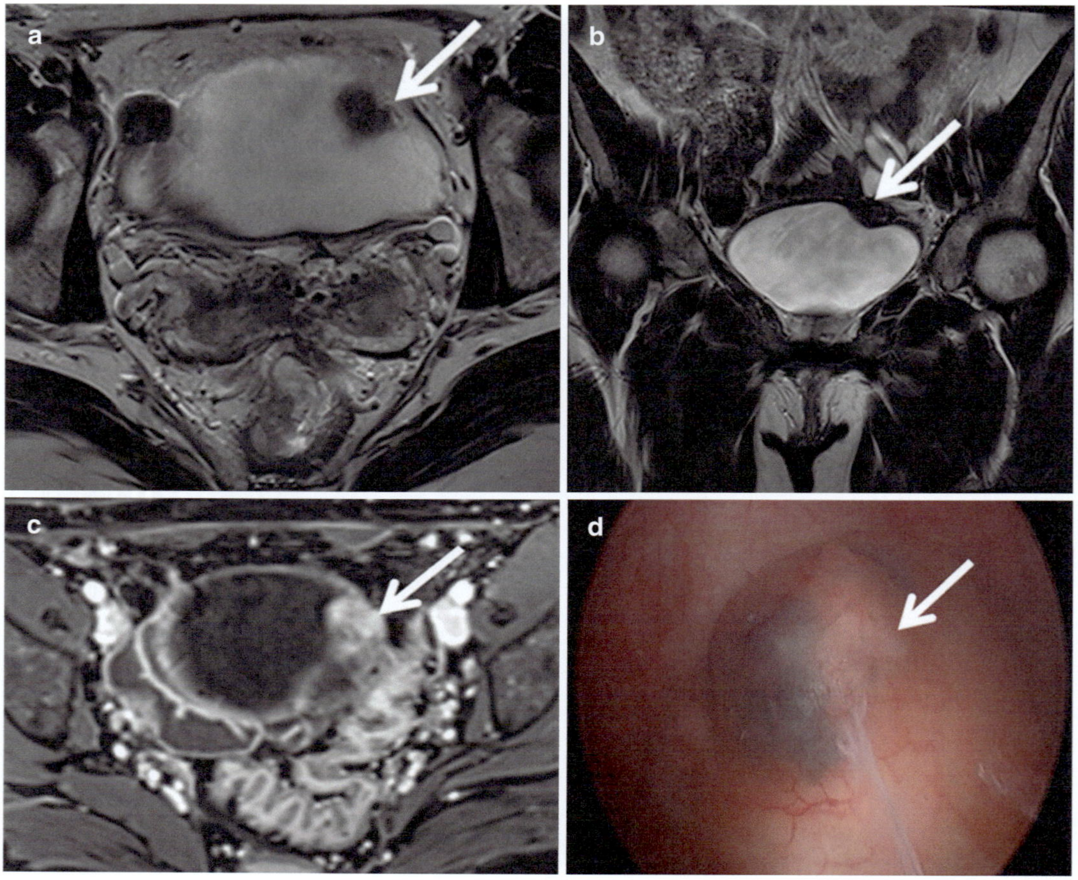

Fig. 5.3 Bladder endometriosis on MRI with operative correlation: 36-year-old patient with dysmenorrhea undergoing preoperative MRI for surgical planning. Axial T2W (**a**), coronal T2W (**b**), and axial postcontrast (**c**) images show a T2W hypointense nodule at the left anterolateral bladder wall (arrow), which enhanced upon contrast administration. In this patient with severe multicompartment endometriosis, this was considered to represent deep endometriosis of the bladder dome. Intraoperative cystoscopy (**d**) was performed for ureteral stent placement, which demonstrated the corresponding submucosal nodule with a purplish coloration, which is typically seen with endometriosis nodules. Notably, the mucosa is preserved over the deep endometriosis nodules, another feature that helps to distinguish it from urothelial malignancy

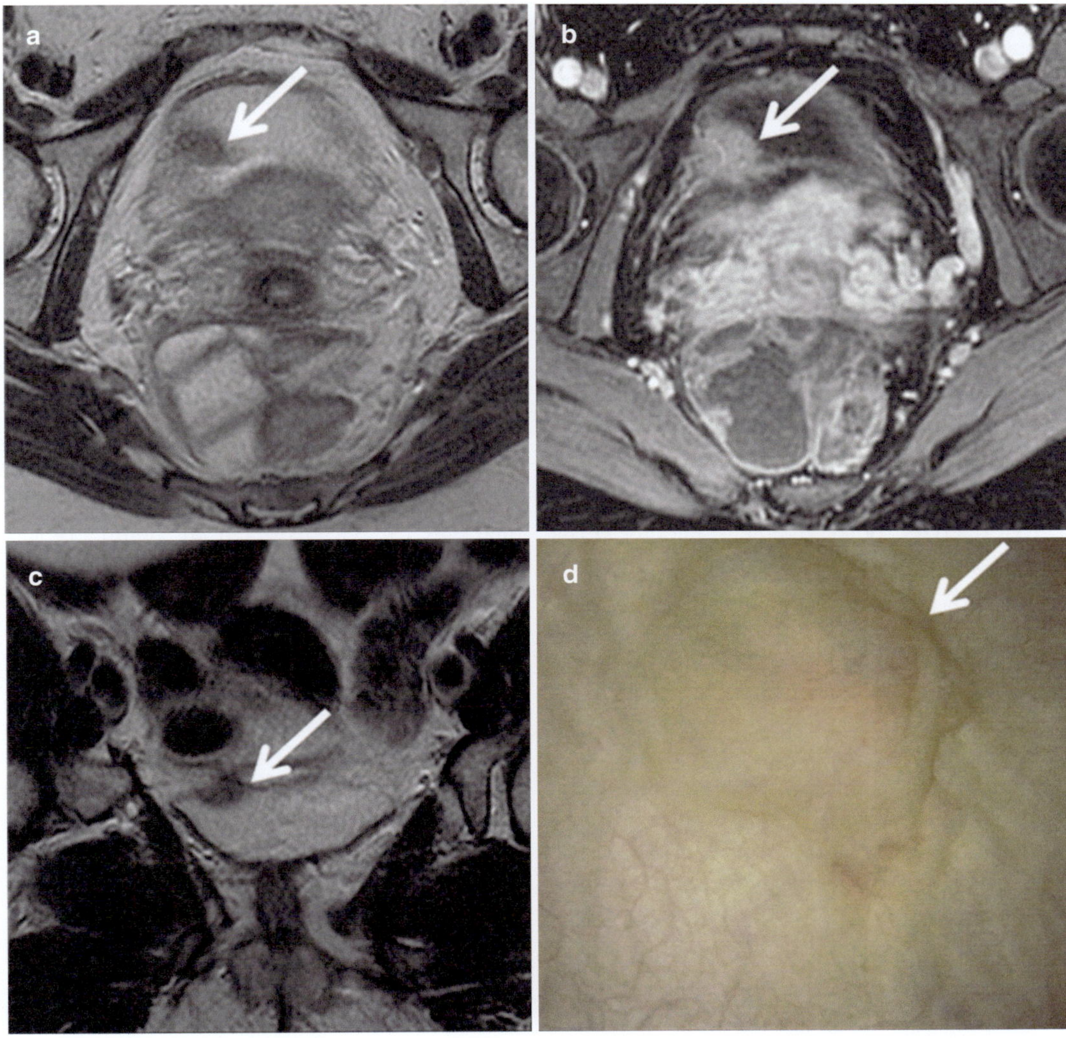

Fig. 5.4 Bladder endometriosis on MRI with operative correlation: 32-year-old patient with painful micturition and a history of endometriosis. Axial T2W (**a**), axial T1W postcontrast (**b**) and coronal T2W (**c**) images demonstrate a T2 hypointense bladder nodule, which enhances upon contrast administration. The focal, full-thickness bladder wall thickening suggests full-thickness muscle involvement. Cystoscopy (**d**) shows an extra-mucosal indentation on the bladder wall without any mucosal involvement. Lesion was surgically resected and pathology proven to represent the deep endometriosis of the bladder wall

5.3 Round Ligament Endometriosis

5.3.1 Anatomical and Clinical Considerations

The round ligament of the uterus originates from the gubernaculum. It is a band of fibromuscular tissue that originates from the uterine horns below the fallopian tubes, is covered proximally by the broad ligament, travels through the inguinal canal, and inserts into the labia majora. It is responsible for anchoring the uterus in an anteverted position in the pelvis. The round ligament has an intra-pelvic portion and an extra-pelvic portion. The extra-pelvic part of the round ligament is in the inguinal region, where it is accompanied by the continued outpouching of the peritoneum, called the canal of Nuck. The round ligament is an infrequent location for deep endometriosis. The prevalence, symptoms, and imaging presentations of and the treatment for the intra- and extra-pelvic portions are different.

For intra-pelvic round ligament endometriosis, the reported prevalence ranges from 4% in patients with endometriosis to 11–14% in patients who have surgical indications for deep endometriosis, with a greater prevalence on the left side [4, 40, 41]. The symptoms are usually nonspecific, and the preoperative diagnosis is based mainly on imaging examinations. A complete and extensive resection of all the visible lesions is usually required to alleviate symptoms and to prevent recurrence.

Extra-pelvic round ligament endometriosis accounts for 0.3–0.6% of patients with endometriosis [42]. Many think that it originates from retrograde menstruation through Nuck's canal or Müllerian remnants tissue [43]. Extra-pelvic round ligament endometriosis is in the inguinal region and altogether constitutes inguinal endometriosis. On the basis of the intraoperative observations of lesion sites, Niitsu et al. categorized inguinal endometriosis into three groups: endometriosis at a hernia sac or hydrocele of Nuck's canal (54%), on the round ligament (36%), and under the skin (10%) [44]. However, given the close relationship between the round ligament and Nuck's canal and given the infiltrative nature of endometriosis, these location differences cannot be diagnosed preoperatively, either via physical palpation or via imaging examination. Therefore, extra-pelvic round ligament endometriosis is generally referred to as inguinal endometriosis or Nuck's canal endometriosis [42, 45–48]. Extra-pelvic round ligament endometriosis is usually seen in women of reproductive age, with an average age of 36 years [46]. The majority of patients present with a unilateral inguinal mass, and half of them report inguinal pain. These symptoms are mostly catamenial, such as an increase in the size and tenderness of the mass during the menstrual period. Other symptoms include dysmenorrhea, lower abdominal pain, and hip pain. Some extra-pelvic round ligament endometriosis lesions are incidental findings during hernia repair [47]. The obliteration of Nuck's canal by endometriosis sometimes occurs, causing the formation of a hydrocele or a hernia of Nuck's canal. Unlike intra-pelvic round ligament endometriosis, a right-side dominance (66%) has been observed for extra-pelvic round ligament endometriosis [45]. The theory of the clockwise intraperitoneal fluid circulation may explain this difference, wherein the endometrial seeding on the right side stays longer before the fluid ascends to the right peritoneal gutter, influenced primarily by gravity. Additionally, the asymmetrical lymphatic drainage in favor of the right inguinal and the protective influence of the sigmoid colon on the left side may further contribute to this [43, 46, 47]. Before treatment, the diagnosis of extra-pelvic round ligament endometriosis can be suspected by finding typical symptoms, via the palpation of a inguinal bulge, and by imaging the inguinal region. The differential diagnosis includes other diseases in the inguinal region, including hernias, lymphadenopathy, abscesses, hematomas, and tumors. Therefore, the diagnosis of extra-pelvic round ligament endometriosis can be confirmed only histologically via fine-needle aspiration or resection and on the basis of finding characteristic endometrial glands with stromal cells within the fibrous connective tissue of the round ligament. Stromal decidualization may occur in pregnancy or with hormonal treatment [47]. The first-line treatment of extra-pelvic round ligament endometriosis is a complete surgical excision, and about one-third of patients would undergo a second surgery [46]. This is why a recent development in radiological interventional procedures (see Chap. 13) has had a high rate of success in this setting. The malignant transformation of extra-pelvic round ligament endometriosis is rare, and the most commonly seen malignant tumors are endometrioid and clear-cell carcinomas [49, 50].

5.3.2 Ultrasonography

5.3.2.1 Intra-Pelvic Round Ligament Endometriosis

Like pelvic deep endometriosis at other sites, transvaginal ultrasound (TVUS) is the first-line imaging modality for the diagnosis of intra-pelvic

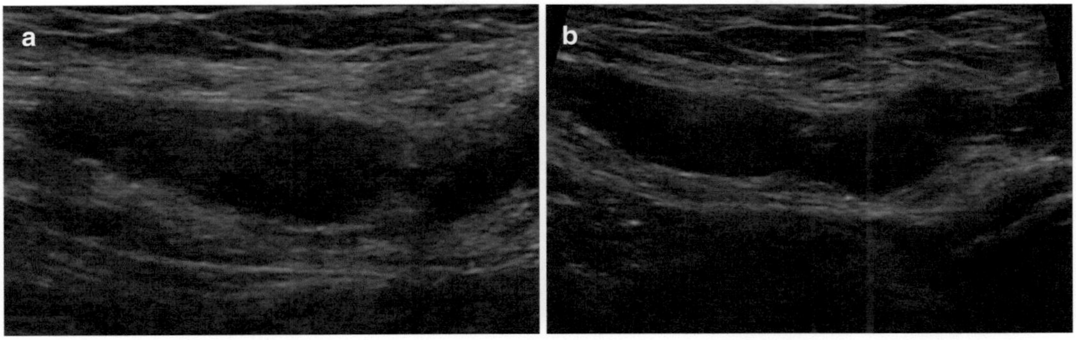

Fig. 5.5 Extra-pelvic round ligament endometriosis on ultrasound: 43-year-old patient presented with a bulge in her inguinal region. Longitudinal transabdominal ultrasound images (**a** and **b**) show two heterogeneous, hypoechoic masses along the course of the right inguinal/round ligament. The imaging features were nonspecific, and hence, a biopsy was performed, which demonstrated endometriosis

round ligament endometriosis. The endometriotic lesion is usually hypoechoic, and small hyperechoic foci or anechoic cysts may be present in larger lesions. The affected round ligament may be shortened, thickened, and/or deviated, which is highly predictive of round ligament endometriosis [40]. No cutoff values have been validated by any consensus with high reproducibility.

5.3.2.2 Extra-Pelvic Round Ligament Endometriosis

Transabdominal ultrasound is the primary method used for the detection and analysis of groin lesions, which can also be used to guide fine-needle aspiration. The sonographic features of extra-pelvic round ligament endometriosis are variable, which can be solid, hypoechoic nodules with internal small hyperechoic foci or anechoic cysts (Fig. 5.5). Sometimes the entire lesion may be cystic, appearing like an endometrioma or a combination of an endometrioma and a cyst [48]. Cyst formation may result from the obliteration of Nuck's canal and/or a hemorrhage, which can present as unilocular or multilocular lesions. The fluid inside the cyst is usually thick and has a ground-glass appearance [51]. On color Doppler sonography, a few foci of internal flow have been identified within the lesions [48]. Pelvic endometriosis is found in most patients with extra-pelvic round ligament endometriosis; however, in a majority of these cases, the intra-pelvic portion of the round ligament is usually uninvolved [52].

5.3.3 Magnetic Resonance Imaging

On MRI, the round ligament can be identified as a pair of thin and consistent structures where the intra-pelvic portion anteromedially courses to the external iliac vessels. A healthy round ligament shows a characteristic "Oreo-cookie" appearance on T2W images with a hyperintense center between two hypointense external lines (Fig. 5.6). It shows a hypointense fibrous signal on T1W images. The accurate description of the lesion location is critical for surgical planning. When performed by experts, MRI shows a sensitivity of 59%, a specificity of 98%, and an overall diagnostic accuracy of 96.2% for round ligament endometriosis [3]. The MRI examination of round ligament endometriosis is usually a part of the overall disease mapping for deep endometriosis, in which T2W imaging without fat suppression in at least two orthogonal planes and T1W imaging with fat suppression in the axial plane are required. T2W imaging with fat suppression, in either the axial or the coronal plane, is recommended to better identify a small amount of free fluid adjacent to the round ligament, which some

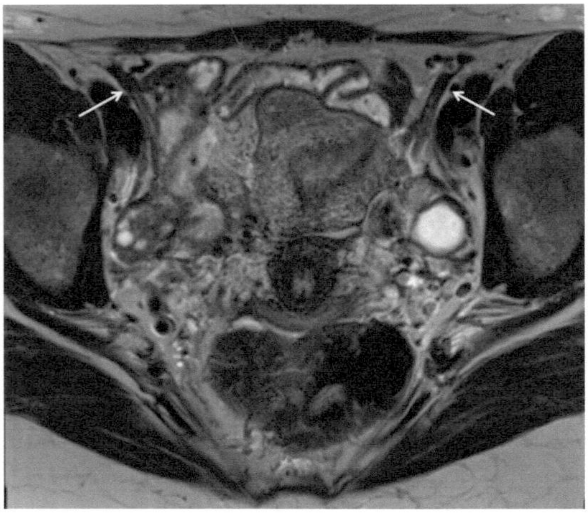

Fig. 5.6 Normal MRI appearance of intra-pelvic round ligament: Axial T2W image shows the normal appearance of the bilateral round ligament with a characteristic "Oreo-cookie" appearance (arrow). The normal round ligament on T2W images is hyperintense inside with hypointense layers outside. The disruption of this appearance is seen with endometriosis of the round ligament

authors think represents an indirect sign of round ligament endometriosis and should prompt evaluation for deep endometriosis plaques [43].

5.3.3.1 Intra-Pelvic Round Ligament Endometriosis

Intra-pelvic round ligament endometriosis exhibits a slight dominance of the left side, and the proximal third of the ligament is the most common location [1, 3, 4]. Affected ligaments may appear thickened, usually more than 1 cm, and can be shortened and irregular, with a nodular appearance [2–4, 40, 45, 53] (Figs. 5.7 and 5.8). No cutoff values have been validated by any consensus with high reproducibility. The asymmetry between the right round ligament and the left round ligament has more diagnostic value than isolated thickness consideration does. The involvement of the proximal ligament adjacent to the uterus may appear as larger lesions with an extension of adjacent deep myometrial

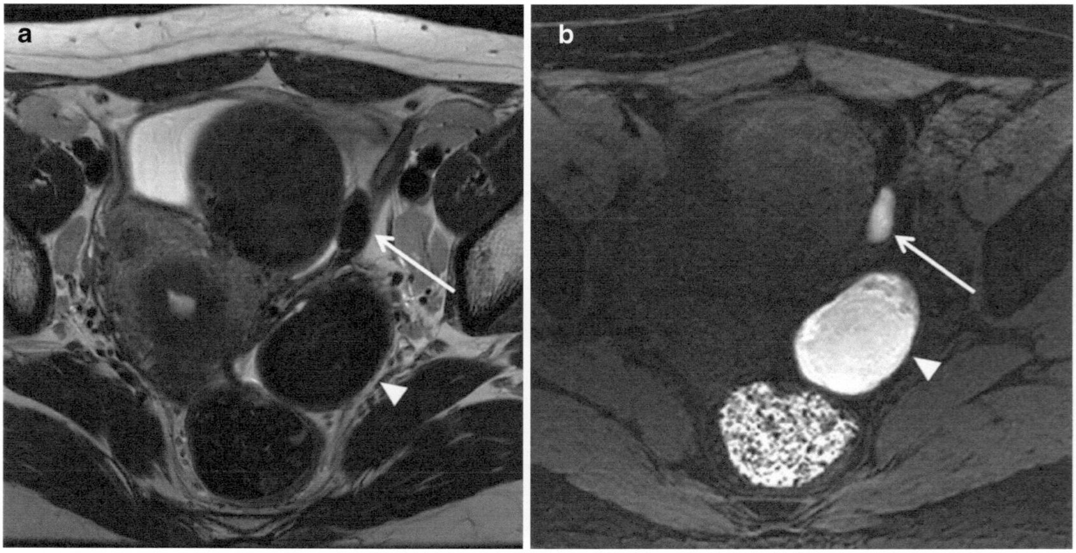

Fig. 5.7 Intra-pelvic round ligament endometriosis on MRI: 33-year-old patient with severe dysmenorrhea undergoing MRI prior to endometriosis surgery. Axial T2W (**a**) and fat-suppressed T1W (**b**) images show a nodular T2W hypointense and T1W hyperintense lesion consistent with deep endometriosis of the proximal third of the left intra-pelvic round ligament (arrow). Also, a left ovarian endometrioma demonstrates T2 shading with T1 hyperintensity and T2 hypointensity (arrowhead)

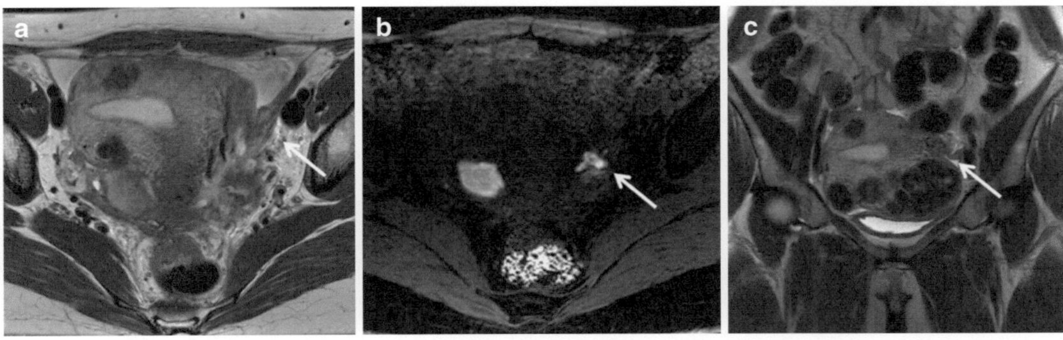

Fig. 5.8 Intra-pelvic round ligament endometriosis on MRI: 36-year-old patient with severe dyspareunia and cyclical abdominal pain undergoing MRI to follow up on findings of endometriosis seen on ultrasound. Axial T2W (**a**), fat-suppressed T1W (**b**), and coronal T2W images (**c**) show that the proximal third of the left round ligament is thickened and irregular (arrow), with a nodular appearance secondary to the extension of adjacent deep endometriosis at the posterior uterine surface. The patient also has multiple myomas and right ovarian endometrioma. Note that the expected healthy appearance of the round ligament is disrupted from deep endometriosis involvement

invasion (Fig. 5.8). Distal involvement at the deep orifice of the inguinal canal adjacent to the epigastric and external iliac vessels can increase surgical complexity [2].

Similar to deep endometriosis of other sites, the signal of round ligament endometriosis varies depending on the presence of stromal tissue, glandular elements, hemorrhage, and inflammatory reactions. Pure fibrous lesions are hypointense on T1W and T2W images; hemorrhagic foci are hyperintense on T1W and/or fat-suppressed T1W images [43]. The most frequent lesions are a mixture of fibrous tissue and multiple small hemorrhagic foci [43].

Extra-Pelvic Round Ligament Endometriosis

Extra-pelvic round ligament endometriosis is most common in the right groin, anterior to the femoral vessel and in continuity with the round ligament. Bilateral involvement is rare [46]. The average size of the lesions has been found to be 2.5 cm, which may extend longitudinally along the axis of the inguinal canal [42, 45]. The borders of these lesions are irregular or have spiculated edges. Extra-inguinal tissues like the abdominis rectus muscle can be involved [45]. This site can also predispose patients to neural endometriosis of the ilioinguinal nerves.

Two patterns of MRI features have been described in extra-pelvic round ligament endometriosis [45]. Most lesions show typical presentations of deep endometriosis, which is a solid nodule or mass with small, scattered cysts and T1W-hyperintense hemorrhagic foci (Fig. 5.9). The solid component is hypo- or iso-intense on T1W and T2W images, and the scattered cysts are usually hyperintense on both T1W and T2W images. The "shading sign" may be seen in these hemorrhagic cysts. The absence of the hemorrhagic foci might be caused by hormonal treatment or pregnancy [45]. The other pattern consists of clusters of hemorrhagic cysts, which are hyperintense on both T1W and T2W images. Enhancement may be homogeneous or heterogeneous depending on the size and components of the lesions. Gadolinium injection is useful in this indication mainly when doubt exists in the main differential diagnosis of desmoid tumors, which are typically enhanced very strongly. Moreover, in endometriotic nodules, the endometrial glands and hemorrhage liquid in the lesions may cause hyperintensity on diffusion-weighted images, which may play a role in the diagnosis of extra-pelvic round ligament endometriosis, especially when other MRI presentations are nonspecific [54]. A significant or increased size, broader invasion into adjacent tissues, and the presence of

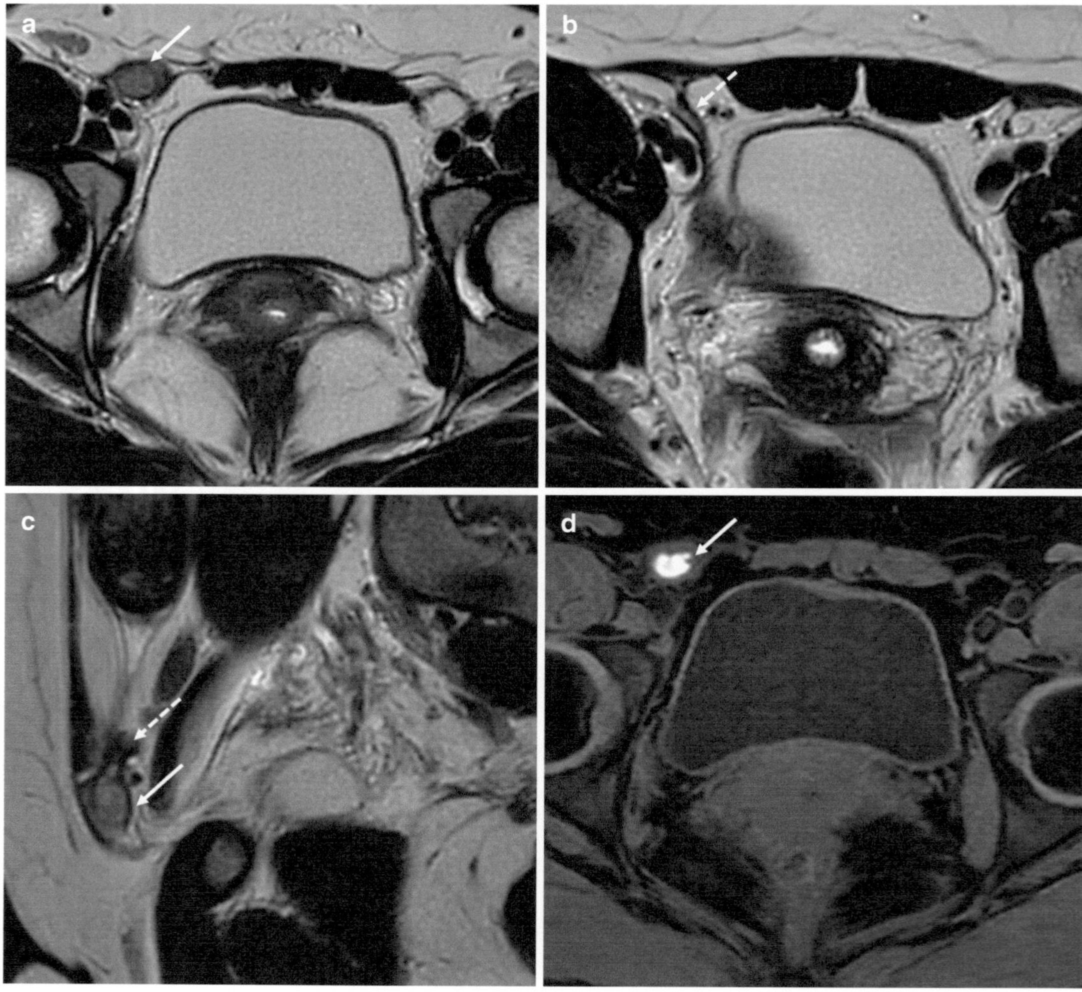

Fig. 5.9 Extra-pelvic round ligament endometriosis on MRI: 35-year-old patient with a right inguinal lump associated with cyclical and exercise-induced pain. Axial T2W (**a** and **b**), sagittal T2W (**c**) and axial fat-suppressed T1W (**d**) images show a solid and cystic nodule (arrows) at the right inguinal canal that is T2W hypointense and T1W hyperintense with hemorrhagic component, and located on the course of the round ligament (dotted arrows)

associated lymph node or distant metastasis may indicate malignant transformation or a differential diagnosis.

5.4 Conclusion

In conclusion, the anterocentral compartment is the least frequently involved compartment for endometriosis and includes the bladder and the proximal part of the round ligament. Although infrequent, the evaluation of this compartment is crucial because underdetection and the resultant incomplete resection of endometriosis may lead the patient to remain symptomatic despite undergoing invasive surgery. In addition, bladder endometriosis can cause urinary symptoms, and appropriate imaging assessment, including the relationship of bladder endometriosis to the ureteral orifices, is necessary for surgical planning.

The distal part of the round ligament that corresponds to the anterolateral compartment may also be cautiously looked at to ensure an adequate assessment of endometriosis in the anterior and anterolateral compartments.

References

1. Jha P, Sakala M, Chamie LP, Feldman M, Hindman N, Huang C, et al. Endometriosis MRI lexicon: consensus statement from the society of abdominal radiology endometriosis disease-focused panel. Abdom Radiol (NY). 2020;45(6):1552–68.
2. Rousset P, Florin M, Bharwani N, Touboul C, Monroc M, Golfier F, et al. Deep pelvic infiltrating endometriosis: MRI consensus lexicon and compartment-based approach from the ENDOVALIRM group. Diagn Interv Imaging. 2023;104(3):95–112.
3. Thomassin-Naggara I, Lamrabet S, Crestani A, Bekhouche A, Wahab CA, Kermarrec E, et al. Magnetic resonance imaging classification of deep pelvic endometriosis: description and impact on surgical management. Hum Reprod. 2020;35(7):1589–600.
4. Thomassin-Naggara I, Monroc M, Chauveau B, Fauconnier A, Verpillat P, Dabi Y, et al. Multicenter external validation of the deep pelvic endometriosis index magnetic resonance imaging score. JAMA Netw Open. 2023;6(5):e2311686.
5. Somigliana E, Vercellini P, Gattei U, Chopin N, Chiodo I, Chapron C. Bladder endometriosis: getting closer and closer to the unifying metastatic hypothesis. Fertil Steril. 2007;87:1287–90.
6. Gabriel B, Nassif J, Trompoukis P, Barata S, Wattiez A. Prevalence and management of urinary tract endometriosis: a clinical case series. Urology. 2011;78:1269–74.
7. Chapron C, Chopin N, Borghese B, Foulot H, Dousset B, Vacher-lavenu MC, et al. Deeply infiltrating endometriosis:pathogenetic implications of the anatomical distribution. Hum Reprod. 2006;21:1839–45.
8. Maccagnano C, Pellucchi F, Rocchini L, Ghezzi M, Scattoni V, Montorsi F, et al. Diagnosis and treatment of bladder endometriosis: state of the art. Urol Int. 2012;89(3):249–58.
9. Agely A, Bolan C, Metcalfe A, VanBuren W, Menias C. Genitourinary manifestations of endometriosis with emphasis on the urinary tract. Abdom Radiol (NY). 2020;45(6):1711–22.
10. Busard MP, Mijatovic V, Lüchinger AB, Bleeker MC, Pieters-van den Bos IC, Schats R, et al. MR imaging of bladder endometriosis and its relationship with the anterior uterine wall: experience in a referral centre. Eur J Radiol. 2012;81(9):2106–11.
11. Wong-You-Cheong JJ, Woodward PJ, Manning MA, Davis CJ. From the archives of the AFIP: inflammatory and nonneoplastic bladder masses: radiologic-pathologic correlation. Radiographics. 2006;26(6):1847–68.
12. Abrao MS, Dias JA Jr, Bellelis P, Podgaec S, Bautzer CR, Gromatsky C. Endometriosis of the ureter and bladder are not associated diseases. Fertil Steril. 2009;91(5):1662–7.
13. Villa G, Mabrouk M, Guerrini M, Mignemi G, Montanari G, Fabbri E, et al. Relationship between site and size of bladder endometriotic nodules and severity of dysuria. J Minim Invasive Gynecol. 2007;14(5):628–32.
14. Leone Roberti Maggiore U, Ferrero S, Candiani M, Somigliana E, Viganò P, Vercellini P. Bladder endometriosis: a systematic review of pathogenesis, diagnosis, treatment, impact on fertility, and risk of malignant transformation. Eur Urol. 2017;71(5):790–807.
15. Gauche Cazalis C, Koskas M, Martin B, Palazzo L, Madelenat P, Yazbeck C. Preoperative imaging of deeply infiltrating endometriosis in: transvaginal sonography, rectal endoscopic sonography and magnetic resonance imaging. Gynecol Obstet Fertil. 2012;40(11):634–41.
16. Tian Z, Zhang YC, Sun XH, Wang Y, Zhao Y, Chang XH, et al. Accuracy of transvaginal ultrasound and magnetic resonance imaging for diagnosis of deep endometriosis in bladder and ureter: a meta-analysis. J Obstet Gynaecol. 2022;42(6):2272–81.
17. Tammaa A, Fritzer N, Lozano P, Krell A, Salzer H, Salama M, et al. Interobserver agreement and accuracy of non-invasive diagnosis of endometriosis by transvaginal sonography. Ultrasound Obstet Gynecol. 2015;46(6):737–40.
18. Thonnon C, Philip CA, Fassi-Fehri H, Bisch C, Coulon A, de Saint-Hilaire P, et al. Three-dimensional ultrasound in the management of bladder endometriosis. J Minim Invasive Gynecol. 2015;22(3):403–9.
19. Young SW, Jha P, Chamié L, et al. Society of radiologists in ultrasound consensus on routine pelvic US for endometriosis. Radiology. 2024;311(1):e232191.
20. Guerriero S, Condous G, van den Bosch T, Valentin L, Leone FP, Van Schoubroeck D, et al. Systematic approach to sonographic evaluation of the pelvis in women with suspected endometriosis, including terms, definitions and measurements: a consensus opinion from the International Deep Endometriosis Analysis (IDEA) group. Ultrasound Obstet Gynecol. 2016;48(3):318–32.
21. Chamié LP. Ultrasound evaluation of deeply infiltrative endometriosis: technique and interpretation. Abdom Radiol (NY). 2020;45(6):1648–58.
22. Collins BG, Ankola A, Gola S, McGillen KL. Transvaginal US of endometriosis: looking beyond the endometrioma with a dedicated protocol. Radiographics. 2019;39(5):1549–68.
23. Savelli L, Manuzzi L, Pollastri P, Mabrouk M, Seracchioli R, Venturoli S. Diagnostic accuracy and potential limitations of transvaginal sonography for bladder endometriosis. Ultrasound Obstet Gynecol. 2009;34(5):595–600.

24. Fedele L, Bianchi S, Zanconato G, Bergamini V, Berlanda N, Carmignani L. Long-term follow-up after conservative surgery for bladder endometriosis. Fertil Steril. 2005;83(6):1729–33.
25. Kinkel K, Frei KA, Balleyguier C, Chapron C. Diagnosis of endometriosis with imaging: a review. Eur Radiol. 2006;16(2):285–98.
26. Chen Y, Han L, Zheng A. An unusual imaging appearance of endometriosis of the bladder. Int J Gynaecol Obstet. 2022;157(1):204–5.
27. Krüger K, Gilly L, Niedobitek-Kreuter G, Mpinou L, Ebert AD. Bladder endometriosis: characterization by magnetic resonance imaging and the value of documenting ureteral involvement. Eur J Obstet Gynecol Reprod Biol. 2014;176:39–43.
28. Martire FG, Russo C, Selntigia A, Siciliano T, Lazzeri L, Piccione E, et al. Transvaginal ultrasound evaluation of the pelvis and symptoms after laparoscopic partial cystectomy for bladder endometriosis. J Turk Ger Gynecol Assoc. 2022;23(3):145–53.
29. Chamié LP, Ribeiro DMFR, Ribeiro GMPAR, Serafini PC. Postoperative imaging findings after laparoscopic surgery for deeply infiltrating endometriosis. Abdom Radiol (NY). 2020;45(6):1847–65.
30. Medeiros LR, Rosa MI, Silva BR, Reis ME, Simon CS, Dondossola ER, et al. Accuracy of magnetic resonance in deeply infiltrating endometriosis: a systematic review and meta-analysis. Arch Gynecol Obstet. 2015;291(3):611–21.
31. Bazot M, Bharwani N, Huchon C, Kinkel K, Cunha TM, Guerra A, et al. European society of urogenital radiology (ESUR) guidelines:MR imaging of pelvic endometriosis. Eur Radiol. 2017;27(7):2765–75.
32. Manganaro L, Fierro F, Tomei A, Irimia D, Lodise P, Sergi ME, et al. Feasibility of 3.0T pelvic MR imaging in the evaluation of endometriosis. Eur J Radiol. 2012;81(6):1381–7.
33. Tong A, VanBuren WM, Chamié L, Feldman M, Hindman N, Huang C, et al. Recommendations for MRI technique in the evaluation of pelvic endometriosis: consensus statement from the Society of Abdominal Radiology endometriosis disease-focused panel. Abdom Radiol (NY). 2020;45(6):1569–86.
34. Rousset P, Bischoff E, Charlot M, Grangeon F, Dubernard G, Paparel P, et al. Bladder endometriosis: preoperative MRI analysis with assessment of extension to ureteral orifices. Diagn Interv Imaging. 2021;102(4):255–63.
35. Bazot M, Gasner A, Lafont C, Ballester M, Daraï E. Deep pelvic endometriosis: limited additional diagnostic value of postcontrast in comparison with conventional MR images. Eur J Radiol. 2011;80(3):e331–9.
36. Takeuchi M, Matsuzaki K, Harada M. Susceptibility-weighted MRI of extra-ovarian endometriosis: preliminary results. Abdom Imaging. 2015;40(7):2512–6.
37. Shenoy-Bhangle AS, Pires-Franco IV, Ray LJ, Cao J, Kilcoyne A, Horvat N, et al. Imaging of urinary bladder and ureteral endometriosis with emphasis on diagnosis and technique. Acad Radiol. 2023;22:S1076-6332(23)00608-6.
38. Busard MP, Mijatovic V, van Kuijk C, Pieters-van den Bos IC, Hompes PG, van Waesberghe JH. Magnetic resonance imaging in the evaluation of (deep infiltrating) endometriosis: the value of diffusion-weighted imaging. J Magn Reson Imaging. 2010;32(4):1003–9.
39. Guerra A, Daraï E, Osório F, Setúbal A, Bendifallah S, Loureiro A, et al. Imaging of postoperative endometriosis. Diagn Interv Imaging. 2019;100(10):607–18.
40. Crispi CP, de Souza CA, Oliveira MA, Dibi RP, Cardeman L, Sato H, et al. Endometriosis of the round ligament of the uterus. J Minim Invasive Gynecol. 2012;19(1):46–51.
41. Redwine DB. Ovarian endometriosis: a marker for more extensive pelvic and intestinal disease. Fertil Steril. 1999;72(2):310–5.
42. Licheri S, Pisano G, Erdas E, Ledda S, Casu B, Cherchi MV, et al. Endometriosis of the round ligament: description of a clinical case and review of the literature. Hernia. 2005;9(3):294–7.
43. Gui B, Valentini AL, Ninivaggi V, Marino M, Iacobucci M, Bonomo L. Deep pelvic endometriosis: don't forget round ligaments. Review of anatomy, clinical characteristics, and MR imaging features. Abdom Imaging. 2014;39(3):622–32.
44. Niitsu H, Tsumura H, Kanehiro T, Yamaoka H, Taogoshi H, Murao N. Clinical characteristics and surgical treatment for inguinal endometriosis in young women of reproductive age. Dig Surg. 2019;36(2):166–72.
45. Gaeta M, Minutoli F, Mileto A, Racchiusa S, Donato R, Bottari A, et al. Nuck canal endometriosis: MR imaging findings and clinical features. Abdom Imaging. 2010;35(6):737–41.
46. Dalkalitsis A, Salta S, Tsakiridis I, Dagklis T, Kalogiannidis I, Mamopoulos A, et al. Inguinal endometriosis: a systematic review. Taiwan J Obstet Gynecol. 2022;61(1):24–33.
47. Mourra N, Cortez A, Bennis M, Guettier C, Zaatari G, Duvillard P, et al. The groin: an unusual location of endometriosis—a multi-institutional clinicopathological study. J Clin Pathol. 2015;68(7):579–81.
48. Yang DM, Kim HC, Ryu JK, Lim JW, Kim GY. Sonographic findings of inguinal endometriosis. J Ultrasound Med. 2010;29(1):105–10.
49. Motooka Y, Motohara T, Honda R, Tashiro H, Mikami Y, Katabuchi H. Radical resection of an endometrioid carcinoma arising from endometriosis in the round ligament within the right canal of Nuck: a case report and literature review. Gynecol Oncol Rep. 2018;24:61–4.
50. Bergamini A, Almirante G, Taccagni G, Mangili G, Viganò P, Candiani M. Endometriosis-associated tumor at the inguinal site: report of a case diagnosed during pregnancy and literature review. J Obstet Gynaecol Res. 2014;40(4):1132–6.

51. Chamié LP, Ribeiro DMFR, Tiferes DA, Macedo Neto AC, Serafini PC. Atypical sites of deeply infiltrative endometriosis: clinical characteristics and imaging findings. Radiographics. 2018;38(1):309–28.
52. Freed KS, Granke DS, Tyre LL, Williams VL, Omert LA. Endometriosis of the extraperitoneal portion of the round ligament: US and CT findings. J Clin Ultrasound. 1996;24(9):540–2.
53. Novellas S, Chassang M, Bouaziz J, Delotte J, Toullalan O, Chevallier EP. Anterior pelvic endometriosis: MRI features. Abdom Imaging. 2010;35(6):742–9.
54. Tokue H, Tsushima Y, Endo K. Magnetic resonance imaging findings of extrapelvic endometriosis of the round ligament. Jpn J Radiol. 2009;27(1):45–7.

Mediocentral Compartment: Torus Uterinum and Proximal Uterosacral Ligaments

6

Adalgisa Guerra, Catarina Janicas, Marta Manso, and Inês Fortuna

6.1 Introduction

As has long been recognized, the uterosacral ligaments (USLs) are crucial structures supporting the uterus and upper third of the vagina, playing a pivotal role in the pathophysiology and treatment of pelvic organ prolapse [1]. Furthermore, the USLs represent the most frequent location of deep pelvic endometriosis (DPE) [2–4], underscoring the importance of understanding their anatomy and recognizing signs of infiltration by DPE.

Numerous efforts have been undertaken to measure and delineate healthy USLs. However, this endeavor has been complicated by the intricate dissection of cadavers [5–7], the somewhat-arbitrary boundaries of resection [6], and the variable visibility of USLs on both transvaginal ultrasound (TVUS) and magnetic resonance imaging (MRI) [8]. The USLs originate from the posterior wall of the cervix and/or vaginal fornix, where they blend with the contralateral ligament and form the torus uterinum. Then, they extend backward around the rectum, forming the lateral borders of the Douglas pouch, and attach to the pelvic sidewall [5–8] (Fig. 6.1). A study conducted by Umek et al. [8], based on the assessment of 70 MRI studies, revealed a noteworthy variety in their origin: 63% of the USLs arose from a plane where both the cervix and the vagina were seen, whereas 33% and 4% arose exclusively from the cervix or the vagina, respectively (Fig. 6.1). Variation was also noted in their insertion: 82% of the USLs attached to the sacrospinous ligament and coccygeus muscle complex; 11% attached to the piriformis muscle, sciatic foramen, or ischial spine; and only 7% attached to the sacrum.

The evolving framework throughout its course adds further complexity to the study and understanding of the USLs [5, 7]. Consistent with this observation, pathologists have categorized the USLs into cervical, intermediate, and sacral segments, all approximately equal in length [5]. The cervical segment primarily comprises densely packed smooth muscle fibers, which maintain continuity with the muscular layer of the cervix, along with small and medium-size vessels. As the ligaments progress posterolaterally into their interme-

A. Guerra (✉)
Department of Radiology, Hospital da Luz Lisboa, Lisbon, Portugal

C. Janicas
Department of Radiology, Unidade Local de Saúde de Lisboa Ocidental, Lisbon, Portugal
e-mail: cjanicas@ulslo.min-saude.pt

M. Manso
Department of Radiology, Hospital Beatriz Ângelo, Loures, Portugal
e-mail: marta.catarino.manso@hbeatrizangelo.pt

I. Fortuna
Department of Gynaecology and Obstetrics, Hospital da Luz Lisboa, Lisbon, Portugal
e-mail: ines.fortuna@hospitaldaluz.pt

I. Thomassin-Naggara (ed.), *Imaging of Endometriosis: A Comparative Guide of US, MRI and Surgery*, https://doi.org/10.1007/978-3-031-82750-1_6

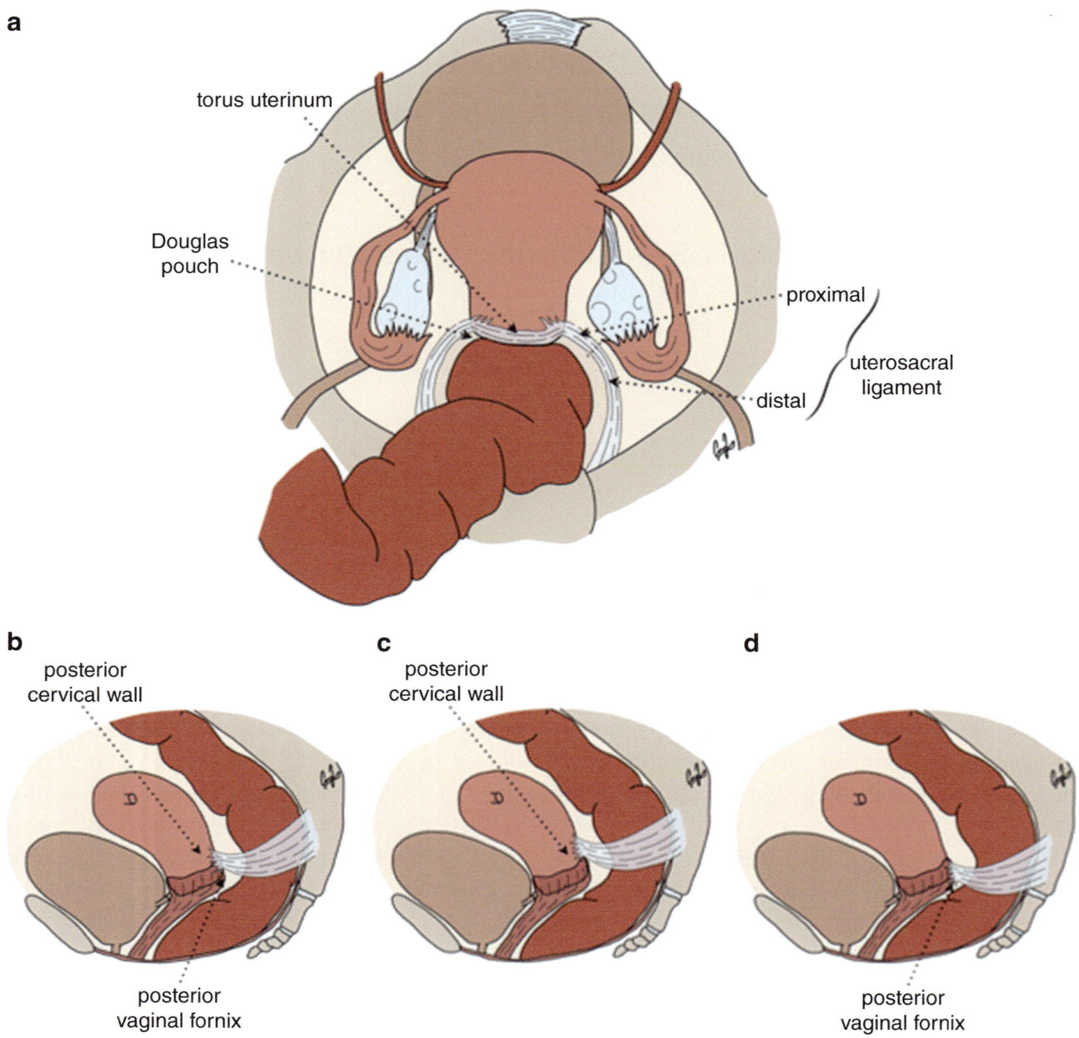

Fig. 6.1 Healthy anatomy of the torus uterinum and uterosacral ligaments (USLs). (**a**) This schematic illustration of the healthy female pelvis highlights the structures of the mediocentral compartment, namely the torus uterinum and USLs. These ligaments may be divided into proximal and distal portions, with the cutoff recently revised to a distance of 2 cm from the cervix. (**b–d**) Schematic profiles of the pelvis depict the different origins of the USLs, which most frequently arise from (**b**) both the posterior cervical wall and the posterior vaginal fornix, followed by exclusively (**c**) the posterior cervical wall and (**d**) the posterior vaginal fornix

diate segment, the smooth muscle becomes less abundant, the connective tissue become denser, and larger nerve bundles and parasympathetic ganglia begin to emerge. Finally, the sacral segment is characterized by loose connective tissue and surrounding fat, with fewer blood vessels and nerves. Lymphatics are present in both the cervical and intermediate segments, albeit to varying degrees [5]. Although surgeons also adopt the division of the USLs into these three segments, their concerns are distinct. Specifically, they note that the cervical segment exhibits the shortest distance to the pelvic ureter (0.7–1.0 cm) and that the sacral segment is closest to the sacral nerve roots, the latter raising the risk of iatrogenic injury during the manipulation of these segments [6].

Similarly, in line with the recent consensus reached by a focused panel of MRI experts specializing in DPE [9], radiologists classify the USLs as proximal or distal, with the cutoff recently revised to a distance of 2 cm from the cervix (previously 1 cm), corresponding approximately to their horizontal and transverse portion at vaginal level. This classification system relates to the risk of ureteral and nerve involvement, which appears to be minimal in the proximal segment when lesion are not to thick. Given the substantial morbidity associated with USL infiltration by DPE [2, 3, 10], as well as the risk of iatrogenic injury to the inferior hypogastric plexus during laparoscopy [6], which can impact both sexual activity and bladder and bowel function, radiologists must have a comprehensive understanding of the healthy imaging anatomy of the USLs and must accurately interpret the findings of DPE.

This chapter will cover the healthy anatomy of the USLs on both TVUS and MRI, followed by a review of the findings related to DPE and potential pitfalls. Whenever feasible, it will strive to correlate imaging findings with those observed during laparoscopy.

6.2 Imaging Anatomy

6.2.1 Transvaginal Ultrasound

Although numerous articles have meticulously delineated the criteria for identifying and reporting USL infiltration by DPE, very few have elucidated their healthy anatomy on TVUS [11–13]. Additionally, measurements pose challenges regarding reproducibility and validation because different working groups select varied landmarks and employ diverse techniques [11, 14, 15]. Nonetheless, agreement seems to have been reached that a healthy USL should slide freely over the vaginal wall when pressure is applied and also appear as a thin, regular, smooth, homogeneous, and hyperechoic strand, particularly in the presence of pelvic fluid [11–13, 16] (Fig. 6.2).

In addition to having prior knowledge of the course and characteristics of a healthy USL, developing a precise technique for accurately depicting and assessing this ligament is imperative. Although variations are noted in the literature and among different centers [14], we propose the following comprehensive method, considering both a longitudinal approach [17] and a transverse approach [18]:

1. Insert the probe in the posterior vaginal fornix.
2. Set the depth to ensure that the cervix represents two-thirds of the screen and the focus immediately behind the cervix.
3. Orientate the probe to the midsagittal plane and angulate it posteriorly toward the pouch of Douglas (point of reference for the following steps).
4. *Longitudinal approach*
   a. For the left USL, rotate the probe 45° counterclockwise as the USL progressively appears as a homogenous hyperechoic strand.
   b. The same maneuver is performed for the right USL.
4. *Transverse approach*
   a. Rotate the probe 90° counterclockwise to obtain a transverse section of the cervix.
   b. For the left USL, angulate the probe to the left until the uterine vessels are in view; the left USL will appear behind them. The probe can then be rotated by a few degrees to visualize the whole USL on a longitudinal plane, appearing as a hyperechoic stripe starting from the cervix and pointing laterally.
   c. The same maneuvers are performed for the right USL.
5. When evaluating each USL, apply gentle pressure with the probe to assess the sliding sign.

Given the torus uterinum's position in the retrocervical area between the USLs, it can be examined by using the same method. However, it is not distinctly defined by TVUS, due to the challenging assessment of the posterior uterine wall, especially when the uterus is retroverted or retroflexed [19].

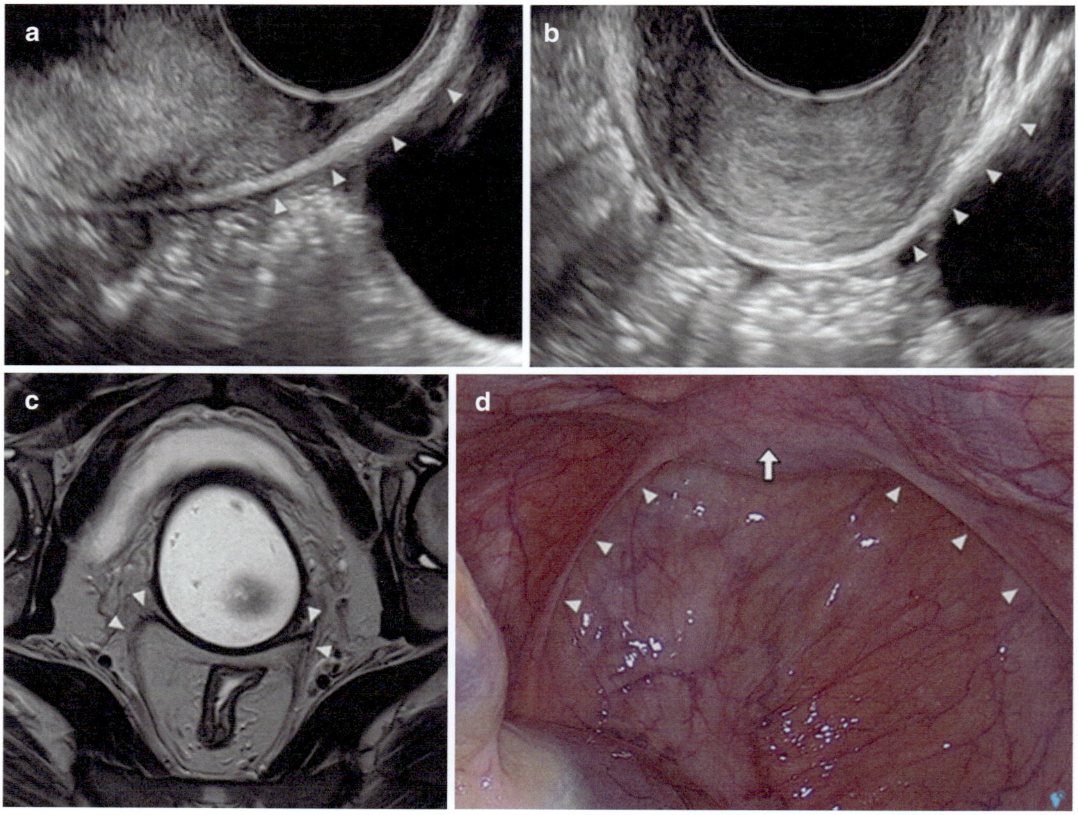

Fig. 6.2 Healthy uterosacral ligaments (USLs) on TVUS and MRI, with laparoscopic correlation. (**a**) Oblique sagittal (**b**) and oblique transverse TVUS images depict the healthy left USL as a hyperechoic homogeneous strand (arrowheads, **a**–**b**). (**c**) On an axial T2-weighted MR image, the USLs are seen as symmetrical, thin, low-signal-intensity lines (arrowheads, **c**) arising from the posterior wall of the cervix and extending backward around the rectum, here almost at the junction with the mesorectal fascia. (**d**) Laparoscopy, performed due to an unrelated condition, reveals symmetrical and fan-shaped USLs (arrowheads, **d**), which blend in the posterior cervical wall to form a smooth torus uterinum (arrow, **d**)

6.2.2 MRI

MRI allows a more straightforward and precise assessment of the USLs, especially their distal segment and the surrounding structures [8]. Although the literature has delinated criteria for USL infiltration by DPE, scant consensus has been reached on its healthy appearance and thickness. Therefore, rather than relying solely on measurements, greater emphasis should be placed on the regularity and symmetry of these ligaments for the time being [9]. With an adequate MRI acquisition protocol, the USLs are identifiable in 87% of studies, manifesting as symmetric, low-signal-intensity strands on T2-weighted (T2W) images [8] (Fig. 6.2). The current ESUR protocol guidelines [20] for the assessment of DPE include sagittal and axial TSE T2-weighted images, axial T1-weighted (T1W) images, and an additional thin-section (2.5–3 mm) oblique axial T2-weighted sequence for the evaluation of the USLs. The axial oblique plane is oriented along one USL or both USLs if visible on sagittal TSE T2-weighted MR images. When the USLs are not visible, the axial oblique plane is oriented perpendicularly to the cervix [21, 22], as illustrated in Fig. 6.3. A significant predominance of subperitoneal fat over connective tissue, a limited distance between the cervix and the sacrum, the enlargement of the uterus, the exces-

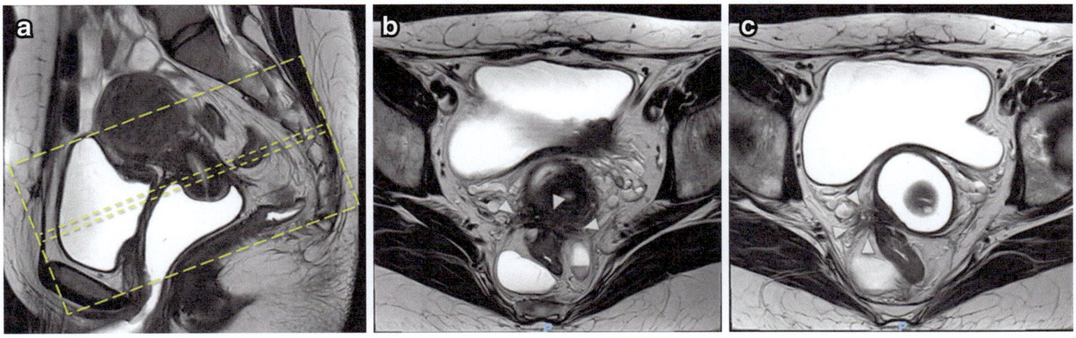

Fig. 6.3 Acquisition of thin-section oblique axial T2-weighted MR sequence to assess uterosacral ligament (USL) infiltration by DPE. (**a**) Sagittal T2-weighted MR image and (**b–c**) oblique axial T2-weighted MR images at the level of (**b**) cervix and (**c**) vaginal fornix. To depict the torus uterinum and USLs accurately, the thin-section oblique axial sequence must be oriented along one USL or both USLs, or it must be oriented perpendicular to the cervix (dashed box, **a**). In this patient, a spiculated nodule (arrowheads) is seen infiltrating the torus uterinum (**b**), right USL, and anterior rectal wall (**c**)

sive distension of the rectum, and the dilation of the uterine vessels might hamper obtaining an accurate visualization of the USLs [8].

The USLs should be visible from their origin to their insertion, although this may vary under the anatomical variations described by Umek et al. [8], as alluded to in the first section of this chapter. Conversely, both the torus uterinum and the retrocervical area, a virtual subperitoneal space located posteriorly to the cervix and in continuity with the rectovaginal septum, should remain imperceptible [23] because their visualization implies infiltration by DPE. Because the USLs and torus uterinum are overlaid by the peritoneum, forming the pouch of Douglas, the presence of ascites may aid in identifying adhesions [10, 23].

6.2.3 Laparoscopy

Laparoscopy allows the direct visualization of the pelvic mediocentral compartment structures. With the camera directed toward the posterior uterine wall, the torus uterinum can be examined in the midline, which is positioned behind the supravaginal cervix [24] and which displays a thin and smooth surface in the absence of disease (Fig. 6.2). For an optimized view, a uterine manipulator can be employed to bring the uterus to an anteverted position.

Laterally and immediately inferiorly to the torus uterinum, the healthy USLs appear as fan-shaped, symmetric, smooth, and regular structures, continuous with the cardinal ligaments and paracolpos. They are free from the adnexa and the rectal wall, defining the lateral boundaries of the pouch of Douglas, spanning along the entire lateral border of the sacral region. As previously mentioned, the USLs are in proximity to the ureters and the hypogastric nerves, which always remain lateral to them [25].

6.3 Imaging Features of Deep Pelvic Endometriosis with Laparoscopic Correlation

As noted earlier, the USLs and torus uterinum have been identified as the most common sites of DPE in the pelvis, with rates of up to 70% in some series [2–4]. Additionally, they are the only sites of involvement in up to 80% of patients [3], underscoring the importance of an accurate assessment via either TVUS or MRI.

6.3.1 Transvaginal Ultrasound

Although the overall accuracy of TVUS in diagnosing DPE is high, the accuracy in detecting lesions in the USLs is less certain. A meta-analysis on the detection of USL endometriosis using TVUS has shown an overall pooled sensitivity of 60% and a specificity of 95% [26]. A recent prospective study by Ros et al. [27] describes a sensitivity of 96.6% and 83.9% and a specificity of 82.1% and 89.4% for detecting the infiltration of the USLs and the torus uterinum, respectively.

Although no consensus has been reached on the threshold for USL thickening on TVUS, likely due to the high variability in measurement methods, the 2016 International Deep Endometriosis Analysis (IDEA) consensus recommends measuring at the USL origin in the transverse plane [28]. According to Chowdary et al., the diffuse thickening of the uterosacral ligaments (USLs) is defined as a measurement of over 3 mm [29], and Bazot et al. [11] identified the nodular thickening of the USLs with a mean thickness of 8.6 mm, ranging from 5 to 14 mm.

As stated by Maple et al. [14] in their systematic review, the following findings are considered indicative of torus uterinum and USL infiltration by DPE: hypoechoic linear thickening with regular margins and hypoechoic nodules with regular, irregular, or stellate margins (Figs. 6.4 and 6.5). These structures are usually fixed to the surrounding pelvic structures and will be tender when pressure is applied. El-Maadawy et al. [30] have also described two signs associated with bilateral USL infiltration, which they have desig-

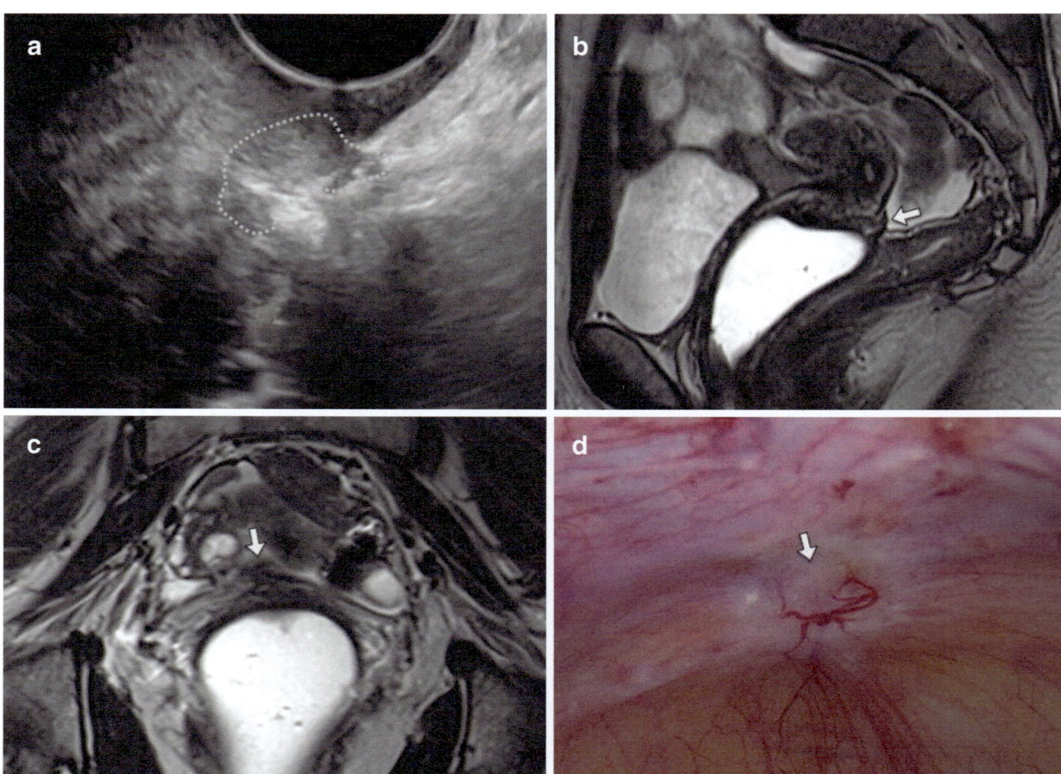

Fig. 6.4 Pelvic deep endometriosis with nodular thickening of the right uterosacral ligament (USL). (**a**) Oblique sagittal TVUS reveals an irregular heterogeneous nodule in the right proximal USL (dotted line). (**b**) In sagittal and (**c**) oblique coronal T2-weighted MR images, it corresponds to a hypointense nodule in the right proximal USL (white arrow, **b**–**c**). (**d**) Laparoscopy also clearly depicts this nodule in the right proximal USL (white arrow, **d**)

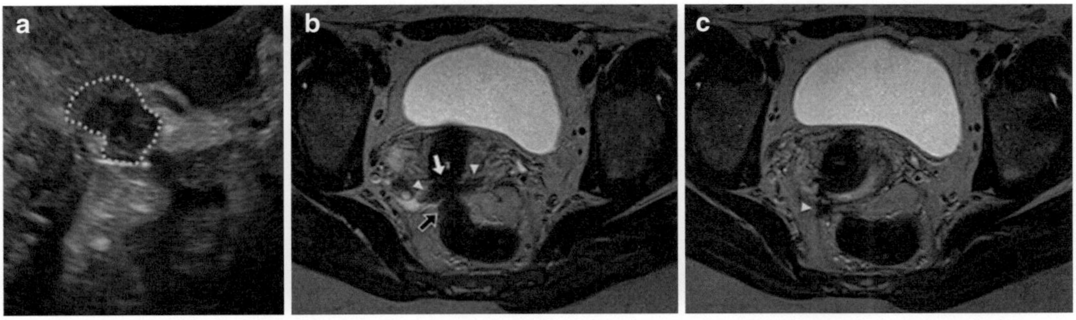

Fig. 6.5 Deep pelvic endometriosis with nodular thickening of the torus uterinum and uterosacral ligaments (USLs). (**a**) Oblique transverse TVUS image depicts a nodule with irregular margins in the right USL (dotted line). (**b–c**) Oblique axial T2-weighted MR images at the level of the torus uterinum and (**b**) posterior vaginal fornix (**c**) reveal a spiculated thickening of the torus uterinum (white arrow) and both proximal USLs (arrowheads), more prominent in the right USL (**c**), where the lesion takes a more nodular spiculated appearance. In addition, a focal contact with the anterior rectal wall (black arrow, **b**) is shown in continuity with the lesion in the torus uterinum

nated as the butterfly and tram-track configurations. The former is identified in the transverse plane and indicates the bilateral infiltration of the USLs and torus uterinum (Fig. 6.6). On the other hand, the tram-track configuration is perceived in the sagittal plane and corresponds to USL and rectal wall infiltration by parallel hypoechoic lesions, which are intervened by hyperechoic chronic inflammatory changes. Nevertheless, the reproducibility of these two signs has yet to be validated.

Multiple preoperative classification systems concerning DPE staging via TVUS have been described. We highlight the recently updated ENZIAN classification, which extends the previous ENZIAN score to incorporate all types of endometrioses, grading uterosacral lesions in the B compartment (mediolateral axis) according to lesion size (<1 cm, 1–3 cm, or >3 cm). Although the torus uterinum is not mentioned, the authors include the retrocervical area in the A compartment (craniocaudal axis), also grading it according to size [31, 32].

6.3.2 MRI

MRI's pooled sensitivity and specificity for torus uterinum and USL infiltration by DPE were determined as 86% and 84%, respectively, indicating higher accuracy than that of TVUS [20].

The diagnosis of DPE relies on identifying areas of fibrosis, which display a signal intensity similar to that of pelvic muscle on T1-weighted and T2-weighted images, occasionally displaying contrast enhancement. USL and torus uterinum lesions typically manifest as nodules of low signal intensity on T2-weighted images, exhibiting regular, irregular, indistinct, or stellate margins [23] (Figs. 6.4, 6.5 and 6.6) or sometimes only regular asymetric thickening (Fig. 6.7). In addition, hemorrhagic foci may be present, identified as hyperintense foci on T1-weighted or fat-suppressed T1-weighted images (Fig. 6.8) or small hyperintense cavities on T2-weighted images, bringing specific signs [2].

Until recently, consensus was lacking on the threshold for USL thickening on MRI. The ENDOVALIRM research group [9] and ESUR now considers definite infiltration if the USL is abnormal in two orthogonal planes, exhibiting a spiculated (with retraction) and/or nodular appearance, or exhibiting the presence of hemorrhagic foci regardless of the thickness. On the contrary, any asymmetry and/or linear smooth thickening, irregular margins, and/or a

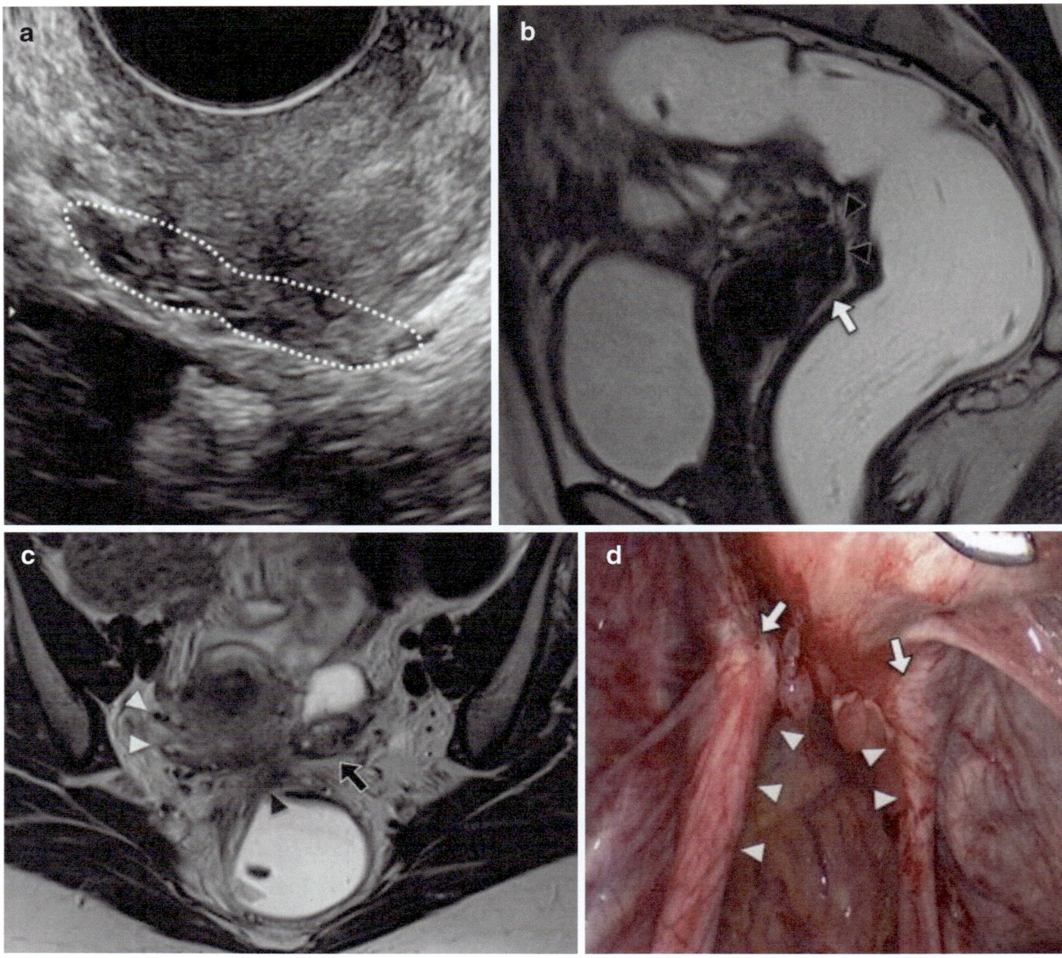

Fig. 6.6 Deep pelvic endometriosis of the torus uterinum and uterosacral ligaments (USLs), with infiltration of the rectovaginal septum. (**a**) Axial TVUS image, at the level of the retrocervical area and posterior vaginal fornix, shows a hypoechogenic spiculated nodule that infiltrates the torus uterinum and both proximal USLs (dotted line, **a**), assuming a butterfly-like configuration. (**b**) Sagittal and (**c**) oblique axial T2-weighted MR images confirm the presence of a hypointense spiculated nodule in the torus uterinum and proximal USLs. It invades the rectovaginal septum (white arrow, **b**), leading to the upward retraction of the posterior vaginal fornix; invades the right parametrium (white arrowheads, **c**); and fixates the left adnexa (black arrow, **c**). In addition, it infiltrates the mesorectal fat (black arrowheads, **b–c**), although with no signs of rectal infiltration. (**d**) Laparoscopy reveals a retractile, fibrotic, infiltrative nodule in the torus uterinum (white arrows, **d**) that distorts both proximal USLs (white arrowheads, **d**)

pseudonodular appearance (defined as present in only one plane) are considered equivocal and nonspecific. Therefore, irregular, pseudonodular, and/or fibrotic smooth thickening are considered as uncertain diagnoses and must be associated with other features for endometriosis to be considered as positive.

The infiltration of the torus uterinum is considered in cases where a mass or thickening is observed in the midportion of the posterior cervix (Fig. 6.5), following the same criteria used for the thickening of the USLs. In most cases of DPE, the proximal portion of the USLs and the torus uterinum are intertwined, such that when the

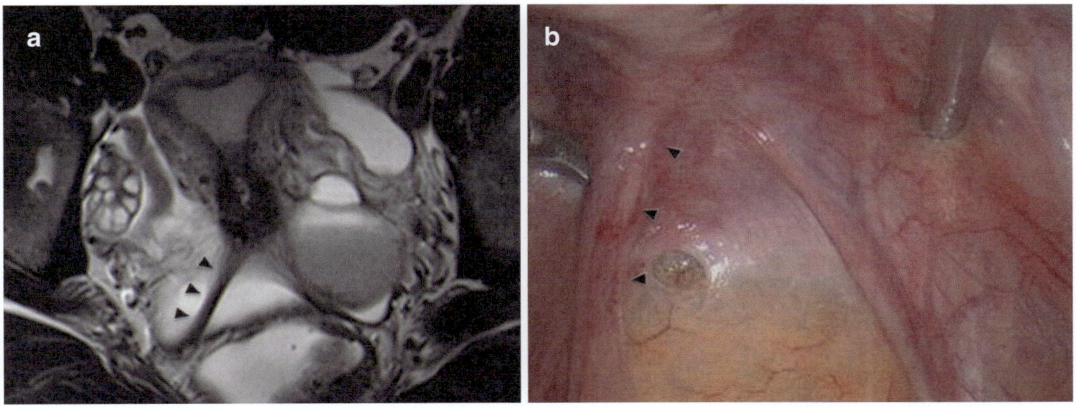

Fig. 6.7 Deep pelvic endometriosis with regular thickening of the right uterosacral ligament (USL). (**a**) Oblique axial T2-weighted MR image reveals a hypointense, smooth, and regular thickening of the right USL (arrowheads, **a**), best depicted by the presence of ascites in the pouch of Douglas. (**b**) Laparoscopy confirms the smooth thickening of the right USL (arrowheads, **b**), which is highlighted by comparison with the healthy left USL

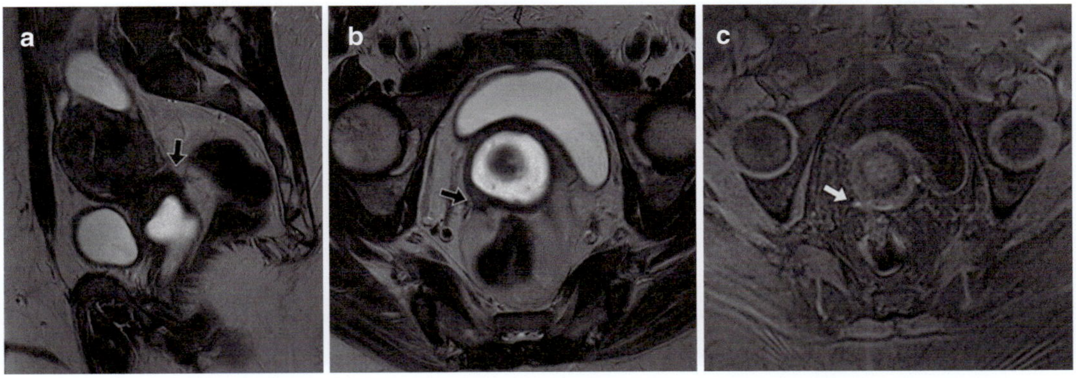

Fig. 6.8 Hemorrhagic deep pelvic endometriosis of the right uterosacral ligament (USL). (**a**) Sagittal and (**b**) oblique axial T2-weighted MR images show a hypointense spiculated nodule in the proximal portion of the right USL (black arrow, **a–b**). (**c**) Oblique axial fat-saturated T1-weighted MR image reveals a hyperintense focus (white arrow, **c**) in the location of the spiculated nodule, in keeping with hemorrhagic content

USLs and torus uterinum are infiltrated bilaterally, it is commonly referred to as an arciform abnormality [20] (Fig. 6.9).

Lesions of significant size in the mediocentral compartment may extend into the adjacent pelvic structures, namely in the mediolateral, posterocentral, and posterolateral compartments. Commonly infiltrated structures include the vaginal fornices, rectovaginal septum, parametria (Fig. 6.6), and rectum [23, 28, 33]. Concerning posterocentral extension, distinguishing between lesions that either contact the rectum (Fig. 6.9) or infiltrate the mesorectal fat and rectal serosa (Fig. 6.10) from rectal endometriosis with infiltration of the muscularis propria is crucial (Fig. 6.11). This differentiation is pivotal because rectal endometriosis may require the segmental resection of the affected segment instead of rectal shaving. On T2-weighted images, the infiltration of the rectum by DPE presents as hypointense focal wall thickening, which should be described in terms of length, wall thickness, and the degree of circumferential invasion, allowing for accurate

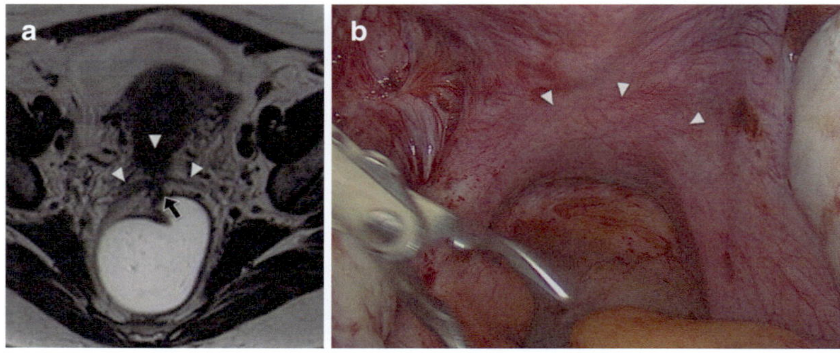

Fig. 6.9 Deep pelvic endometriosis with an arciform abnormality of the torus uterinum and uterosacral ligaments (USLs). (**a**) Oblique axial T2-weighted MR image shows an irregular thickening of the torus uterinum and USLs (arrowheads, **a**), in keeping with an arciform abnormality. (**b**) In laparoscopy, these findings correlate with the regular thickening of the torus uterinum and USLs (arrowheads, **b**). In addition, MR shows the lesion contacting the rectal wall (black arrow, **a**), with no infiltration

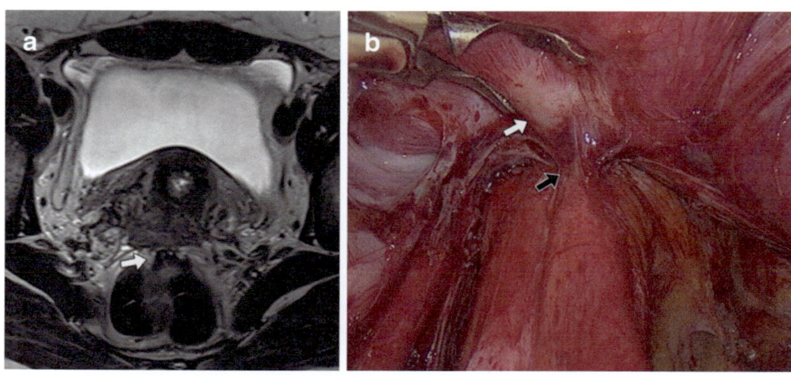

Fig. 6.10 Deep pelvic endometriosis of the torus uterinum with infiltration of the rectal serosa. (**a**) Oblique axial T2-weighted MR image reveals a nodular thickening of the torus uterinum with infiltration of the mesorectal fat and rectal serosa (white arrow, **a**), apparently sparing the muscularis propria and, therefore, not fulfilling the criteria for rectal endometriosis. (**b–c**) Laparoscopy shows the nodular lesion in the torus uterinum (white arrow, **b**) infiltrating the rectal serosa (black arrow, **b**), which was resected via rectal shaving

surgical planning [9]. Given the complex surgical resection of these lesions, the distance to the endocervical canal should also be specified [9, 20].

Finally, adhesions are seen as spiculated low-signal-intensity strands between the organs on both T1-weighted and T2-weighted images or are detected by indirect signs such as a distortion of the healthy anatomy [34] (Fig. 6.12). Mediocentral DPE-associated adhesions can lead to a distortion of healthy pelvic anatomy and a frozen pelvis, with the complete obliteration of the retrouterine excavation by a block of tissue, as well as the obliteration of the pouch of Douglas [20] (Fig. 6.13).

According to the dPEI classification [35], when only the USL and/or the torus are involved due to DPE, the disease is considered as a mild form with a small risk of postoperative complications (score 1), the shortest operation duration, and the shortest hospital stay. The detection of DPE, with DPE located only in the USL and the torus, may be operated by nontertiary centers because the risk of injuries to the inferior hypogastric plexus is quite low.

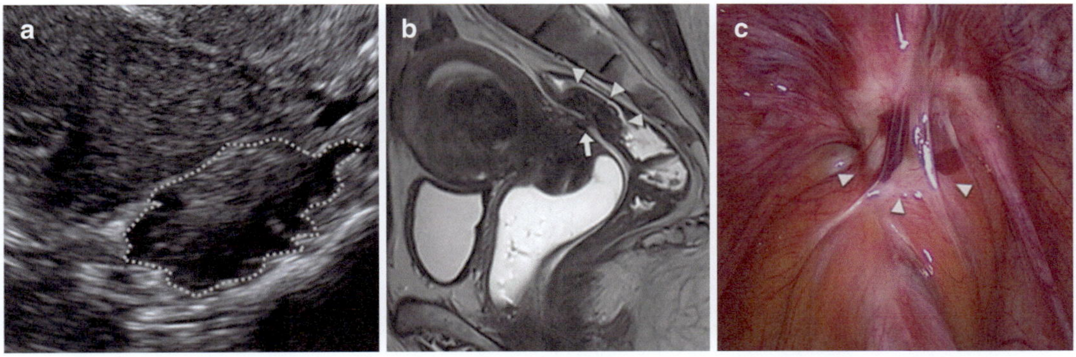

Fig. 6.11 Deep pelvic endometriosis of the torus uterinum and rectosigmoid transition. (**a**) Oblique transverse TVUS image shows hypoechoic focal thickening of the anterior colorectal wall (dotted, **a**) near the torus uterinum, highly suspicious of rectal endometriosis. (**b**) Sagittal T2-weighted MR image better depicts the nodular thickening of the torus uterinum (white arrow, **b**) with extension to the posterocentral compartment and infiltration of the anterior colorectal wall (arrowheads, **b**), leading to the focal thickening of the muscularis propria and submucosal edema. (**c**) Laparoscopy confirms colorectal infiltration by the lesion in the torus uterinum (arrowheads, **c**), therefore requiring segmental resection

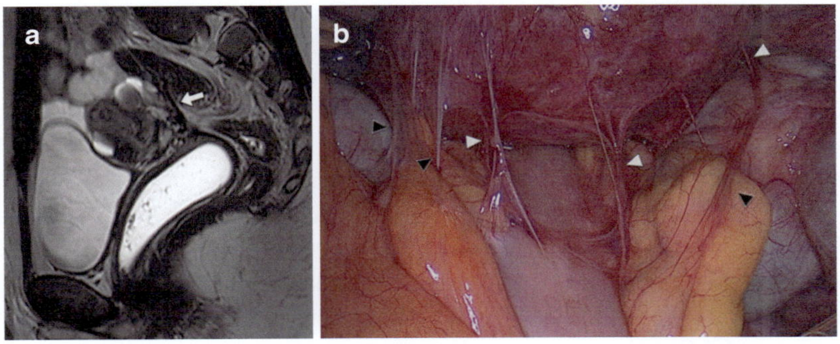

Fig. 6.12 Deep pelvic endometriosis (DPE) with adhesions in the mediocentral compartment. (**a**) Sagittal T2-weighted MR image shows hypointense strands (white arrow, **a**) between the posterior uterine wall and the rectosigmoid transition, in keeping with pelvic adhesions and highly suspicious of DPE. (**b**) Laparoscopy better depicts these endometriotic changes, showing multiple filmy (black arrowheads, **b**) and dense adhesions (white arrowheads, **b**) surrounding the pelvic structures

6.3.3 Laparoscopy

Laparoscopy findings of DPE have been described, classified, and staged over the past 30 years by using various reporting systems developed for different objectives. However, consensus has yet to be reached on the best reporting system [36]. The well-known revised American Society for Reproductive Medicine (ASRM) score [37] can be applied to pelvic lesions involving the torus uterinum and USLs, accounting for superficial and deep lesions according to their size (<1 cm, 1–3 cm, or >3 cm), as well as filmy or dense adhesions and the obliteration of the pouch of Douglas. Nevertheless, this classification system has not been developed for presurgical staging. On the other hand, as previously discussed, the modified ENZIAN classification system classifies lesions from the USLs and retrocervical area into different compartments, grading them according to size [32].

In keeping with the revised ASRM score [37], the morphological appearances of DPE in the torus uterinum and USLs include regular thickening (Figs. 6.7 and 6.9), nodular infiltration (Fig. 6.4), and retraction (Figs. 6.6 and 6.13) [25,

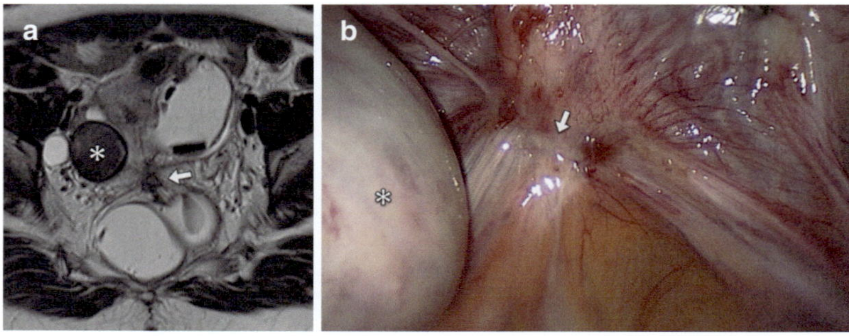

Fig. 6.13 Deep pelvic endometriosis with obliteration of the pouch of Douglas. (**a**) Oblique axial T2-weighted MR image reveals a spiculated nodule in the torus uterinum and both uterosacral ligaments (white arrow, **a**), which fixate the right adnexa, rectum, and sigmoid colon, thereby causing the obliteration of the pouch of Douglas. Note the presence of an endometrioma in the right ovary (asterisk, **a**). (**b**) Laparoscopy correlates with these imaging findings, showing the obliteration of the pouch of Douglas by the central spiculated nodule (white arrow, **b**) and the right-sided endometrioma (asterisk, **b**)

37]. These findings are associated, on laparoscopy, with the presence of superficial implants, which are classified as "red" (red, red-pink, and clear lesions), "white" (white and yellow-brown lesions and peritoneal defects), or "black" (black and blue lesions). Filmy or dense adhesions to surrounding structures may also be seen [25, 37] (Fig. 6.12). In more severe cases, the USL lesions can extend to the surrounding compartments, leading to distortions of healthy pelvic anatomy, the invasion of the rectum and parametria, and the obliteration of the pouch of Douglas (Figs. 6.10, 6.11, and 6.13).

6.4 Pitfalls and Anatomical Variations

Pitfalls in the evaluation of USLs and torus uterinum may relate to both patient and technical imaging factors. In patients with prior surgery or previous pelvic infections, resulting in residual fibrosis, adhesions, and distorted anatomy, the primary challenge lies in differentiating fibrotic or scar tissue from an evolving lesion. Postsurgical aspects range from almost healthy to fibrotic sequelae that manifest as adhesions, bands, or linear tracks within the dissection planes of pelvic surgery. This differentiation can be particularly challenging on TVUS because these conditions often present similar findings. However, lesion-size evolution along studies, rectal wall invasion, and the onset of symptoms may be used as discriminating features. On MRI, resections of the sequelae of USLs can appear as hypointense linear bands on T2-weighted images, exhibiting a darker signal intensity compared to fibrosis caused by DPE (Fig. 6.14). In patients without prior surgery, USL infiltration by endometriosis is suggested by irregular or nodular thickening. However, in a postoperative context, these criteria lack specificity and should be accompanied by consistent clinical symptoms to diagnose DPE recurrence confidently [38]. This phenomenon is also observed at laparoscopy where the USL may be thickened and rigid and may mimic the endometriotic location. That is why most authors retain the necessity of having at least one pathological analysis of a location with endometriosis to positively diagnose the disease.

Other patient-related pitfalls include the presence of additional imaging findings, such as large leiomyomas or endometriomas, preventing the clear visualization of the pouch of Douglas and proximal USLs. In addition, a retroflexed uterus may impair the precise visualization of a retrocervical plaque (Fig. 6.15).

The misinterpretation of the images by the radiologist can also be a pitfall in itself. For example, USL infiltration should be considered equivocal if the thickness is 3–5 mm and when its irregular and/or pseudonodular appearance is only seen in one plane (Fig. 6.16). To definitively

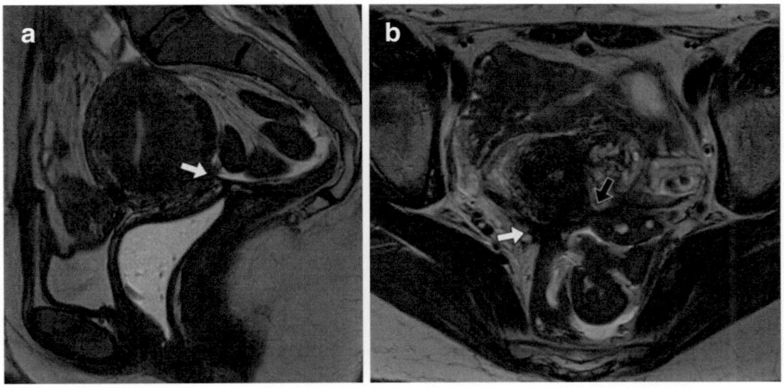

Fig. 6.14 Postsurgical fibrosis mimicking deep pelvic endometriosis (DPE) in a patient previously submitted to a laparoscopic resection of DPE lesions. (**a**) Sagittal and (**b**) oblique axial T2-weighted MR images reveal multiple adhesions and strikingly hypointense fibrotic bands. This results in the distortion of the pelvic anatomy, namely the upward retraction of the posterior vaginal fornix and anterior rectal wall (white arrow, **a**–**b**) and the fixation of the left adnexa to the posterior wall of the cervix (black arrow, **b**). The absence of hemorrhagic foci on T1-weighted images (not shown), as well as the linear morphology and hypointensity of these bands, suggests postsurgical fibrosis instead of DPE recurrence. Reprinted with permission from Ref. [38]

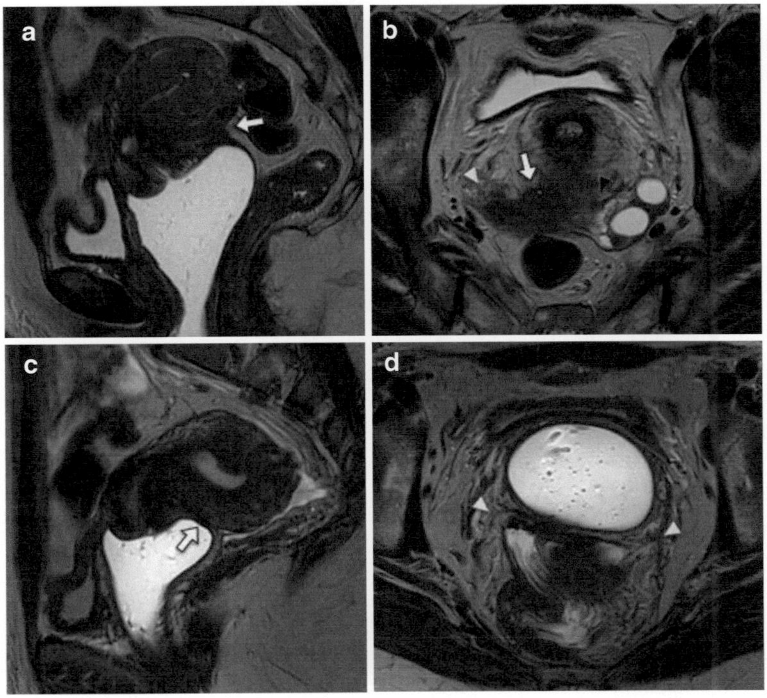

Fig. 6.15 Retroflexed uterus hindering an accurate evaluation of the torus uterinum. (**a**, **c**) Sagittal and (**b**, **d**) oblique axial T2-weighted MR images from two patients. (**a**–**b**) In the first case, although the assessment of the torus uterinum is limited, a hypointense nodule (white arrow, **a**) is seen infiltrating the posterior vaginal fornix and the posterior wall of the uterus. This nodule is probably fixing the uterus in this position, which highly suggests the presence of deep pelvis endometriosis (DPE) and external adenomyosis. The oblique axial image confirms the presence of a nodule in the torus uterinum and uterosacral ligaments (USLs) (white arrow, **b**) that infiltrates the right parametrium (white arrowhead, B) and fixes the left adnexa (black arrowhead, **b**). (**c**–**d**) In opposition, the MR images of the second patient reveal an intact fat plane between the torus uterinum and the vaginal fornix (white arrow, **c**), which safely excludes DPE in this location. The evaluation of oblique axial images supports the absence of DPE by revealing symmetric thin USLs (white arrowheads, **d**)

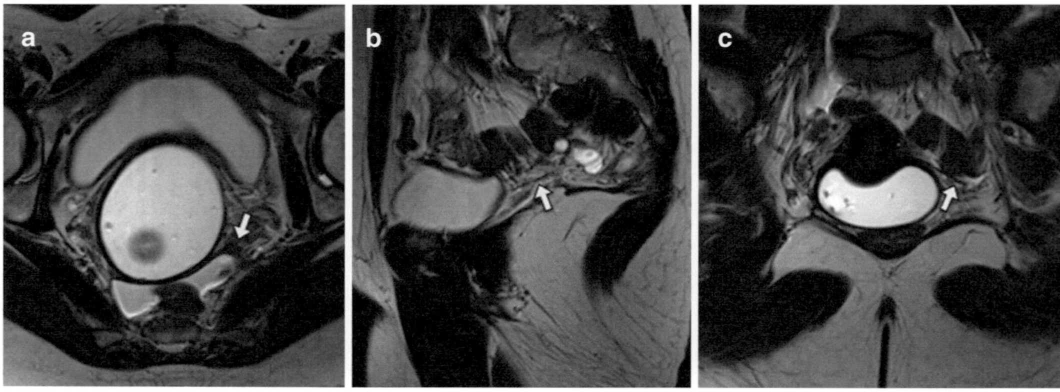

Fig. 6.16 Artifactual thickening of the left uterosacral ligament (USL) mimicking deep pelvic endometriosis (DPE). (**a**) Oblique axial T2-weighted MR image simulates the regular thickening of the left USL (arrow, **a**). However, a subsequent evaluation of the (**b**) sagittal and (**c**) oblique coronal T2-weighted images reveals that this impression is given by overlapping with the sigmoid colon (arrow, **b**–**c**), thus confirming the healthy appearance of the left USL and the artifactual nature of this finding

diagnose endometriosis in these cases, including a thin-section oblique axial T2-weighted sequence in the protocol is crucial, or to assess the multiplanar three-dimensional (3D) T2-weighted images carefully, looking on a T1W sequence for hemorrhagic implants or nodules is crucial.

Finally, endometriotic USL thickening must be differentiated from the thickened appearance of USLs due to anatomical variants, regional vein structures, fibrosis, or a misinterpretation of the images. This is why a 3D T2W sequence is very useful in clinical practice. Therefore, one must keep in mind the nonspecific nature of T2-hypointense findings in the absence of hemorrhagic implants or nodules [39].

6.5 Conclusion

In summary, understanding the anatomy and imaging characteristics of the USLs and torus uterinum is essential for accurately diagnosing and managing DPE. Despite the challenges in delineating the healthy anatomy and detecting infiltration by DPE, advancements in TVUS and MRI have improved diagnostic accuracy. A careful consideration of anatomical variations, technical nuances, and potential pitfalls is crucial for optimal patient care and surgical planning.

References

1. Donaldson K, Huntington A, De Vita R. Mechanics of uterosacral ligaments: current knowledge, existing gaps, and future directions. Ann Biomed Eng. 2021;49:1788–804.
2. Bazot M, Darai E, Hourani R, Thomassin I, Cortez A, Uzan S, Buy JN. Deep pelvic endometriosis: MR imaging for diagnosis and prediction of extension of disease. Radiology. 2004;232:379–89.
3. Chapron C, Fauconnier A, Vieira M, Barakat H, Dousset B, Pansini V, Vacher-Lavenu MC, Dubuisson JB. Anatomical distribution of deeply infiltrating endometriosis: surgical implications and proposition for a classification. Hum Reprod. 2003;18:157–61.
4. Redwine DB. The distribution of endometriosis in the pelvis by age groups and fertility. Fertil Steril. 1987;47:173–5.
5. Campbell RM. The anatomy and histology of the sacrouterine ligaments. Am J Obstet Gynecol. 1950;59:1–12.
6. Vu D, Haylen BT, Tse K, Farnsworth A. Surgical anatomy of the uterosacral ligament. Int Urogynecol J. 2010;21:1123–8.
7. Blaisdell FE. The anatomy of the sacro-uterine ligaments. Anat Rec. 1917;12:1–42.
8. Umek WH, Morgan DM, Ashton-Miller JA, DeLancey JO. Quantitative analysis of uterosacral ligament origin and insertion points by magnetic resonance imaging. Bone. 2004;103:447–51.
9. Rousset P, Florin M, Bharwani N, Touboul C, Monroc M, Golfier F, Nougaret S, Thomassin-Naggara I. Deep pelvic infiltrating endometriosis: MRI consensus lexicon and compartment-based approach from

the ENDOVALIRM group. Diagn Interv Imaging. 2023;104:95–112.
10. Fratelli N, Scioscia M, Bassi E, Musola M, Minelli L, Trivella G. Transvaginal sonography for preoperative assessment of deep endometriosis. J Clin Ultrasound. 2013;41:69–75.
11. Bazot M, Thomassin I, Hourani R, Cortez A, Darai E. Diagnostic accuracy of transvaginal sonography for deep pelvic endometriosis. Ultrasound Obstet Gynecol. 2004;24:180–5.
12. Millischer AE, Salomon LJ, Santulli P, Borghese B, Dousset B, Chapron C. Fusion imaging for evaluation of deep infiltrating endometriosis: feasibility and preliminary results. Ultrasound Obstet Gynecol. 2015;46:109–17.
13. Yin S, Lin Q, Xu F, Xu J, Zhang Y. Diagnosis of deep infiltrating endometriosis using transvaginal ultrasonography. Front Med. 2020;7:567929.
14. Maple S, Chalmers KJ, Bezak E, Henry K, Parange N. Ultrasound characteristics and scanning techniques of uterosacral ligaments for the diagnosis of endometriosis: a systematic review. J Ultrasound Med. 2023;42:1193–209.
15. Ohba T, Mizutani H, Maeda T, Matsuura K, Okamura H. Evaluation of endometriosis in uterosacral ligaments by transrectal ultrasonography. Hum Reprod. 1996;11:2014–7.
16. Bazot M, Detchev R, Cortez A, Amouyal P, Uzan S, Daraï E. Transvaginal sonography and rectal endoscopic sonography for the assessment of pelvic endometriosis: a preliminary comparison. Hum Reprod. 2003;18:1686–92.
17. Leonardi M, Condous G. A pictorial guide to the ultrasound identification and assessment of uterosacral ligaments in women with potential endometriosis. Australas J Ultrasound Med. 2019;22:157–64.
18. Savelli L, Ambrosio M, Salucci P, Raimondo D, Arena A, Seracchioli R. Transvaginal ultrasound features of normal uterosacral ligaments. Fertil Steril. 2021;116:275–7.
19. Bazot M, Daraï É. Endométriose. In: Bazot M, Tardivon A, editors. Imagerie de la femme: gynecologie. Paris: Lavoisier; 2017. p. 417–88.
20. Bazot M, Bharwani N, Huchon C, et al. European society of urogenital radiology (ESUR) guidelines: MR imaging of pelvic endometriosis. Eur Radiol. 2017;27:2765–75.
21. Thomassin-Naggara I, Lamrabet S, Crestani A, Bekhouche A, Wahab CA, Kermarrec E, Touboul C, Daraï E. Magnetic resonance imaging classification of deep pelvic endometriosis: description and impact on surgical management. Hum Reprod. 2020;35:1589–600.
22. Bazot M, Gasner A, Ballester M, Daraï E. Value of thin-section oblique axial T2-weighted magnetic resonance images to assess uterosacral ligament endometriosis. Hum Reprod. 2011;26:346–53.
23. Loubeyre P, Petignat P, Jacob S, Egger JF, Dubuisson JB, Wenger JM. Anatomic distribution of posterior deeply infiltrating endometriosis on MRI after vaginal and rectal gel opacification. Am J Roentgenol. 2009;192:1625–31.
24. Baggish M. Pelvic anatomy from the laparoscopic view. In: Baggish M, Karram M, editors. Atlas of pelvic anatomy and gynecologic surgery. 5th ed. Philadelphia: Elsevier; 2020. p. 1277–82.
25. Puntambekar S, Nanda SM, Parikh K. Laparoscopic pelvic anatomy in females: applied surgical principles. Singapore: Springer; 2019. https://doi.org/10.1007/978-981-13-8653-4.
26. Gerges B, Li W, Leonardi M, Mol BW, Condous G. Optimal imaging modality for detection of rectosigmoid deep endometriosis: systematic review and meta-analysis. Ultrasound Obstet Gynecol. 2021;58:190–200.
27. Ros C, de Guirior C, Mension E, Rius M, Valdés-Bango M, Tortajada M, Matas I, Martínez-Zamora M, Gracia M, Carmona F. Transvaginal ultrasound for diagnosis of deep endometriosis involving uterosacral ligaments, torus uterinus and posterior vaginal fornix: prospective study. Ultrasound Obstet Gynecol. 2021;58:926–32.
28. Guerriero S, Condous G, van den Bosch T, et al. Systematic approach to sonographic evaluation of the pelvis in women with suspected endometriosis, including terms, definitions and measurements: a consensus opinion from the International Deep Endometriosis Analysis (IDEA) group. Ultrasound Obstet Gynecol. 2016;48:318–32.
29. Chowdary P, Stone K, Ma T, Readman E, McIlwaine K, Druitt M, Ellett L, Cameron M, Maher P. Multicentre retrospective study to assess diagnostic accuracy of ultrasound for superficial endometriosis—are we any closer? Aust New Zeal J Obstet Gynaecol. 2019;59:279–84.
30. El-Maadawy SM, Alaaeldin N, Nagy CB. Role of preoperative ultrasound mapping in the surgical management of deep infiltrating endometriosis: a prospective observational study. Egypt J Radiol Nucl Med. 2021;52:159. https://doi.org/10.1186/s43055-021-00526-w.
31. Hudelist G, English J, Thomas AE, Tinelli A, Singer CF, Keckstein J. Diagnostic accuracy of transvaginal ultrasound for non-invasive diagnosis of bowel endometriosis: systematic review and meta-analysis. Ultrasound Obstet Gynecol. 2011;37:257–63.
32. Keckstein J, Saridogan E, Ulrich UA, et al. The #Enzian classification: a comprehensive non-invasive and surgical description system for endometriosis. Acta Obstet Gynecol Scand. 2021;100:1165–75.
33. Bazot M, Lafont C, Rouzier R, Roseau G, Thomassin-Naggara I, Daraï E. Diagnostic accuracy of physical examination, transvaginal sonography, rectal endoscopic sonography, and magnetic resonance imaging to diagnose deep infiltrating endometriosis. Fertil Steril. 2009;92:1825–33.
34. Maciel C, Ferreira H, Djokovic D, Kyaw Tun J, Keckstein J, Rizzo S, Manganaro L. MRI of endometriosis in correlation with the #Enzian classification:

applicability and structured report. Insights Imaging. 2023;14:120.

35. Thomassin-Naggara/Rousset et al. JAMA Netw Open. 2023;6(5):e2311686. https://doi.org/10.1001/jamanetworkopen.2023.11686.
36. Vermeulen N, Abrao MS, Einarsson JI, et al. Endometriosis classification, staging and reporting systems: a review on the road to a universally accepted endometriosis classification. J Minim Invasive Gynecol. 2021;28:1822–48.
37. Birmingham A. Revised American Society for reproductive medicine classification of endometriosis: 1996. Fertil Steril. 1997;67:817–21.
38. Guerra A, Daraï E, Osório F, Setúbal A, Bendifallah S, Loureiro A, Thomassin-Naggara I. Imaging of postoperative endometriosis. Diagn Interv Imaging. 2019;100:607–18.
39. Ruaux E, VanBuren WM, Nougaret S, Gavrel M, Charlot M, Grangeon F, Bolze P-A, Thomassin-Naggara I, Rousset P. Endometriosis MR mimickers: T2-hypointense lesions. Insights Imaging. 2024;15:20.

7 Mediocentral Compartment: Vaginal Endometriosis and Rectovaginal Septum

Marie Florin and Yohann Dabi

7.1 Introduction

The incidence of vaginal endometriosis is recorded in the literature as ranging from 11% to 50%. [1, 2] It is frequently associated with the extensive posterior infiltrative involvement of the uterosacral ligaments, torus uterinum, rectovaginal septum, rectum, and parametrium.

A preoperative diagnosis of vaginal endometriosis is crucial for several reasons. First, it allows for anticipating the surgical gestures and difficulties that could occur during surgery. The quality of preoperative assessment is well known to influence the surgical excision quality and minimize the risk of incomplete excision or unforeseen procedures. [3] Second, it can significantly modify the preoperative counseling, especially in cases of multiple-compartment lesions. Indeed, it can impact the risk of preoperative stoma by decreasing the risk of digestive fistula [4]. Eventually, vaginal infiltration significantly impacts the risk of postoperative dysuria, even if the literature remains unclear about whether it is a marker of severe endometriosis or vaginal infiltration by itself.

M. Florin
Hôpital Tenon, Paris, France
e-mail: marie.florin@aphp.fr

Y. Dabi (✉)
Sorbonne University - Department of Gynecology, Obstetric and Reproductive Medicine, Paris, France
e-mail: yohann.dabi@aphp.fr

The posterior vaginal fornix is the primary site for vaginal involvement, often arising from the inferior extension of a retrocervical lesion [2]. Exceptionally, the anterior wall or distal vaginal location can be affected, especially after a surgery such as episiotomy. Vaginal endometriosis appears as a thickening wall with or without a cystic implant, which can be hemorrhagic on imaging examination.

7.2 Anatomical Definition

7.2.1 Rectovaginal Septum Endometriosis

The rectovaginal septum (RVS) is a retroperitoneal structure situated between the posterior vaginal wall and the anterior surface of the rectum [5]. It originates at the base of the pouch of Douglas and extends downward to the apex of the perineal body. It can be visualized more clearly by using perineal fluid, which highlights the reflection of the peritoneum (Fig. 7.1).

The definition of endometriosis of the rectovaginal septum is controversial. Some authors use the term *RVS deep infiltrating endometriosis (DIE)* and others *rectovaginal DIE* [6–8]. The rectovaginal septum is an anatomical individual structure, whereas the rectovaginal areas include the rectum, vagina, and RVS [8]. Furthermore, the definition of rectovaginal endometriosis lacks

I. Thomassin-Naggara (ed.), *Imaging of Endometriosis: A Comparative Guide of US, MRI and Surgery*, https://doi.org/10.1007/978-3-031-82750-1_7

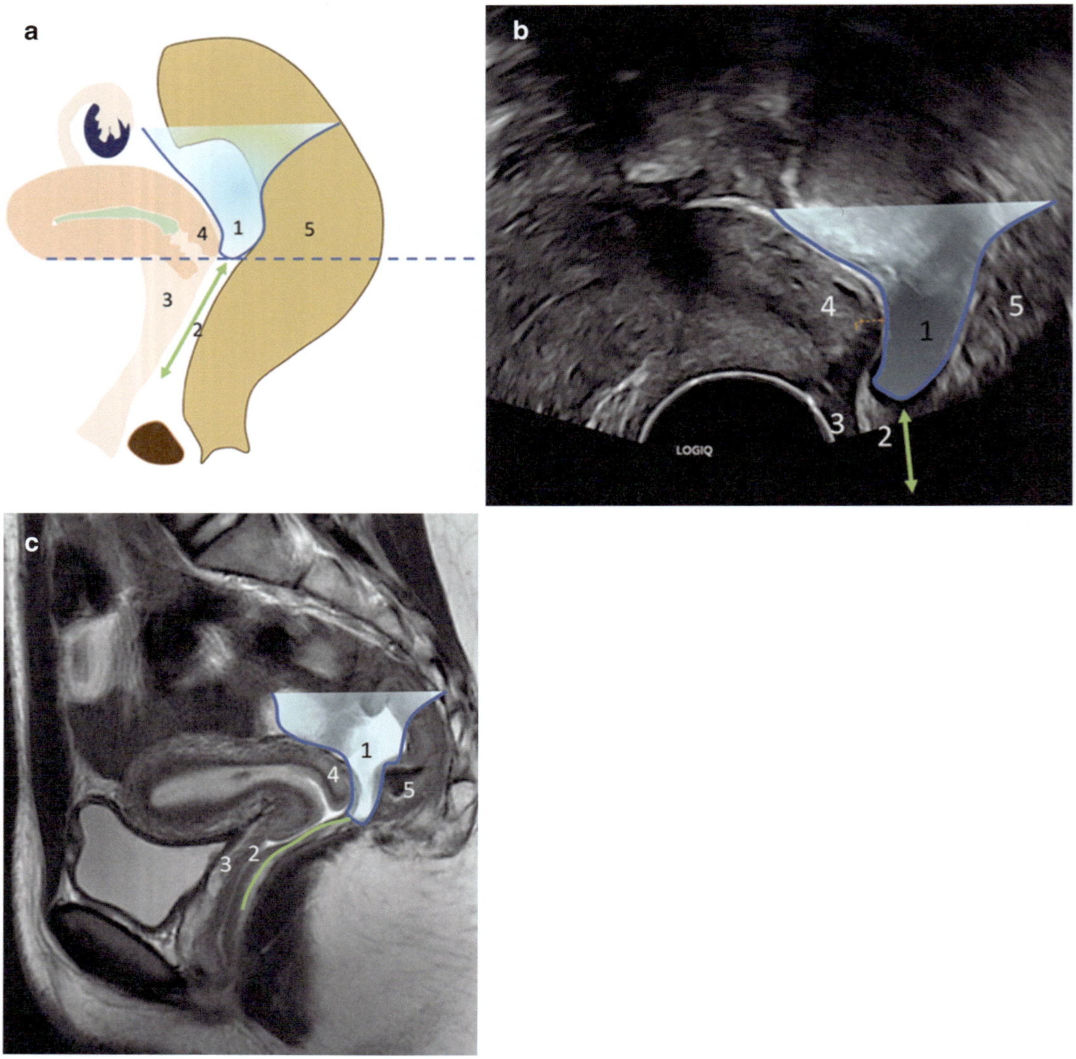

Fig. 7.1 Schematic drawing (**a**), ultrasound image (**b**), and sagittal T2 turbo spin echo (TSE) sequences (**c**) illustrate the definition of the rectovaginal septum (RVS). The RVS (2) is indicated by the double-headed green arrow, between the posterior vaginal wall (3) and the anterior rectum wall (5), positioned anatomically below the blue line marking the lower border of the posterior lip of the cervix (4) on the schematic drawing. The upper boundary of the RVS is identified where the blue line intersects with the lower border of the posterior lip of the cervix. The caudal end of the peritoneum (1) at the lower margin of the rectouterine peritoneal pouch (the cul-de-sac of Douglas) is represented

consistency. It's been characterized as endometriotic lesions that penetrate both the rectum and the posterior vaginal fornix, potentially extending into the rectovaginal septum. Alternatively, some describe it as nodules infiltrating primarily the RVS, possibly extending into the vagina and/or the rectum [8]. Isolated rectovaginal septum endometriosis is rare.

Suspicion of the involvement of the RVS arises when a DIE nodule is observed in the rectovaginal space below the line delineated by the lower border of the posterior lip of the cervix, beneath the peritoneum (Fig. 7.2) [9]. RVS DIE typically extends from the posterior vaginal wall, the anterior rectal wall, or both the posterior vaginal wall and the anterior rectal wall.

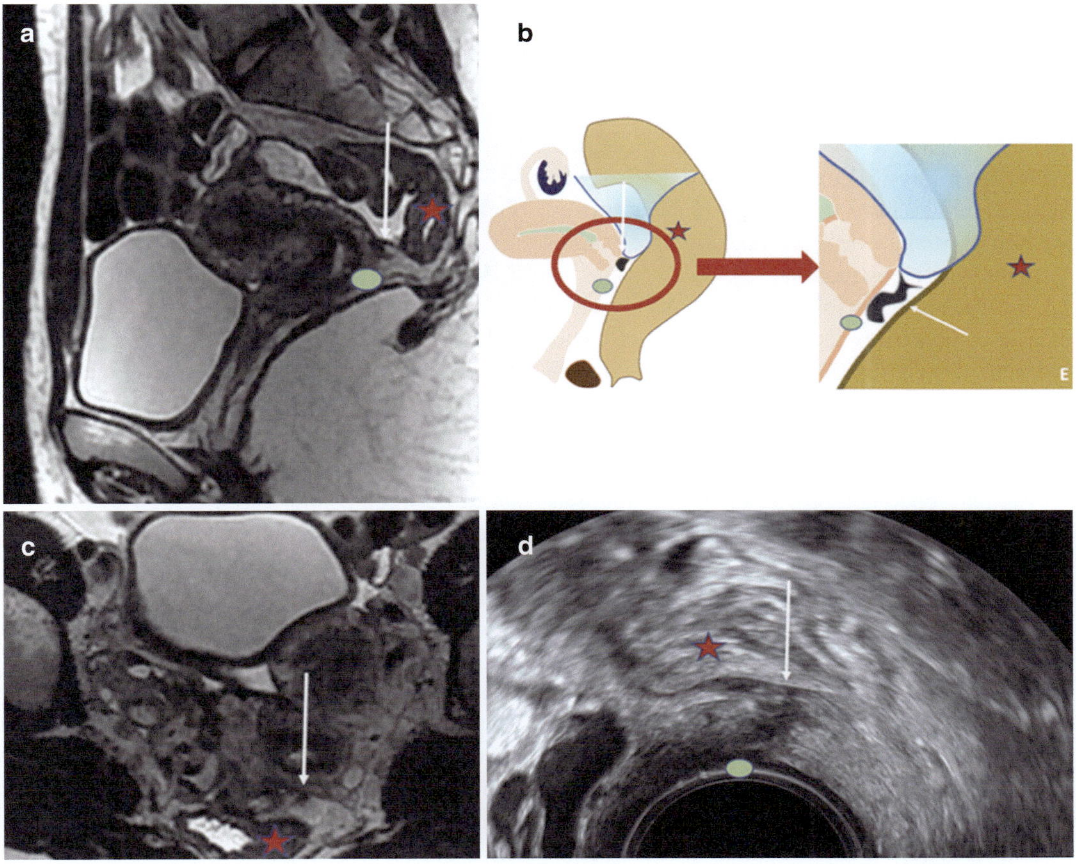

Fig. 7.2 Schematic drawings (**d** and **e**), ultrasound images (**c**): axial (**a**) and (**b**) sagittal MRI sequences demonstrating isolated deep infiltrating endometriosis (white arrow) in the rectovaginal septum (RVS). Red star is the rectum; green circle is the vagina

7.2.2 Vaginal Endometriosis

The posterior vaginal fornix is predominantly affected in cases of vaginal involvement, typically originating from the inferior extension of an extensive retrocervical lesion with uterosacral parameters and rectum involvement. In rare instances, the anterior wall or distal vaginal region may also be affected.

The vaginal wall has three layers:

- The inner layer, called the mucosa, is composed of squamous cells. It is also called the epithelium.
- The middle layer, called the muscularis, is made up of muscular tissue.
- The outer layer, called the adventitia, is composed of connective tissue. The need to perform a partial colpectomy is related to the thickness of vaginal involvement, especially the involvement of the inner and/or middle layer.

7.3 Value of Clinical Examination

Although no symptom has been specifically associated with vaginal endometriosis and although patients with vaginal lesions often report similar symptoms to those with deep infiltrating endometriosis, deep dyspareunia is one of the most often reported symptoms. [10] Vaginal location is one of the DPE locations that is easily accessible to clinical examination, which has been well demonstrated as a factor that reduces the time to diagnosis [10, 11]. The ability to a detect vaginal nodule is related to the moment in the menstrual cycle when physical examination is performed. Several studies have demonstrated an improvement in the diagnostic relevance of pelvic examination during menstruation [12].

The diagnostic performance of physical examination is marked by its excellent specificity and low sensitivity (30–50%) [13] and is why a normal clinical examination does not rule out the diagnosis. [14] Indeed, a "positive" clinical examination is very relevant [13].

Vaginal endometriosis can be diagnosed through speculum examination by identifying a typical blue nodule in the posterior vaginal fornix. Other signs can be identified, such as cervix deviation or retraction or even irregularity in the vaginal wall or a bleeding lesion upon examination.

Vaginal examination is also the first step in any surgical intervention for endometriosis under general anesthesia. Indeed, the clinical examination during consultation may be interrupted due to pain and be incomplete. Moreover, some patients may refuse the examination during consultation. Literature data are completely lacking on the performance of examination under general anesthesia versus consultation for the diagnosis of vaginal involvement. The examination under general anesthesia allows for assessing the transfixing or nontransfixing nature of the lesion via vaginal touch (vaginal mucosa involvement).

Thus, given the quite low sensitivity of physical examination, it needs to be correlated with the results of transvaginal ultrasonography and MRI. Recently, a study tested the ability of physical examination, ultrasonography, and MR imaging to diagnose the different DPE locations. [15] Regarding vaginal locations, this study demonstrated the high sensitivity of MRI but the high specificities of transvaginal ultrasonography and physical examination. The authors concluded that the best model to correctly diagnose vaginal endometriosis was to have two techniques of the three (pelvic examination (PE), transvaginal ultrasound (TVUS), and magnetic resonance imaging (MRI)) be positive to affirm vaginal endometriosis (an accuracy value of 82.6%, a sensitivity of 50%, and a specificity of 90.9%).

7.4 Imaging Techniques

7.4.1 Vaginal Endometriosis

7.4.1.1 TVUS

The involvement of the posterior vaginal fornix is challenging to identify on ultrasound (US), with a sensitivity of approximately 30% in the literature [9]. Normal vaginal thickness is measured between 3 and 5 mm (Fig. 7.3). Vaginal involvement is characterized by a thickening of more than 5 mm of the posterior vaginal fornix or by the presence of a nodule in the hypoechoic layer of the vaginal wall (Fig. 7.4). The nodule can be homogenous or with possible hyper- or hypoechoic cystic lesions. The presence of cysts behind the uterine cervix is extremely specific but difficult to assess. [9] Indeed, the main differential diagnoses are Naboth cysts, which are very common. The vaginal involvement ultrasound diagnostic is very subtle and requires a high level of expertise [16]. For this reason, significant variability abounds among studies on the diagnostic performance of ultrasound in detecting vaginal endometriosis [17–19].

Expanding the vagina allows a better exploration of the vaginal wall, especially to detect microcysts, thickening, and adjacent anatomical structures (Fig. 7.5). The sonovaginography can be useful to improve diagnostic performance, particularly in conjunction with clinical examination [17, 19]. Although systematic vaginal opacification is not recommended, it can increase sensitivity in patients with inconclusive first-line sonography. To conduct gel contrast sonovaginography, 20–50 mL of ultrasound gel is introduced into the posterior vaginal fornix by using a 20 mL plastic syringe. This gel facilitates an acoustic window, enabling a "standoff" view of the structures within the posterior compartment.

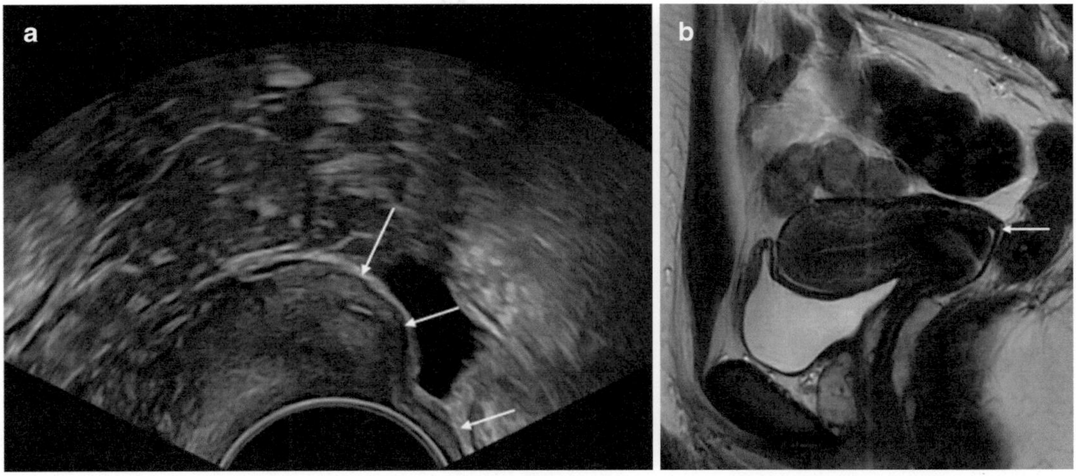

Fig. 7.3 Endovaginal ultrasound (**a**) and sagittal T2 TSE MRI (**b**) showing a healthy vaginal posterior wall with a thickness <5 mm

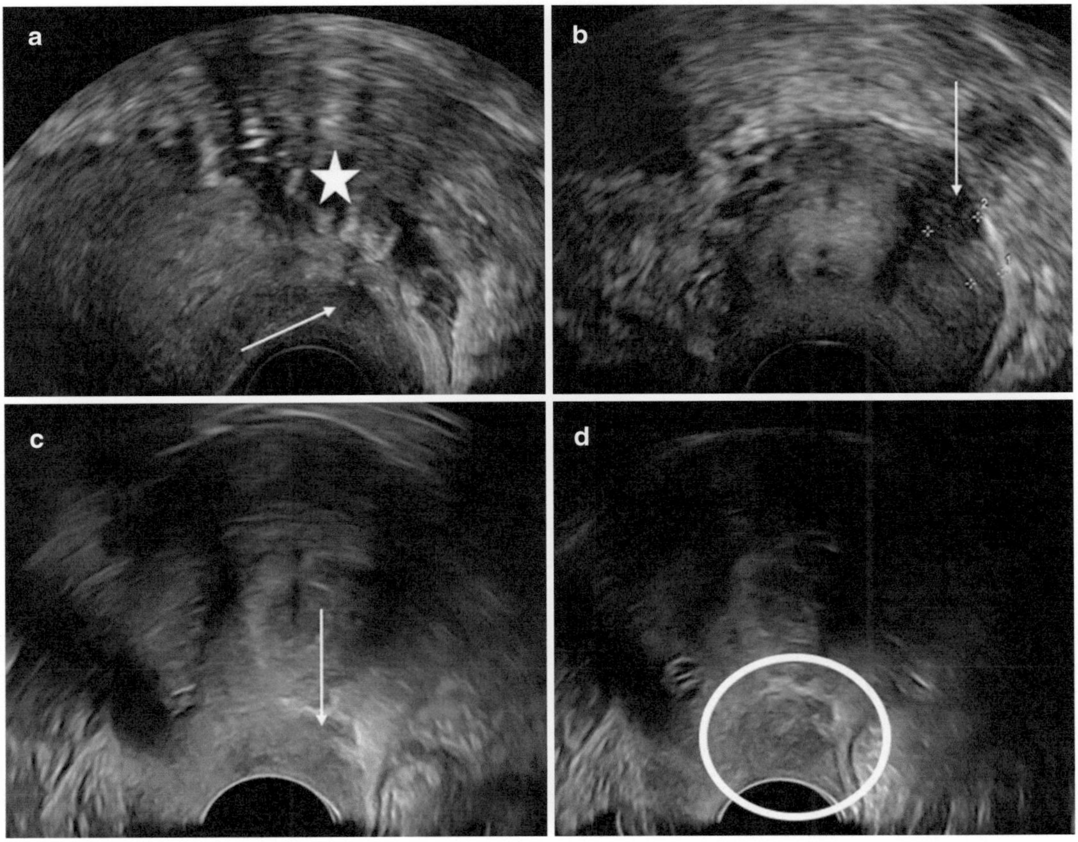

Fig. 7.4 Endovaginal ultrasound (**a** and **b**) Sagittal US showing the vaginal posterior involvement of deep endometriosis (arrows) with extension of the rectosigmoid wall (star). It also shows a >5 mm thickening of the wall of the posterior vaginal. (**c** and **d**) Sagittal US showing a large nodule in the posterior vaginal wall (arrow and circle)

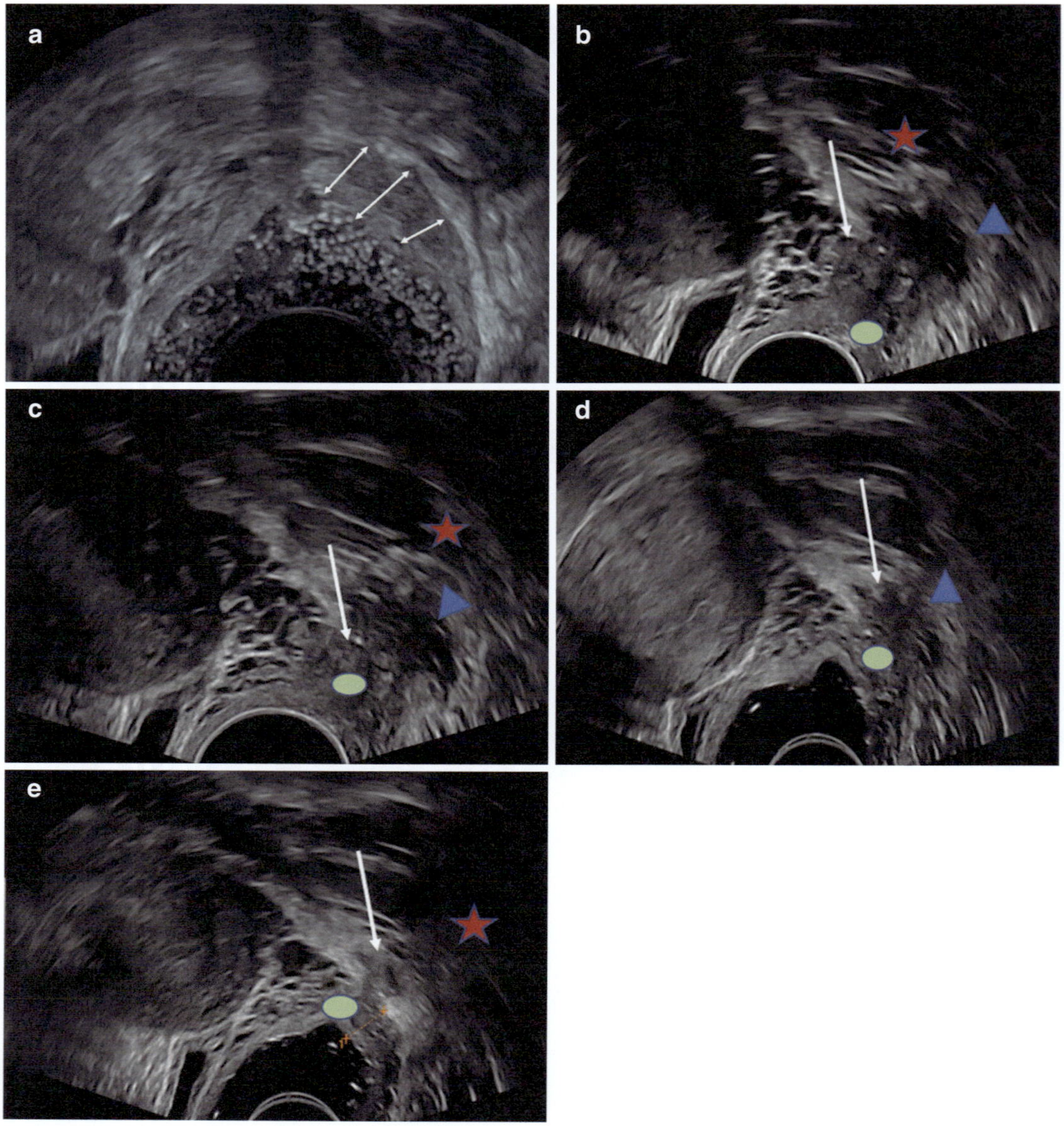

Fig. 7.5 (**a**) Sonovaginography showing vaginal opacification, which expands the vagina and allows a better visualization of posterior vaginal wall thickening. Endovaginal ultrasound (**b** and **c**) Sagittal US showing vaginal posterior involvement of deep endometriosis (arrows). The vagina endometriosis extending to rectal muscularis (blue head arrow), torus, left uterosacral ligament and proximal parametrium. Red star is the rectum; green circle is the vagina. It also shows a >5 mm thickening of the wall of the posterior vaginal. (**e** and **d**) show the same lesions via sonovaginography

7.4.1.2 MRI

Vaginal posterior fornix endometriosis appears as a nodule or a thickening of the posterior vaginal wall with the appearance of a supernumerary cervix. The presence of hemorrhagic (hypersignal T1) or cystic (hypersignal T2) implants is very specific [2], but this "classical" presentation is not the most frequently encountered (Fig. 7.6). Vaginal endometriosis involves a lesion above the level of the pouch of Douglas, whereas the rectovaginal septum involves one below that level.

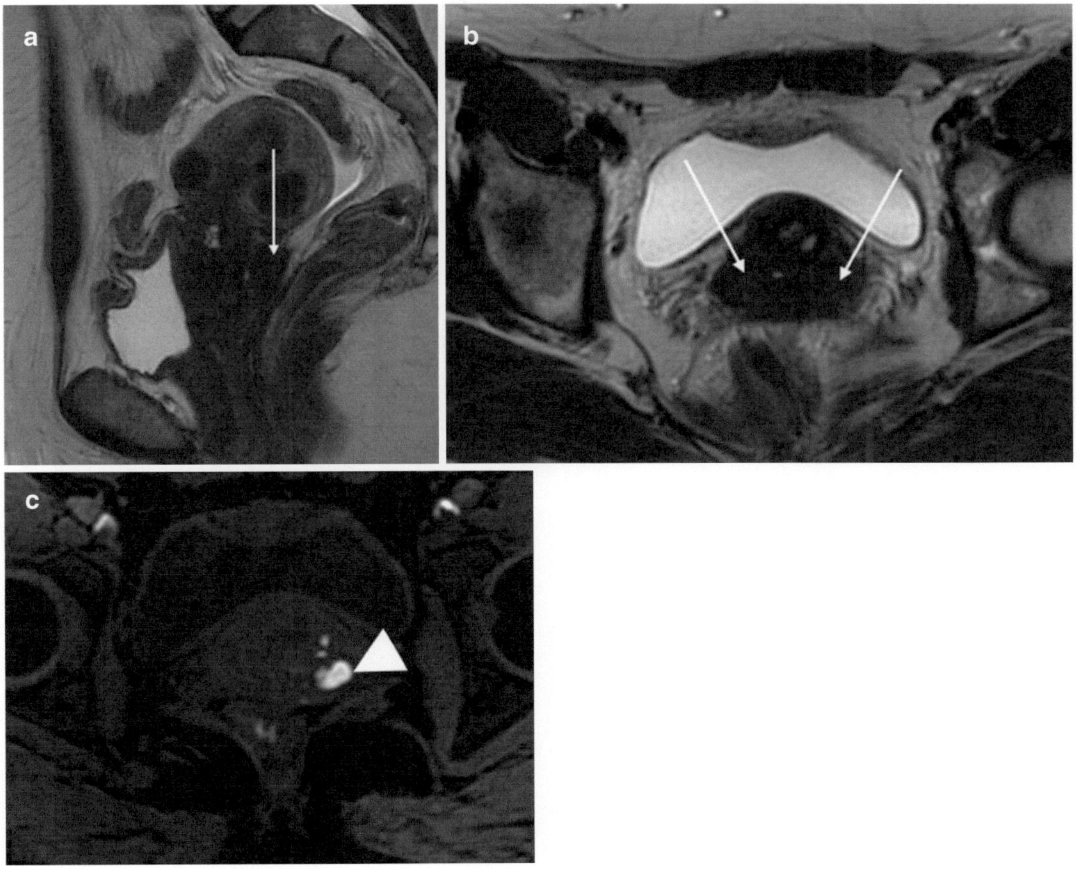

Fig. 7.6 (**a**) Sagittal T2 TSE sequence MRI showing a vaginal posterior nodule (arrow) with the appearance of a supernumerary cervix. (**b**) Axial T2 TSE sequence MRI showing a vaginal posterior nodule (arrow). (**c**) Axial T1 fat-saturated sequence MRI showing hemorrhagic implants (head arrow) in the vaginal wall in hypersignal T1

Researching the associated lesion—such as the involvement of the torus uterinum, uterosacral ligament, rectum, or parametrium endometriosis, which increases the risk of postoperative complications, particularly in the rectovaginal fistula—is crucial [20]. In cases of large, hemicircumferential, or lateral lesions, resection may result in dysuria, due to the proximity of the inferior hypogastric plexus and the potential for alteration. Thus, length, thickness, and circumference must be included in the MRI report (Fig. 7.7). [21]

The vaginal walls typically collapse, making evaluation challenging, and the spontaneous visualization of the rectovaginal septum is equally inconsistent. The lesions of deep pelvic endometriosis (DPE) typically manifest as infiltrating masses, creating a continuum among various anatomical structures that distort pelvic anatomy, blurring the normally distinct compartments. These lesions are composed primarily of fibrous tissue. Therefore, imaging must be capable of detecting the prevalent and widespread fibrotic component, which appears markedly hypointense on T2-weighted MRI images. The MRI signal characteristics of the vaginal and rectal walls closely resemble those of fibrous lesions [2]. Consequently, an inherent challenge hampers detecting and assessing deep pelvic endometriosis lesions. That's why in the event of any suspicion of vaginal involvement, vaginal opacification may be useful to improve

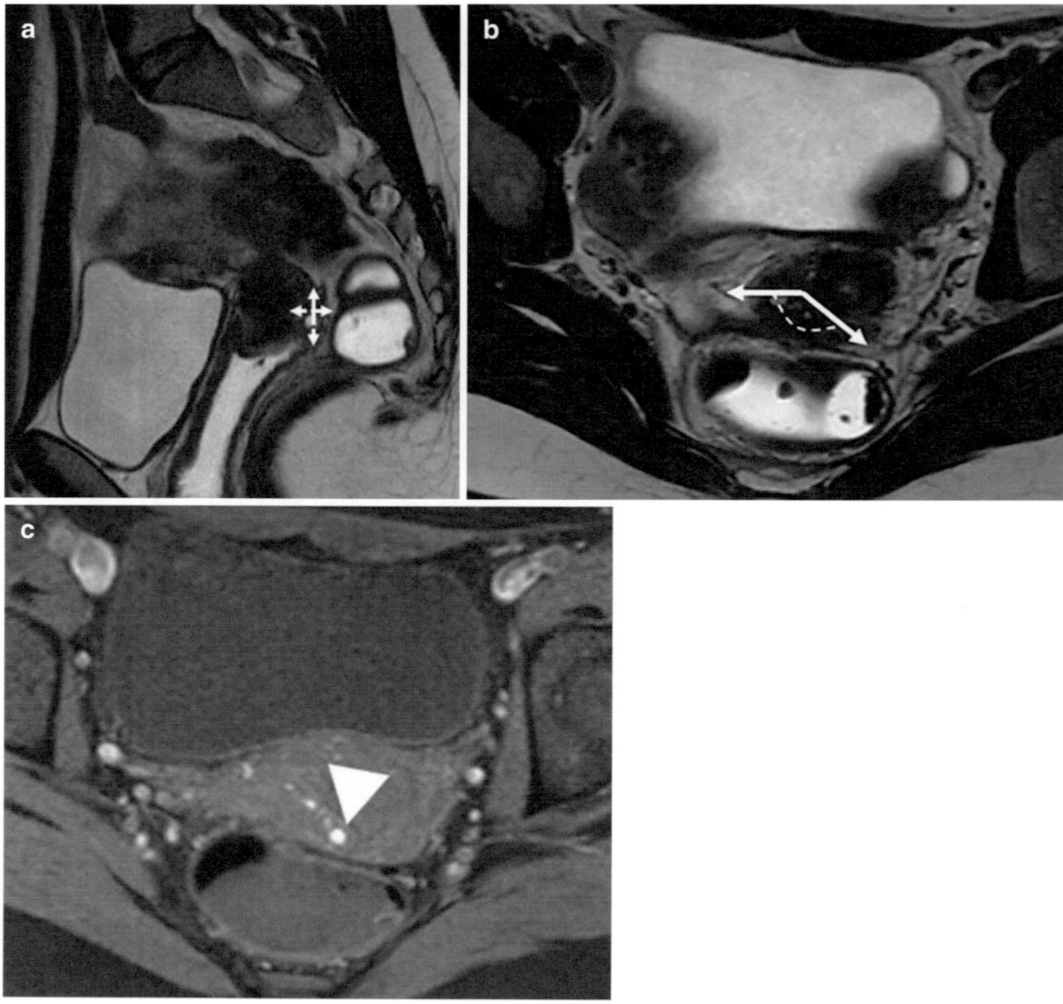

Fig. 7.7 (**a**) Sagittal T2 TSE sequence MRI showing a vaginal posterior nodule with length and thickness. Cystic (hypersignal T2) implants appear in hypersignal T2. (**b**) Axial T2 TSE sequence MRI showing a vaginal posterior nodule with circumference. (**c**) Axial T1 fat-saturated sequence MRI showing hemorrhagic cysts (head arrow) in the vaginal wall

diagnostic accuracy, particularly in less-experienced readers [22]. Today, using sonographic gel for vaginal opacification is considered an optional method for assessing deep pelvic endometriosis [23].

In the literature, MRI demonstrates superior diagnostic performance in detecting vaginal endometriosis compared to ultrasound, especially due to its higher sensitivity [20, 24, 25]. Regarding MR protocol, many techniques are under debate: First, vaginal opacification has been proposed to improve vaginal endometriosis, especially for less-experienced radiologists [22]. Second, other authors have shown that three-dimensional (3D) T2-weighted sequences allowed the better detection of vaginal endometriosis [26]. Third, gadolinium injection has been promoted by some authors, whereas others have demonstrated the absence of added value, regardless of the expertise level of the readers (Fig. 7.8). [27]

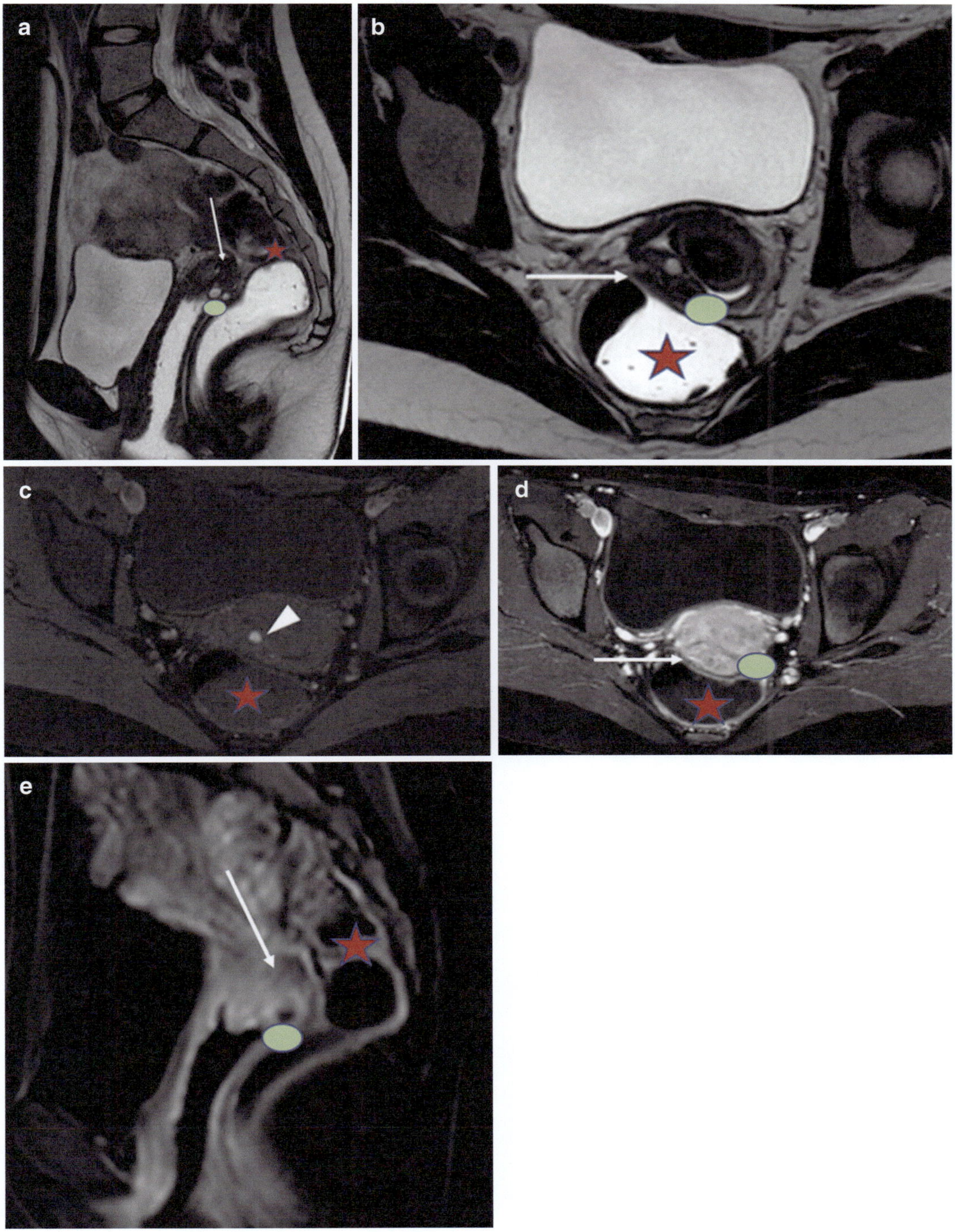

Fig. 7.8 (**a**) Sagittal T2 TSE sequence MRI showing a vaginal posterior nodule (arrow) with cyst implants. (**b**) Axial T2 TSE sequence MRI showing a vaginal posterior nodule (arrow). (**c**) Axial T1 fat-saturated sequence MRI showing hemorrhagic implants (head arrow) in the vaginal wall in hypersignal T1. (**d** and **e**) (axial and sagittal, respectively) Gadolinium-enhanced T1 sequence showing the vaginal nodule of DIE (arrow) enhanced, but it does not improve diagnostic performance. Red star is the rectum; green circle is the vagina

Recently, a large multicentric study was conducted comparing the different protocols for the diagnosis of different DPE locations [28], where the authors demonstrated among a cohort of 571 women that vaginal opacification does not improve the detection of vaginal nodules but decreases the detection of torus/USL nodules. In fact, the distension of the posterior fornix may decrease the fatty rectouterine space, which is really helpful when diagnosing nodules on the torus/USL. In this study, no impact of gadolinium injection was noted, but the number of women who underwent gadolinium injection was low. Finally, a new consensus from the European Society of Urogenital Radiology was reached, where more than 80% of the included experts did not recommend gadolinium injection in this setting (ESUR 2025).

Nabothian cysts are the main differential diagnosis of vaginal endometriosis because they appear as either a single cystic lesion or multiple cystic lesions within the fibrous cervical stroma, appearing contiguous and round with well-defined boundaries [29]. Multiple Nabothian cysts exhibit posterior acoustic enhancement on ultrasound. These cysts demonstrate intermediate or slightly high signal intensity on T1-weighted images and display prominent high signal intensity on T2-weighted images (Fig. 7.9).

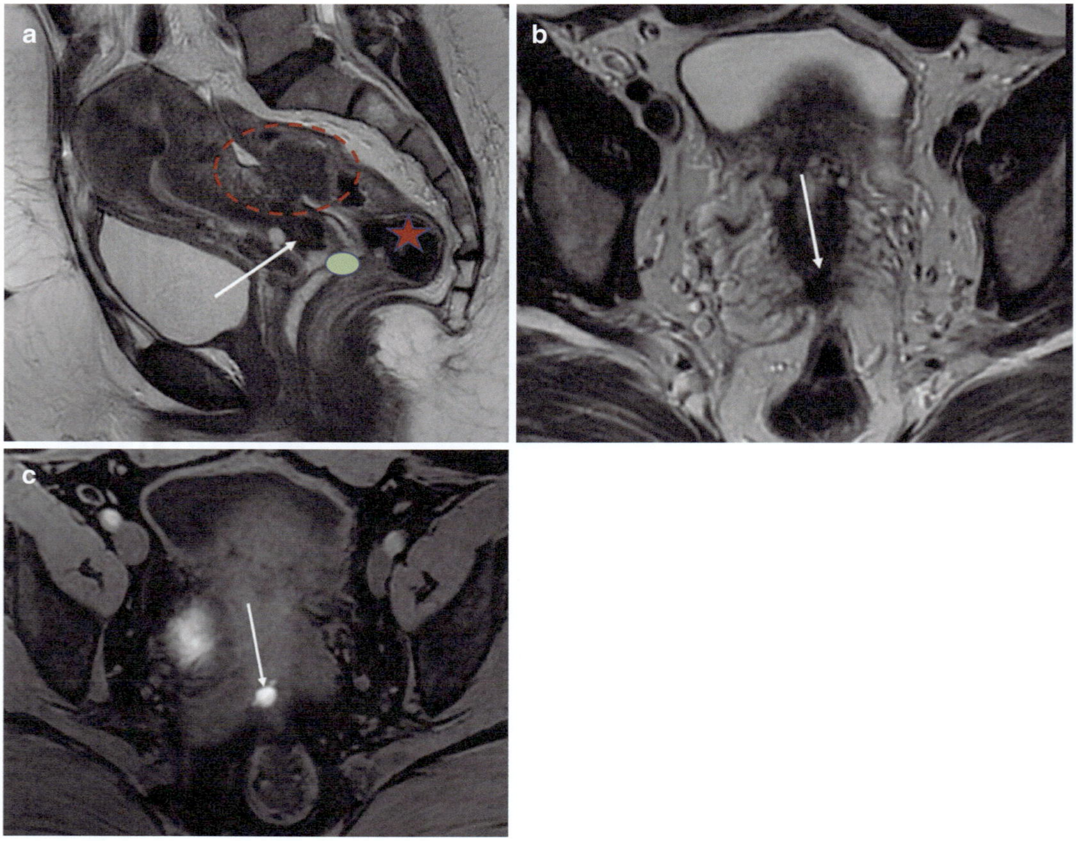

Fig. 7.9 (**a**) Sagittal T2 TSE sequence MRI showing a vaginal posterior nodule (arrow) with an extensive posterior DIE in the rectosigmoid wall junction (red circle). This nodule is a Nabothian cyst. (**b**) Axial T2 TSE sequence MRI showing the vaginal posterior nodule (arrow). (**c**) Axial T1 fat-saturated sequence MRI showing the hypersignal T1 nodule in vagina (Nabothian cyst). Red star is the rectum; green circle is the vagina

7.4.2 Rectovaginal Endometriosis

7.4.2.1 TVUS

On ultrasound, detecting the involvement of the vagino rectal septum (VRS) must be performed in the sagittal view with the vagina in front and the wall of the upper rectum behind. The diagnosis of RVS DIE is performed with the absence of the normal hyperechoic layer between the vagina and rectum, attributed to the presence of a DIE nodule (Fig. 7.10) [8]. The use of sonovaginography improves the detection of RVS DIE (Figs. 7.11 and 7.12) [18, 19]. Usually, RVS involvement is suspected in the presence of extensive endometriosis extending to the torus, uterosacral ligament, vagina, and parametrium.

7.4.2.2 MRI

On MRI, RVS involvement is reflected by the presence of a hyposignal T2 nodule under the reflection of the peritoneum behind the uterine cervix (Fig. 7.13). The dimensions of the RVS DIE nodule should be documented in three orthogonal planes, and the distance between the lower margin of the lesion and the anal verge should be measured. This practice should be followed regardless of whether the DIE is confined solely to the vagina or rectum or if it involves the vagina, RVS, and rectum. The surgical management of low RVS lesions is linked to significant complications, such as fistula formation [6, 25].

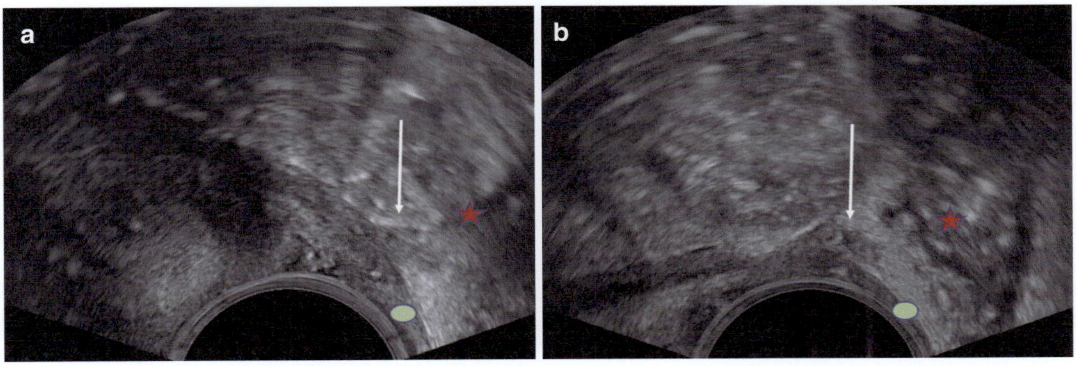

Fig. 7.10 Sagittal (**a**) and coronal (**b**) ultrasound showing a small nodule of DIE in the RVS (white arrow) infiltrating the hyperechoic fat plane of the anterior mesorectum. Red star is the rectum; green circle is the vagina

Fig. 7.11 Coronal (**a**) and sagittal (**b**) sonovaginography showing a nodule of DIE in the RVS (white arrow). Red star is the rectum; green circle is the vagina

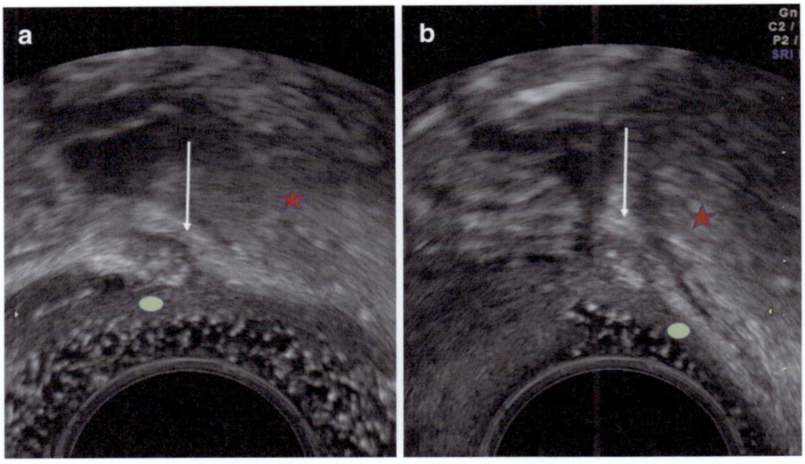

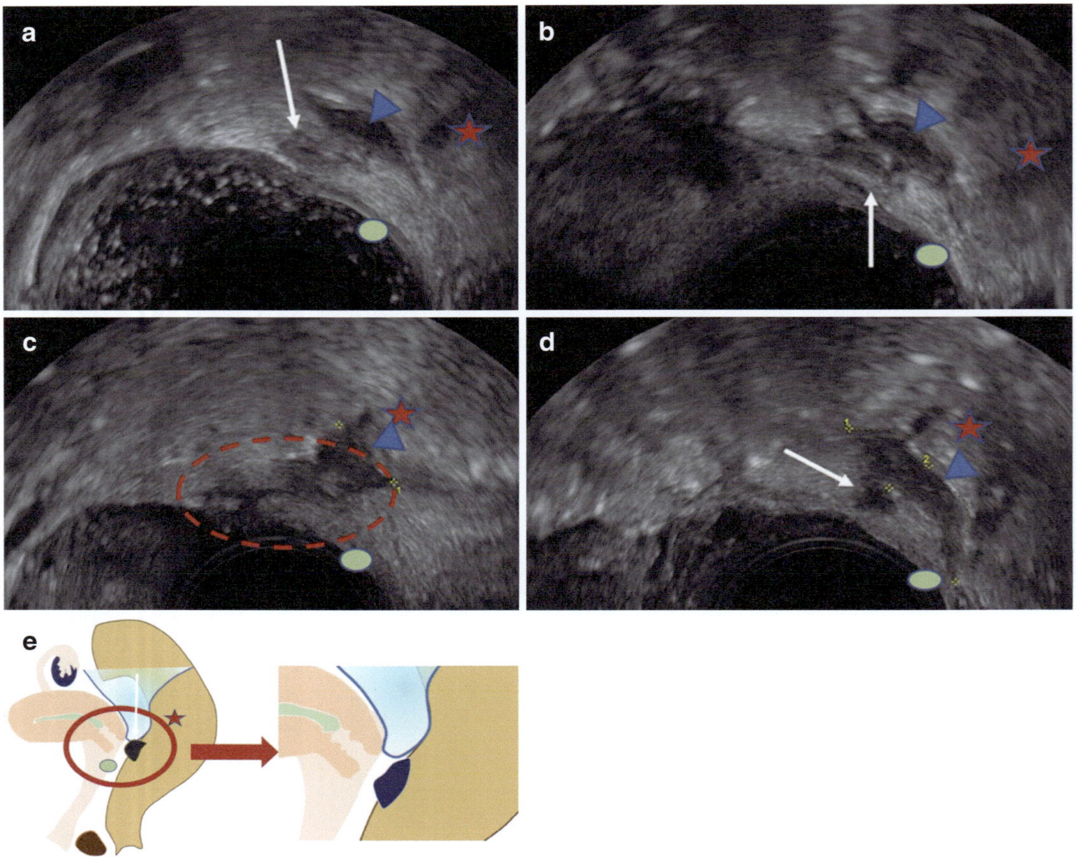

Fig. 7.12 Extensive posterior and lateral DIE via sonovaginography with vaginal gel (**a** and **b**) and ultrasound without vaginal gel (**c** and **d**). It also shows an RVS endometriosis (white arrow) extending to the rectal muscularis (blue head arrow), torus, left uterosacral ligament, and proximal parametrium (red circle). Red star is the rectum; green circle is the vagina

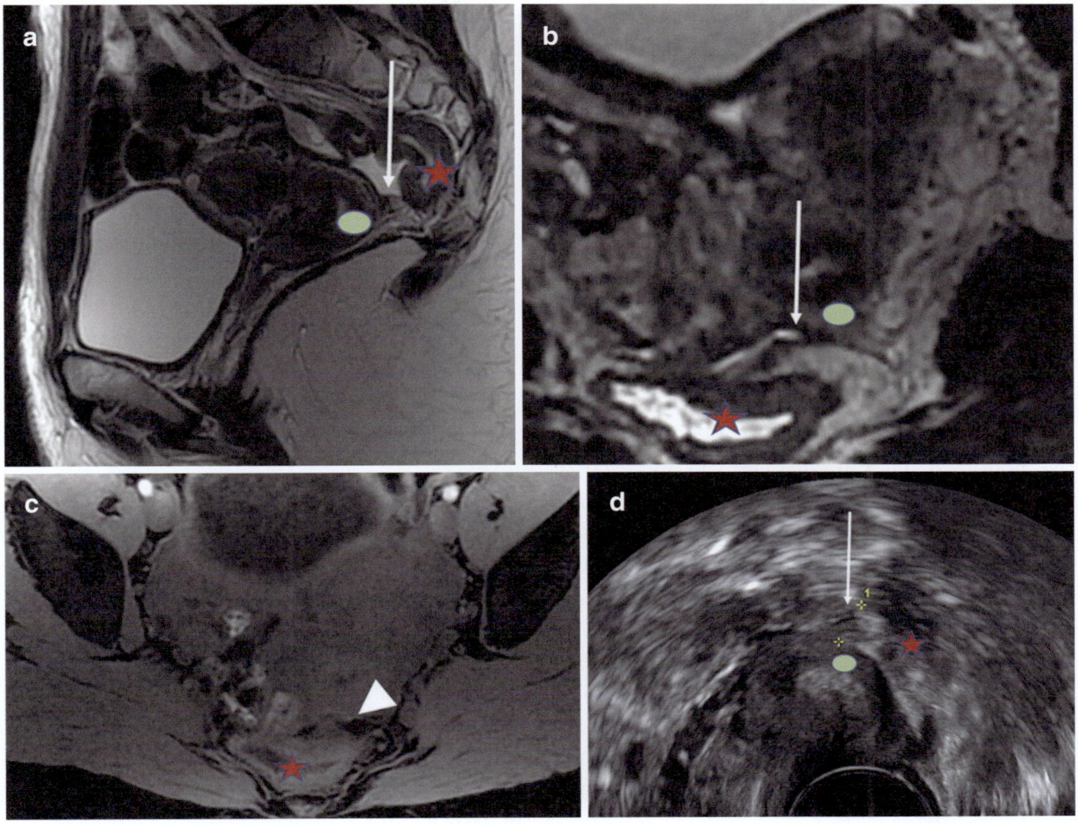

Fig. 7.13 (**a**) Sagittal, (**b**) axial T2 TSE, and (**c**) T1 fat-saturated MRI sequences and (**d**) ultrasound images showing isolated deep infiltrating endometriosis (white arrow) in the rectovaginal septum (RVS). Red star is the rectum; green circle is the vagina. Hemorrhagic implant in RVS on T1 sequence (head arrow). The case of Madame O. This is the case of consulting Miss. O on the management of deep infiltrating endometriosis. She has one child whom she delivered vaginally. She complains mostly about intense invalidating dysmenorrhea with dyspareunia, diarrhea, and painful defecation with rectal bleeding. At physical examination, the speculum examination under general anesthesia had the aspect displayed in Fig. 7.14

7.5 Surgical Management

The following are the key elements to know before surgery for endometriosis involving a vaginal lesion:

1. Regarding the endometriosis, other localizations of the disease, especially rectal endometriosis; its position; the size of the rectal lesion; and the involvement of the anterior compartment.
2. Regarding the vaginal lesion, the total size of the lesion, the size of the lesion completely infiltrating the three layers of the vagina, and the location of the lesion on the vagina.

The gold standard surgical approach for endometriosis resection is the minimally invasive route. Initial exploration in the case of objective vaginal involvement often identifies a filled/inaccessible Douglas pouch. Confirming the infiltrating nature at the vaginal level and the need for colpectomy is often possible after initial adhesiolysis, where bilateral ureterolysis allows for pediculating the lesions on the uterine body.

Surgery on vaginal nodules comes with two main challenges: First, related to the detection of the vaginal location in the posterior fornix, which is crucial on preoperative imaging because the surgery of a vaginal location significantly increases the risk of de novo dysuria [30]. This is why the detection of vaginal endometriosis adds one additional point to the dPEI score. In fact, adjacent to the posterior vaginal fornix are located the fibers of the inferior hypogastric plexus, which forms a triangle with a posterior basis in the rectal fascia and extends anteriorly to the innervate uterus and the bladder. When a vaginal nodule has to be removed, especially when the nodule is laterally located, an increase in nerve injuries occurs. Second, nodules in the rectovaginal septum are related due to the importance of the rectovaginal cleavage. In over 90% of cases, the rectovaginal septum begins below the lower part of the Douglas pouch in line with the middle third of the vagina [31], whereas deep lesions almost always involve the upper third of the vagina. These nodules are not lesions of the rectovaginal septum per se but could deserve the term *rectovaginal* when they infiltrate both the rectum and the vagina.

Surgical access to this area is essential because it allows for identifying potential vaginal involvement on one hand and rectal involvement on the other hand. Thus, successful cleavage is necessary downstream of the lesions (in healthy tissue). Regarding the lesions, two options are available:

1. In **pass "through,"** a portion of the lesions is "left" on the uterine body and the vagina, whereas the other part is left on the rectum. Each lesion is then removed "independently." The use of a vaginal candle allows, on the one hand, for confirming vaginal involvement if it was not clinically transfixing (visible on speculum examination) and, on the other hand, for restricting the portion justifying partial colpectomy. This vaginal "shaving" step is technical, but its mastery limits the indications for colpectomy. This step also determines the depth of the involvement of the layers of the vaginal wall.
2. In the **monobloc approach**, the lesions are medialized progressively, and then cleavage between the lesion and the healthy vagina is performed as described earlier. Partial colpectomy, carrying the transfixing portion, is performed, and the lesion is pediculated on the rectum. The rectovaginal cleavage is then continued downstream of the lesion. The lesion is then excised—with rectal shaving if necessary—to circumscribe the area infiltrating the rectal muscularis, which would justify discoid or segmental resection if it were extensive.

Figures 7.14, 7.15, 7.16, 7.17 and 7.18 illustrate the case of Mrs. O and the correlation between surgery and imaging.

Techniques for tissue interposition to cover vaginal stitching for fistula risk

For a long time, a postoperative stoma was systematically used to decrease the risk of fistula in patients undergoing digestive resection associated or not with vaginal excision. The cohort of 1102 patients reported by Roman et al. included 37 patients with bowel fistulae (3.4%), of whom 23 (62.2%) were found to have rectovaginal fistulae and 14 (37.8%) leakage. The more recent works by Roman et al. [32] have found no difference in the rate of postoperative fistula according to the realization of stoma during surgery. Obviously, improvement in surgical techniques as well as the use of robotic surgery could also have contributed to the decreased risk of postoperative fistula. Also, several techniques have been developed to attempt to reduce the risk of postoperative fistula. Our team reported the technique of tissue interposition of either the mesorectum flap or the prevesical flap to "cover" the site of anastomosis [33]. These techniques are simple to perform, they do not significantly increase the operative duration, and no fistula has been observed in our department since their routine

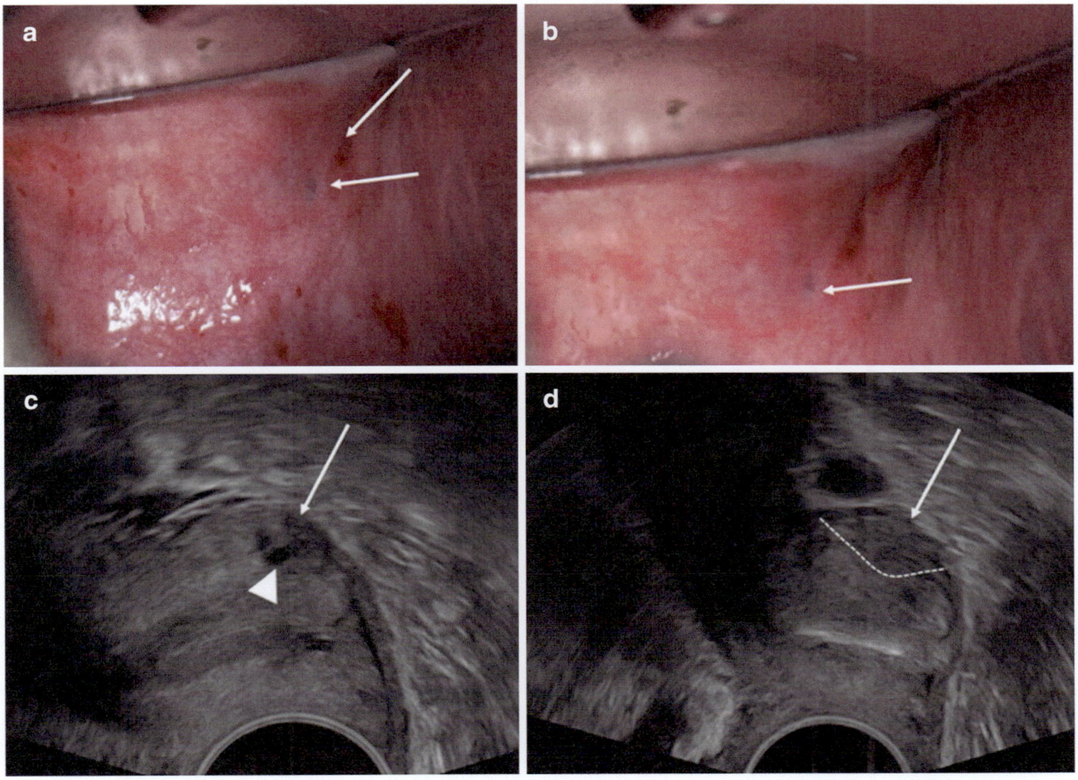

Fig. 7.14 (**a** and **b**) Physical examination with speculum examination showing hemorrhagic cyst red and blue on vaginal wall (arrows). (**c** and **d**) Sagittal endovaginal ultrasound showing the vaginal endometriosis nodule (arrow) with cyst implant (head arrow)

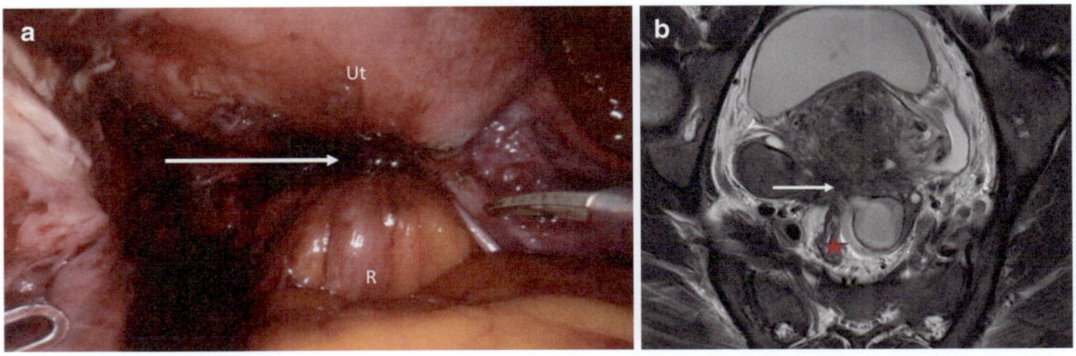

Fig. 7.15 First step of the surgery: exploratory phase with imagery correlation (**a**) Rectal impaction on the posterior face of the uterus. At this moment, vaginal infiltration can be confirmed or evaluated. (**b**) Axial T2 TSE sequence MRI showing the rectal impaction on the posterior face of the uterus (arrow). Red star is the rectum

incorporation in such patients began. Also, radiologists must specify whether infiltration of the mesorectum is or isn't present and the circumference of the rectal lesion, if any, which could limit the availability of such techniques.

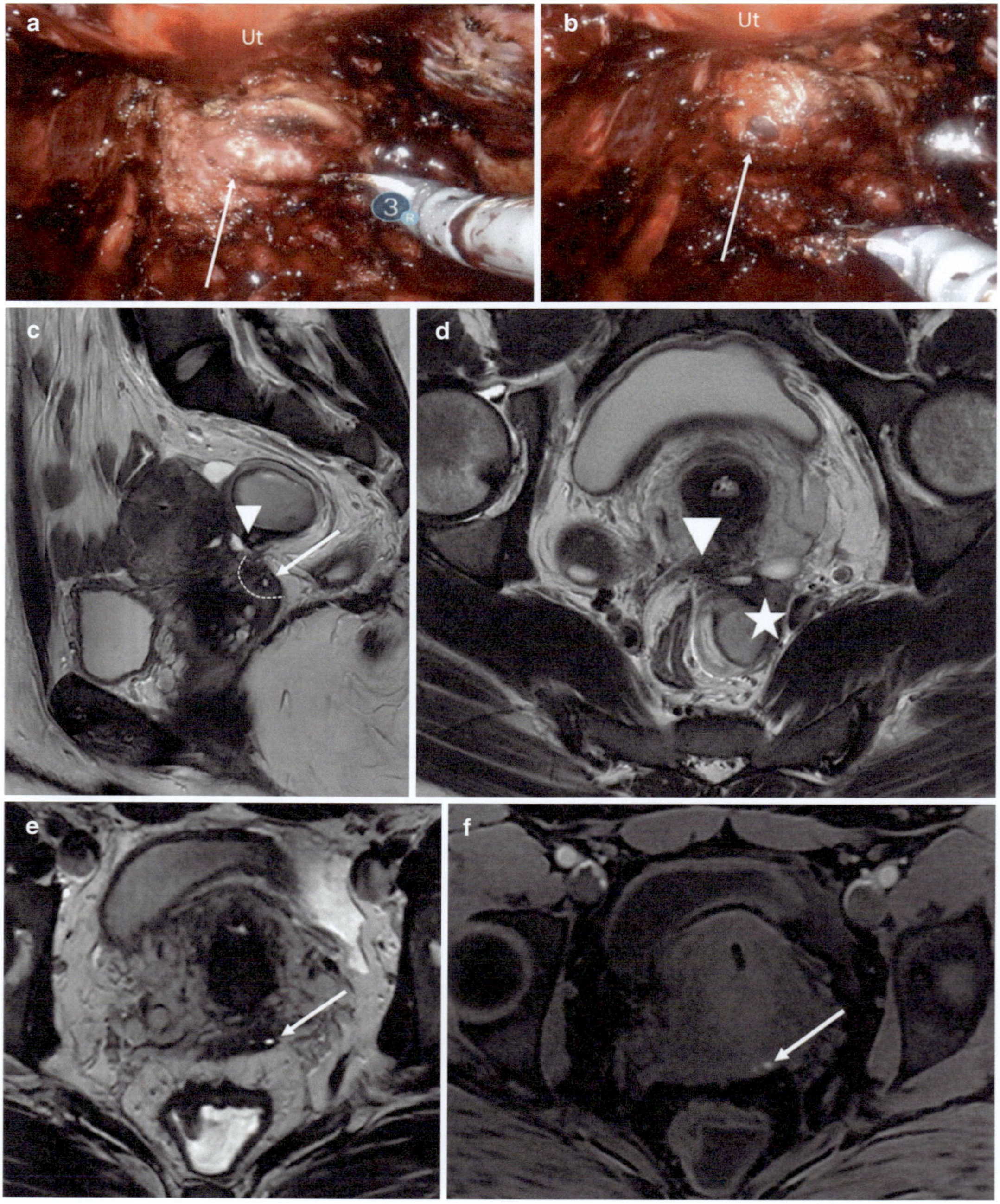

Fig. 7.16 Second step of the surgery with imagery correlation (**a**) Following adhesiolysis and the liberation of the rectum, vaginal shaving is required to delimitate the infiltrating portion. Here, the arrow is pointing to the vaginal exposure thanks to a vaginal. (**b**) The infiltrating portion of the vaginal endometriosis is delimited to allow restricted and tailored colpectomy. (**c**) Sagittal T2 TSE sequence MRI showing a posterior vaginal nodule with cyst implant (arrow). IT shows associated posterior involvement, visible here with a thickening of the torus (head arrow). (**d** and **e**) Axial T2 TSE sequence MRI showing vaginal endometriosis with cyst implant (arrow). It shows the posterior involvement of torus, uterosacral ligaments, and proximal parametrium (head arrow). The left ovary is retracted and adherent to the uterus with an endometrioma (star). (**f**) Axial T1 fat-saturated sequence MRI showing vaginal endometriosis with hemorrhagic implants (arrow)

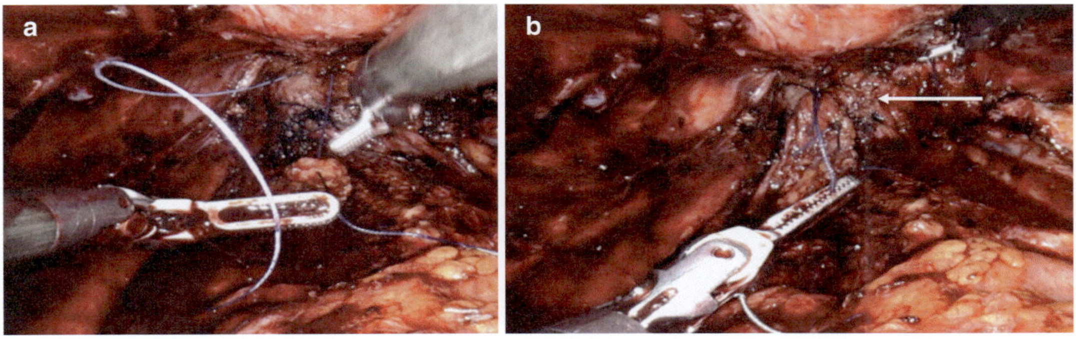

Fig. 7.17 The last step of surgery To decrease the risk of postoperative fistula when patients undergo concomitant rectal resection, several techniques have been attempted. In this case, the mesorectum flap is used to cover the vaginal stitches (**a** and **b**) and avoid having the two scars (vaginal and rectal) face each other

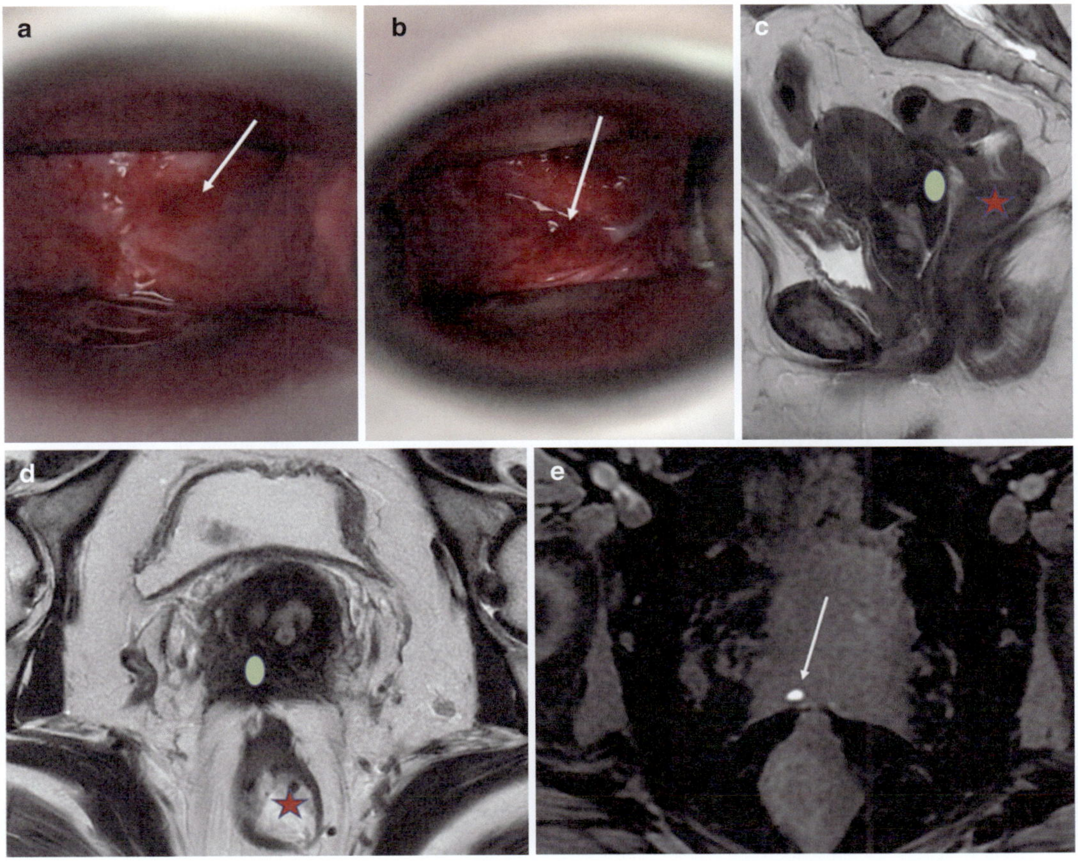

Fig. 7.18 The case of Madame S. with vaginal endometriosis involvement (**a** and **b**) Physical examination with speculum examination showing hemorrhagic cyst red and blue on vaginal wall (arrows). (**c** and **d**) Sagittal and axial T2 TSE showing the vaginal endometriosis nodule (green circle) with cyst implant (arrow) on axial T1 Fat-Sat (FS). Red star is the rectum. (**e**) Axial T1 FS with vaginal hemorrhagic cyst

7.6 Conclusion

Vaginal endometriosis presents unique diagnostic and surgical challenges due to its often-extensive involvement with surrounding structures, such as the rectovaginal septum, rectum, and uterosacral ligaments. Preoperative diagnosis is essential to anticipate surgical difficulties, improve excision quality, and tailor patient counseling. Clinical examination, although highly specific, has limited sensitivity and must be complemented by imaging techniques like TVUS and MRI for accurate diagnosis.

Surgical management prioritizes minimally invasive approaches, paying particular attention to preserving nerve function and minimizing the risk of postoperative complications such as fistula. Advanced imaging and surgical techniques continue to evolve, improving outcomes for patients with this complex condition.

References

1. Chapron C, Fauconnier A, Vieira M, et al. Anatomical distribution of deeply infiltrating endometriosis: surgical implications and proposition for a classification. Hum Reprod. 2003;18(1):157–61. https://doi.org/10.1093/humrep/deg009.
2. Bazot M, Darai E, Hourani R, et al. Deep pelvic endometriosis: MR imaging for diagnosis and prediction of extension of disease. Radiology. 2004;232(2):379–89. https://doi.org/10.1148/radiol.2322030762.
3. Leonardi M, Singh SS, Murji A, et al. Deep endometriosis: a diagnostic dilemma with significant surgical consequences. J Obstet Gynaecol Can. 2018;40(9):1198–203. https://doi.org/10.1016/j.jogc.2018.05.041.
4. Kondo W, et al. Complications after surgery for deeply infiltrating pelvic endometriosis. BJOG. 2011;118(3):292–8. PubMed. Accessed January 7, 2024. https://pubmed.ncbi.nlm.nih.gov/21083863/.
5. Bazot M, Detchev R, Cortez A, Amouyal P, Uzan S, Daraï E. Transvaginal sonography and rectal endoscopic sonography for the assessment of pelvic endometriosis: a preliminary comparison. Hum Reprod. 2003;18(8):1686–92. https://doi.org/10.1093/humrep/deg314.
6. Martin DC, Batt RE. Retrocervical, retrovaginal pouch, and rectovaginal septum endometriosis. J Am Assoc Gynecol Laparosc. 2001;8(1):12–7. https://doi.org/10.1016/s1074-3804(05)60543-9.
7. Guerriero S, Condous G, van den Bosch T, et al. Systematic approach to sonographic evaluation of the pelvis in women with suspected endometriosis, including terms, definitions and measurements: a consensus opinion from the International Deep Endometriosis Analysis (IDEA) group. Ultrasound Obstet Gynecol. 2016;48(3):318–32. https://doi.org/10.1002/uog.15955.
8. Reid S, Condous G. The issues surrounding the pre-operative TVS diagnosis of rectovaginal septum endometriosis. Australas J Ultrasound Med. 2014;17(1):2–3. https://doi.org/10.1002/j.2205-0140.2014.tb00082.x.
9. Bazot M, Thomassin I, Hourani R, Cortez A, Darai E. Diagnostic accuracy of transvaginal sonography for deep pelvic endometriosis. Ultrasound Obstet Gynecol. 2004;24(2):180–5. https://doi.org/10.1002/uog.1108.
10. Agarwal SK, Chapron C, Giudice LC, et al. Clinical diagnosis of endometriosis: a call to action. Am J Obstet Gynecol. 2019;220(4):354.e1–354.e12. https://doi.org/10.1016/j.ajog.2018.12.039.
11. Soliman AM, Fuldeore M, Snabes MC. Factors associated with time to endometriosis diagnosis in the United States. J Womens Health (Larchmt). 2017;26(7):788–97. https://doi.org/10.1089/jwh.2016.6003.
12. Koninckx PR, Meuleman C, Oosterlynck D, Cornillie FJ. Diagnosis of deep endometriosis by clinical examination during menstruation and plasma CA-125 concentration*†. Fertil Steril. 1996;65(2):280–7. https://doi.org/10.1016/S0015-0282(16)58086-8.
13. Bazot M, Lafont C, Rouzier R, Roseau G, Thomassin-Naggara I, Daraï E. Diagnostic accuracy of physical examination, transvaginal sonography, rectal endoscopic sonography, and magnetic resonance imaging to diagnose deep infiltrating endometriosis. Fertil Steril. 2009;92(6):1825–33. https://doi.org/10.1016/j.fertnstert.2008.09.005.
14. Becker CM, et al. ESHRE guideline: endometriosis. Hum Reprod Open. 2022;2022(2):hoac009. PubMed. Accessed February 1, 2024. https://pubmed.ncbi.nlm.nih.gov/35350465/.
15. Roditis A, Florin M, Rousset P, et al. Accuracy of combined physical examination, transvaginal ultrasonography, and magnetic resonance imaging to diagnose deep endometriosis. Fertil Steril. 2023;119(4):634–43. https://doi.org/10.1016/j.fertnstert.2022.12.025.
16. Bazot M, Daraï E, Biau DJ, Ballester M, Dessolle L. Learning curve of transvaginal ultrasound for the diagnosis of endometriomas assessed by the cumulative summation test (LC-CUSUM). Fertil Steril. 2011;95(1):301–3. https://doi.org/10.1016/j.fertnstert.2010.08.033.
17. Hudelist G, Oberwinkler KH, Singer CF, et al. Combination of transvaginal sonography and clinical examination for preoperative diagnosis of pelvic endometriosis. Hum Reprod. 2009;24(5):1018–24. https://doi.org/10.1093/humrep/dep013.

18. Saccardi C, Cosmi E, Borghero A, Tregnaghi A, Dessole S, Litta P. Comparison between transvaginal sonography, saline contrast sonovaginography and magnetic resonance imaging in the diagnosis of posterior deep infiltrating endometriosis. Ultrasound Obstet Gynecol. 2012;40(4):464–9. https://doi.org/10.1002/uog.11102.
19. Dessole S, Farina M, Rubattu G, Cosmi E, Ambrosini G, Nardelli GB. Sonovaginography is a new technique for assessing rectovaginal endometriosis. Fertil Steril. 2003;79(4):1023–7. https://doi.org/10.1016/s0015-0282(02)04952-x.
20. Thomassin-Naggara I, Lamrabet S, Crestani A, et al. Magnetic resonance imaging classification of deep pelvic endometriosis: description and impact on surgical management. Hum Reprod. 2020;35(7):1589–600. https://doi.org/10.1093/humrep/deaa103.
21. Rousset P, Florin M, Bharwani N, et al. Deep pelvic infiltrating endometriosis: MRI consensus lexicon and compartment-based approach from the ENDOVALIRM group. Diagn Interv Imaging. 2023;104(3):95–112. https://doi.org/10.1016/j.diii.2022.09.004.
22. Chassang M, Novellas S, Bloch-Marcotte C, et al. Utility of vaginal and rectal contrast medium in MRI for the detection of deep pelvic endometriosis. Eur Radiol. 2010;20(4):1003–10. https://doi.org/10.1007/s00330-009-1627-8.
23. Bazot M, Bharwani N, Huchon C, et al. European society of urogenital radiology (ESUR) guidelines: MR imaging of pelvic endometriosis. Eur Radiol. 2017;27(7):2765–75. https://doi.org/10.1007/s00330-016-4673-z.
24. Hottat N, Larrousse C, Anaf V, et al. Endometriosis: contribution of 3.0-T pelvic MR imaging in preoperative assessment--initial results. Radiology. 2009;253(1):126–34. https://doi.org/10.1148/radiol.2531082113.
25. Del Frate C, Girometti R, Pittino M, Del Frate G, Bazzocchi M, Zuiani C. Deep retroperitoneal pelvic endometriosis: MR imaging appearance with laparoscopic correlation. Radiographics. 2006;26(6):1705–18. https://doi.org/10.1148/rg.266065048.
26. Bazot M, Stivalet A, Daraï E, Coudray C, Thomassin-Naggara I, Poncelet E. Comparison of 3D and 2D FSE T2-weighted MRI in the diagnosis of deep pelvic endometriosis: preliminary results. Clin Radiol. 2013;68(1):47–54. https://doi.org/10.1016/j.crad.2012.05.014.
27. Bazot M, Gasner A, Lafont C, Ballester M, Daraï E. Deep pelvic endometriosis: limited additional diagnostic value of postcontrast in comparison with conventional MR images. Eur J Radiol. 2011;80(3):e331–9. https://doi.org/10.1016/j.ejrad.2010.12.006.
28. Thomassin-Naggara I, Zoua CS, Bazot M, et al. Diagnostic MRI for deep pelvic endometriosis: towards a standardized protocol? Eur Radiol. 2024;34(12):7705–15. https://doi.org/10.1007/s00330-024-10842-0.
29. Park SB, et al. Multilocular cystic lesions in the uterine cervix: broad spectrum of imaging features and pathologic correlation. AJR Am J Roentgenol. 2010;195(2):517–23. PubMed. Accessed February 25, 2024. https://pubmed.ncbi.nlm.nih.gov/20651212/.
30. Kondo W, Bourdel N, Tamburro S, et al. Complications after surgery for deeply infiltrating pelvic endometriosis. BJOG. 2011;118(3):292–8. https://doi.org/10.1111/j.1471-0528.2010.02774.x.
31. Kuhn RJ, Hollyock VE. Observations on the anatomy of the rectovaginal pouch and septum. Obstet Gynecol. 1982;59(4):445–7.
32. Roman H, Braund S, Hennetier C, et al. Combined cystoscopic-abdominal vs. abdominal only route for complete excision of large deep endometriosis nodules infiltrating the supratrigonal area of the bladder: a comparative study. J Minim Invasive Gynecol. 2024;31(4):295–303. https://doi.org/10.1016/j.jmig.2024.01.007.
33. Hini JD, Ferrier C, Owen C, et al. Interposing lateral pelvic peritoneum between the vaginal and digestive scares during a surgical colorectal resection for endometriosis, without associated hysterectomy. Gynecol Obstet Fertil Senol. 2020;48(5):457–9. https://doi.org/10.1016/j.gofs.2020.03.004.

8 Mediocentral Compartment: Uterus: External Adenomyosis

Rosemarie Forstner

8.1 Introduction

Adenomyosis and endometriosis are defined by the presence and growth of ectopic endometrial tissue (glands and stroma) within the myometrium or outside of the uterus, respectively [1, 2]. They present the benign, estrogen-dependent conditions of uncertain pathogenesis, sharing both histological and clinical features [3]. Affected women are of premenopausal age and often suffer from considerable impairment to their quality of life and reproductive dysfunction [4]. Overlapping symptoms constitute chronic pelvic pain, dysmenorrhea, dyspareunia, and abnormal uterine bleeding [5, 6]. However, as has been well documented, approximately 30% of women with proven adenomyosis or endometriosis may remain asymptomatic [7, 8].

Although most authors consider adenomyosis and endometriosis as separate conditions, other authors rather consider these as different phenotypes of the same disease [9, 10]. Adenomyosis comprises a spectrum of diseases that present with different phenotypes [2, 3, 11]. Hypothesized mechanisms to induce adenomyosis include autotraumatization with chronic injury and tissue repair at the junctional zone (JZ), metaplasia of stem cells from Mullerian remnants, and retrograde menstruation with the migration of ectopic endometrial cells [2].

Internal adenomyosis can present as a focal lesion or as diffuse lesions in the inner myometrium or can replace the entire myometrium, with or without surrounding the hypertrophied myometrium [12]. External adenomyosis is limited to the outer myometrium, and it may result from endometriosis growing through the uterine serosa into the uterus. This "from the outside to the inside" theory has been supported by the presence of the site- specific phenotypes of posterior and anterior focal adenomyosis [13].

The strong association between deep infiltrative endometriosis (DIE) and adenomyosis ranging from approximately 20–50% has been confirmed both in imaging studies and in hysterectomy specimens [14–16]. Of note, the recently recognized entity of posterior external adenomyosis is almost always seen in association with DIE in the posterior compartment or with DIE of the gastrointestinal system [17].

R. Forstner (✉)
Department of Radiology, University Hospital Salzburg, Paracelsus Medical University, Salzburg, Austria
e-mail: R.Forstner@salk.at

I. Thomassin-Naggara (ed.), *Imaging of Endometriosis: A Comparative Guide of US, MRI and Surgery*, https://doi.org/10.1007/978-3-031-82750-1_8

8.2 General Aspects of External Adenomyosis

Synonyms or often interchangeably used terms: external adenomyosis, extrinsic adenomyosis, anterior or posterior focal adenomyosis, deep infiltrative endometriosis of the uterus, serosal implants of the uterus in DIE, subtype 2 adenomyosis in the Kishi classification, and subtype 3 in the Morphological Uterus Sonographic Assessment (MUSA) classification of adenomyosis

Adenomyotic areas in the outer periphery of the uterus that are discontinuous from the junctional zone have been introduced into the MR imaging literature as a separate entity of external respectively extrinsic adenomyosis [18–20]. Whether it presents a manifestation of deep infiltrative endometriosis with serosal and outer myometrial involvement or whether it is rather a subtype of adenomyosis that is closely linked with deep infiltrating endometriosis remains a matter of debate [2, 5, 18, 19, 21–23]. Most publications of MRI findings in the gynecologic literature favor the term *extrinsic adenomyosis* over *external adenomyosis*. A synonymous entity often described in association with DIE is focal adenomyosis of the outer myometrium (FOAM) [13].

The term *external adenomyosis* is not used explicitly in the US literature, but it is an element of the US scoring system published by Lazzeri et al. [24]. In 2019, the MUSA (Morphological Uterus Sonographic Assessment) group published a uniform US classification and reporting system to be used for describing morphological variations of adenomyosis and its extent [25] (Fig. 8.1a, b). Adenomyosis is stratified by the anterior and posterior locations and by its location within different layers of the myometrium. External adenomyosis with the involvement of the outer myometrium constitutes the type 3 subtype [11, 25].

Clinical presentation, histopathology, and cell biology insights underline the close association between external adenomyosis and deep endometriosis [3]. Biomarker expression analysis on epithelial cell markers and stromal cell markers also links external adenomyosis to DIE, whereas internal adenomyosis seems to present a distinct entity [26].

The pathognomonic feature of external adenomyosis is the presence of endometrial glands and stroma with muscular reactive hyperplasia within the outer myometrium, and the junctional zone is not involved [3, 27]. Typical are damage to the uterine surface and the extension of adenomyosis from the outer periphery toward the inner myometrium [20]. In contradistinction to internal adenomyosis, the junctional zone is intact. However, external adenomyosis can also occur with other phenotypes of adenomyosis [4, 18].

The site of the uterine involvement defines the presence of external adenomyosis as an anterior type or a posterior type [18]. In lateral deep pelvic endometriosis, concomitant external adenomyosis may be found along the lateral uterine walls [3, 23].

Different mechanisms of pathogenesis have been postulated for internal adenomyosis and for external adenomyosis as well as for posterior external adenomyosis and for anterior external adenomyosis [3, 20, 28]. Most authors agree that posterior external adenomyosis results from the secondary invasion of endometrial implants through the uterine serosa to the outer myometrium [2, 5, 11, 27]. Furthermore, the coexistence of DIE and external adenomyosis has shown to present an independent risk for complications in laparoscopic surgery for deep endometriosis [29]. Thus, knowing their sites; extent, including the depth of myometrial involvement; and severeness is an important criterion for treatment decisions [5, 27].

8.2.1 Posterior External Adenomyosis

Posterior external adenomyosis constitutes the vast majority (>90%) of external adenomyosis, and it is typically seen in younger age and in nulligravid women [17, 19]. It is located in the posterior subserosal myometrium and is typically associated with DIE of the posterior compart-

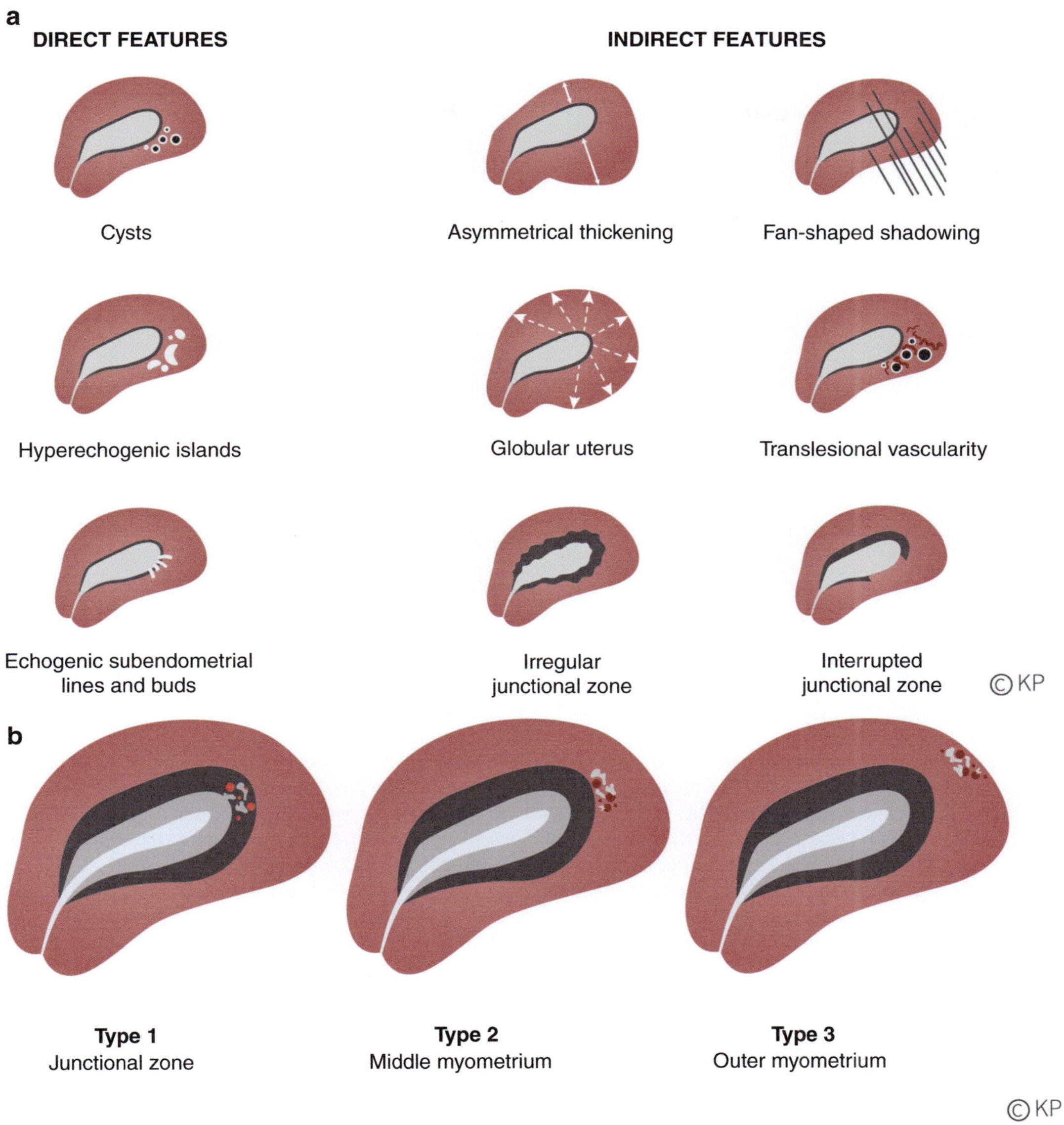

Fig. 8.1 MUSA criteria for TVUS of adenomyosis. (**a**) Schematic display of Morphological Uterus Sonographic Assessment (MUSA) features of uterine adenomyomas. Adapted from Harmsen et al. [12]. (**b**) Uterine layer infiltration according to the sonographic classification and reporting system for diagnosing adenomyosis. Adapted from van den Bosch et al. [25]

ment and with ovarian endometriomas [12, 17, 30] (Fig. 8.2). In this setting, endometriomas are large and carry a high risk of recurrence after surgery, in both the early period and a later follow-up period [17]. In one study, the rate of external adenomyosis in patients with recurrent endometrioma was as high as 48% [17]. DIE lesions associated with external adenomyosis involve the rectum, the pouch of Douglas, or the upper vagina; tend to be multiple and large; and are associated with higher American Society of Reproductive Medicine (ASRM) scores [5, 17]. In a series of 100 patients with large (>3 cm) deep endometriotic nodules at vaginal examina-

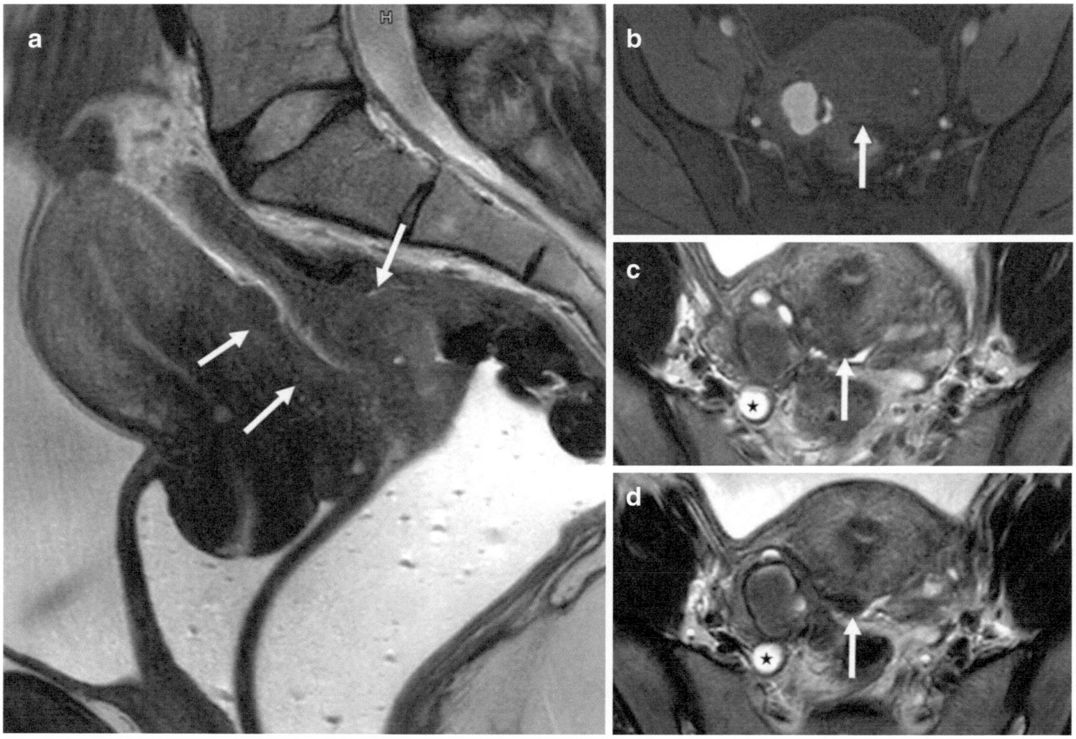

Fig. 8.2 Posterior external adenomyosis associated with extensive DIE of the rectum, posterior fornix, and bilateral endometriomas with retractile fibrosis. Sagittal T2 (**a**) and transaxial T2WIs at two levels (**c** and **d**) show external adenomyosis as an ill-defined low-SI mass at the outer cervix and uterus (arrow in **c**) with a well-delineated nodule at its superior aspect (arrow in d) that is associated with DIE of the anterior wall of the rectum (arrow in **a**). On T1 FS (**b**), no hemorrhagic elements are seen in external adenomyosis in contradistinction to the adjacent endometriomas. Dilated right ureter (*)

tion, posterior external adenomyosis was found in 97% [31]. Compared to women with internal adenomyosis, women with external adenomyosis tend to be younger and more likely to show coexisting endometriosis, more severe pain, and fertility impairment [17, 32]. This was also confirmed by a study correlating various clinical data, MRI features, and histopathological findings obtained via endoscopy in different types of adenomyosis and recurrent endometriomas. The external type of adenomyosis was found significantly more often (48%) than other types of adenomyosis were. In 233 patients with recurrent endometriosis, the external type, the intrinsic type, the indeterminate type (according to the Kishi classification) and no adenomyosis were reported in 112, 55, 47, and 66 patients, respectively [17]. The duration of antihormonal treatment was also longer for the patients with external adenomyosis [17]. External myometrial adenomyosis, typically associated with multiple and more-extensive manifestations of DIE, has been reported as a poor prognostic criterion and indicative of extensive surgery [27].

8.2.2 Anterior External Adenomyosis

Compared to the posterior type, anterior external adenomyosis is much rarer, at 5–8% [18]. It is less commonly associated with endometriomas and seems also less commonly linked with DIE of the bladder and gastrointestinal tract. The association of DIE of the anterior compartment is high and ranges from 50% to 94% [33–35].

Particularly, when evaluating DIE of the bladder or of the proximal round ligaments, the coex-

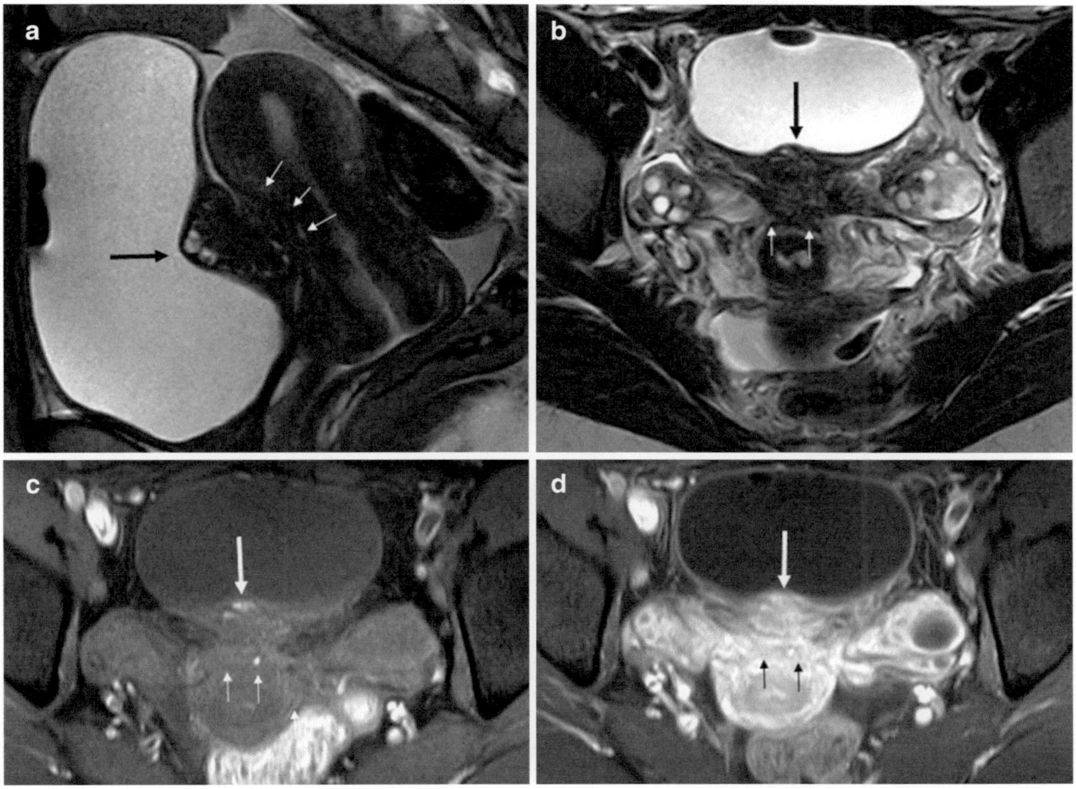

Fig. 8.3 MRI of anterior external adenomyosis associated with DIE of bladder. Sagittal and transaxial T2WIs show a nodule (arrow) with an impression in the bladder wall in continuity with an ill-defined bandlike lesion of the adjacent outer myometrium (thin arrows) that is 2 cm in length. T2WIs demonstrate predominantly low-SI and small peripheral hyperintense foci (**a** and **b**). Some of these have high SI on T1 FS, typical of hemorrhagic contents (**c**). Gadolinium (Gd) T1 FS shows contrast enhancement of both DIE and external adenomyosis (**d**)

istence of both entities should be carefully investigated [21, 34]. Anterior external adenomyosis manifests as predominantly fibrous lesions with an hourglass configuration, in contiguity with DIE of the bladder dome, or next to subperitoneal DIE nodules along the uterovesical junction [35]. Sizes range from 9 to 50 mm, with a mean size of 24 ± 14 mm [34]. Typically, the outer myometrium is involved, though growth to the junctional zone is rare [35] (Fig. 8.3). In a study of 32 patients with DIE of the bladder, anterior external adenomyosis was found in 68%, but only 18% (4/32) had adenomyosis extending to the junctional zone [34]. Rousset et al. underlined the importance of reporting the depth of myometrial invasion (including the distance to the endometrial cavity) and differentiated between moderate and severe types [34]. This information may be relevant in surgery planning—e.g., for the prediction of the feasibility of complete resection or for estimating the risk of recurrence [34]. In one small series, a more aggressive surgery featuring the excision of the myometrium resulted in a significantly lower risk of recurrence for bladder endometriosis [36].

8.3 Imaging Findings in External Adenomyosis

External adenomyosis refers to deep infiltrating endometriosis that arises within the subserosal myometrium and extends more or less toward the inner myometrium, but with an inconspicuous junctional zone. It is characterized by ill-defined nodular masses, where the epicenter in the outer myometrium displays the imaging characteristics of adenomyomas/focal adenomyosis, and in the vast majority of cases, it is in proximity to other deep infiltrating endometrioses in the anterior or, more commonly, is in the posterior compartment or adjacent to ovarian endometriomas [17, 19]. The depth of myometrial thickness involvement by the adenomyotic nodules corresponds to a *moderate* manifestation (limited to the subserosal external myometrium), and an extension up to the junctional zone corresponds to a *severe* manifestation [34] (Fig. 8.4).

External adenomyosis can be isolated or found in combination either with other benign uterine

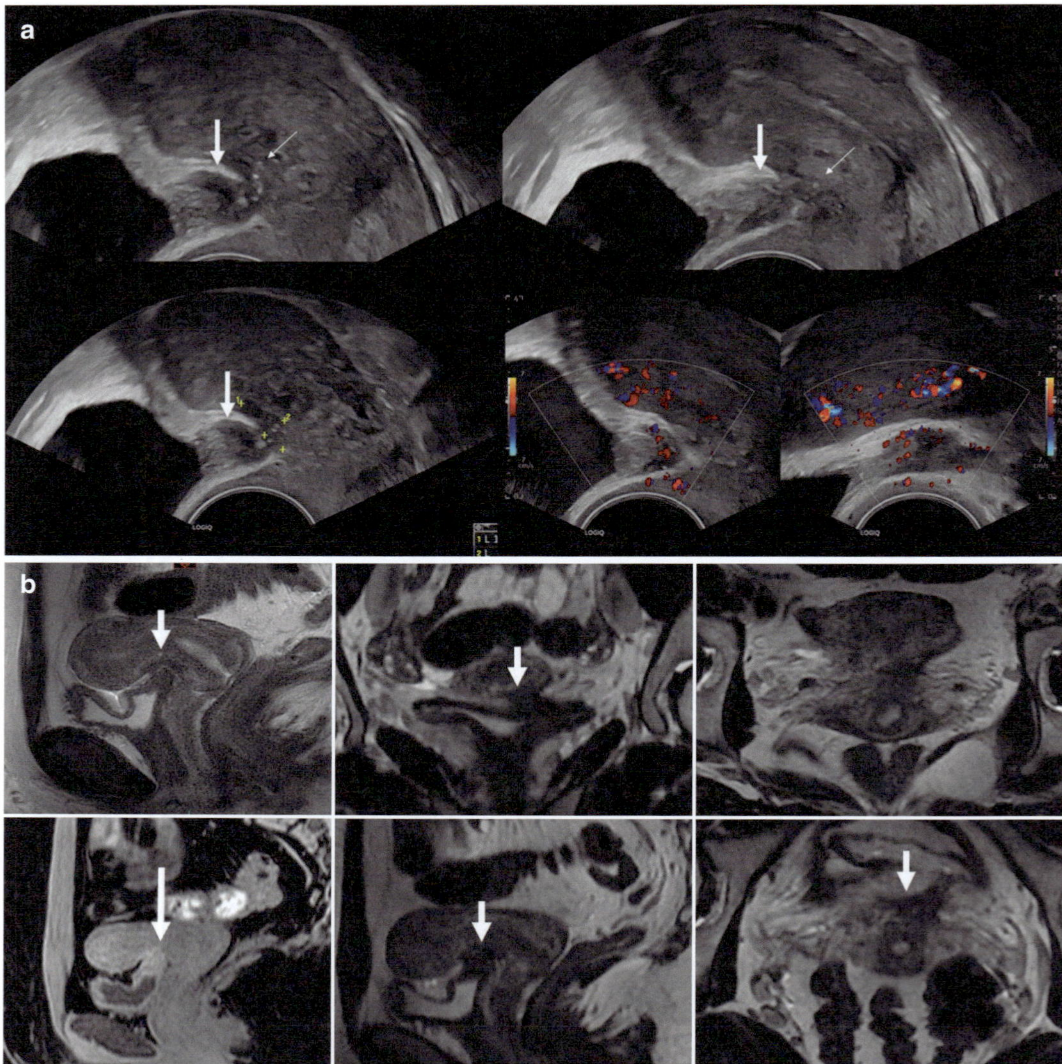

Fig. 8.4 A 29-year-old presenting with dysuria and chronic pelvic pain. US and MRI show DIE of the bladder in continuity with anterior external adenomyosis. (**a**) TVUS shows DIE of the posterior third of the bladder dome and the left uterovesical pouch (arrow) extending to the outer myometrium, which displays an ill-defined outer margin (thin arrow). This corresponds to a moderate manifestation of external adenomyosis. (**b**) DIE presents as a low-SI lesion along the posterior third of the bladder and the left uterovesical pouch with continuous extension to the outer uterine contour (arrow). It displays low SI on multiplanar T2WIs and is slightly hyperintense on T1FS (long arrow)

conditions, such as internal adenomyosis, including diffuse adenomyosis and adenomyoma, or with leiomyomas [18, 33]. In an MRI series of 100 patients presenting with large DIE and external posterior adenomyosis, the posterior aspect of the uterus and the cervix were involved more often (39% and 40%, respectively) than the cervicovaginal area (20%), whereas external adenomyosis involving both the uterus and the cervix was seen in only 1% [31].

In anterior external adenomyosis, involvement with DIE may be continuous with DIE, typically of the bladder along the vesicouterine pouch, or no direct communication may be seen [35].

8.3.1 MRI Findings in External Adenomyosis

The MRI features of external adenomyosis include a focal irregular thickening of the anterior or the posterior outer contour of the uterus with/without its extension to the inner myometrium but with an intact JZ [18, 27] (Figs. 8.5 and 8.6). External adenomyosis is considered a location of deep infiltrating endometriosis in the mediocentral compartment [27]. It is best visualized on sagittal T2-weighted images (T2Wis) as a solid mass of the outer myometrium (Figs. 8.3 and 8.5). Due to its low signal intensity (SI) on

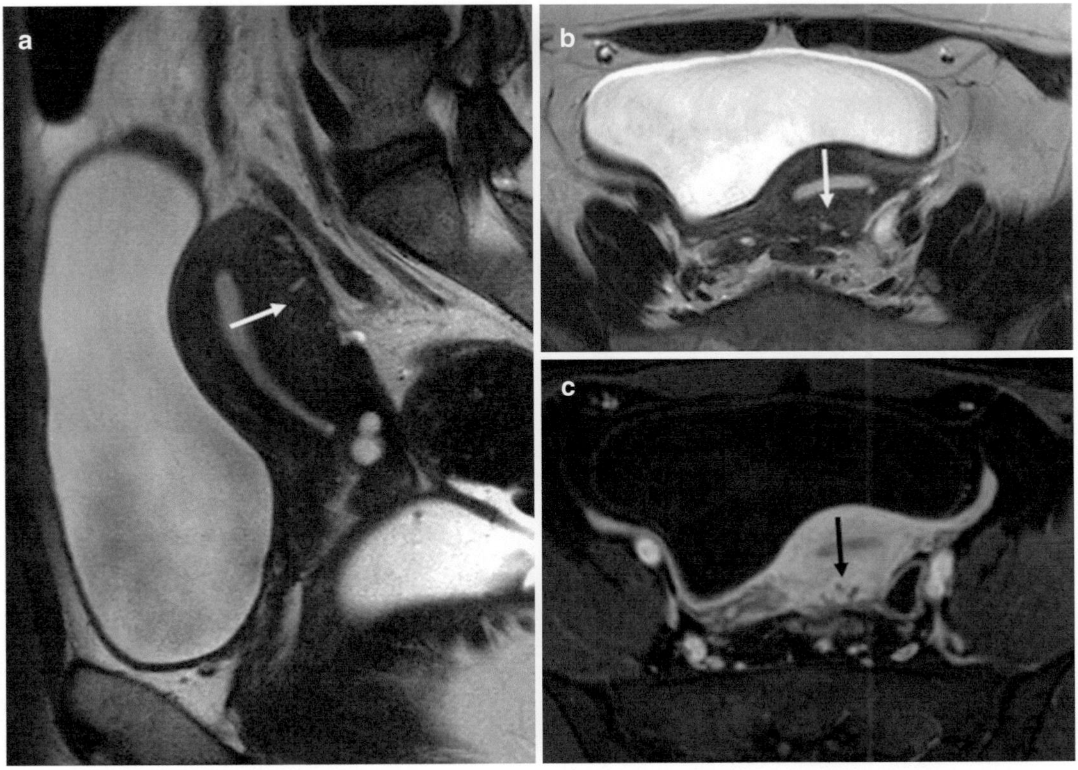

Fig. 8.5 A 34-year-old with history of surgery for endometriomas and DIE in the posterior compartment. Sag T2 WI shows diffuse thickening of the posterior uterine wall and a normal junctional zone (**a**). External adenomyosis (arrow) is slightly hyperenhancing on the Gd T1FS image (**c**) and is poorly defined toward the inner myometrium on sagittal and transaxial T2 images (a and b) and displays peripheral linear cystic areas. The outer contour is irregular and adhesions to the adjacent rectum are seen (**b** and **c**)

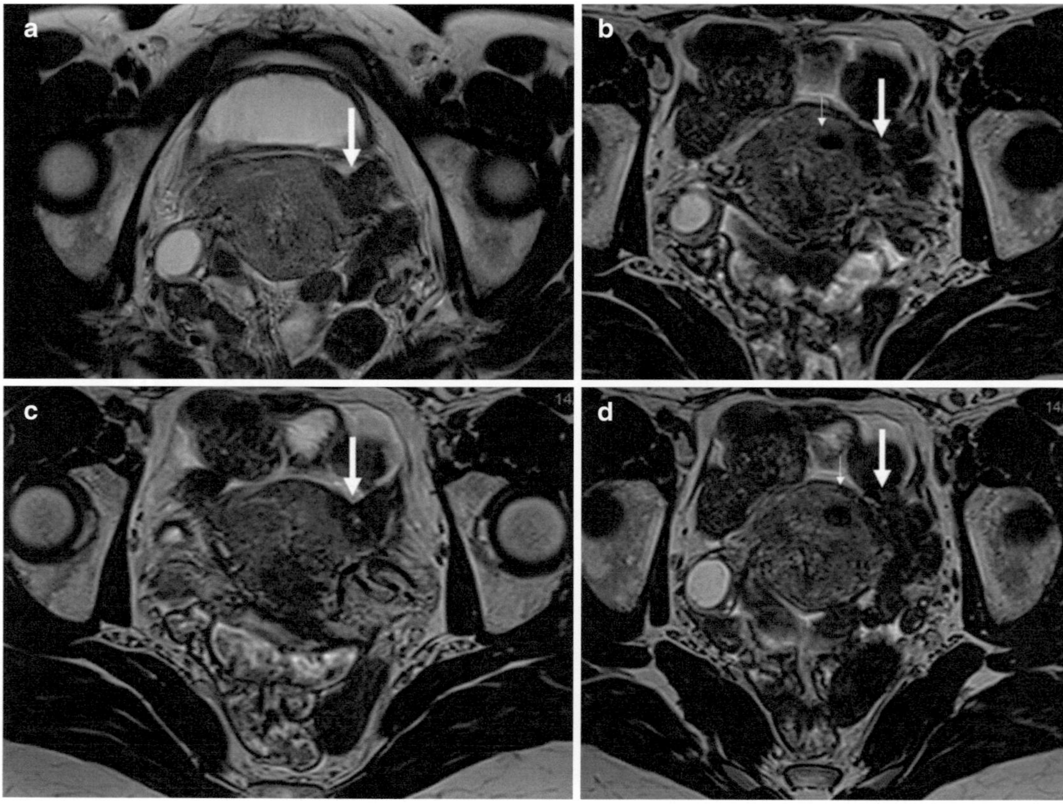

Fig. 8.6 External adenomyosis and unilateral endometriosis of round ligament in a 40-year-old female with history of surgery for endometriosis. Transaxial T2WIs show left sided thickening of the central aspect of the left round ligament. The adjacent outer uterus shows a hypointense bandlike lesion of low SI (arrow). The other myometrium is unremarkable except for a well-delineated mural leiomyoma (small arrow)

T2WIs, differentiating it from adjacent fibrous endometriotic plaques in the anterior or posterior compartment may be difficult [27]. In contrast to uterine leiomyomas, the margins are not well delineated. Furthermore, heterogeneous borders and myometrial cysts may be seen in external adenomyosis (Figs. 8.5 and 8.7) [18]. These range from 2 to 9 mm in size, and they may display high SI on T2WIs and may display T1 hyperintense hemorrhagic foci. The high SI of blood on T1 and on T1 fat saturation (FS) presents a highly specific feature of adenomyosis [37] (Fig. 8.7).

A high association exists between posterior external adenomyosis and deep endometriosis of the rectum, and the cul-de-sac is obliterated in most cases [17, 19]. A tear-drop deformity of the usually round contour of the rectum due to endometriotic adhesions is frequently seen in coexistence with external adenomyosis [19] (Fig. 8.8).

Typical of anterior external adenomyosis is a T2 hypointense nodular mass with ill-defined borders on the outer myometrium at the level of uterine isthmus with or without continuity with DIE of the adjacent bladder [35]. In contrast, external adenomyosis may be associated with deep infiltrating endometriosis involving the bladder basis, the vesicouterine pouch, or the pouch of Douglas and thus would be associated with a high risk of surgery [38, 39].

According to the ENDOVALIRM lexicon and classification, external adenomyosis is consid-

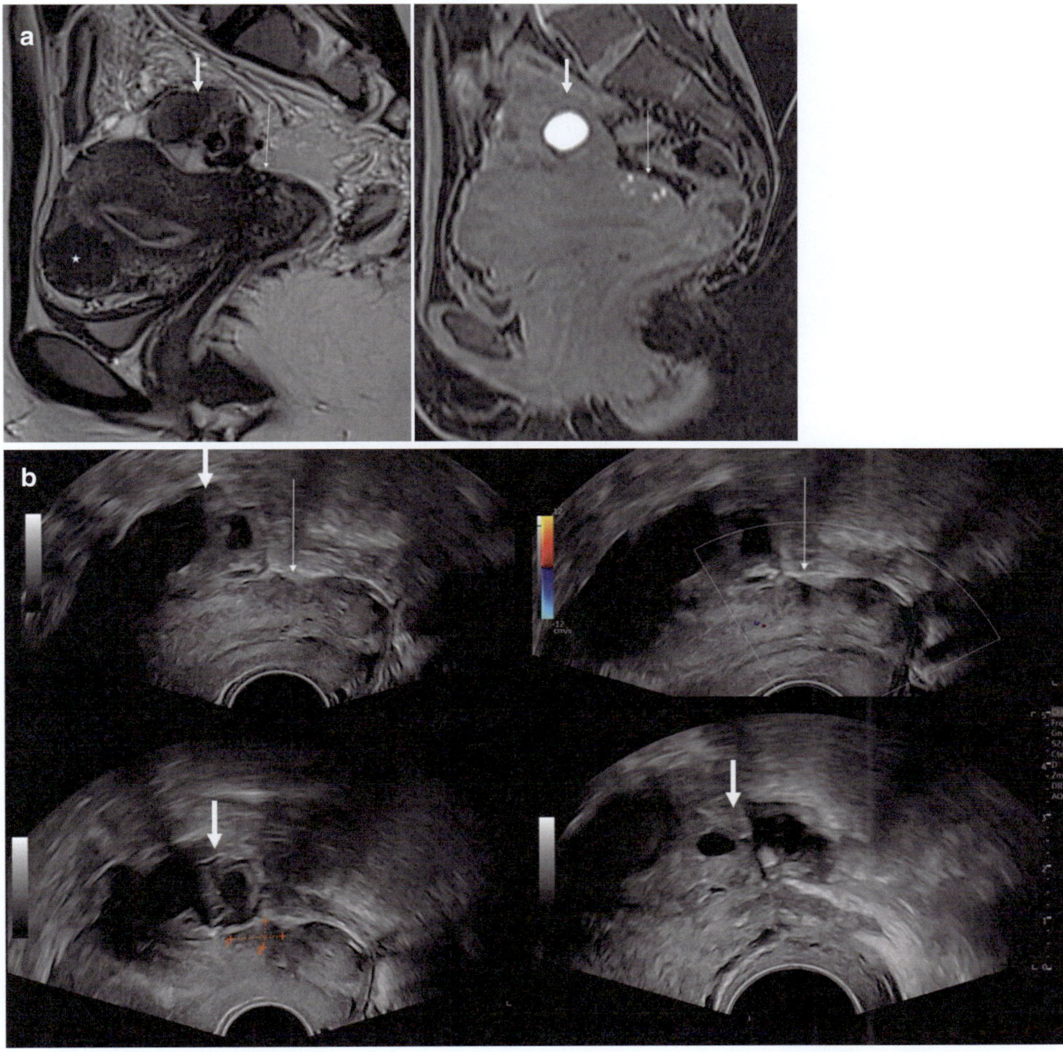

Fig. 8.7 MRI (**a**) and TVUS (**b**) in in a 39-year-old woman with posterior external adenomyosis and endometrioma with history of infertility, chronic pelvic pain, and dyspareunia. (**a**) Sagittal T2-weighted fat-saturated images (T2WFSIs) and T1-weighted fat-saturated images (T1SFSIs) show an endometrioma in the retrouterine location (arrow). The posterior aspect of the adjacent torus uterinus shows irregular contours on T2WIs (long arrow). High-SI foci on T1 FS (long arrow) representing hemorrhagic elements facilitate the diagnosis of external adenomyosis. (**b**) The corresponding TVUS also demonstrates the irregular contour at the posterior outer shell of the uterus. It is hypopvascular on color Doppler imaging (long arrow). See also the endometrioma (arrow)

ered as a location in the mediocentral compartment and counts as one point for either type of location (anterior or posterior location) [27, 39]. This location was described in the ENDOVALIRM cohort in 27.4% (166/605) of women, including the posterior location in 72%, the anterior location in 21%, and anteroposterior nodules in 7%. External adenomyosis was associated with internal adenomyosis in only 27.1% (45/166) of cases, whereas internal adenomyosis was associated with external adenomyosis in 31.4% (45/143). These elements support the theory that internal adenomyosis and external adenomyosis are different diseases.

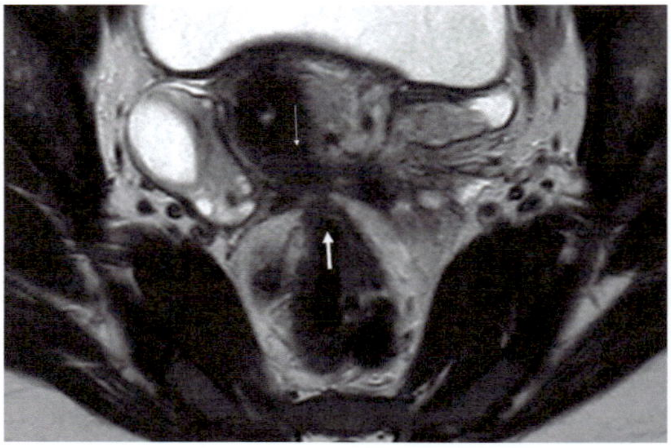

Fig. 8.8 Tear-drop deformity of the rectum. A tear-drop deformity of the rectum (arrow) is shown adjacent to external adenomyosis (thin arrow) and DIE of the uterosacral ligaments

8.3.2 Differential Diagnosis

The hallmark of an internal adenomyosis diagnosis is a thickness of the junctional zone (JZ) that is at least 12 mm (Figs. 8.9 and 8.10). However, the thickness of the junctional zone as a single criterion should be used with caution because this criterion is only an indirect sign of the disease (a reaction to the abnormal location of endometrial tissue in the myometrium) [18]. This sign has a sensitivity between 63% and 70% and a specificity between 88% and 96% [40–42]. The only specific direct sign of internal adenomyosis is the presence of hemorrhagic cysts with high

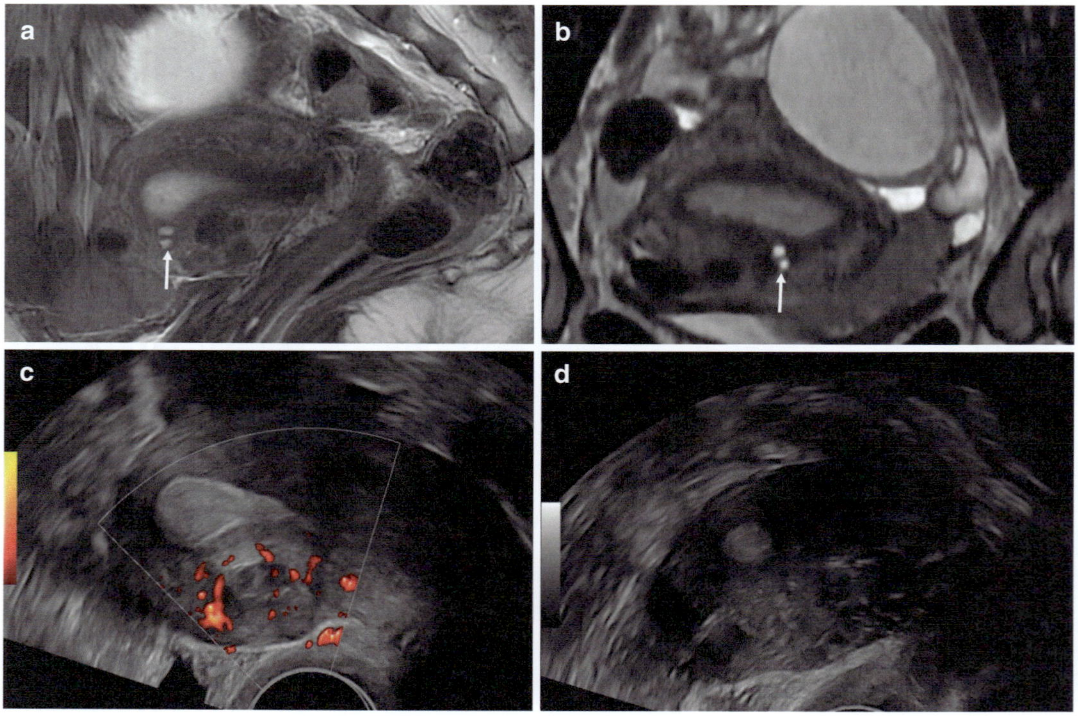

Fig. 8.9 Internal adenomyosis and mural leiomyomas of the anterior uterine wall shown on MRI and TVUS. Internal adenomyosis is characterized as a thickening of the junctional zone and high-SI foci seen on T2WIs (arrow). Adjacent well-delineated low-SI mural nodules present leiomyomas (**a** and **b**). Due to the coexistence of leiomyomas, the differentiation of these entities is more challenging in TVUS. The anterior uterine wall is asymmetrically widened, and an ill-delineated junctional zone and hyperechogenic areas can be identified (**d**). Translesional vascularity is typical for adenomyosis, and leiomyomas may be surrounded by vessels (**c**)

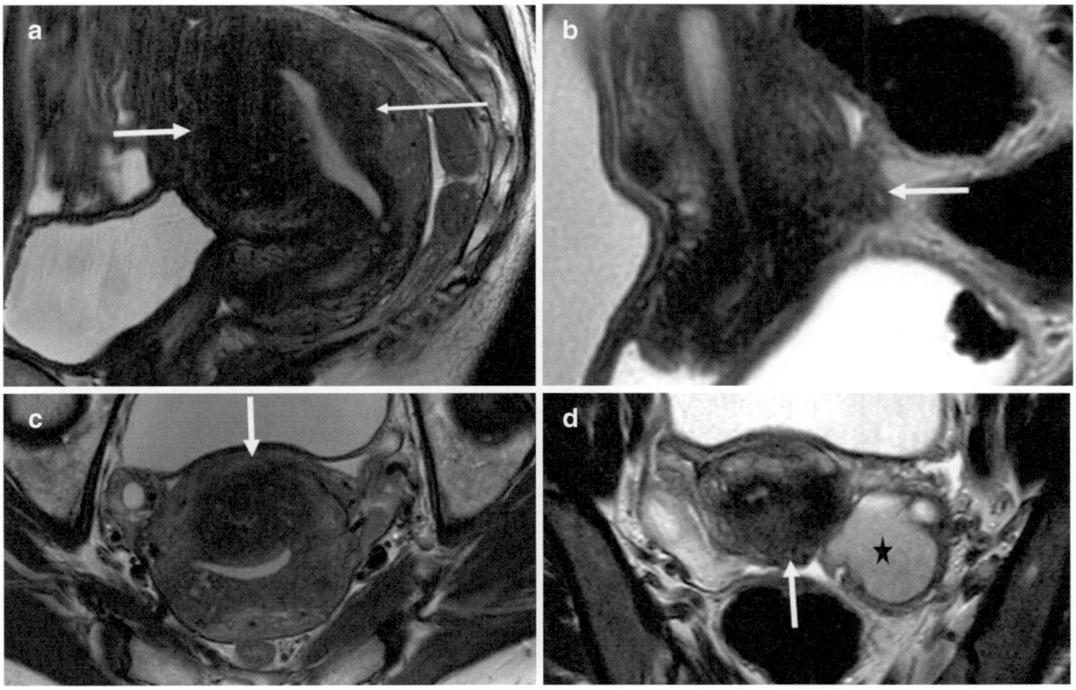

Fig. 8.10 Different types of adenomyosis in two female patients. Sagittal and transaxial T2WIs demonstrate an adenomyoma of the anterior wall and internal adenomyosis of the posterior wall (arrows in **a** and **c**). The adenomyoma is well delineated toward the outer myometrium, and the posterior junctional zone is irregularly thickened (**c**). Both are of low SI on T2WIs and display small areas of high SI. Posterior external adenomyosis adjacent to an endometrioma (*) is shown (**b** and **d**). It is located within and along the posterior contour of the uterus. It is poorly defined and displays low SI extending to near the junctional zone (**d**)

T1-weighted (T1W) signal or cysts with high T2W signal in the myometrium. This feature of tiny disseminated myometrial cysts or hemorrhagic foci has a sensitivity of 50% and a specificity of 98% [40–42]. Thus, in the absence of this direct sign, additional indirect signs are needed to affirm internal adenomyosis. This includes focal/diffuse myometrial bulkiness and/or the ratio of a junctional zone/myometrium thickness of more than 40%, and it includes a difference of the junctional zone thickness (JZ maximum–JZ minimum) that is greater than 5 mm [18, 40, 43]. The latter yielded a sensitivity of 70% and a specificity of 85% for adenomyosis [41]. Internal adenomyosis is described as focal or diffuse with a symmetrically or asymmetrically thickened myometrium.

Another form of internal adenomyosis is named adenomyomas. Although the imaging features of the mass on T1WIs and T2WIs may be similar, adenomyomas present as ill-delineated adenomyotic masses that are contained within the uterine wall (Fig. 8.10). This entity corresponds to focal adenomyosis and does not have true borders. They may display some mass effect, but even at large sizes, their mass effect to adjacent structures is small—e.g., the uterine cavity is smaller in leiomyomas. Moreover, in focal adenomyosis or leiomyoma, myometrial vessels go through the lesion. Subserosal adenomyomas may present with similar imaging features as those of external adenomyosis. The differentiation from leiomyomas is crucial because during hysteroscopic resection, the absence of borders may mislead the surgeon and risk uterine perforation.

Leiomyomas in subserosal or outer myometrial locations can be clearly distinguished due to their strong delineation, their evident mass effect, and the presence of peripheral vessels that are not seen in adenomyomas. The "claw sign" and bridging vessels are other imaging features assisting in their differentiation [44]. *Myometrial contraction* that is a common physiological phenomenon can mimic pathological conditions such as focal or sometimes diffuse internal or external adenomyosis. Regarding external adenomyosis, it appears as a pseudonodular T2-hypointense aspect at the level of the serosa. The key finding to differentiate between these conditions is to compare T2WIs from two different planes to assess for partial or complete resolution, as contractions typically improve or resolve between sequences.

8.3.3 US Findings in External Adenomyosis

External adenomyosis was introduced into the MRI literature as focal adenomyosis of the outer myometrium associated with DIE. No larger series assessing the role of US in external anterior or posterior adenomyosis exists [18]. However, external adenomyosis is within the range of transvaginal ultrasonography (TVUS) findings seen in DIE, particularly with advanced manifestations of posterior compartment DIE [19, 31]. Di Donato et al. reported a prevalence of adenomyosis of 21.8% in 1618 cases of surgically proven endometriosis [45]. Thus, when assessing deep endometriosis, a specific search for the presence of this new category of adenomyosis should be performed. This issue has recently been integrated in the ENZIAN classification, which provides a comprehensive assessment of endometriosis and associated findings and incorporates the general presence of adenomyosis [46]. External adenomyosis corresponds to type 3 in the TVUS classification of adenomyosis in the Morphological Uterus Sonographic Assessment (MUSA) classification (Fig. 8.1). Here, myometrial layer involvement constitutes one of the seven categories, and the myometrium is divided into inner (type 1), middle (type 2), and outer (subserosal, type 3) layers [18, 25].

US findings indicative of external adenomyosis constitute focal adenomyosis at the outer uterine shell (Fig. 8.11). They manifest as adenomyotic

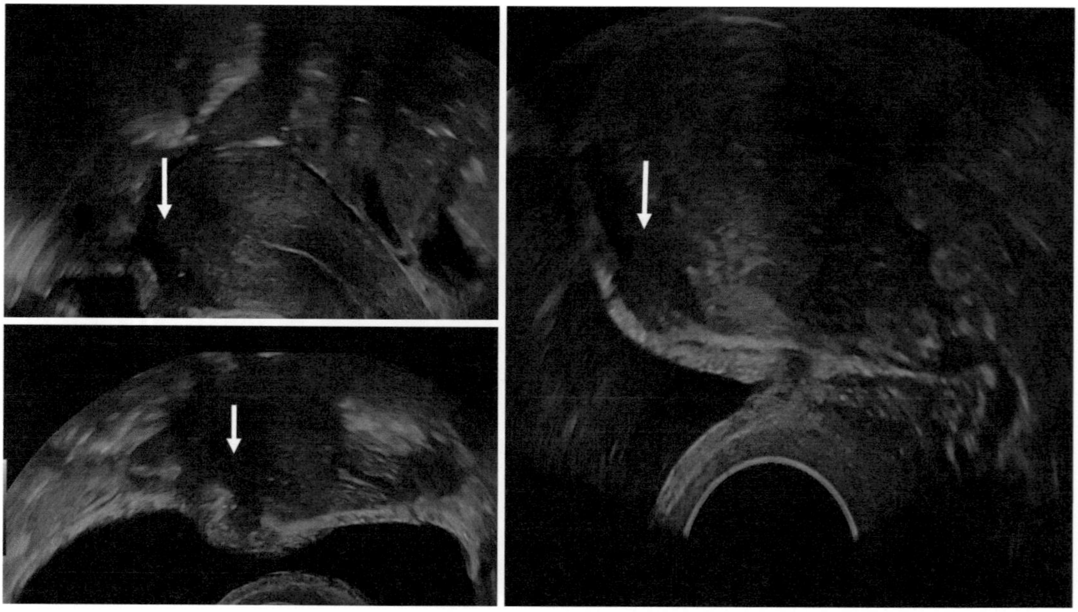

Fig. 8.11 TVUS in the external anterior of the uterus in a 32-year-old female patient with history of chronic pelvic pain, dysuria, and dyspareunia. The TVUS image of anterior external adenomyosis shows an ill-defined elliptical hypoechoic mass of the outer anterior myometrium displaying uterine and extrauterine extension (arrow). The bladder and uterovesical pouch were unremarkable

lesions with an elliptical shape and ill- defined margins [47]. Furthermore, outer myometrial border irregularities and heterogeneity on power Doppler analysis may be identified, and myometrial cysts and radial vessels may also be identified [18, 48]. In posterior external adenomyosis, hypoechoic infiltrative, spherical infiltrative, or nodular areas in the outer uterine wall may be seen adjacent to DIE of the rectum or DIE of the rectovaginal pouch or large endometriomas (Fig. 8.7). Exacoustos et al. reported the ultrasound features of 43 adolescents with adenomyosis and found that the posterior uterine wall (58%) and the outer myometrial layer (93%) were the most commonly affected areas. Furthermore, in 44% of this population, at least one site of pelvic endometriosis was also seen [49]. Particularly, in extensive posterior deep endometriosis, a meticulous assessment of the outer contour of the uterus is warranted [18]. Typical sites to search for external adenomyosis include the posterior inferior aspect of the uterus and the cervix and less commonly the cervicovaginal junction [31]. External adenomyosis may also be seen adjacent to large endometriomas [17]. Furthermore, the question mark sign in combination with the clinical finding of uterine tenderness has shown to be strongly associated with DIE and adenomyosis [48, 50]. The question mark sign correlates with the position of the uterus fixed in retroflexion and is caused by adhesions and DIE lesions as well as adenomyosis of the posterior uterus [51]. Other findings include the obliteration of the pouch of Douglas and the attachment of the posterior uterine wall to DIE. At this level, the absence of the organ-sliding phenomenon of the adjacent structures will be found [49].

Anterior external adenomyosis can be diagnosed in irregular hypoechoic lesions of the outer myometrium surface at the level of the inferior uterine segment (Fig. 8.4). It is often seen in combination with foci of DIE of the bladder dome, of the vesicouterine pouch, or of the round ligaments.

8.3.4 Differential Diagnosis

8.3.4.1 Focal Internal Adenomyosis and Adenomyoma

Diffuse expansion with indistinct margins of the JZ toward the adjacent myometrium is the hallmark of adenomyosis. Less commonly, focal adenomyosis can be found, either isolated or more commonly in conjunction with other types of adenomyosis [2, 18]. Owing to ambiguous definitions, the distinction between focal adenomyosis and adenomyoma is challenging, and they are also often used interchangeably. Some authors use the border of the surrounding myometrium as a criterion for their differentiation. Thus, focal adenomyosis presents circumscribed adenomyotic lesions where more than 25% of their circumference is surrounded by a healthy myometrium [25]. It is termed *adenomyoma* if it is distinctly demarcated and surrounded by a hypertrophic myometrium [25].

8.3.4.2 Leiomyomas

Differentiation between leiomyomas and adenomyomas has important therapeutic implications. Although differentiating between leiomyomas and diffuse adenomyosis is usually feasible, its differential diagnosis from well-defined adenomyomas or the differentiation of adenomyomas and leiomyomas with cystic degeneration may be difficult [5] (Fig. 8.9). Fibroids are typically well-defined round lesions that can display a broad spectrum of internal echogenicity and may also have calcifications. Power Doppler is very useful in the differential diagnosis between leiomyomas and focal adenomyosis. Leiomyomas display circular flow along the pseudocapsule. The absence of internal vascularization favors leiomyomas, whereas focal adenomyosis and adenomyomas show diffuse vascularity within their lesions [48, 52]. However, a US assessment of adenomyosis is limited, particularly in the presence of large fibroids or large uteri with multiple fibroids [53].

8.4 Conclusion

The term *external adenomyosis* is commonly used to describe the external invasion of the outer myometrium with variable depths of invasion into the myometrium by ectopic endometrial tissue, where this term refers to adenomyosis in which endometrial tissue invades the intact junctional zone. This phenomenon is highly associated with DIE or with endometriomas. Because the term *external adenomyosis* is a source of confusion with internal adenomyosis and because these two pathologies present different entities, the term *myometrial deep infiltrative endometriosis* should be preferred. Internal adenomyosis should be considered as an associated pathology with DIE and be systematically described. External adenomyosis should be considered as a location within the myometrium of DIE (mediocentral location).

Acknowledgments I express many thanks to Professor Isabelle Thomassin-Naggara, Paris, for helping me with US and MRI cases.

References

1. Bergeron C, Amant F, Ferenczy A. Pathology and physiopathology of adenomyosis. Best Pract Res Clin Obstet Gynaecol. 2006;20:511–21.
2. Chapron C, Vannuccini S, Santulli P, Abrão MS, Carmona F, Fraser IS, Gordts S, Guo SW, Just PA, Noël JC, Pistofidis G, Van den Bosch T, Petraglia F. Diagnosing adenomyosis: an integrated clinical and imaging approach. Hum Reprod Update. 2020;26:392–411.
3. Habiba M, Guo SW, Benagiano G. Are adenomyosis and endometriosis phenotypes of the same disease process? Biomol Ther. 2023;14(1):32i.
4. Bourdon M, Santulli P, Marcellin L, Maignien C, Maitrot-Mantelet L, Bordonne C, Plu Bureau G, Chapron C. Adenomyosis: an update regarding its diagnosis and clinical features. J Gynecol Obstet Hum Reprod. 2021;50:102228.
5. Marcellin L, Santulli P, Bourdon M, Maignien C, Campin L, Lafay-Pillet MC, Millischer AE, Bordonne C, Borghese B, Dousset B, Chapron C. Focal adenomyosis of the outer myometrium and deep infiltrating endometriosis severity. Fertil Steril. 2020;114:818–27.
6. Van den Bosch T, Van Schoubroeck D. Ultrasound diagnosis of endometriosis and adenomyosis: state of the art. Best Pract Res Clin Obstet Gynaecol. 2018;51:16–24. https://doi.org/10.1016/j.bpobgyn.2018.01.013.
7. Pados G, Gordts S, Sorrentino F, Nisolle M, Nappi L, Daniilidis A. Adenomyosis and infertility: a literature review. Medicina. 2023;59(9):1551.
8. Zondervan KT, Becker CM, Missmer SA. Endometriosis. N Engl J Med. 2020;382:1244–56.
9. Koninckx PR, Martin DC. Deep endometriosis: a consequence of infiltration or retraction or possibly adenomyosis externa? Fertil Steril. 1992;58:924–8.
10. Zegers-Hochschild F, Adamson GD, Dyer S, Racowsky C, de Mouzon J, Sokol R, Rienzi L, Sunde A, Schmidt L, Cooke ID, Simpson JL, van der Poel S. The international glossary on infertility and fertility care, 2017. Hum Reprod. 2017;32:1786–801.
11. Tellum T, Munro MG. Classifications of adenomyosis and correlation of phenotypes in imaging and histopathology to clinical outcomes: a review. Curr Obstet Gynecol Rep. 2022;11:1–11.
12. Harmsen MJ, Van den Bosch T, de Leeuw RA, Dueholm M, Exacoustos C, Valentin L, Hehenkamp WJK, Groenman F, De Bruyn C, Rasmussen C, Lazzeri L, Jokubkiene L, Jurkovic D, Naftalin J, Tellum T, Bourne T, Timmerman D, Huirne JAF. Consensus on revised definitions of Morphological Uterus Sonographic Assessment (MUSA) features of adenomyosis: results of modified Delphi procedure. Ultrasound Obstet Gynecol. 2022;60:118–31.
13. Chapron C, Tosti C, Marcellin L, Bourdon M, Lafay-Pillet MC, Millischer AE, et al. Relationship between the magnetic resonance imaging appearance of adenomyosis and endometriosis phenotypes. Hum Reprod. 2017;32:1393–401. https://doi.org/10.1093/humrep/dex088.
14. Di Donato N, Montanari G, Benfenati A, Leonardi D, Bertoldo V, Monti G, Raimondo D, Seracchioli R. Prevalence of adenomyosis in women undergoing surgery for endometriosis. Eur J Obstet Gynecol Reprod Biol. 2014;181:289–93.
15. Naftalin J, Hoo W, Pateman K, Mavrelos D, Holland T, Jurkovic D. How common is adenomyosis? A prospective study of prevalence using transvaginal ultrasound in a gynaecology clinic. Hum Reprod. 2012;12:3432–9.
16. Weiss G, Maseelall P, Schott LL, et al. Adenomyosis a variant, not a disease? Evidence from hysterectomized menopausal women in the Study of Women's Health Across the Nation (SWAN). Fertil Steril. 2009;91:201–6.
17. Sun M, Xu P, Zou G, Wang J, Zhu L, Zhang X. Extrinsic adenomyosis is associated with postoperative recurrence of ovarian endometrioma. Front Med (Lausanne). 2022;12(8):815628. https://doi.org/10.3389/fmed.2021.815628.
18. Bazot M, Daraï E. Role of transvaginal sonography and magnetic resonance imaging in the diagnosis of uterine adenomyosis. Fertil Steril. 2018;109:389–97.
19. Kishi Y, Suginami H, Kuramori R, Yabuta M, Suginami R, Taniguchi F. Four subtypes of adenomyosis assessed by magnetic resonance imaging and their

specification. Am J Obstet Gynecol. 2012;207:114.e1–7.
20. Zhang M, Bazot M, Tsatoumas M, et al. MRI of adenomyosis: where are we today? Curr Obstet Gynecol Rep. 2022;11:225–37.
21. Jha P, Sakala M, Chamie LP, Feldman M, Hindman N, Huang C, Kilcoyne A, Laifer-Narin S, Nicola R, Poder L, Shenoy-Bhangle A, Tong A, VanBuren W, Taffel MT. Endometriosis MRI lexicon: consensus statement from the society of abdominal radiology endometriosis disease-focused panel. Abdom Radiol (NY). 2020;45:1552–68.
22. Siegelman ES, Oliver ER. MR imaging of endometriosis: ten imaging pearls. Radiographics. 2012;32:1675–91.
23. Chamié LP, Blasbalg R, Pereira RM, Warmbrand G, Serafini PC. Findings of pelvic endometriosis at transvaginal US, MR imaging, and laparoscopy. Radiographics. 2011;31(4):E77–100.
24. Lazzeri L, Morosetti G, Centini G, Monti G, Zupi E, Piccione E, et al. A sonographic classification of adenomyosis: interobserver reproducibility in the evaluation of type and degree of the myometrial involvement. Fertil Steril. 2018;110:1154–61.
25. Van den Bosch T, de Bruijn AM, de Leeuw RA, Dueholm M, Exacoustos C, Valentin L, Bourne T, Timmerman D, Huirne JAF. Sonographic classification and reporting system for diagnosing adenomyosis. Ultrasound Obstet Gynecol. 2019;53:576–82.
26. Khan KN, Fujishita A, Koshiba A, Kuroboshi H, Mori T, Ogi H, et al. Biological differences between intrinsic and extrinsic adenomyosis with coexisting deep infiltrating endometriosis. Reprod Biomed Online. 2019;39:343–53.
27. Rousset P, Florin M, Bharwani N, Touboul C, Monroc M, Golfier F, Nougaret S, Thomassin-Naggara I, ENDOVALIRM Group. Deep pelvic infiltrating endometriosis: MRI consensus lexicon and compartment-based approach from the ENDOVALIRM group. Diagn Interv Imaging. 2023;104(3):95–112.
28. Leyendecker G, Bilgicyildirim A, Inacker M, Stalf T, Huppert P, Mall G, Böttcher B, Wildt L. Adenomyosis and endometriosis. Re-visiting their association and further insights into the mechanisms of auto-traumatisation. An MRI study. Arch Gynecol Obstet. 2015;291:917–32.
29. Gracia M, de Guirior C, Valdés-Bango M, et al. Adenomyosis is an independent risk factor for complications in deep endometriosis laparoscopic surgery. Sci Rep. 2022;12:7086.
30. Larsen SB, Lundorf E, Forman A, Dueholm M. Adenomyosis and junctional zone changes in patients with endometriosis. Eur J Obstet Gynecol Reprod Biol. 2011;157:206–11.
31. Donnez J, Dolmans MM, Fellah L. What if deep endometriotic nodules and uterine adenomyosis were actually two forms of the same disease? Fertil Steril. 2019;111:454–6.
32. Bourdon M, Oliveira J, Marcellin L, Santulli P, Bordonne C, Maitrot Mantelet L, et al. Adenomyosis of the inner and outer myometrium are associated with different clinical profiles. Hum Reprod. 2021;36:349–57.
33. Marcellin PS, Bortolato S, Morin C, Millischer AE, Borghese B, Chapron C. Anterior focal adenomyosis and bladder deep infiltrating endometriosis: is there a link? J Minim Invasive Gynecol. 2018;25:896–901.
34. Rousset P, Bischoff E, Charlot M, Grangeon F, Dubernard G, Paparel P, Lega JC, Golfier F. Bladder endometriosis: preoperative MRI analysis with assessment of extension to ureteral orifices. Diagn Interv Imaging. 2021;102:255–63.
35. Busard MP, Mijatovic V, Lüchinger AB, Bleeker MC, Pieters-van den Bos IC, Schats R, van Kuijk C, Hompes PG, van Waesberghe JH. MR imaging of bladder endometriosis and its relationship with the anterior uterine wall: experience in a tertiary referral centre. Eur J Radiol. 2012;81:2106–11.
36. Fedele L, Bianchi S, Zanconato G, Bergamini V, Berlanda N, Carmignani L. Long-term follow-up after conservative surgery for bladder endometriosis. Fertil Steril. 2005;83:1729–33.
37. Celli V, Dolciami M, Ninkova R, Ercolani G, Rizzo S, Porpora MG, Catalano C, Manganaro L. MRI and adenomyosis: what can radiologists evaluate? Int J Environ Res Public Health. 2022;19:5840.
38. Bazot M, Daraï E, Benagiano GP, Reinhold C, Favier A, Roman H, Donnez J, Bendifallah S. ENDO_STAGE magnetic resonance imaging: classification to screen endometriosis. J Clin Med. 2022;11:2443.
39. Thomassin-Naggara I, Monroc M, Chauveau B, et al. Multicenter external validation of the deep pelvic endometriosis index magnetic resonance imaging score. JAMA Netw Open. 2023;6(5):e2311686.
40. Bazot M, Cortez A, Darai E, Rouger J, Chopier J, Antoine JM, et al. Ultrasonography compared with magnetic resonance imaging for the diagnosis of adenomyosis: correlation with histopathology. Hum Reprod. 2001;16:2427–33.
41. Margit Dueholm M, Lundorf E, Hansen ES, Solgård Sørensen J, Ledertoug S, Olesen F. Magnetic resonance imaging and transvaginal ultrasonography for the diagnosis of adenomyosis. Fertil Steril. 2001;76:588–94.
42. Reinhold C, McCarthy S, Bret PM, Mehio A, Atri M, Zakarian R, Glaude Y, Liang L, Seymour RJ. Diffuse adenomyosis: comparison of endovaginal US and MR imaging with histopathologic correlation. Radiology. 1996;199(1):151–8.
43. Tellum T, Matic GV, Dormagen JB, Nygaard S, Viktil E, Qvigstad E, Lieng M. Diagnosing adenomyosis with MRI: a prospective study revisiting the junctional zone thickness cutoff of 12 mm as a diagnostic marker. Eur Radiol. 2019;29:6971–81.
44. Kubik-Huch RA, Weston M, Nougaret S, Leonhardt H, Thomassin-Naggara I, Horta M, Cunha TM, Maciel C, Rockall A, Forstner R. European Society of Urogenital Radiology (ESUR) guidelines: MR imaging of leiomyomas. Eur Radiol. 2018;28:3125–37.

45. Di Donato N, Montanari G, Benfenati A, Leonardi D, Bertoldo V, Monti G, Raimondo D, Seracchiol R. Prevalence of adenomyosis in women undergoing surgery for endometriosis. Eur J Obstet Gynecol Reprod Biol. 2014;181:289–93.
46. Keckstein J, Saridogan E, Ulrich UA, et al. The #Enzian classification: a comprehensive non-invasive and surgical description system for endometriosis. Acta Obstet Gynecol Scand. 2021;100:1165–75.
47. Lazzeri L, Di Giovanni A, Exacoustos C, Tosti C, Pinzauti S, Malzoni M, Petraglia F, Zupi E. Preoperative and postoperative clinical and transvaginal ultrasound findings of adenomyosis in patients with deep infiltrating endometriosis. Reprod Sci. 2014;21:1027–33.
48. Exacoustos C, Manganaro L, Zupi E. Imaging for the evaluation of endometriosis and adenomyosis. Best Pract Res Clin Obstet Gynaecol. 2014;28:655–81.
49. Exacoustos C, Lazzeri L, Martire FG, Russo C, Martone S, Centini G, Piccione E, Zupi E. Ultrasound findings of adenomyosis in adolescents: type and grade of the disease. J Minim Invasive Gynecol. 2022;29:291–299.e1.
50. Di Donato N, Bertoldo V, Montanari G, Zannoni L, Caprara G, Seracchioli R. Question mark form of uterus: a simple sonographic sign associated with the presence of adenomyosis. Ultrasound Obstet Gynecol. 2015;46:126–7.
51. Zannoni L, Ambrosio M, Raimondo D, Arena A, Del Forno S, Borghese G, Paradisi R, Seracchioli R. Question mark sign and transvaginal ultrasound uterine tenderness for the diagnosis of adenomyosis: a prospective validation. J Ultrasound Med. 2020;39:1405–12.
52. Chiang CH, Chang MY, Hsu JJ, et al. Tumor vascular pattern and blood flow impedance in the differential diagnosis of leiomyoma and adenomyosis by color doppler sonography. J Assist Reprod Genet. 1999;16:268–75.
53. Champaneria R, Abedin P, Daniels J, Balogun M, Khan KS. Ultrasound scan and magnetic resonance imaging for the diagnosis of adenomyosis: systematic review comparing test accuracy. Acta Obstet Gynecol Scand. 2010;89:1374–84.

9 Posterocentral Compartment (Rectum)

Pascal Rousset, Edouard Ruaux, Pierre-Adrien Bolze, Eddy Cotte, Isabelle Thomassin-Naggara, and François Golfier

9.1 Introduction

The posterocentral compartment includes the rectum and rectosigmoid junction, excluding the sigmoid above them. The mesorectum belongs to the mediocentral compartment, whereas the fascia recti, also known as visceral fascia or mesorectal fascia, is part of the posterolateral compartment [1].

Bowel endometriosis is by definition deep endometriosis (DE). It is characterized by the presence of endometrial-like tissue infiltrating at least the muscularis propria, resulting in smooth muscle hyperplasia and fibrosis. Serosal involvement is categorized as superficial endometriosis. Rectal endometriosis (RE) represents one of the most severe forms of the condition, occurring in 5–12% of cases, with rates exceeding 30% in some expert centers [2]. Patients with pelvic endometriosis at other sites, such as ovarian endometriomas kissing the ovaries, torus, and/or vagina, are more likely to have rectal involvement. Therefore, in patients presenting with rectal symptoms and known endometriosis at other sites, the search for rectal involvement should be included in the diagnostic evaluation. Conversely, isolated rectal endometriosis is rare, and the identification of such a lesion should prompt the radiologist to search for additional lesions to ensure complete mapping [3].

Radiologists face the particular task of optimizing imaging for the accurate assessment of the extent of rectal involvement by endometriosis. Rectal endometriosis management is complex, and multidisciplinary team discussion evaluating the risk–benefit balance of options provides the optimal personalized treatment. Thus, an accurate preoperative diagnostic workup is essential in surgical decision-making, in providing patients with informed consent regarding potential treatments (such as hormonal therapies or surgical approaches), and in obtaining adequate consent in the event of surgery. Moreover,

P. Rousset (✉) · E. Ruaux
Department of Radiology, Lyon Sud University Hospital, Hospices Civils de Lyon, Claude Bernard Lyon 1 University, Lyon, France
e-mail: pascal.rousset@chu-lyon.fr; edouard.ruaux@chu-lyon.fr

P.-A. Bolze · F. Golfier
Department of Gynecological and Oncological Surgery, Lyon Sud University Hospital, Hospices Civils de Lyon, Claude Bernard Lyon 1 University, Lyon, France
e-mail: Pierre-adrien.bolze@chu-lyon.fr; francois.golfier@chu-lyon.fr

E. Cotte
Department of Digestive Surgery, Lyon Sud University Hospital, Hospices Civils de Lyon, Claude Bernard Lyon 1 University, Lyon, France
e-mail: eddy.cotte@chu-lyon.fr

I. Thomassin-Naggara
Imageries Radiologiques et Interventionnelles Spécialisées (IRIS), Tenon Hospital, AP-HP, Sorbonne Université, Paris, France
e-mail: isabelle.thomassin@aphp.fr

I. Thomassin-Naggara (ed.), *Imaging of Endometriosis: A Comparative Guide of US, MRI and Surgery*, https://doi.org/10.1007/978-3-031-82750-1_9

when surgery is decided on, the resources to be deployed can be better anticipated, in particular the assistance of a colorectal/general surgeon when needed.

9.2 Practical Epidemiology of Rectosigmoid Endometriosis Lesions

The prevalence of bowel endometriosis is not exactly defined and is estimated to affect 3.8% to 37% of patients with endometriosis [4]. Although most cases invade the rectosigmoid colon, bowel endometriosis can involve any portion of the gastrointestinal tract, from very rare stomach lesions to common rectal endometriosis [5]. RE occurs in approximately 10% of DE patients [2]. In about 70% of cases, bowel endometriosis is associated with other DEs, ones that require specific procedures for the genitals or urinary tract [2].

By definition, 100% of patients with RE exhibit muscular involvement. However, submucosal involvement has been reported in 34% of cases, with infiltration into the mucosa observed in only 10% of rectal lesions [6]. Moreover, when infiltrated, the mucosa is histologically only focally involved [7]. Bowel endometriosis is often multifocal. Small satellite lesions, <2 cm within the main nodule, have been reported in as many as 62% of patients with bowel endometriosis (BE). Larger lesions, typically >2 cm away from main lesion, have been reported in 38% of rectal lesions (e.g., distinct rectal and sigmoid lesions or rectal and ileocecal nodules) [6].

Transvaginal ultrasonography (TVUS) and magnetic resonance imaging (MRI) provide similar accuracy for the diagnosis of rectosigmoid endometriosis. But pelvic MRI provides substantial advantages over sonography for the comprehensive detailed mapping of bowel endometriosis and surrounding lesions in the preoperative period.

Surgical options for RE depend on multiple parameters, including location, length, depth [8], circumference, multicentricity, multifocality, and distance between the lower part of the rectosigmoid lesion and the anal verge [9]. Lesions in the other compartments of the pelvis or in the abdomen have also to be considered. Surgical procedures typically include the partial- or full-thickness disc excision of the bowel wall lesion and segmental resection; they will be described in this chapter. A successful surgical treatment with good short- and long-term outcomes for the patient is largely dependent on a high level of confidence between an experienced multidisciplinary surgical team and an expert radiologist, who can provide precise information for effective surgical planning.

9.3 Clinical Symptoms of Rectosigmoid Endometriosis

Surgical decision-making for colorectal endometriosis is based primarily on symptoms such as dyschezia, dyspareunia, tenesmus, constipation, diarrhea, and rectal bleeding, typically with catamenial resurgence. Symptoms associated with the other localizations of endometriosis should also be addressed. More importantly, patients should be asked to evaluate the intensity of each painful symptom, using a visual analogic score or a numerical scale for example. However, an evaluation of the type and severity of painful symptoms is not sufficient. To improve the quality and security of care, the consequences of endometriosis and its symptoms on all aspects of daily life must be assessed, using validated questionnaires, such as the 12-item Short-Form Health Survey (SF12) [10]. Finally, the detection of a central sensitization syndrome is also crucial to improve surgical decision-making in colorectal endometriosis [11].

9.4 Challenge and Decision-Making for Surgery

In almost all patients with DE, including rectosigmoid endometriosis, hormone treatment and analgesics are the necessary first steps outside infertility, and surgery will not be initially indicated. Hormone treatment is known to reduce severe endometriosis-associated pain, even if efficacy, along with side effects, are highly individual [12]. Although an up-front indication for surgery can be advocated in cases of severe lumen narrowing by large sigmoid lesions, RE is exceptionally associated with such a risk, unlike some rectosigmoid junction lesions. The identification of preocclusive symptoms is considered as a reasonable indication for surgery to prevent an ill-defined but severe risk of acute occlusion.

Severe resistance and intolerance to different medical treatments are usual indications for surgery. Deep alteration in personal or professional quality of life by noncontrolled painful symptoms is the usual complaint of patients seeking surgical advice. Most of them, although already aware of the potential complications of bowel surgery, put these serious risks in the background, favoring the improvement of their severe symptoms through surgery. Risks of complications should be exposed as clearly as possible. Using preoperative imaging classification can help in evaluating the likelihood of surgical complications so that patients can have all the relevant information. While the ENZIAN classification demonstrates a good estimation of operative time [13], the validation of the deep Pelvic Endometriosis Index (dPEI) magnetic resonance imaging score shows its ability to predict operative time altogether with postoperative complication risks and de novo voiding function [14, 15].

The indication for surgery with the aim of improving fertility lacks consensus due to the absence of randomized studies. A high level of evidence is lacking, and a strong recommendation for surgery could not be made, even in the latest 2022 ESHRE guidelines [16]. No compelling evidence indicates that surgery for DE, including RE, improves spontaneous fertility. Additionally, surgery prior to in vitro fertilization (IVF) has not been associated with a confirmed improvement in reproductive outcomes [12, 16]. Moreover, severe recurring pain upon the cessation of hormonal treatment for conception can be an indication for surgery, regardless of fertility outcomes. For instance, avoiding sexual intercourse due to severe dyspareunia can strongly limit spontaneous fertility. Decision-making regarding surgery in infertile patients should therefore consider evaluations of severe pain and individual preferences, alongside providing patients with thorough information about the lack of strong evidence for the benefits of surgery and the specific complications associated with bowel surgery.

9.4.1 Technical Procedures for Rectosigmoid Endometriosis

As stated by the Consensus on the Recording of Deep Endometriosis Surgery (CORDES), three surgical techniques have been described for bowel endometriosis as defined by at least the infiltration of the muscular layer (Fig. 9.1) [17]. Partial-thickness discoid excision consists of the selective excision of an RE lesion without entering the bowel lumen, which requires the closure

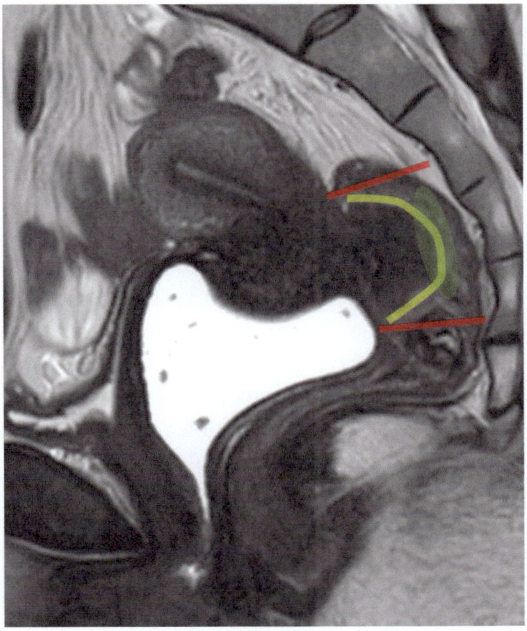

Fig. 9.1 Schematic representation of the three surgical techniques for removing a rectal lesion. T2-weighted MR image in the sagittal plane shows a schematic representation of the three surgical procedures for rectal lesions: partial-thickness disc excision (yellow line), full-thickness disc excision (green spot), and segmental resection (red lines)

of the muscular defect without a mucosa defect. Full-thickness discoid excision consists of the selective excision of the RE lesion with opening of the bowel lumen, followed by the closure of the bowel wall, which can be either open full-thickness excision followed by manual closure or closed full-thickness excision with a stapler. Segmental resection and reanastomosis include the resection of a bowel segment with reanastomosis by any means. The term *bowel "shaving"* is therefore not intended for real bowel endometriosis but rather only for superficial peritoneal endometriosis, and it consists of the superficial excision or ablation of the serosa and subserosa endometriosis, without requiring suturing. It will not be addressed in this chapter.

9.4.2 Criteria for Technical Procedure Selection

To date, no consensus has been reached on the procedure to be adopted between partial-thickness disc excision, full-thickness disc excision, and segmental resection with reanastomosis for RE. All techniques have been reported to improve pain, bowel symptoms, and quality of life if all endometriosis lesions can be completely removed. French guidelines stated as a level of evidence that surgery for colorectal endometriosis improves the intensity of gynecological, digestive, and general symptoms as well as quality of life, without being able to predict the duration of this effectiveness [12]. All techniques have been associated with a relatively low level of severe bowel complications, and a recent meta-analysis reported a global 1.5% risk of rectovaginal fistula and 1.2% risk of intraabdominal fistula [18]. A high level of evidence for choosing a conservative over a radical procedure, and vice versa, is lacking, and the type of procedure is often a matter of surgeon experience. Remarkably, the 2022 ESHRE guidelines group decided not to make any conclusions or recommendations on the technique to be used [16].

Some data favor the most conservative approach as a reasonable strategy. A recent meta-analysis demonstrated that shaving (now termed *partial-thickness disc excision*) was less associated with postoperative complications and that full-thickness disc excision could be the technique of choice for large bowel infiltration. Rectal shaving was indeed less associated with rectovaginal fistula than with full-thickness disc excision (OR = 0.19, 95% CI 0.10–0.36, $p < 0.00001$) and segmental colorectal resection (OR = 0.26, 95% CI 0.15–0.44, $p < 0.00001$). No difference was found in the occurrence of rectovaginal fistula between full-thickness disc excision and segmental colorectal resection [18].

A 3 cm length of the RE lesion is often reported as a cutoff between the conservative approach and the segmental resection, and preoperative MRI can give an accurate estimation of this size. However, limiting preoperative imaging to this simplistic information has not been adopted, because increasing the experience of the surgeon progressively pushes the limits of disc excision [19]. Moreover, MRI can give much-more-precise information that the surgeon can rely on to anticipate the choice for the procedure. As stated before, Rousset et al. demonstrated that RE lesion circumference ≥ 38% was highly predictive of segmental resection (OR = 60.4, 95% CI 12.3–296.2, $p < 0.001$) and that the combination of this sign with a thickness ≥ 14 mm was even more highly predictive of segmental resection, with an accuracy of 90.2 (95% CI 79.8–96.3, $p < 0.0001$) [20]. Whatever the performance of preoperative imaging criteria, a gray zone will remain that should probably favor partial- and full-thickness disc excision procedures over segmental resection, due to fewer short-term complications [21]. As a result, the majority of RE surgeries could accurately be anticipated with a conservative procedure, whereas segmental resection should be limited either to nodules with important thickness and circumference values on MRI (as described above) or when the completeness of surgical excision cannot be ascertained preoperatively.

9.4.3 Main Steps of Partial-Thickness Disc Excision

Partial-thickness discoid excision consists of the excision of the RE lesion without entering the bowel lumen, which requires the mandatory closure of the muscular defect (Fig. 9.2). The laparoscopic approach is almost always possible, with robotic assistance when possible, to allow for a more ergonomic and precise gesture (Fig. 9.3). The posterior lesions of the retrocervical area, including the uterine torus, uterosacral ligament (USL), and/or vagina, are first excised, when necessary, and left attached to the anterior bowel wall before the mobilization of the rectum is performed and the healthy rectovaginal septum entered. The healthy bowel wall is circumscribed as much as possible to the RE lesion by separating the lateral rectal ligaments so that they are usually anteriorly retracted toward the lesion. The superficial fatty tissue located orally and aborally to the lesion is then removed. These steps should allow a clear identification of approximately 1 cm of healthy bowel wall all around the lesion, for the later precise and strong suturing of the muscular defect.

The excision of the lesion begins at its oral end, using scissors to tightly enter the rectal layers, deep enough to progressively remove the whole thickness of the RE lesion. Cold scissors prevent any diathermic lesions that could induce the postoperative perforation of the bowel wall. All fibrous lesions should be removed from the rectal wall. Ensuring a good distinction of fibrous abnormal tissue from the underlying soft normal layer is usually recognized when cutting is easy and soft under the lesion, whereas hard cutting is typical of nonadequate intralesional excision. Surgeons must be aware that the depth of rectal layer involvement by the lesion is usually not homogeneous, with the deepest infiltration in the middle of the nodule. The risk of opening the rectal lumen therefore increases from the upper part of the lesion to its center and then decreases from its center to the aboral limit. Because the accuracy of TVUS, MRI, and RES in differentiating muscularis from submucosal and mucosal infiltration is not satisfactory [22, 23] and because the quality of the surgical view is not always optimal, the bowel lumen can be unexpectedly and unnecessarily opened, transforming a partial-thickness in full-thickness disc excision. Although laparotomy has been progressively abandoned in favor of laparoscopy, partly because of the high magnification of the latter, allowing more-precise section, the even-higher magnification and the three-dimensional (3D) vision allowed with robotic surgery, together with its tools' precision and ergonomic comfort, increase one's ability to distinguish the RE lesion from the underlying uninvolved layers. Even if not strictly proven, improvement in the quality of vision and gestures with robotic surgery will likely allow complete partial-thickness disc excision to be carried out more frequently with the most conservative approach toward underlying noninvolved bowel layers. After the removal of the lesion from the rectal wall, bowel filling with a solution of blue ink helps in identifying the degree of rectal wall weakness and of an unexpected mucosal leak. Bowel wall suture is then typically performed using PDS 3/0, with either continuous or interrupted suture. A clear initial identification of a healthy rectal wall around the lesion is crucial for a safe suture.

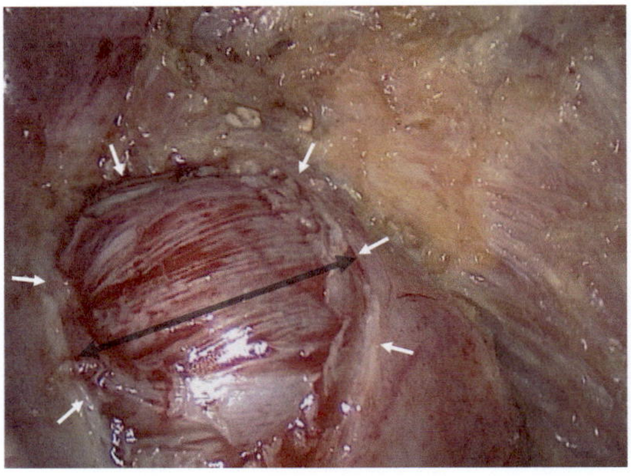

Fig. 9.2 Surgical view of anterior rectal wall partial-thickness disc excision. Laparoscopic surgical view showing the limits of the rectal muscular defect (white arrows) and the circular muscular layer (double-headed black arrow) uncovered after excision of the lesion involving the rectal longitudinal layer

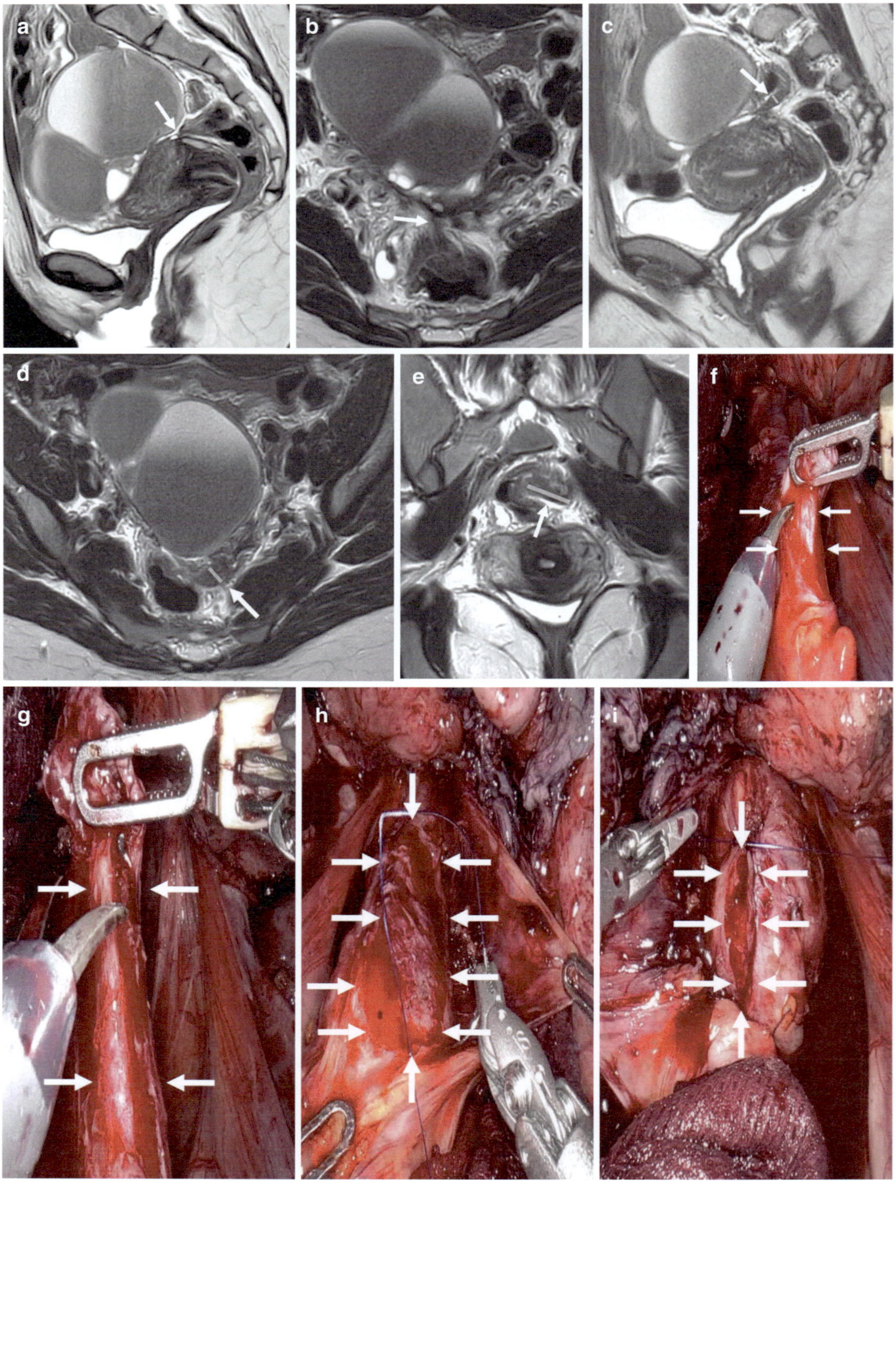
a
b
c
d
e
f
g
h
i

9.4.4 Main Steps of Full-Thickness Disc Excision

The open full-thickness disc excision of a RE lesion removes the whole thickness of the involved rectal wall (Fig. 9.4), usually with scissors, by opening the bowel lumen, followed by manual closure. A laser can also be used instead of scissors. It includes the same first steps as those for partial-thickness excision, including a meticulous healthy bowel wall identification around the lesion and then the deep excision, with cold scissors, of the submucosa and mucosa before the manual closure of the opened rectal wall. Opening and excising the mucosa are strictly necessary for the complete removal of RE lesions in a minority of patients because infiltration into the mucosa occurs in only 10% of RE lesions [6]. Again, the unintended opening of the rectal lumen is possible for lesions involving only the muscular layers of the rectum, and the quality of vision of the surgical field as allowed by robotic surgery probably reduces such a preoperative event. The quality of bowel wall suture is even more crucial because leakage through the suture could be responsible for a postoperative pelvic abscess or fistula. A tight running suture is typically performed with PDS 3/0, and a leakage test, with a solution of blue ink, for instance, is mandatory at the end of the procedure.

The closed full-thickness disc excision of a RE lesion uses a stapler for the removal of the whole thickness of the involved rectal wall. It includes the mobilization of the rectum from the posterior infiltration of the retrocervical aera, including uterine torus, USL, and/or vagina, when necessary, and entering the healthy rectovaginal septum. Retrocervical lesions are separated from the rectal lesion posteriorly and sent for pathology review. Lateral rectal ligaments are separated from the rectal wall for the identification of the healthy bowel wall around the lesion remaining on the anterior part of the rectum. The most exophytic part of the rectal wall lesion is removed. A transrectal mechanic stapler is then introduced into the rectal lesion. Two stitches previously placed apart from the nodule allow the lesion to be guided into the opened stapler. The closure of the device allows the full-thickness disc excision of the lesion. An air leakage test is then performed. This technic minimizes peritoneal contamination when compared to the open full-thickness procedure and possibly the risk of postoperative abscess formation or fistula. On the other hand, it does not allow for a tailored surgery and could be considered as an overtreatment for the majority of RE lesions that do not include the rectal mucosa.

Fig. 9.3 Partial-thickness robotic disc excision of rectal endometriosis: (**a**) Sagittal and (**b**) axial T2-weighted MR images show adhesion between the torus and the anterior serosa of the upper rectum (arrows), consisting of a focal rectal wall attraction but without wall thickening. This space was freed via adhesiolysis without an underlying rectal lesion at surgery. (**c**) Sagittal, (**d**) axial, and (**e**) coronal T2-W MR images show a rectal lesion (arrows) with a thickness of 6 mm (line on **c**), a transverse axis of 10 mm (line on **d**), and length of 15 mm (line on **e**). (**f**) Robotic surgery view after dissection showing the beginning of procedure by entering the anterior rectal longitudinal muscular layer with cold scissors at the upper extremity of the lesion. (**g**) Robotic surgery view after dissection showing the lifting of the lesion away from the underlying healthy muscular layer, progressing towards the distal end of the lesion. (**h**) Robotic surgery view after dissection showing the suturing of the rectal wall, beginning at the uppermost point of the muscular defect. (**i**) Robotic surgery view after dissection showing the placing of a stitch at the distal end of the defect before meticulously closing the rectal wall with a running suture. White arrows on (**f**, **g**, **h**, and **i**) indicate the limits of rectal muscular defect

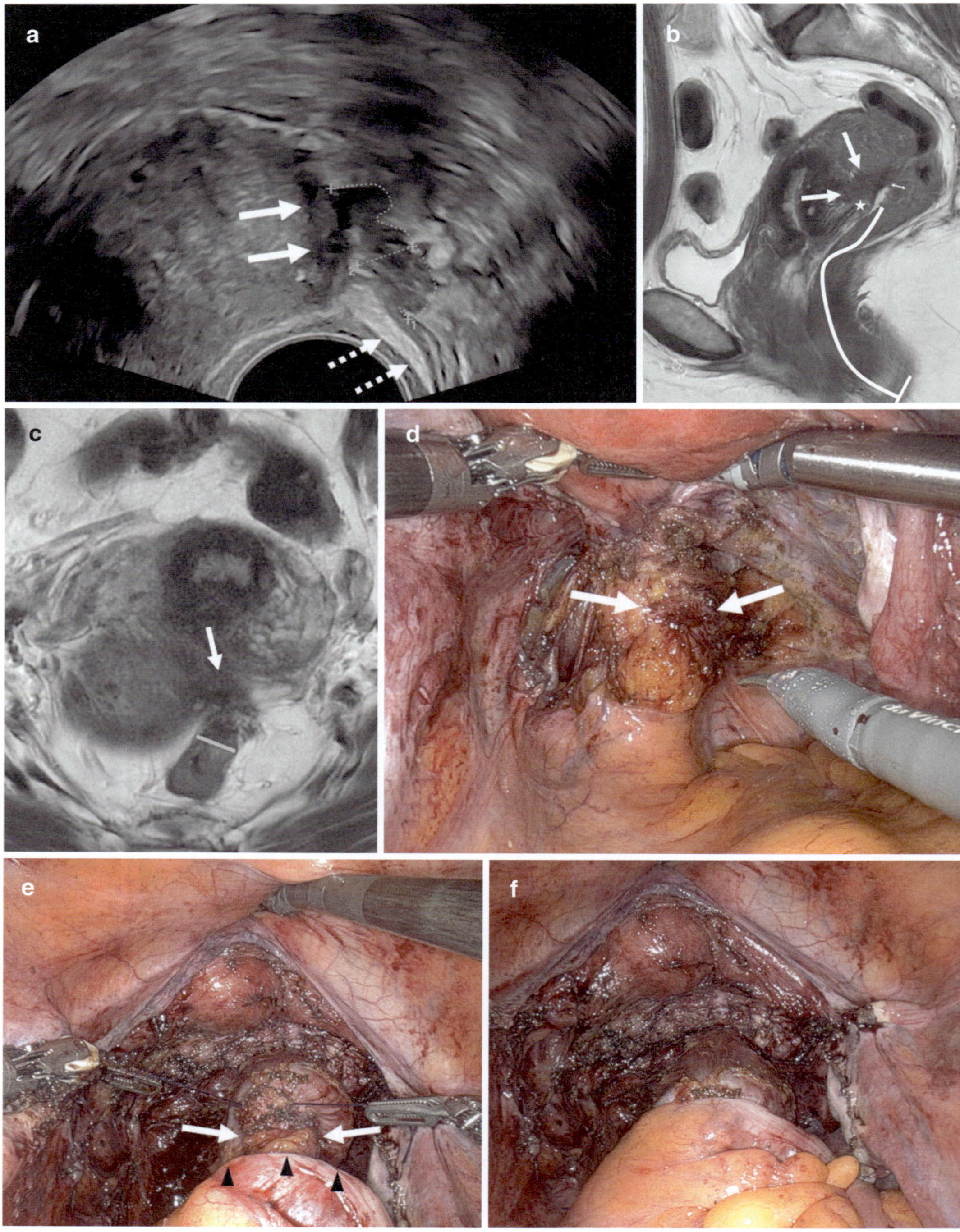
a
b
c
d
e
f

9.4.5 Main Steps of Segmental Colorectal Resection and Reanastomosis

Conventional or robotic-assisted laparoscopy is performed for the vast majority of patients, and laparotomy can be decided on in difficult situations and in case of some preoperative complications (Figs. 9.5 and 9.6). After bilateral ureterolysis, laterorectal spaces are entered until the inferior limit of the retrocervical lesions has been reached. Torus uterinum, vaginal, and USL lesions are excised when necessary and the healthy rectovaginal septum developed until the inferior limit of the rectal lesion has been reached. Laterally, sacrorectal septum (also called posterolateral parametrium) lesions, frequently associated when segmental resection is necessary, are also excised. Lateral rectal ligaments and the mesorectum are separated close to the bowel wall, allowing the complete mobilization and preparation of the bowel. The left paracolic gutter has been opened previously. The distal rectum is then cut with a stapler and extracted through a limited 4 cm suprapubic transverse or lateral oblique incision. The upper end of the rectum is then cut after checking for unexpected multifocal lesions. The anvil is placed and the colon reintroduced into the peritoneal cavity. A termino-terminal transanal colorectal anastomosis is then performed with a circular stapler. Further mobilization of the rectum featuring the separation of the inferior mesenteric artery may be necessary to allow an anastomosis free of tension. An air leakage test is performed. All the incisions are then closed. A temporary defunctioning stoma, typically a Turnbull ileostomy, can be decided on to prevent anastomosis leakage from developing into severe complications [24]. This decision depends on the distance between both the level of the anastomosis and the concomitant opening of the vagina when necessary, on one hand, and on the level of the bowel anastomosis, on the other. The beliefs of the surgeon strongly participate in this decision, with probably a more conservative approach with increasing experience and confidence, except when ultralow colorectal or even coloanal anastomoses are necessary.

Fig. 9.4 Rectal closed full-thickness disc excision: (**a**) Sagittal TVUS image shows a lesion of the upper rectum located above the level of the torus, behind external adenomyosis lesions (long arrows), 8 mm thick and 3.6 cm long, using a curvilinear line. Note the absence of the posterior vaginal fornix (dashed arrows). (**b**) Sagittal and (**c**) axial T2-weighted MR images show a rectal lesion located 10 cm (curved line) from the anal margin (white line) (measure note shown) with a thickness of 9 mm (double-headed arrow), a transverse axis of 12 mm (white line), and a length of 32 mm (measures note shown), located behind external adenomyosis lesions (arrows). Note the absence of posterior vaginal fornix involvement (star). (**d**) Robotic surgery view before dissection of lesion of the anterior rectal wall (white arrows). (**e**) Robotic surgery view showing circular stapler opened inside the rectum. Note the two stitches guiding the lesion between the stapler jaws. White arrow heads: anvil shaft. Black arrowheads: anvil shape in the upper rectum. (**f**) Robotic surgery view showing side-to-side anastomosis performed with full-thickness excision of the anterior rectal wall lesion

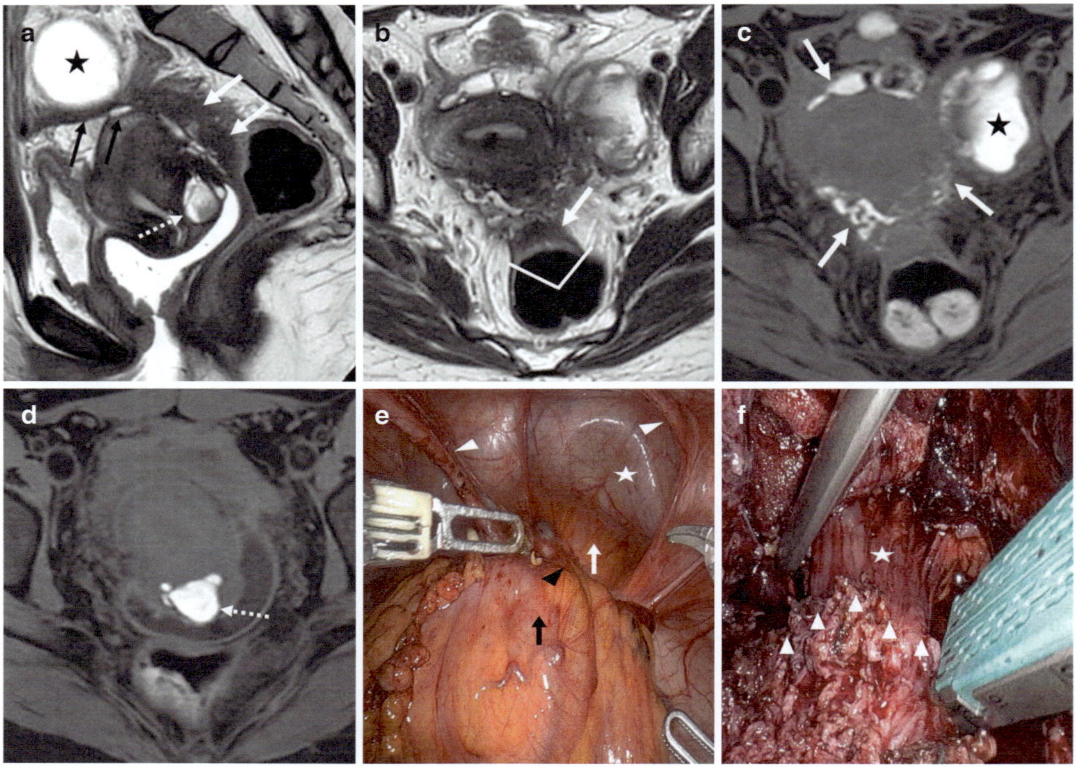

Fig. 9.5 Segmental resection of rectal endometriosis: (**a**) Sagittal T2-weighted MR image shows a rectal lesion (white arrows) located 10 cm from the anal margin, with a thickness of 14 mm and a length of 8 cm (measures note shown) as the rectal lesion continues on the rectosigmoid junction (black arrows) in contact with the left ovary (star). (**b**) Axial T2-weighted MR image shows the rectal lesion (arrow) with a transverse axis of 24 mm (measure note shown) and a circumference of 85°. (**c**) Axial at the level of the pouch of Douglas and (**d**) at the level of the cervix fat-suppressed T1-weighted MR images reveals diffuse T1-hyperintense endometriotic cystic lesions (arrows); superficial and deep endometriosis lesions, including the posterior part of the cervix (dashed arrow on **d** and **a**); and a left ovarian endometrioma (star). (**e**) Robotic surgery view showing preoperative initial aspect of a 10 cm mid and upper rectum endometriosis lesion. White arrowheads: umbilical arteries. Star: bladder peritoneum. White arrow: upper rectum covering uterus. Black arrowhead: striction of rectosigmoid junction. Black arrow: normal distal sigmoid. (**f**) Robotic surgery view showing robot-assisted colorectal segmental resection of a 10 cm mid and upper rectal endometriosis lesion. Arrowheads: lower limit of mid-rectum lesion. Star: healthy mid-rectum prepared for resection with a stapler

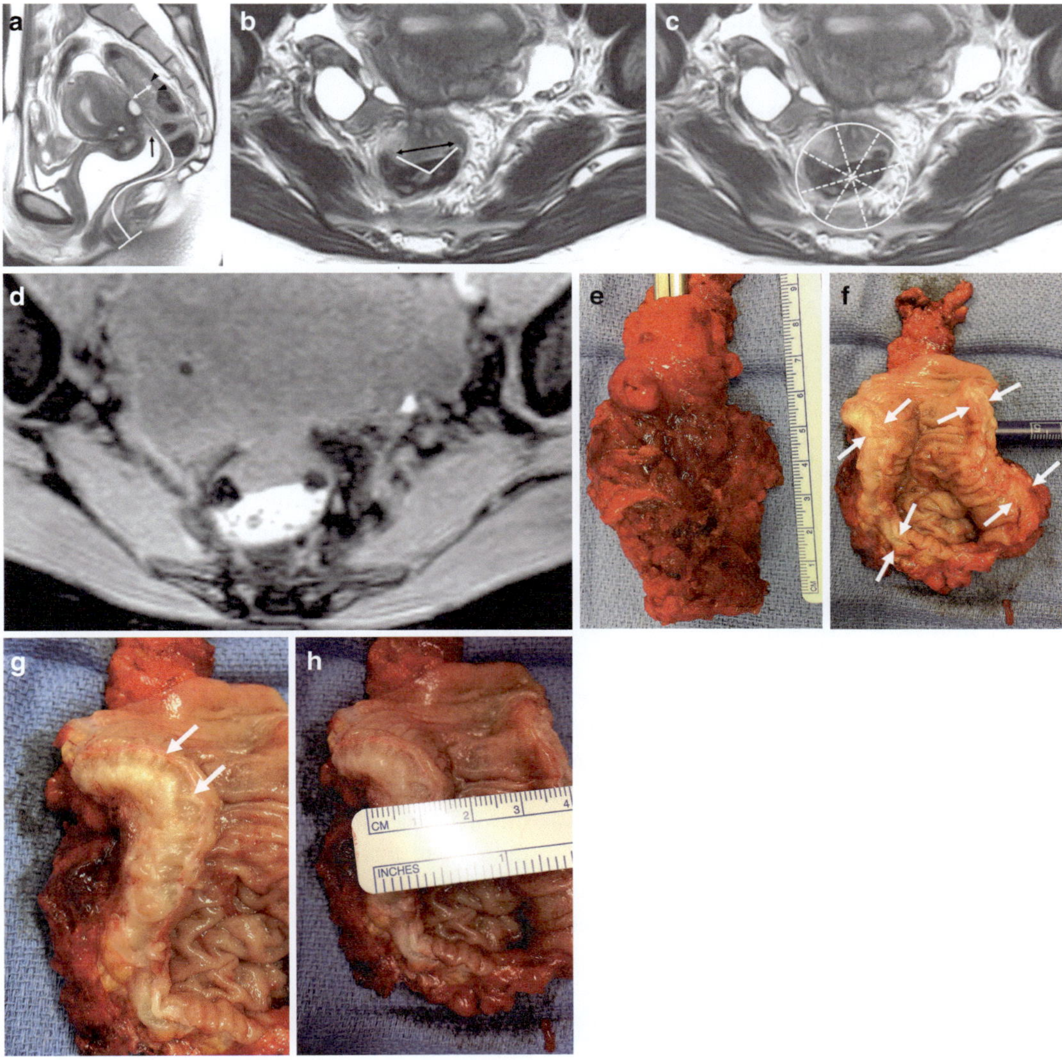

Fig. 9.6 Segmental resection of rectal endometriosis: (**a**) Sagittal T2-weighted MR image shows a rectal lesion located 10 cm (curved line) from the anal margin (white line) (measure note shown), with a thickness of 15 mm (double-headed arrow) (measure note shown). Note the submucosal oedema as a high signal intensity of the lesion on the luminal side (arrowheads), and note the lack of involvement of the vaginal fornix (arrow). (**b**) Axial T2-weighted MR image shows the measure of the transverse axis (double-headed arrow) and a circumference of 96°. (**c**) Axial T2-weighted MR image shows the segmentation in eight radii to evaluate the circumference of the rectal involvement and shows the involvement of three radii. (**d**) Axial fat-suppressed T1-weighted MR image reveals no T1-hyperintense foci. (**e**) Macroscopic view after segmental rectal resection with a 6 cm anterior lesion. (**f**) Macroscopic view showing longitudinal anterior opening of the rectal segment. Arrows: thickening of rectal wall. (**g**) Macroscopic view showing rectal wall fibrous aspect. Arrows: Submucosal oedema between mucosa and involved muscularis. (**h**) Macroscopic view showing a 14 mm thickening of the rectal wall

9.5 Imaging Diagnosis of Rectal Endometriosis

9.5.1 Transvaginal Ultrasonography

TVUS is currently considered the first-line technique for primary diagnosis in patients suspected of having bowel endometriosis [25, 26]. TVUS offers several advantages over other imaging techniques. It is highly available and well tolerated by patients even if the prerequisite is a skilled operator, whose services are relatively inexpensive compared to the cost of MRI. It shows reliable reproducibility compared to MRI and cannot detect intestinal nodules located beyond the sigmoid region, because they fall outside the TVUS field.

9.5.1.1 Patient Preparation and Transvaginal Ultrasonography Techniques

Patient education is crucial in the diagnostic process. Instructions, including bowel preparation if required by the radiologist, bladder filling, and the maneuvers performed during ultrasound (US) examinations, have to be provided to patients by all those involved in the care process.

Some radiologists require bowel preparation, typically a rectal enema administered a few hours prior to the exam (Fig. 9.7). This preparation helps eliminate fecal residues and gas in the rectosigmoid colon, thereby enhancing the detection of bowel lesions and allowing the evaluation of the bowel up to 25–30 cm, and it is less accurate for sigmoid lesion [25, 27]. Patient compliance with bowel preparation is generally high, and adverse effects are minimal, though some patients experience mild abdominal cramps and/or hypotension. However, the society of radiologists in ultrasound that convened a multidisciplinary panel of experts recommended no bowel preparation [28]. A recent study has shown that bowel preparation does not significantly enhance the accuracy of TVUS in diagnosing RE. Additionally, it does not improve the performance of TVUS either in diagnosing submucosal infiltration or multifocal disease or in estimating the size and distance of nodules from the anal verge [29].

A modified approach known as rectal water-contrast transvaginal ultrasonography (RWC-TVUS) has been developed (Fig. 9.7). Although bowel cleansing is typically recommended before RWC-TVUS, evidence supporting its impact on exam performance is lacking [30]. This technique involves injecting saline solution (100 to 350 mL) into the rectosigmoid, which may cause discomfort but is generally well tolerated. RWC-TVUS has shown promise in diagnosing RE more accu-

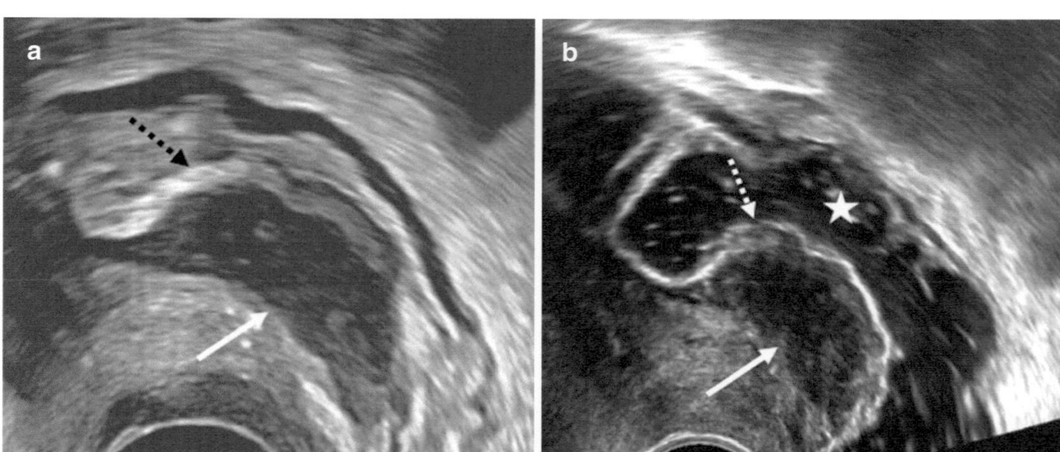

Fig. 9.7 TVUS with and without rectal water opacification: (**a**) Sagittal and (**b**) sagittal images after water opacification (star) show a large rectal lesion (arrows). Hyperechoic submucosal edema (dashed arrows), likely attributed to prior bowel preparation with enema, appears more pronounced without water opacification in (**a**)

rately than traditional TVUS and is also effective in identifying significant intestinal stenosis [31]. However, systematic reviews and meta-analysis have not revealed significant differences in the performance of nonenhanced TVUS versus enhanced TVUS in diagnosing RE, though some have suggested that enhanced techniques are more suitable as secondary investigations to evaluate the depth of endometriosis infiltration into the intestinal wall or the presence of rectal stenosis [32, 33].

Three-dimensional transvaginal ultrasonography (3D TVUS) is also applicable for deep endometriosis assessment, offering volumetric reconstruction and multiple viewing planes, including the elusive coronal plane, which is challenging to obtain when using two-dimensional (2D) TVUS alone [34].

9.5.1.2 Transvaginal Ultrasonography Findings

Ultrasound allows for a visualization of all five layers of the bowel wall, including the mucosa, submucosa, muscularis propria, and serosa (Fig. 9.8) [35]. Rectal lesions typically appear anteriorly between the 10 and 2 o'clock positions, behind the uterus and/or at the level of rectovaginal septum. They often present as irregular hypoechogenic masses with blurred margins, penetrating the rectal wall and replacing the normal muscularis propria. Cystic components are rare.

The International Deep Endometriosis Analysis (IDEA) group has established consensus terminology, definitions, and measurements for describing the sonographic features of various endometriosis phenotypes. Rectosigmoid nodules can exhibit various morphological appearances (Figs. 9.9 and 9.10), such as classically a hypoechoic nodule retraction and adhesions called the "Indigenous headdress" or "moose antler" signs [36]. These nodules may also display a "comet" shape with a thinner part at one end. They can be restricted to the muscle layer or infiltrate the underlying submucosal layer. Mucosal infiltration is rare.

Nodules situated below the insertion level of the uterosacral ligaments on the uterine cervix are categorized as lower (subperitoneal) anterior rectal lesions, whereas those above this insertion point are classified as upper anterior rectal lesions. Lesions located at the level of the uterine fundus are designated as rectosigmoid junction

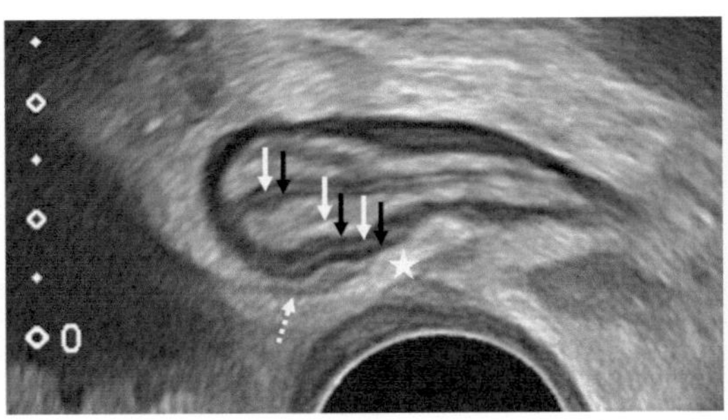

Fig. 9.8 Normal typical layered structure of the rectal wall on TVUS. Sagittal TVUS image shows the typical layered structure of the rectal wall: starting with the first hyperechoic layer, representing the mucosa, followed by the hypoechoic layer, corresponding to the muscularis mucosae. Next, the hyperechoic submucosa is visible, succeeded by the hypoechoic internal layer of muscularis propria and then by the hyperechoic interface between the hypoechoic internal and external layers of muscularis propria. Of note, the hyperechoic space anterior to the rectum (star) denotes the fat of the anterior mesorectum, which is situated beneath the pouch of Douglas and which is identified by the hypoechoic peritoneal reflection (dashed arrow)

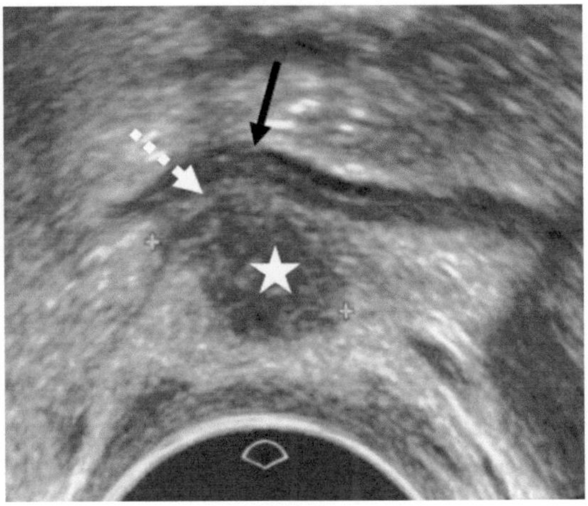

Fig. 9.9 Serosal rectal lesion. Sagittal TVUS image shows a nodular lesion (star) against the rectal wall with a hyperechoic interface (dashed arrow) and a normal aspect of the muscularis propria of the rectal wall (black arrow). This space was freed via adhesiolysis without an underlying rectal lesion at surgery

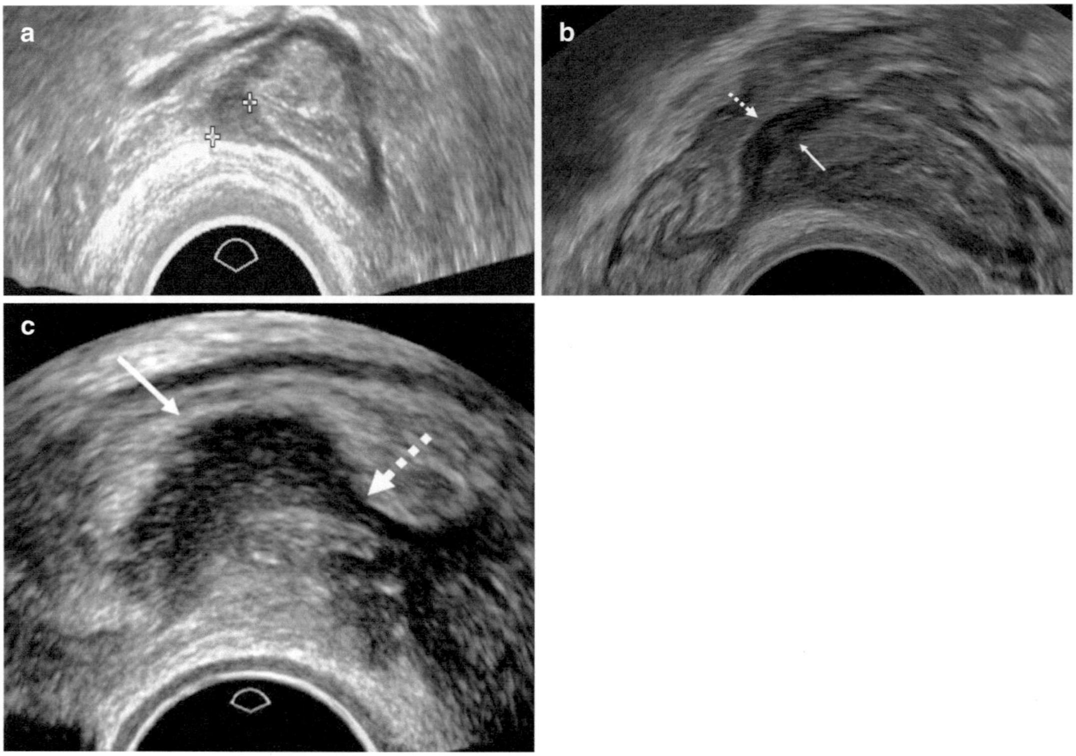

Fig. 9.10 Three lesions on TVUS resected via the three surgical techniques: (**a**) Sagittal TVUS image shows a centimetric rectal lesion removed via partial-thickness disc excision of rectal endometriosis. (**b**) Sagittal TVUS image shows a 2 cm long rectal lesion within the full thickness of the muscularis propria (arrow) and no submucosal involvement (dashed arrow) removed via full-thickness disc excision of rectal endometriosis. (**c**) Sagittal TVUS image shows a large rectal lesion involving the submucosae (long arrow) removed via segmental resection. Note the "comet" shape with a thinner part at one end (dashed arrow)

lesions, whereas those positioned above the uterine fundus are designated as anterior sigmoid lesions. The peritoneal reflection (Fig. 9.8) serves as a landmark for assessing the distance between the lesion and the anal border because it is typically situated approximately 8–9 cm from the anal verge.

According to IDEA consensus, the diameters of rectosigmoid nodules should be recorded in three orthogonal planes, and the distance from the lower margin of the most caudal lesion to the anal verge should be measured. Additionally, bowel lesions may present as isolated and multifocal (involving multiple lesions within the same segment).

9.5.1.3 Transvaginal Ultrasonography Performance

The efficacy of TVUS in diagnosing RE heavily relies on the expertise of the examiner. Nevertheless, evidence suggests that the learning curve for identifying the involvement of the rectosigmoid could be relatively brief [37, 38].

A Cochrane review evaluating the accuracy of imaging tests for endometriosis identified TVUS as meeting the criteria for the SPIN (specific positive test results rule in the disease) triage test, indicating its proficiency in diagnosing RE [39]. TVUS exhibited a sensitivity of 90% (95% CI, 82–97%) and a specificity of 96% (95% CI, 94–99%) across 14 studies involving 1616 participants [39]. Guerriero et al. conducted a systematic review and meta-analysis to assess the accuracy of TVUS in diagnosing deep endometriosis of the rectosigmoid colon; 19 studies involving 2639 patients, of whom 992 had RE, were analyzed [33]. The pooled sensitivity, specificity, LR+, and LR− of TVUS for detecting RE were 91%, 97%, 33.0, and 0.10, respectively. Notably, significant heterogeneity was observed among the studies, attributed mainly to variations in the prevalence of RE across different populations. A recent systematic review and meta-analysis by Gerges et al. showed an overall sensitivity and specificity of 89% and 97%, respectively [32].

Although TVUS may demonstrate superior accuracy in detecting superficial rectal endometriosis, both TVUS (Fig. 9.9) and MRI exhibit nearly identical sensitivity, specificity, and accuracy values in diagnosing deep rectal lesions [40]. A recent systematic review and meta-analysis further confirmed the comparable diagnostic performance of TVUS and MRI, with pooled values for sensitivity and specificity of 90% and 96%, respectively, for both modalities [41].

In addition to direct imaging findings, several "soft markers" have been identified as indirect signs of rectosigmoid involvement. Notably, the presence of "kissing ovaries" and the presence of the "sliding sign" have been associated with RE [42]. The term *kissing ovaries* refers to ovaries that are wholly or partially joined and stabilized behind the uterus within the pouch of Douglas [43]. This sign has a significantly higher prevalence of bowel endometriosis in patients with kissing ovaries compared to those without (18.5% vs. 2.5%). The uterine sliding maneuver can assess adhesions within the pouch of Douglas. By applying pressure with a transvaginal probe, the immobility of the rectum against the uterus and posterior cervix/vaginal fornix can be observed. However, the sonographer should explain this maneuver to the patient before proceeding and remain attentive to the patient's discomfort or even pain, notably if the sonographer experiences difficulty in placing the transducer in the posterior fornix. The term *sliding sign negative* suggests possible adhesions and the endometriotic involvement of these structures. Conversely, the sliding of the rectum against the uterine wall is termed *sliding sign positive*. A prospective multicenter study evaluated the utility of a negative sliding sign in predicting rectal endometriosis, demonstrating its usefulness with an accuracy of 93%, sensitivity of 85%, and specificity of 96% [44].

Despite its utility, and in addition to operator dependence, TVUS has some other limitations, such as a depth resolution that offers a poor visualization of extra-pelvic endometriosis and bowel lesions proximal to the rectosigmoid due to reverberation artifacts from bowel gases. Additionally, difficulty in performing the TVUS scan in patients with vaginal tenderness, coexistent pelvic pathology as large uterine fibroids or immobility, a high patient body mass index, or bowel involvement above the rectosigmoid junction may hinder TVUS accuracy.

9.5.2 MRI

MRI is a second-line technique in DE diagnosis, essentially due to cost and availability. In contrast to TVUS, it exhibits a higher sensitivity and higher accuracy, with an overall evaluation of the pelvic cavity, including multifocality, lesions above the rectosigmoid junction, and lateral compartments.

9.5.2.1 Indication

In patients with prior inconclusive TVUS results, MRI is presently endorsed as a secondary diagnostic modality in the preoperative assessment of deep endometriosis, mainly due to the narrower field of view of TVUS [45]. MRI can also serve as a primary investigative tool in women exhibiting a high clinical suspicion of intestinal endometriosis, notably with rectosigmoid symptoms. Since the landmark study by Bazot et al. [46], MRI has become widely adopted for diagnosing DE and is acknowledged as the optimal imaging modality, providing a comprehensive roadmap of DE crucial for preoperative decision-making.

9.5.2.2 MRI Protocol

The MR magnet's strength can be either 1.5 T or 3 T. Patient preparation should encompass comprehensive instructions and the elucidation of the procedure to ensure enhanced patient adherence and, consequently, improved image quality. Fasting for 3–4 h prior to the examination is recommended. Using an antiperistaltic agent is recommended as the most effective strategy for minimizing bowel motion artifacts unless contraindicated (e.g., in cases of pregnancy, allergies, or pheochromocytoma). Limited data preclude definitive recommendations on the use of intravenous gadolinium chelate for evaluating intestinal endometriosis [47].

Bowel preparation prior to pelvic MRI is not commonly addressed in most studies. Bowel preparation varies when employed. Notably, bowel enema, rectal suppository pills, or water are frequently utilized [48]. Some authors advocate bowel preparation as "best practice" for detecting pelvic bowel endometriosis, arguing that it provides a better visualization of the digestive wall and enhances the quality of MRI interpretation with fewer artifacts, notably when using a 3D T2-weigthed sequence [49].

Rectal opacification has been suggested as an "option" for assessing RE. Typically, two types of contrast media can be employed (sonographic gel or water) [50]. Discrepancies exist in the literature regarding the utility of rectal opacification in diagnosing RE. Whereas some publications advocate for rectal opacification, contending that it provides a better contrast between the rectal lumen and the wall [51], others argue that it is ineffective, especially in intestinal endometriosis, citing reasons such as time consumption, patient discomfort, movement artifacts, and rectosigmoid colon spasm [52]. Additionally, the rectal progression of viscous sonographic gel may be impeded by stool presence or may fail to achieve complete rectal opacification due to passive low pressure against stenosis, resulting in inadequate lesion distension. In this context, prior bowel preparation seems preferable.

9.5.2.3 MRI Findings and Performances

A diagnosis of RE is indicated on T2-weighted sequences by the presence of an iso- or hypointense (relative to myometrium) nodular or mass-like thickening of the bowel wall, accompanied by the obliteration of the normal hypointense signal of the wall, suggestive of fibrosis and muscular hypertrophy (Figs. 9.3, 9.6, and 9.11) [46]. Sometimes cystic or hemorrhagic foci on T2-weighted images (T2WIs) or T1-weighted images (T1WIs) are present (Fig. 9.11). The degree of thickening, typically exceeding 3 mm, can vary, appearing minimally in a linear pattern or as a mass. Although the disappearance of fatty space between the uterus and rectosigmoid or the obliteration of the Douglas pouch may draw attention to the rectal wall, they are insufficient for diagnosis.

On axial sequences, a triangular appearance with a posterior base facing the digestive wall and an anterior apex converging toward the uterus are highly indicative. MRI findings characteristic of rectal endometriosis include the "fan-shaped" and "mushroom cap" appearances [48]. The "fan-shaped" appearance involves fan-shaped bowel wall thickening with hypointense T2-weighted signal (similar to muscle) and slightly high signal intensity on the mucosal side [48]. The "mushroom cap" appearance refers to the focal thickening of the rectal wall's resembling the head of an umbrella, often associated with hypertrophy of the muscularis propria and smooth muscle hyperplasia (Fig. 9.12) [23].

Systematic reviews and meta-analysis comparing the accuracy of TVUS and MRI have revealed similar performance values for the two imaging techniques in diagnosing RE [25, 41, 53]. However, the reported sensitivity and specificity of MRI for RE have been reported to range from 63% to 98% and 89% to 100%, respectively [41]. Variations in sensitivity could be attributed to differences in MRI protocols, where studies lacking antiperistaltic drugs, bowel preparation, and administration have reported significantly lower sensitivities [54]. Nevertheless, a recent

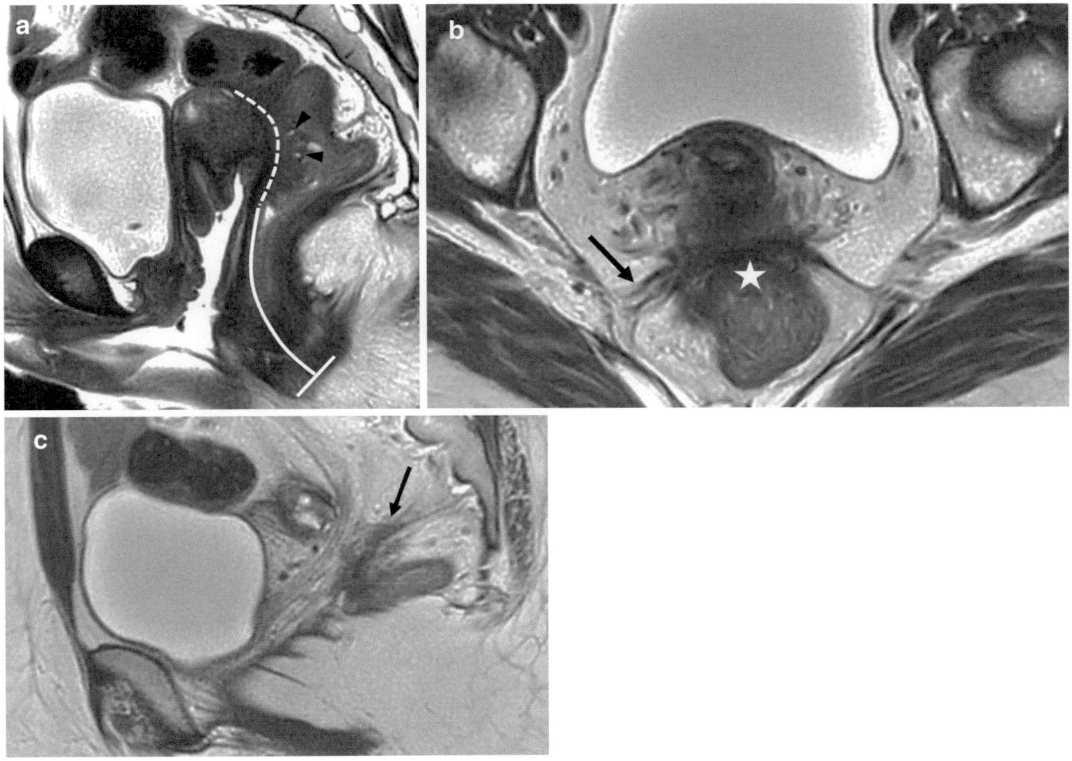

Fig. 9.11 Segmental resection of rectal endometriosis: (**a**) Sagittal T2-weighted MR image shows a rectal lesion located 7 cm (curved line) from the anal margin (white line) (measure note shown), with a length of 52 mm using a curve line (dashed line) and 50 mm by adding together the linear measurement following the curve of the lesion. Note the presence of microcysts within the lesion (arrowheads). (**b**) Axial and (**c**) sagittal T2-weighted MR images show nodular infiltration into the torus, extending to the right sacrorectal septum (also called posterolateral parametrium) (arrows) and the anterior rectal wall (star)

systematic review and meta-analysis by Gerges et al. showed overall sensitivity and specificity values of 86% and 96%, respectively [32].

Additionally, a challenge lies in differentiating thin rectal DE from simple adhesions with adjacent structures, such as the uterus. While TVUS remains more sensitive but less specific than MRI, both modalities are accurate in determining the presence of an infiltrative rectal nodule and differentiating these cases from superficial serosal involvement (Figs. 9.3 and 9.8) [55].

Few mimickers of rectosigmoid involvement exist, primarily identified by the presence of endoluminal feces, thick-content diverticula (coprolith), and, more rarely, colorectal cancer or pelvic actinomycosis [56].

9.5.3 The MRI/TVUS Fusion Technique

Fusion imaging combines MRI and US images, offering real-time visualization and high tissue contrast [57]. The MRI/TVUS fusion technique could be useful in clinical practice because it can enhance the detection of abnormalities by interchangeably utilizing the strengths of both imaging modalities (Fig. 9.13) [58]. No consensus has been reached on the optimal requirements, due to the limited number of published works on this technique [58]. Beyond its educational value in refining the learning curve, this technique may also serve as a valuable second-line treatment for more-precise lesion characterization, especially in

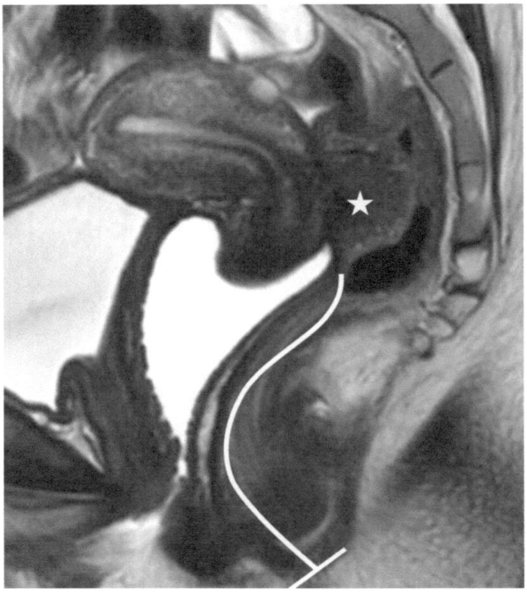

Fig. 9.12 Segmental resection of rectal endometriosis. The sagittal T2-weighted MR image shows a rectal lesion (star) located 9 cm (white curved line) from the anal margin (white line), and with a thickness of 16 mm (measure not shown). Note the submucosal edema as a high signal intensity of the lesion on the luminal side

assessing the depth of infiltration within the rectal wall. Notably, a drawback of this approach is the requirement of two separate exams instead of one.

9.5.4 Rectal Endoscopy

A recent meta-analysis comparing the diagnostic performances of TVUS, rectal endoscopic ultrasound (REUS), and MRI in detecting deep endometriosis found that REUS exhibits similar accuracy to that of the other techniques, with overall sensitivity, specificity, and accuracy values of 92%, 98%, and 99%, respectively [32]. However, REUS is more invasive, and TVUS or MRI should be favored as the initial investigative modality due to its lower invasiveness compared to that of REUS.

Thus, REUS may serve as a supplementary technique, often employed to resolve ambiguous cases identified via TVUS and/or MRI [59, 60]. In cases where TVUS or MRI reveals bowel involvement, REUS may not be necessary. However, when symptoms strongly indicate rectosigmoid involvement in patients without evi-

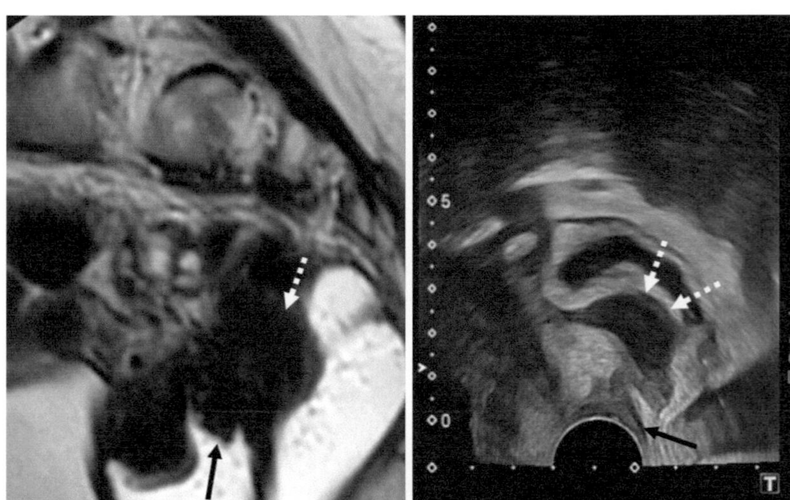

Fig. 9.13 Image fusion between real-time US and MR images. Sagittal T2-weighted MR (left) and TVUS (right) images show a rectal lesion of the middle rectum. The posterior vaginal fornix involvement is better seen on an MR image (black arrows), whereas the rectal infiltration up to the submucosae is better evaluated on TVUS (dashed arrow)

dent intestinal lesions on TVUS and/or MRI, REUS becomes more imperative to exclude bowel invasion [61].

The procedure is typically performed with a flexible tube, without general anesthesia, and is generally well tolerated. REUS allows the differentiation of bowel wall layers, with lesions presenting as rounded or triangular hypoechoic infiltrative areas thickening the intestinal wall. However, a notable limitation of REUS is its restricted ability to evaluate only the distal part of the rectosigmoid. Moreover, TVUS or MRI should always complement REUS to assess the presence of additional lesions [62].

9.5.5 Computerized Tomography (CT) Enema and Barium Enema

Another imaging modality utilized for detecting endometriosis is multidetector computerized tomography enema (MDCT-e). This involves distending the colon with water during MDCT imaging. Although traditionally used for imaging colorectal cancer, MDCT-e has been increasingly adopted for diagnosing bowel endometriosis due to recent insights into intestinal wall involvement. Bowel cleansing is typically required before this examination, and colonic distention is achieved by injecting warm water into the anal canal after administering an antiperistaltic agent for intestinal hypotonization [63]. Iodine contrast material is then administered, followed by computerized tomography (CT) acquisition in the venous phase.

MDCT-e is generally well tolerated by patients and offers a good visualization of the bowel wall. Endometriosis involvement typically manifests as a nodular lesion with contrast enhancement infiltrating the colon or rectosigmoid wall. The absence of a fat plane between the bowel wall and the nodule suggests infiltration into the intestinal muscularis propria [64]. One advantage of MDCT-e is its ability to assess the entire bowel, allowing for differential diagnosis from other pathologies, such as inflammatory disease.

However, due to the radiation exposure associated with MDCT-e, which averages between 12 and 15.8 mSv, caution must be exercised in determining its necessity, especially given the high-risk age group of female subjects vulnerable to radiation-related damage. Additionally, the administration of iodinated contrast material may pose risks of adverse reactions. Consequently, MDCT-e is not routinely employed as a first-line investigation for patients suspected of having RE and is used more favorably for a complete study of the digestive tract when indicated [25].

The double-contrast barium enema (DCBE) was historically employed as the primary diagnostic tool for bowel endometriosis, but its usage has declined due to advancements in CT-based approaches. This technique entails the injection of barium, followed by allowing air into the rectosigmoid colon, necessitating bowel preparation beforehand. Barium is administered while the patient lies in a left-side-down lateral position, and after intestinal hypotonization, air from the room is insufflated into the colon [65].

In a prospective study comparing the accuracy of DCBE and TVUS in diagnosing RE, TVUS demonstrated superior performance [66]. However, DCBE and MDCT-e offer a comprehensive overview of the entire colon, enabling the diagnosis of endometriotic lesions located proximally to the sigmoid colon, such as cecal lesions.

9.6 Preoperative Key Imaging Findings to Report

The detection of a rectal lesion constitutes merely the initial phase in apprising the surgeon and is insufficient in delineating the surgical approach. Subsequent to detection, giving an analytical description of the lesion becomes imperative. The evaluation of rectal endometriosis poses considerable challenges, particularly for nonspecialized radiologists. Although a dearth of expertise may compromise specificity, the utilization of structured reporting significantly enhances sensitivity compared to that of routine readings. Therefore, a specialized report holds promise in refining and standardizing clinical practice [67].

For gynecologist surgeons, various critical factors necessitate assessment, encompassing precise lesion localization, proximity to the anal margin, lesion count, dimensions, depth, the circumferential extent of rectal involvement, and concomitant deep endometriotic lesions. The efficacy of surgical intervention for rectal endometriosis, alongside the selection of an appropriate surgical approach (segmental resection or partial or complete discoid resection), hinges on the accurate identification of imaging findings when determining the course of surgical treatment. With more-precise information at hand, the surgeon can offer comprehensive informed consent and judiciously allocate resources, which involves collaborating with a colorectal surgeon when necessary. Furthermore, a meticulous MRI analysis can serve as a navigational aid during the surgical procedure given that rectal and perirectal involvements may largely elude direct visualization [68]. This aspect is crucial from the patient's perspective because high-quality imaging facilitates tailored and precise information dissemination, thereby fostering informed decision-making.

9.6.1 Distance to the Anal Verge

The distance to the anal verge, defined as the space between the inferior margin of the lowest bowel lesion and the anal verge, warrants careful evaluation due to its significant impact on surgical outcomes. The involvement of the lower rectum has been well established to correlate with a heightened risk of anastomotic leakage, pelvic abscess formation, and rectovaginal fistula, particularly when colpectomy is necessary, often necessitating the adoption of a systematic defunctioning stoma by most surgeons. Additionally, the resection of the lower rectum is associated with a higher incidence of postoperative de novo digestive symptoms.

Any assessment of this distance proves challenging via ultrasound, although reference points such as the rectovaginal septum, the lower lip of the posterior cervix, and the anal margin provide some guidance, with a sequential measurement approach [69]. However, evaluation using MRI is notably simpler and more precise. The definition of the distinct segments of the rectum is crucial in this context: the lower rectum spans from 0 to 5 cm from the anal verge, the mid rectum from 5 to 10 cm, and the upper rectum from 10 to 15 cm. Lesions localized above 15 cm or at the site of the sigmoid colon's origin are categorized at the rectosigmoid junction [20, 70, 71]. On MRI, the anal verge typically corresponds, on a paramedian sagittal view, to the lower end of the external anal sphincter (Figs. 9.4, 9.6, 9.11, 9.12, and 9.14) [70]. The distance can be assessed by summing linear measurements along the rectal curvature or employing a curvilinear approach (Figs. 9.4, 9.6, 9.11, 9.12, and 9.14) [20]. Notably, rectal opacification may affect measurements, potentially elongating the distance due to rectal distension, consequently often placing the lesion farther from the anal margin.

Considering the relationship to the peritoneal reflection is also crucial for preoperative planning, aiding in delineating whether the lesion lies above, at, or below the peritoneal reflection line (Fig. 9.14) [72, 73]. However, estimating this line may be challenging due to potential variations caused by the rectal and Douglas cul-de-sac symphysis associated with rectal lesions.

9.6.2 Lesion Sizes

The assessment of lesion size and bowel involvement in endometriosis holds paramount importance. Despite the absence of a clear consensus on the preferred surgical techniques for colorectal resection in endometriosis, an accurate evaluation of lesion size is critical. Both TVUS and MRI have shown strong correlation with postsurgical specimen measurements. However, two factors may influence this correlation: rectal opacification, which distends the lumen and stretches the rectal wall, and significant retraction within rectosigmoid lesions, which can lead to an overestimation of lesion thickness and an underestimation of lesion length.

9.6.2.1 The Length

The length of lesions can be measured by using either a sum of linear measurements following

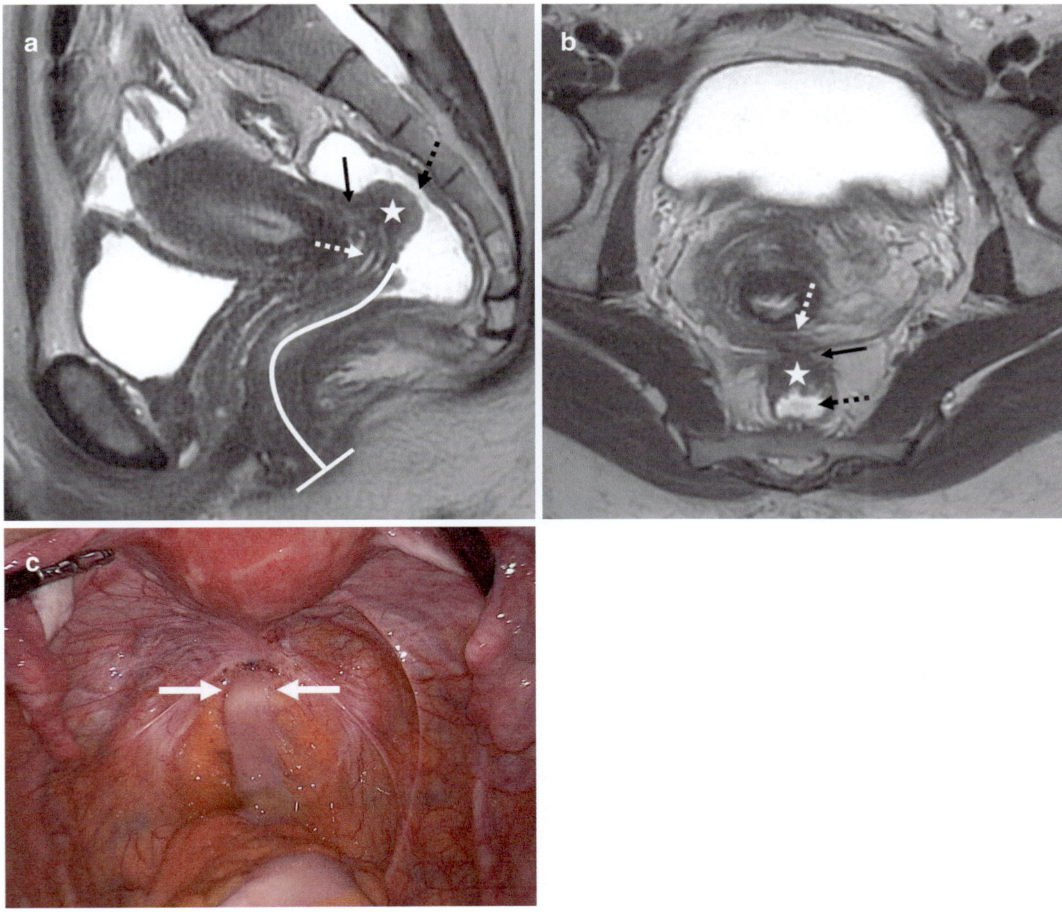

Fig. 9.14 Segmental resection of rectal endometriosis: (**a**) Sagittal and (**b**) axial T2-weighted MR images show rectal lesion (stars) located 9 cm from the anal margin using the curved line and bulging in the rectal lumen, which is responsible for stenosis (black dashed arrows) and which has a thickness of 14 mm, and a submucosal edema with a circumference of 50% (measure note shown). Note the symphysis of the Douglas pouch (arrows), the lesion being at the level of the peritoneal reflection. Note the absence of posterior vaginal fornix involvement (white dashed arrows). (**c**) Laparoscopic surgical view showing an abnormal angulation of the rectum (white arrows) attracted toward the torus uterinum, indicating the presence of a lesion not limited to the USL ligaments. Note the inadequate evaluation of the lesion in relation to subperitoneal development, demonstrating the critical role of preoperative MRI. The patient had a segmental resection. Submucosal involvement on the pathology report was in accordance with MRI analysis

the curve for elongated lesions or a curvilinear approach on sagittal T2-weighted images, or T2WIs (Figs. 9.3 and 9.11). Rectal partial-thickness disc excision, which involves excising the serosa and partially the muscularis without opening the bowel lumen, is reserved primarily for lesions ≤3 cm in size, although some authors have extended its application to longer lesions [20, 74, 75]. Indeed, this size cutoff remains somewhat arbitrary in surgical practice, as certain lesions larger than 3 cm may still be amenable to partial-thickness disc excision, particularly if they are not excessively lengthy or wide and infiltrate only the external muscular layer [76, 77].

9.6.2.2 Transverse Axis

Measuring the transverse axis is more feasible on MRI compared to TVUS because axial slices cannot be obtained with TVUS. It is assessed on axial T2-weighted images (Fig. 9.4), or on coronal T2-weighted images when necessary to evaluate the involvement of the rectosigmoid junction. Lesions that are excessively wide, taking into account both circumference and potential retraction, may necessitate a segmental resection to prevent a significant distortion of the bowel axis and subsequent wall stricture [78].

9.6.2.3 Thickness

Thickness is evaluated by measuring the thicker nodular portion from its luminal side, at best excluding any mucosal/submucosal edema if present, to its anterior border (Figs. 9.4 and 9.6). In cases of extensive retrocervical masses, the anterior border of the rectal lesion is often determined by the slightly T2 hyperintense dividing line between the rectal nodule and the torus uterinum and/or determined by posterior vaginal fornix involvement because such nodules must be excluded from the measurement of the rectal lesion.

Rousset et al. identified a cutoff size of 14 mm correlated with segmental resection, whereas Scardapane et al. found a cutoff size of >11 mm on MR colonography [20]. However, MR colonography clearly distends the rectum, which may result in the stretching of the lesion and thus a slightly thinner measurement [36].

On TVUS, Malzoni et al. reported a mean thickness of identified bowel nodules as 13.4 mm ± 4.8 mm (mean ± standard deviation) for lesions removed via segmental resection and 5.8 mm ± 2.7 mm for those removed via nodulectomy, with all the shaved nodules having a thickness of ≤7 mm [79].

9.6.3 Circumference

Measuring circumference is more feasible on MRI than on TVUS because axial slices cannot be obtained with TVUS. However, 3D TVUS with axial reconstruction may offer assistance. Similar to the assessment of the transverse axis, bowel circumference involvement is evaluated on axial T2-weighted images, or it is evaluated on coronal T2-weighted images when necessary for the evaluation of the rectosigmoid junction. This can be achieved by dividing the rectal wall into eight radii, each accounting for 12.5%, or more easily by utilizing a 360-degree scale (Figs. 9.5, 9.6, and 9.15). The presence of rectal opacification may slightly modify the circumference evaluation.

Rousset et al. demonstrated that a circumference ≥ 3/8 radii (approximately 40%) was one of the two most predictive signs of segmental resec-

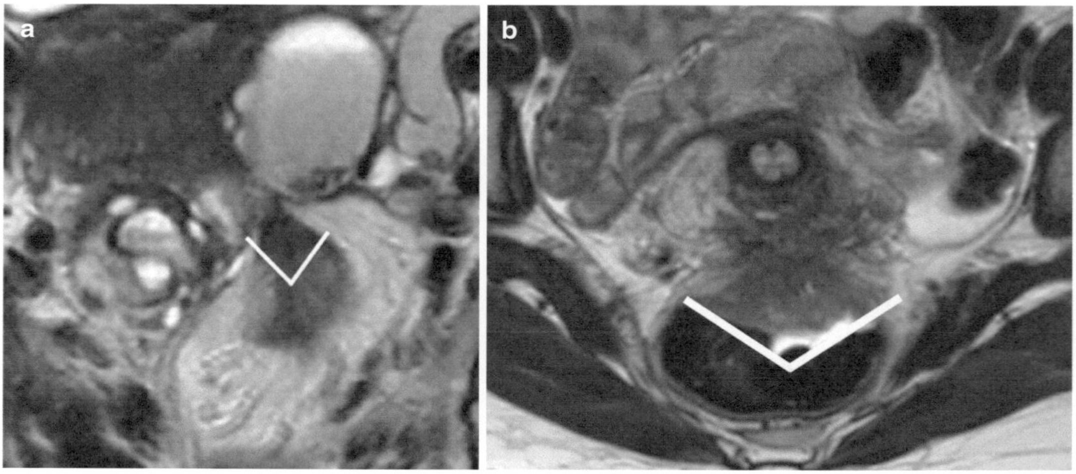

Fig. 9.15 Two lesions with different circumferential involvement on MRI resected via the two surgical techniques: (**a**) Axial T2-image shows a circumferential involvement of 70° (20%) in a patient who underwent a partial-thickness disc excision of rectal endometriosis. Note the presence of bilateral kissing ovaries. (**b**) Axial T2-image shows a circumferential involvement of 140° (≈40%) in a patient who underwent a segmental resection of rectal endometriosis

tion, with an odds ratio of 60.4 (95% CI 12.3–296.2), $p < 0.001$ (Fig. 9.15). The combination of this sign with a thickness ≥ 14 mm predicted segmental resection with an accuracy of 90.2% (95% CI 79.8–96.3, $p < 0.0001$) [20].

In addition to circumference evaluation, the use of rectal opacification aids in assessing the extent of stenosis. Scardapane et al. evaluated the degree of stenosis between the nodule and adjacent normal bowel diameter in degrees, demonstrating that a stenosis >30% accurately predicted bowel resection [80]. Rectal water-contrast transvaginal ultrasonography can also assess the degree of stenosis, facilitated by the use of 3D imaging [81].

9.6.4 Depth of Infiltration

Assessing the depth of infiltration within the various layers of the rectal wall is a crucial yet challenging aspect, particularly given the potential variability in depth across the extent of the lesion, with deeper infiltration more commonly observed at the center of the lesion. Both TVUS and MRI are adept at identifying infiltrative rectal nodules and distinguishing them from superficial serosal plaques (Figs. 9.3 and 9.10) [73]. MRI is valuable for detecting rectal endometriosis but may be less accurate in detecting submucosal/mucosal involvement compared to TVUS (Fig. 9.13) or RES. However, it remains difficult, and studies have not reported satisfactory accuracy values for TVUS or MRI in differentiating endometriotic infiltration into each bowel wall layer, particularly in distinguishing muscularis lesions from submucosal and mucosal lesions [22, 23]. TVUS tends to overestimate depth, whereas MRI may underestimate it.

The significance of a high-signal T2WI suggesting mucosal/submucosal edema at the lumen side of the rectal lesion is uncertain (Figs. 9.6 and 9.12), with differing interpretations among authors. Some consider it indicative of muscularis damage, and others view it as extension to the submucosa with associated submucosal edema [22, 23]. However, this sign may converge to be an indirect sign of deep muscularis propria infiltration within at least the internal muscular layer of the rectal wall.

In a study by Rousset et al., almost all the lesions with a nodular thickness ≥ 14 mm and/or a circumference ≥3/8 radius (38%) demonstrated deep infiltration [20]. These signs could thus serve as indirect indicators of deep infiltration, as supported by the surgical study of Abrao et al., which demonstrated that when lesions extended more deeply than the submucosal layer in segmentally resected specimens, the affected bowel circumference exceeded 40% [78].

9.6.5 Associated Lesions

Certain pararectal lesions associated with rectal lesions may predict the need for segmental resection. Especially for these associated lesions, pelvic MRI is essential compared to TVUS because it allows for a more comprehensive mapping of the lesions.

Involvement of the sacrorectal septum (also called the posterolateral parametrium) is identified on T2-weighted images by the loss of the normal appearance of the subperitoneal pararectal cellular sheet, behind the uterosacral ligament, with a thickening of the fascia recti extending posteriorly from the rectovaginal septum (Fig. 9.11) [82]. Of note, this type of involvement is part of the posterolateral compartment. In a study by Rousset et al., sacrorectovaginal septum involvement was the only pararectal sign statistically correlated with segmental resection [20]. This may be attributed to the association of this type of involvement with large and extensive lesions that may necessitate nonconservative procedures. The complete resection of such lesions entails extensive excision in the mesorectum and fascia recti, compromising the rectal vascular supply and rectal innervation due to the resection of the inferior hypogastric plexus, which lies at the anterior and upper part of the fascia recti. Therefore, this MRI sign is important not only to indicate the risk of segmental resection but also to anticipate increased potential morbidity with functional rectal and bladder disorders due to the resection of one or both inferior hypogastric plexuses [83–86].

Conversely, although more frequently associated with large rectal involvement, other perirectal involvements, such as the vaginal fornix, parametrium, or ureter, may complicate the procedure and the technique but can technically be removed without impairing rectal conservation and may not preclude a partial-thickness disc excision on the rectal lesion when feasible [20, 76].

The cloverleaf sign, formed by at least three organs converging in the center due to constrictive adhesions from DE, has been associated with a higher likelihood of bowel resection [87]. However, notably, sigmoid involvement, which typically requires resection due to its mobile nature, was also included in the study. Nonetheless, perirectal involvements should still be reported because they may complicate surgery, and the concomitant involvement of the posterior vaginal fornix may necessitate a temporary ileostomy in the case of rectal segmental resection to prevent rectovaginal fistula formation.

9.6.6 Multiple Lesions

Rectosigmoid lesions may occur as multiple lesions, and the detection of one lesion should prompt the radiologist to diligently search for additional lesions. Pelvic MRI, more so than TVUS, enables the detection of the multifocal involvement of the digestive tract (Fig. 9.16). Intestinal deep infiltrating endometriosis can manifest as multifocal (multiple lesions on the same segment) or multicentric (multiple lesions affecting several bowel segments). The distance between lesions should be documented and may influence the surgical strategy. For instance, two lesions within 2 cm proximity may be addressed with the same procedure, whereas two lesions situated more than 2 cm apart may require different types of resections, potentially combining partial-thickness disc excision or complete discoid resection techniques [88].

What's more, in the case of rectosigmoid lesions, up to a third of patients may present right-sided digestive lesions, ileal and/or caecal and/or appendicular [89]. These are difficult to detect on pelvic MRI [90], and may require further investigation by MR enterography [89], more favorably than by CT enema [91]. In fact, MR enterography provides favorable anterograde opacification for exploration of the small intestine, and is radiation-free. CT should be avoided in young patients whenever possible, due to the associated radiation exposure, being consistent

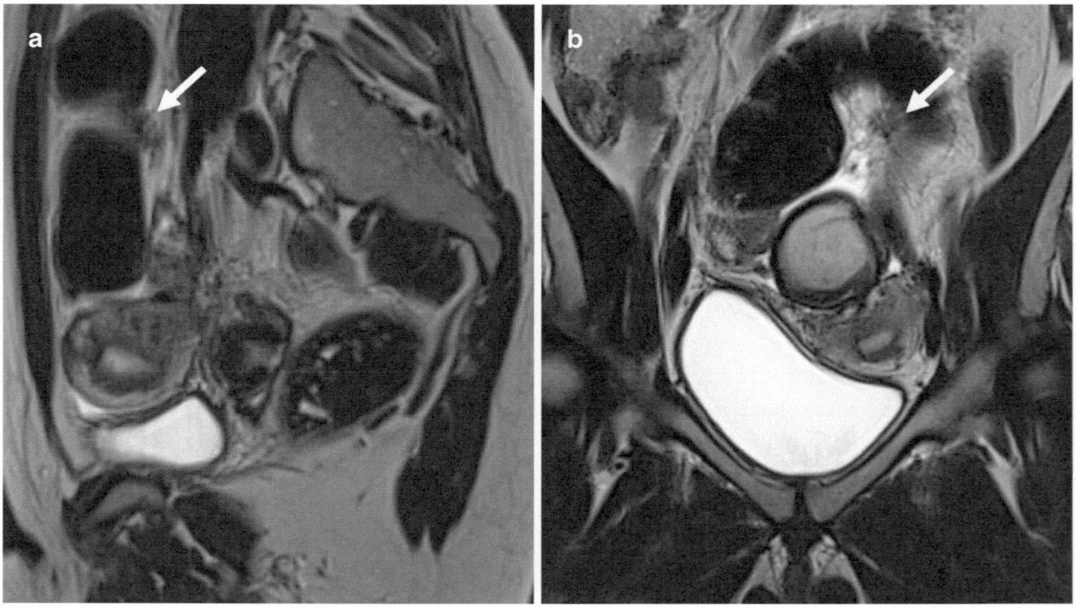

Fig. 9.16 Rectosigmoid multifocal lesions: (**a**) Sagittal and (**b**) coronal T2-weighted MR images show a small sigmoid lesion (arrows) unseen on previous TVUS in a patient with a rectal lesion

with the ALARA principle [92]. The number of lesions, the distance between lesions, the appendicular, caecal or ileal location, the distance to the ileocaecal valve, the size of lesions and any upstream distension should be described.

9.7 Conclusion

The complexity of endometriosis has been well illustrated by cases involving the rectum and rectosigmoid junction. This highlights the necessity for close collaboration between radiologists and surgeons to ensure thorough diagnostic investigations and effective treatment planning.

Surgical intervention, in appropriate cases, involves meticulous preoperative planning, comprehensive patient counseling, and collaboration with a multidisciplinary surgical team when necessary. TVUS and/or MRI play crucial roles in preoperative evaluation, facilitating a patient-centered approach. This approach is supported by standardized reporting, which aids surgeons in selecting the most suitable surgical techniques for lesion removal.

References

1. Rousset P, Florin M, Bharwani N, Touboul C, Monroc M, Golfier F, et al. Deep pelvic infiltrating endometriosis: MRI consensus lexicon and compartment-based approach from the ENDOVALIRM group. Diagn Interv Imaging. 2023;104(3):95–112.
2. Chapron C, Fauconnier A, Vieira M, Barakat H, Dousset B, Pansini V, et al. Anatomical distribution of deeply infiltrating endometriosis: surgical implications and proposition for a classification. Hum Reprod. 2003;18(1):157–61.
3. Hajati A, Hajati O. A review of more than 2000 cases of site-specific pelvic endometriosis rates by MRI: a guide to minimizing under/overdiagnosis non-invasively. Insights Imaging. 2022;13(1):129.
4. Remorgida V, Ferrero S, Fulcheri E, Ragni N, Martin DC. Bowel endometriosis: presentation, diagnosis, and treatment. Obstet Gynecol Surv. 2007;62(7):461–70.
5. Rzewuska N, Kunicki M, Mechsner S, Kordowitzki P. Rare clinical presentation of postmenopausal endometriosis: a new perspective. Aging Dis. 2023;15:2361.
6. Kavallaris A, Köhler C, Kühne-Heid R, Schneider A. Histopathological extent of rectal invasion by rectovaginal endometriosis. Hum Reprod. 2003;18(6):1323–7.
7. Anaf V, El Nakadi I, Simon P, Van de Stadt J, Fayt I, Simonart T, et al. Preferential infiltration of large bowel endometriosis along the nerves of the colon. Hum Reprod. 2004;19(4):996–1002.
8. Redwine DB, Wright JT. Laparoscopic treatment of complete obliteration of the cul-de-sac associated with endometriosis: long-term follow-up of en bloc resection. Fertil Steril. 2001;76(2):358–65.
9. Possover M, Diebolder H, Plaul K, Schneider A. Laparascopically assisted vaginal resection of rectovaginal endometriosis. Obstet Gynecol. 2000;96(2):304–7.
10. Gandek B, Ware JE, Aaronson NK, Apolone G, Bjorner JB, Brazier JE, et al. Cross-validation of item selection and scoring for the SF-12 health survey in nine countries: results from the IQOLA project. International quality of life assessment. J Clin Epidemiol. 1998;51(11):1171–8.
11. Cardaillac C, Levesque A, Riant T, Mortier A, Neunlist M, Perrouin-Verbe MA, et al. Evaluation of a scoring system for the detection of central sensitization among women with chronic pelvic pain. Am J Obstet Gynecol. 2023;229(5):530.e1–530.e17.
12. Collinet P, Fritel X, Revel-Delhom C, Ballester M, Bolze PA, Borghese B, et al. Management of endometriosis: CNGOF/HAS clinical practice guidelines—short version. J Gynecol Obstet Hum Reprod. 2018;47(7):265–74.
13. Haas D, Chvatal R, Habelsberger A, Schimetta W, Wayand W, Shamiyeh A, et al. Preoperative planning of surgery for deeply infiltrating endometriosis using the ENZIAN classification. Eur J Obstet Gynecol Reprod Biol. 2013;166(1):99–103.
14. Thomassin-Naggara I, Monroc M, Chauveau B, Fauconnier A, Verpillat P, Dabi Y, et al. Multicenter external validation of the deep pelvic endometriosis index magnetic resonance imaging score. JAMA Netw Open. 2023;6(5):e2311686.
15. Thomassin-Naggara I, Lamrabet S, Crestani A, Bekhouche A, Wahab CA, Kermarrec E, et al. Magnetic resonance imaging classification of deep pelvic endometriosis: description and impact on surgical management. Hum Reprod. 2020;35(7):1589–600.
16. Becker CM, Bokor A, Heikinheimo O, Horne A, Jansen F, Kiesel L, et al. ESHRE guideline: endometriosis. Hum Reprod Open. 2022;2022(2):hoac009.
17. Vanhie A, Meuleman C, Tomassetti C, Timmerman D, D'Hoore A, Wolthuis A, et al. Consensus on recording deep endometriosis surgery: the CORDES statement. Hum Reprod. 2016;31(11):2660.
18. Bendifallah S, Puchar A, Vesale E, Moawad G, Daraï E, Roman H. Surgical outcomes after colorectal surgery for endometriosis: a systematic review and meta-analysis. J Minim Invasive Gynecol. 2021;28(3):453–66.
19. Abo C, Bendifallah S, Jayot A, Nyangoh Timoh K, Tuech JJ, Roman H, et al. Discoid resection for colorectal endometriosis: results from a prospective cohort from two French tertiary referral centres. Colorectal Dis. 2019;21(11):1312–20.

20. Rousset P, Buisson G, Lega JC, Charlot M, Gallice C, Cotte E, et al. Rectal endometriosis: predictive MRI signs for segmental bowel resection. Eur Radiol févr. 2021;31(2):884–94.
21. Mabrouk M, Raimondo D, Altieri M, Arena A, Del Forno S, Moro E, et al. Surgical, clinical, and functional outcomes in patients with Rectosigmoid endometriosis in the Gray zone: 13-year long-term follow-up. J Minim Invasive Gynecol. 2019;26(6):1110–6.
22. Brusic A, Esler S, Churilov L, Chowdary P, Sleeman M, Maher P, et al. Deep infiltrating endometriosis: can magnetic resonance imaging anticipate the need for colorectal surgeon intervention? Eur J Radiol. 2019;121:108717.
23. Busard MPH, van der Houwen LEE, Bleeker MCG, Pieters van den Bos IC, Cuesta MA, van Kuijk C, et al. Deep infiltrating endometriosis of the bowel: MR imaging as a method to predict muscular invasion. Abdom Imaging. 2012;37(4):549–57.
24. Coletta D, De Padua C, Iannone I, Puzzovio A, Greco PA, Patriti A, et al. Defunctioning ileostomy to prevent the anastomotic leakage in colorectal surgery. The state of the art of the different available types. Front Surg. 2022;9:866191.
25. Condous G, Gerges B, Thomassin-Naggara I, Becker C, Tomassetti C, Krentel H, et al. Non-invasive imaging techniques for diagnosis of pelvic deep endometriosis and endometriosis classification systems: an International Consensus Statement. Ultrasound Obstet Gynecol. 2024;64:129–44.
26. Ferrero S, Barra F, Scala C, Condous G. Ultrasonography for bowel endometriosis. Best Pract Res Clin Obstet Gynaecol. 2021;71:38–50.
27. Young SW, Dahiya N, Patel MD, Abrao MS, Magrina JF, Temkit M, et al. Initial accuracy of and learning curve for transvaginal ultrasound with bowel preparation for deep endometriosis in a US Tertiary Care Center. J Minim Invasive Gynecol. 2017;24(7):1170–6.
28. Young SW, Jha P, Chamié L, Rodgers S, Kho RM, Horrow MM, et al. Society of Radiologists in ultrasound consensus on routine pelvic US for endometriosis. Radiology. 2024;311(1):e232191.
29. Ferrero S, Scala C, Stabilini C, Vellone VG, Barra F, Maggiore ULR. Transvaginal sonography with vs without bowel preparation in diagnosis of rectosigmoid endometriosis: prospective study. Ultrasound Obstet Gynecol. 2019;53(3):402–9.
30. Ferrero S, Barra F, Stabilini C, Vellone VG, Leone Roberti Maggiore U, Scala C. Does bowel preparation improve the performance of rectal water contrast transvaginal ultrasonography in diagnosing Rectosigmoid endometriosis? J Ultrasound Med. 2019;38(4):1017–25.
31. Valenzano Menada M, Remorgida V, Abbamonte LH, Nicoletti A, Ragni N, Ferrero S. Does transvaginal ultrasonography combined with water-contrast in the rectum aid in the diagnosis of rectovaginal endometriosis infiltrating the bowel? Hum Reprod. 2008;23(5):1069–75.
32. Gerges B, Li W, Leonardi M, Mol BW, Condous G. Optimal imaging modality for detection of rectosigmoid deep endometriosis: systematic review and meta-analysis. Ultrasound Obstet Gynecol. 2021;58(2):190–200.
33. Guerriero S, Ajossa S, Orozco R, Perniciano M, Jurado M, Melis GB, et al. Accuracy of transvaginal ultrasound for diagnosis of deep endometriosis in the rectosigmoid: systematic review and meta-analysis. Ultrasound Obstet Gynecol. 2016;47(3):281–9.
34. Guerriero S, Saba L, Ajossa S, Peddes C, Angiolucci M, Perniciano M, et al. Three-dimensional ultrasonography in the diagnosis of deep endometriosis. Hum Reprod. 2014;29(6):1189–98.
35. Atkinson NSS, Bryant RV, Dong Y, Maaser C, Kucharzik T, Maconi G, et al. How to perform gastrointestinal ultrasound: anatomy and normal findings. World J Gastroenterol. 2017;23(38):6931–41.
36. Guerriero S, Condous G, van den Bosch T, Valentin L, Leone FPG, Van Schoubroeck D, et al. Systematic approach to sonographic evaluation of the pelvis in women with suspected endometriosis, including terms, definitions and measurements: a consensus opinion from the international deep endometriosis analysis (IDEA) group. Ultrasound Obstet Gynecol. 2016;48(3):318–32.
37. Eisenberg VH, Alcazar JL, Arbib N, Schiff E, Achiron R, Goldenberg M, et al. Applying a statistical method in transvaginal ultrasound training: lessons from the learning curve cumulative summation test (LC-CUSUM) for endometriosis mapping. Gynecol Surg. 2017;14(1):19.
38. Piessens S, Healey M, Maher P, Tsaltas J, Rombauts L. Can anyone screen for deep infiltrating endometriosis with transvaginal ultrasound? Aust N Z J Obstet Gynaecol. 2014;54(5):462–8.
39. Nisenblat V, Bossuyt PMM, Farquhar C, Johnson N, Hull ML. Imaging modalities for the non-invasive diagnosis of endometriosis. Cochrane Database Syst Rev. 2016;2(2):CD009591.
40. Alborzi S, Poordast T, Askary E, Javedanmehr M, Shahraki MH, Alborzi S, et al. Evaluation and comparison of the accuracy of transvaginal ultrasound and MRI for the diagnosis of deep rectal endometriosis: a cross-sectional study. Int J Gynaecol Obstet. 2023;161(2):586–93.
41. Moura APC, Ribeiro HSAA, Bernardo WM, Simões R, Torres US, D'Ippolito G, et al. Accuracy of transvaginal sonography versus magnetic resonance imaging in the diagnosis of rectosigmoid endometriosis: systematic review and meta-analysis. PLoS One. 2019;14(4):e0214842.
42. Guerriero S, Ajossa S, Pascual MA, Rodriguez I, Piras A, Perniciano M, et al. Ultrasonographic soft markers for detection of rectosigmoid deep endometriosis. Ultrasound Obstet Gynecol. 2020;55(2):269–73.
43. Ghezzi F, Raio L, Cromi A, Duwe DG, Beretta P, Buttarelli M, et al. « kissing ovaries »: a sonographic sign of moderate to severe endometriosis. Fertil Steril. 2005;83(1):143–7.

44. Hudelist G, Fritzer N, Staettner S, Tammaa A, Tinelli A, Sparic R, et al. Uterine sliding sign: a simple sonographic predictor for presence of deep infiltrating endometriosis of the rectum. Ultrasound Obstet Gynecol. 2013;41(6):692–5.
45. Bazot M, Bharwani N, Huchon C, Kinkel K, Cunha TM, Guerra A, et al. European society of urogenital radiology (ESUR) guidelines: MR imaging of pelvic endometriosis. Eur Radiol. 2017;27(7):2765–75.
46. Bazot M, Darai E, Hourani R, Thomassin I, Cortez A, Uzan S, et al. Deep pelvic endometriosis: MR imaging for diagnosis and prediction of extension of disease. Radiology. 2004;232(2):379–89.
47. Bazot M, Gasner A, Lafont C, Ballester M, Daraï E. Deep pelvic endometriosis: limited additional diagnostic value of postcontrast in comparison with conventional MR images. Eur J Radiol. 2011;80(3):e331–9.
48. Yoon JH, Choi D, Jang KT, Kim CK, Kim H, Lee SJ, et al. Deep rectosigmoid endometriosis: "mushroom cap" sign on T2-weighted MR imaging. Abdom Imaging. 2010;35(6):726–31.
49. Thomassin-Naggara I, Rousset P, Touboul C, Razakamanantsoa L, Manganaro L. Reasons why it is time to change imaging guidelines on endometriosis. Eur Radiol. 2024;34:6175.
50. Chassang M, Novellas S, Bloch-Marcotte C, Delotte J, Toullalan O, Bongain A, et al. Utility of vaginal and rectal contrast medium in MRI for the detection of deep pelvic endometriosis. Eur Radiol. 2010;20(4):1003–10.
51. Takeuchi H, Kuwatsuru R, Kitade M, Sakurai A, Kikuchi I, Shimanuki H, et al. A novel technique using magnetic resonance imaging jelly for evaluation of rectovaginal endometriosis. Fertil Steril. 2005;83(2):442–7.
52. Hottat N, Larrousse C, Anaf V, Noël JC, Matos C, Absil J, et al. Endometriosis: contribution of 3.0-T pelvic MR imaging in preoperative assessment—initial results. Radiology. 2009;253(1):126–34.
53. Guerriero S, Saba L, Pascual MA, Ajossa S, Rodriguez I, Mais V, et al. Transvaginal ultrasound *vs* magnetic resonance imaging for diagnosing deep infiltrating endometriosis: systematic review and meta-analysis. Ultrasound Obstet Gynecol. 2018;51(5):586–95.
54. Abrao MS, Gonçalves MO, Dias JA, Podgaec S, Chamie LP, Blasbalg R. Comparison between clinical examination, transvaginal sonography and magnetic resonance imaging for the diagnosis of deep endometriosis. Hum Reprod. 2007;22(12):3092–7.
55. Sloss S, Mooney S, Ellett L, Readman E, Ma T, Brouwer R, et al. Preoperative imaging in patients with deep infiltrating endometriosis: an important aid in predicting depth of infiltration in rectosigmoid disease. J Minim Invasive Gynecol. 2022;29(5):633–40.
56. Ruaux E, VanBuren WM, Nougaret S, Gavrel M, Charlot M, Grangeon F, et al. Endometriosis MR mimickers: T2-hypointense lesions. Insights Imaging. 2024;15(1):20.
57. Millischer AE, Salomon LJ, Santulli P, Borghese B, Dousset B, Chapron C. Fusion imaging for evaluation of deep infiltrating endometriosis: feasibility and preliminary results. Ultrasound Obstet Gynecol. 2015;46(1):109–17.
58. Bazot M, Spagnoli F, Guerriero S. Magnetic resonance imaging and ultrasound fusion technique in gynecology. Ultrasound Obstet Gynecol. 2022;59(2):141–5.
59. Rossi L, Palazzo L, Yazbeck C, Walker F, Chis C, Luton D, et al. Can rectal endoscopic sonography be used to predict infiltration depth in patients with deep infiltrating endometriosis of the rectum? Ultrasound Obstet Gynecol. 2014;43(3):322–7.
60. Bazot M, Bornier C, Dubernard G, Roseau G, Cortez A, Daraï E. Accuracy of magnetic resonance imaging and rectal endoscopic sonography for the prediction of location of deep pelvic endometriosis. Hum Reprod. 2007;22(5):1457–63.
61. Kim A, Fernandez P, Martin B, Palazzo L, Ribeiro-Parenti L, Walker F, et al. Magnetic resonance imaging compared with rectal endoscopic sonography for the prediction of infiltration depth in colorectal endometriosis. J Minim Invasive Gynecol. 2017;24(7):1218–26.
62. Noventa M, Scioscia M, Schincariol M, Cavallin F, Pontrelli G, Virgilio B, et al. Imaging modalities for diagnosis of deep pelvic endometriosis: comparison between trans-vaginal Sonography, rectal endoscopy sonography and magnetic resonance imaging. A head-to-head meta-analysis. Diagnostics. 2019;9(4):225.
63. Ferrero S, Biscaldi E, Vellone VG, Venturini PL, Maggiore ULR. Computed tomographic colonography vs rectal water- contrast transvaginal sonography in diagnosis of rectosigmoid endometriosis: a pilot study. Ultrasound Obstet Gynecol. 2017;49(4):515–23.
64. Biscaldi E, Ferrero S, Leone Roberti Maggiore U, Remorgida V, Venturini PL, Rollandi GA. Multidetector computerized tomography enema versus magnetic resonance enema in the diagnosis of rectosigmoid endometriosis. Eur J Radiol. 2014;83(2):261–7.
65. Ribeiro HSAA, Ribeiro PA, Rossini L, Rodrigues FC, Donadio N, Aoki T. Double-contrast barium enema and transrectal endoscopic ultrasonography in the diagnosis of intestinal deeply infiltrating endometriosis. J Minim Invasive Gynecol. 2008;15(3):315–20.
66. Savelli L, Manuzzi L, Coe M, Mabrouk M, Di Donato N, Venturoli S, et al. Comparison of transvaginal sonography and double-contrast barium enema for diagnosing deep infiltrating endometriosis of the posterior compartment. Ultrasound Obstet Gynecol. 2011;38(4):466–71.
67. Jaramillo-Cardoso A, Shenoy-Bhangle A, Garces-Descovich A, Glickman J, King L, Mortele KJ. Pelvic MRI in the diagnosis and staging of pelvic endometriosis: added value of structured reporting and expertise. Abdom Radiol. 2020;45(6):1623–36.

68. Bazot M, Daraï E. Role of transvaginal sonography and magnetic resonance imaging in the diagnosis of uterine adenomyosis. Fertil Steril. 2018;109(3):389–97.
69. Aas-Eng MK, Dauser B, Lieng M, Diep LM, Leonardi M, Condous G, et al. Transvaginal sonography accurately measures lesion-to-anal-verge distance in women with deep endometriosis of the rectosigmoid. Ultrasound Obstet Gynecol. 2020;56(5):766–72.
70. Han YE, Park BJ, Sung DJ, Kim MJ, Han NY, Sim KC, et al. How to accurately measure the distance from the anal verge to rectal cancer on MRI: a prospective study using anal verge markers. Abdom Radiol. 2021;46(2):449–58.
71. D'Souza N, Balyasnikova S, Tudyka V, Lord A, Shaw A, Abulafi M, et al. Variation in landmarks for the rectum: an MRI study. Colorectal Dis. 2018;20(10):O304–9.
72. Sim KC, Park BJ, Kim MJ, Sung DJ, Han NY, Han YE, et al. Accuracy of MRI for predicting anterior peritoneal reflection involvement in locally advanced rectal cancer: a comparison with operative findings. Abdom Radiol. 2022;47(2):508–16.
73. Aas-Eng MK, Lieng M, Dauser B, Diep LM, Leonardi M, Condous G, et al. Transvaginal sonography determines accurately extent of infiltration of rectosigmoid deep endometriosis. Ultrasound Obstet Gynecol. 2021;58(6):933–9.
74. Perandini A, Perandini S, Montemezzi S, Bonin C, Bellini G, Bergamini V. Defining probabilities of bowel resection in deep endometriosis of the rectum: prediction with preoperative magnetic resonance imaging. J Obstet Gynaecol Res. 2018;44(2):292–7.
75. Roman H, Bubenheim M, Huet E, Bridoux V, Zacharopoulou C, Collinet P, et al. Baseline severe constipation negatively impacts functional outcomes of surgery for deep endometriosis infiltrating the rectum: results of the ENDORE randomized trial. J Gynecol Obstet Hum Reprod. 2019;48(8):625–9.
76. Roman H, Moatassim-Drissa S, Marty N, Milles M, Vallée A, Desnyder E, et al. Rectal shaving for deep endometriosis infiltrating the rectum: a 5-year continuous retrospective series. Fertil Steril. 2016;106(6):1438–1445.e2.
77. Roman H, Bubenheim M, Huet E, Bridoux V, Zacharopoulou C, Daraï E, et al. Conservative surgery versus colorectal resection in deep endometriosis infiltrating the rectum: a randomized trial. Hum Reprod. 2018;33(1):47–57.
78. Abrão MS, Podgaec S, Dias JA, Averbach M, Silva LFF, Marino de Carvalho F. Endometriosis lesions that compromise the rectum deeper than the inner muscularis layer have more than 40% of the circumference of the rectum affected by the disease. J Minim Invasive Gynecol. 2008;15(3):280–5.
79. Malzoni M, Casarella L, Coppola M, Falcone F, Iuzzolino D, Rasile M, et al. Preoperative ultrasound indications determine excision technique for bowel surgery for deep infiltrating endometriosis: a single, high-volume center. J Minim Invasive Gynecol. 2020;27(5):1141–7.
80. Scardapane A, Lorusso F, Francavilla M, Bettocchi S, Fascilla FD, Angelelli G, et al. Magnetic resonance colonography may predict the need for bowel resection in colorectal endometriosis. Biomed Res Int. 2017;2017:5981217.
81. Philip CA, Bisch C, Coulon A, Maissiat E, de Saint-Hilaire P, Huissoud C, et al. Three-dimensional sonorectography: a new transvaginal ultrasound technique with intrarectal contrast to assess colorectal endometriosis. Ultrasound Obstet Gynecol. 2015;45(2):233–5.
82. Buy JN, Ghossain M. Secondary Mullerian system. In: Buy JN, Ghossain M, editors. Gynecological imaging: a reference guide to diagnosis. Berlin, Heidelberg: Springer; 2013. p. 439–505. https://doi.org/10.1007/978-3-642-31012-6_17.
83. Ceccaroni M, Clarizia R, Bruni F, D'Urso E, Gagliardi ML, Roviglione G, et al. Nerve-sparing laparoscopic eradication of deep endometriosis with segmental rectal and parametrial resection: the Negrar method. A single-center, prospective, clinical trial. Surg Endosc. 2012;26(7):2029–45.
84. Ruffo G, Sartori A, Crippa S, Partelli S, Barugola G, Manzoni A, et al. Laparoscopic rectal resection for severe endometriosis of the mid and low rectum: technique and operative results. Surg Endosc. 2012;26(4):1035–40.
85. Nezhat C, Falik R, McKinney S, King LP. Pathophysiology and management of urinary tract endometriosis. Nat Rev Urol. 2017;14(6):359–72.
86. Tosti C, Pinzauti S, Santulli P, Chapron C, Petraglia F. Pathogenetic mechanisms of deep infiltrating endometriosis. Reprod Sci. 2015;22(9):1053–9.
87. Härmä K, Binda A, Ith M, Poellinger A, Siegenthaler F, Heverhagen J, et al. Cloverleaf sign in pelvic magnetic resonance imaging for deep infiltrating endometriosis: association with longer operation times, greater blood loss, and higher rates of bowel resection. Invest Radiol. 2020;55(1):53–9.
88. Abrão MS, Petraglia F, Falcone T, Keckstein J, Osuga Y, Chapron C. Deep endometriosis infiltrating the recto-sigmoid: critical factors to consider before management. Hum Reprod Update. 2015;21(3):329–39.
89. Rousset P, Peyron N, Charlot M, Chateau F, Golfier F, Raudrant D, et al. Bowel endometriosis: preoperative diagnostic accuracy of 3.0-T MR enterography–initial results. Radiology. 2014;273(1):117–24.
90. Belghiti J, Thomassin-Naggara I, Zacharopoulou C, Zilberman S, Jarboui L, Bazot M, et al. Contribution of Computed Tomography Enema and Magnetic Resonance Imaging to Diagnose Multifocal and Multicentric Bowel Lesions in Patients With Colorectal Endometriosis. J Minim Invasive Gynecol. 2015;22(5):776–84.
91. Woo S, Suh CH, Kim H. Diagnostic performance of computed tomography for bowel endometriosis: A systematic review and meta-analysis. Eur J Radiol. 2019;119:108638.
92. Nisenblat V, Bossuyt PM, Farquhar C, Johnson N, Hull ML. Imaging modalities for the non-invasive diagnosis of endometriosis. Cochrane Database Syst Rev 2016; 2:CD009591.

10 Antero-, Medio-, and Posterolateral Compartments: Parametrium

Cyril Touboul, Isabelle Thomassin-Naggara, Yohann Dabi, Emile Darai, and Pascal Rousset

10.1 Introduction

The lateral compartment is a critical location of endometriosis for symptoms and complications because it may involve multiple structures located in the parametrium, such as the ureter, uterine artery, hypogastric artery and nerves, and inferior hypogastric plexus (or pelvic plexus). The prevalence of this location is likely low, lower than 15% in a series of patients who underwent surgery for complex deep infiltrating endometriotic (DIE) disease [1, 2]. However, the description of this location is preoperatively crucial to inform patients of the necessity of a resection such as parametrectomy, which is associated with a high risk of postoperative complications [3]. Such resections are linked to the risk of ureteral injury causing the possibility of ureteral fistula and/or urinary or anorectal dysfunction due to nerve injury. In addition, missing the description of this location on preoperative imaging may lead to discovering the lesions preoperatively and to more-extensive or inadequate surgery because the initial laparoscopic view doesn't allow a comprehensive visualization of the complete extension. This is also a cause of preoperative misinformation for patients. Usually, patients with parametrial involvement more often report—in addition to traditional dysmenorrhea and dyspareunia—dysuria due to the loss of urinary feeling or voiding troubles and digestive symptoms such as irritable bowel syndrome. They also report paresthesia with burning sensations and posterior leg irradiation.

Classically, the parametrium is defined as the tissue surrounding the uterine artery. However, many denominations have been used to designate this area, especially to define the parametrium in cervical cancer [4]. In patients with endometriosis, this is also a classical location of the disease [1]. The main difference with the lateral parametrium involved in cervical cancer is that endometriotic infiltration into the parametrium could be lateral but is mainly posterior, surrounding the distal uterosacral ligament. Less frequently, endometriotic infiltration can involve the anterior parametrium and in this case may be associated with ureteral or bladder lateral involvement. Here we will define the specificities of the endometriotic parametrium and the therapeutic impact of this involvement.

C. Touboul (✉) · Y. Dabi · E. Darai
Department of Gynecologic Surgery, Tenon University Hospital—APHP, Sorbonne University, Paris, France

GRC endometriose C3E, Sorbonne University, Paris, France
e-mail: cyril.touboul@aphp.fr

I. Thomassin-Naggara
Imageries Radiologiques et Interventionnelles Spécialisées (IRIS), Tenon Hospital, AP-HP, Sorbonne Université, Paris, France

P. Rousset
Department of Radiology, Lyon Sud University Hospital, Hospices Civils de Lyon, Claude Bernard Lyon 1 University, Lyon, France

I. Thomassin-Naggara (ed.), *Imaging of Endometriosis: A Comparative Guide of US, MRI and Surgery*, https://doi.org/10.1007/978-3-031-82750-1_10

10.2 Surgical Definitions

10.2.1 Anatomical Description

The classical anatomical description of the parametrium was initially carried out in the cervical cancer literature and was used in endometriosis descriptions. On the basis of embryological and anatomical dissections, Hockel showed in 2005 [5] that the parametrium appeared to consist of two structures: (1) the mesometrium, composed of lymphofatty tissue accompanying the uterine artery and located laterally, and (2) the infraureteral parametrium, spreading backward and caudally in a plane close to the uterosacral ligaments and extending to the presacral visceral pelvic fascia. This description led to defining the lateral supraureteral parametrium and the posterior infraureteral parametrium, followed by the uterosacral ligaments or the so-called visceral pelvic fascia [4]. This description is crucial for endometriosis, in which posterior parametrium involvement is much more common than lateral parametrium involvement. The ureter is a critical anatomic landmark to individualize these two areas (Fig. 10.1). The ureter is part of the lateral parametrium and can be preserved by dissecting the crossing area with the uterine artery (Fig. 10.2). The anterior parametrium is involved in cases of persistent disease above this crossing area, when the ureter is entering in vesical trigona, just beneath external bladder pillar. After opening the paravesical space, the anterior parametrium is located medially and may be associated with the ureteral and/or vesical walls laterally.

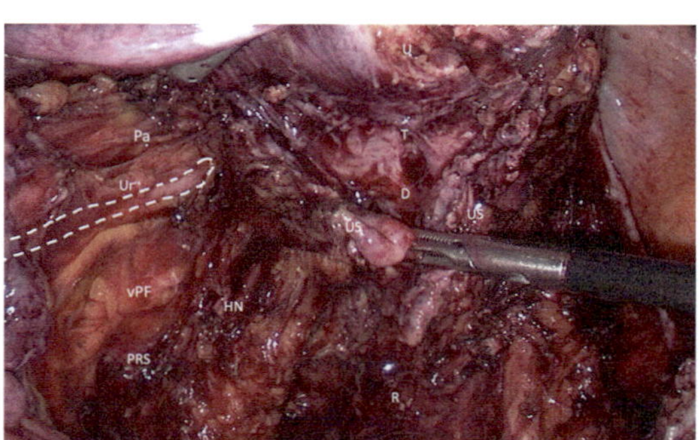

Fig. 10.1 Surgical anatomy of the pelvis: laparoscopic posterior view. Left uterosacral ligament is pulled medially with laparoscopic forceps and the ureter is limiting the visceral pelvic fascia below and the lateral parametrium above. *Ur* ureter, *Pa* parametrium, *vPF* visceral pelvic fascia, *HN* hypogastric nerve, *US* uterosacral ligament, *T* torus, *D* Douglas pouch, *U* uterus, *R* rectum

Many appellations are used to designate this region, but some authors have proposed unified terminology [6]. We therefore chose to use the terms *parametrium*, *anterior parametrium*, *lateral parametrium*, *paracervix*, and *posterior parametrium*, composed of uterosacral ligaments and visceral pelvic fascia (i.e., the sacrorectal blade) (Fig. 10.3). The paravesical and pararectal spaces are also critical dissections needed to distinguish the different parts of the parametrium.

Recently, many authors have described disease-specific endometriotic parametrial involvement [1, 7, 8]. This infiltration usually follows the visceral pelvic fascia (vPF) where the inferior pelvic plexus is located (IPP). Moreover, hypogastric nerve infiltration and inflammation are parts of the pathophysiology of posterior and parametrial DIE, explaining the neurological and urinary symptoms reported by patients.

Having thorough knowledge of the anatomy of the hypogastric plexus and nerve is particularly important for a surgeon because the inferior hypogastric plexus lies along the parametrium, between the uterosacral ligaments and the ureters [9]. This plexus is formed by the convergence of sympathetic and parasympathetic nerves and by visceral afferent fibers, the latter playing a crucial role in the innervation of pelvic organs, including the bladder, rectum, reproductive organs, and pelvic floor muscles.

Surgical procedures on the parametrium require carefully considering the anatomical nuances of the inferior hypogastric plexus, the preservation of nerve function, and multidisciplinary collaboration to achieve optimal outcomes and minimize postoperative complications. Surgeons must possess advanced skills and expertise in pelvic anatomy and surgical techniques to address the complexities associated with interventions in this region. Preoperative imaging may help to evaluate the risk of injuries to this plexus and thus predict the risk of de novo

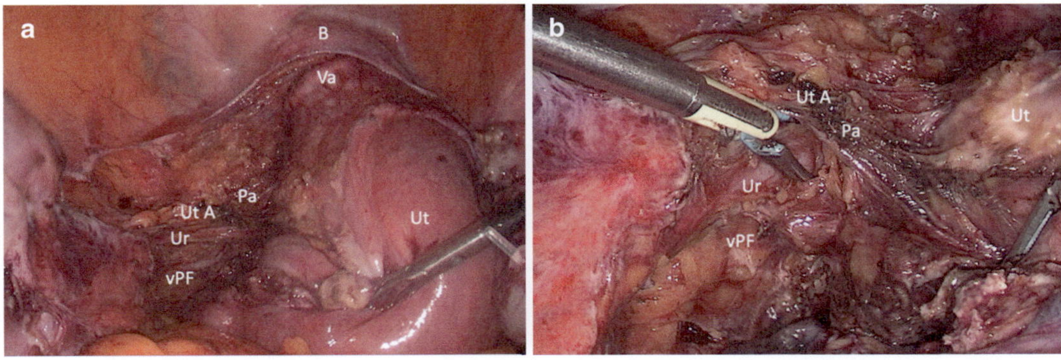

Fig. 10.2 Anatomical description of surgical lateral supraureteral parametrium: (**a**) global view and (**b**) zoom-in view of the crossing area between the ureter and the uterine artery. *Ut A* uterine artery, *Ur* ureter, *Pa* parametrium, *vPF* visceral pelvic fascia, *B* bladder, *Ut* uterus

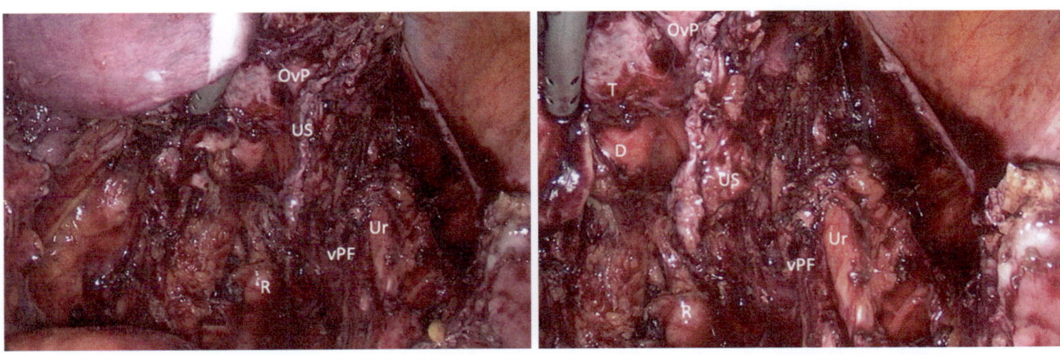

Fig. 10.3 Surgical view of right posterior infraureteral parametrium (uterosacral ligament and visceral fascia). *Ur* ureter, *vPF* visceral pelvic fascia, *US* uterosacral ligament, *T* torus, *D* Douglas pouch, *OvP* ovarian fossae peritoneum, *U* uterus, *R* rectum

voiding dysfunction [2, 10], which is a frequent postoperative complication that must be explained to the patient preoperatively because the impact on their quality of life can be huge.

The inferior hypogastric plexus is situated behind the peritoneum, in front of the sacrum, and medially to the internal iliac vessels. It extends laterally and medially to form the vesical and rectovaginal plexus (Fig. 10.4). This plexus is the convergence of the hypogastric and splanchnic nerves and is implicated in the stimulation of bladder contraction during voiding; in the rectal contraction and relaxation of the internal anal sphincter during defecation; in the innervation of the reproductive organs, influencing sexual arousal and reproductive functions; and in the modulation blood flow, glandular secretion, and smooth muscle contraction within the reproductive system and pelvic floor muscles. Thus, the inferior hypogastric plexus is intimately involved in the regulation of bladder, bowel, reproductive, and sexual functions and in pelvic floor muscle control and blood flow regulation within the pelvic cavity. Dysfunction in the inferior hypogastric plexus can lead to various pelvic disorders and symptoms related to urinary, gastrointestinal, and reproductive health. It lies in the extraperitoneal connective tissue, lateral to the rectum and vagina and beneath the ureter (between the ureter and the levator ani), in the sacrorecto-genital septum (visceral pelvic fascia). Its shape is triangular with a posterior base and its upper angle receives the hypogastric nerve, while the posteroinferior angle receives

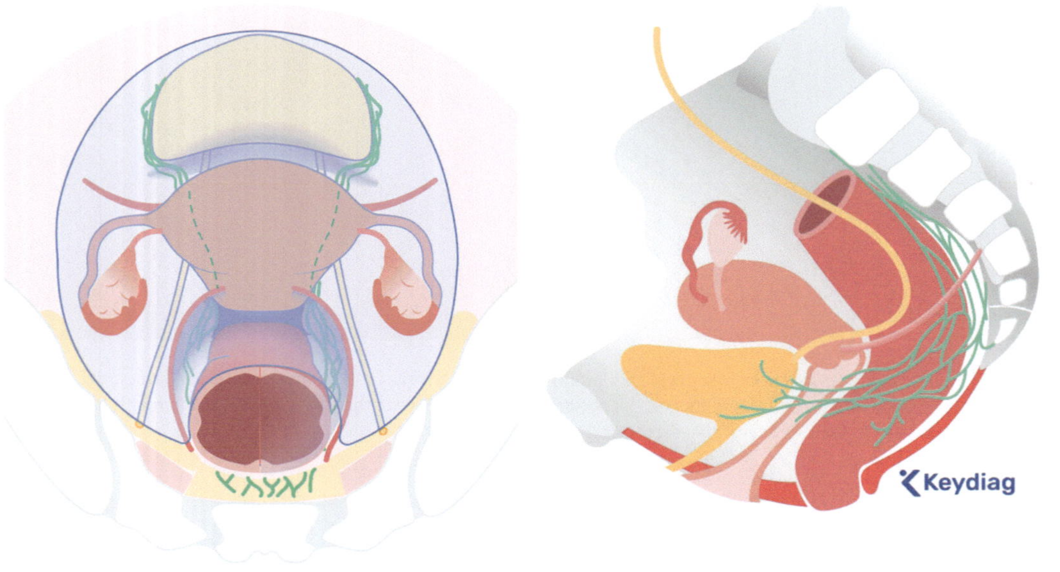

Fig. 10.4 Inferior hypogastric plexus. Its shape is triangular (yellow) with a posterior base, and its upper angle receives the hypogastric nerve, whereas the posteroinferior angle receives the pelvic splanchnic nerves (yellow). Its fibers then spread to reach the rectum, uterus, and bladder. The anteroinferior angle corresponds to the point of intersection between the uterine artery and the ureter. (Source: Thomassin-Naggara et al., Euro Radiol. 2025, in press)

the pelvic splanchnic nerves (Fig. 10.4). Its fibers then spread to reach the rectum, uterus, and bladder. The anteroinferior angle corresponds to the point of intersection between the uterine artery and the ureter. The inferior hypogastric plexux (IHP) is typically found positioned under the deep uterine vein.

10.2.2 Surgical Anatomical Description

Surgical anatomy differs from classical anatomy in that the opening of artificial surgical dissection plans allows for following anatomical structures, thus modifying the point of view of the anatomist. The anatomic description starts with ureteral dissection and the opening of the Latzko pararectal space. The parametrium is the structure located between these opened spaces. Of course, when lateral parametrial endometriosis is diagnosed, the major issue is ureteral involvement. Fortunately, parametrial endometriosis close to the ureter without hydronephrosis is considered to be at a low risk of ureteral involvement and may occur in <0.5% of cases [11]. This can be challenged when the ureter is surrounded by endometriosis, increasing the risk of such involvement. When hydronephrosis is present, the priority should be to place a stent in the ureter and take time to plan the intervention with a multidisciplinary team involving urologists. The hydronephroses can still be caused by compression and not involvement, but it can be difficult to address preoperatively. Various techniques, including ureteral shaving, ureteral resection with end-to-end anastomosis, and ureterovesical reimplantation, are possible.

10.3 Radiological Definitions

Discrepancies between the anatomical terminology used in imaging diagnostics and gynecological surgery is classically reported [12]. The first description of lateral endometriotic locations was performed by Bazot et al., describing on MRI a low-signal-intensity area in T2-weighted MRI sequences, with or without the inclusion of tiny high-signal-intensity spots in the paracervical or paravaginal regions and with or without pelvic wall involvement or ureteral dilatation [1]. In this distinguished paper, the authors suggest a possible difference between proximal parametrial involvement, characterized by a low-signal-intensity area in the paracervical and paravaginal regions on T2-weighted MR imaging, and distal parametrial involvement, exhibiting pelvic wall involvement or ureteral dilatation. Recently, on the basis of the description of surgical anatomy, a French consensus published by the Endoval IRM group proposed to delineate lateral endometriotic locations into two compartments [13]: the mediolateral compartment and the posterolateral compartment (Fig. 10.5). In addition, a third lateral compartment is less frequently involved laterally because it is endometriotic and located medially to the paravesical space and is thus named the anterolateral parametrium.

The mediolateral compartment encompasses the lateral anatomical parametrium, defined as the connective tissue sheet containing blood vessels, the ureter, and the inferior hypogastric plexus (Fig. 10.5). The lateral parametrium extends from the lateral surface of the cervix and vagina to the lateral pelvic wall in the frontal plane. Recently, an addendum dedicated to parametrial description was published to complete the ultrasonographic description of pelvic endometriosis according to IDEA [14]. This group, led by Guerriero et al., described the sonographic features of lateral parametrial invasion as a regularly or irregularly shape (star-shaped) hypoechoic nodule localized at the level of crossing between the ureter and the uterine artery. The authors wrote that well-defined parametrial nodules are more commonly located cranially to the uterine artery, whereas fan-shaped lesions featuring the retraction of the surrounding tissues are more frequently found in a caudal location (the paracervix). In the latter case, ovarian mobility is often reduced [15]. The diagnostic performance of TVUS for the diagnosis of deep endometriotic parametrial involvement in women with suspected deep endometriosis is moderate with a pooled sensitivity of 31% and a pooled specificity of 98% [16]. This is why the exhaustive mapping of DIE disease must be performed via pelvic MRI before DIE surgery (Fig. 10.6).

Regarding MR description, the EndovalIRM group defines this space as lateral to the uterine cervix or vagina and named it the mediolateral parametrium. It is situated between an anterior horizontal line passing anteriorly to the cervix or vagina and a posterior line passing anteriorly to the rectum. Involvement is considered in the presence of nodular tissue infiltration and anatomical distortion, primarily arising from thick lesions in the proximal uterosacral ligament (the frontal segment of the uterosacral ligament, or USL) or lesions in the inferior and posterior part of the broad ligament.

A potential pitfall is that MRI descriptions of subtle findings may correspond only to ovarian fossa involvement or to periovarian infiltration necessitating only peritoneal resection during surgery (Fig. 10.7). Importantly, the extension in this compartment should be described as involving the proximal lateral parametrium or the distal lateral parametrium if the ureter is involved, the descendant part of the uterine artery up to the pelvic wall with its external iliac vessels, and/or the obturator nerves and vessels (Figs. 10.8 and 10.9).

In cases of distal lateral parametrium involvement, MRI descriptions are crucial because parametrectomy featuring the section of the uterine artery, followed by the uncrossing maneuver, may be required for complete DIE removal, posing a higher risk of ureteral injury and urinary/anorectal dysfunction secondary to nerve injury (Fig. 10.10). Note that in cases of kissing ovaries, proximal parametrial assessment may be challenging or overestimated due to local retraction. This condition is associated with moderate-to-severe endometriosis, and parameters are at least partly involved [15].

For ureteral endometriosis, surgical management includes conservative ureterolysis with the removal of adjacent DIE, ureteral shaving with cold scissors, or radical approaches such as ureteral segmental resection and anastomosis or reimplantation. Ureteric involvement due to endometriosis can be extrinsic or intrinsic:

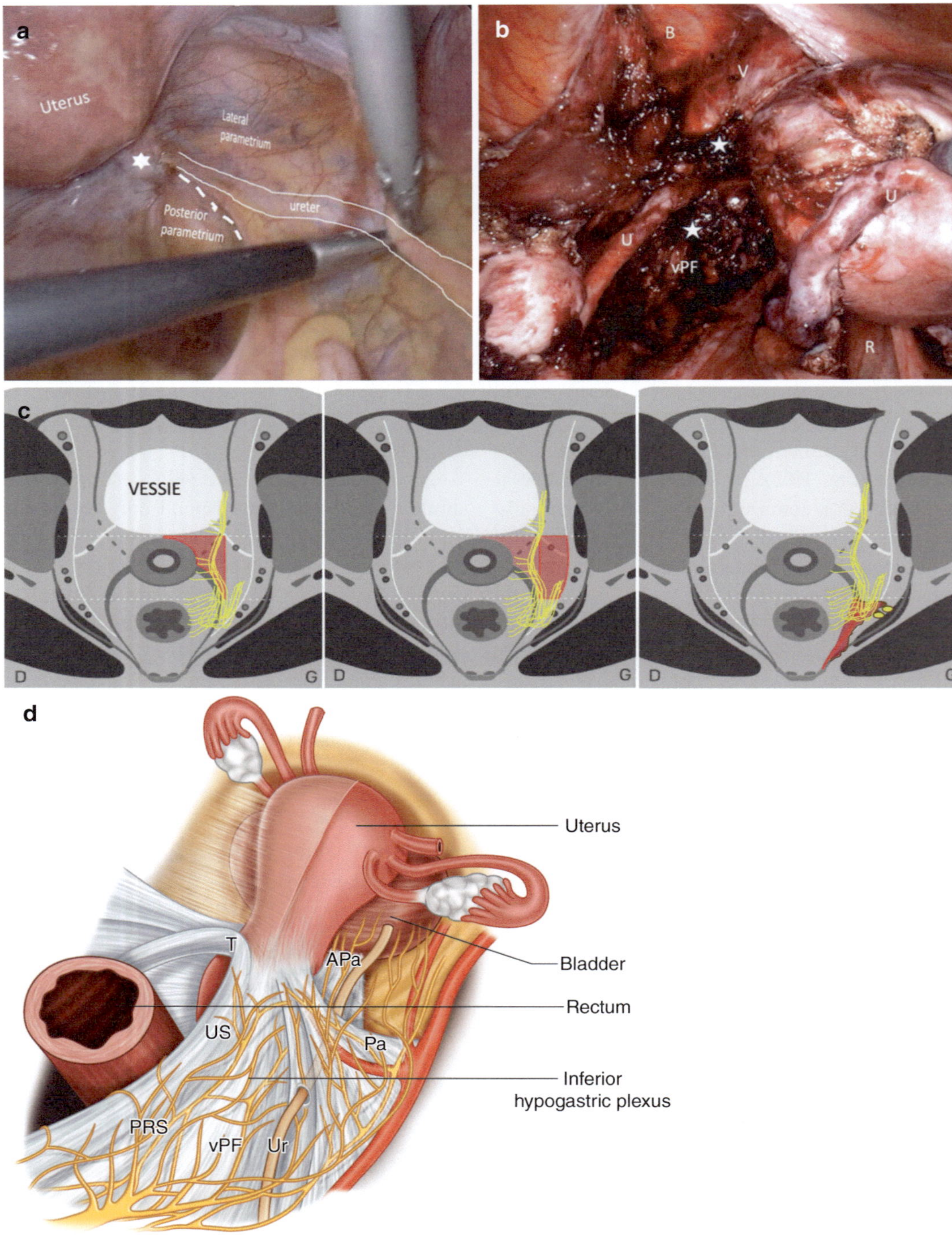
a
Uterus
Lateral parametrium
Posterior parametrium
ureter
b
B
V
U
vPF
U
R
c
VESSIE
D
G
D
G
D
G
d
Uterus
Bladder
Rectum
Inferior hypogastric plexus
T
APa
US
Pa
PRS
vPF
Ur

Extrinsic disease is more common and treated by shaving, whereas intrinsic disease requires segmental ureteric resection (Figs. 10.11 and 10.12).

The second surgical procedure usually requires the presence of a urologist and should be anticipated. Assessing extrinsic or intrinsic involvement remains challenging on imaging, with extrinsic involvement reported in 80% of cases if encasement is <360° and intrinsic in over 50% of cases if encasement is 360°. The length of the involved ureter and the distance from the ureterovesical junction could also aid in guiding surgical management.

The anterolateral compartment comprises the anterior anatomical parametrium and is located medially to the paravesical space and named the anterolateral parametrium. This nodule may come from the lateral round ligament (describe in Chap. 5) or the mediolateral parametrium, or it may be associated with urinary involvement.

The posterolateral compartment comprises the posterior anatomical parametrium, which corresponds to the distal part of the uterosacral ligament (USL) and the sacrorectal septa and to the sacral roots of the greater sciatic foramen (GSF). Both entities may be grouped under what is named the posterolateral parametrium. The distal USL is defined as the portion of the USL with an anteroposterior direction. Involvement is considered isolated when the USL is affected within its plane, constituting the medial roof of the sacrorecto-genital septum (SRGS) (Fig. 10.13).

If infiltration extends beyond the USL plane, it is deemed as invading the sacrorectal septum and finally the SRGS (Fig. 10.14). For surgeons, the boundary is marked by the level of the ureter because the hypogastric plexus is situated within the SRGS beneath the ureter and the deep uterine vein. This septum is distinguished from the mediolateral parametrium (as defined previously), which is positioned posteriorly to the horizontal line passing anteriorly to the rectum and laterally to or encompassing the mesorectal fascia (also called fascia recti) (Fig. 10.15).

Two degrees of MRI involvement are proposed herein, either without or with pelvic wall infiltration (involving internal iliac vessels, sacral roots, and the sciatic nerve). Additionally, the depth of the extension and the distance to the iliococcygeus muscle of the levator ani muscle could also be noted (Fig. 10.16).

The involvement of the SRGS in DIE is crucial to document before surgery to anticipate the heightened risk of rectal and bladder dysfunction resulting from the resection of the inferior hypogastric plexus. The inferior hypogastric plexus, the hypogastric nerve, and the pelvic splanchnic nerves constitute the nervous elements within the pararectal fossa. These nerves play vital roles in urinary, digestive, and sexual functions, necessitating specific neurological management through re-education or neurostimulation.

A significant pitfall that may mimic USL endometriotic location is a postoperative fibrosis of the posterolateral compartment that is diagnosed by using MR imaging due to the very low T2W signal and the absence of hemorrhagic spots on a T1W sequence (Figs. 10.17 and 10.18). Figures 10.19, 10.20, 10.21, 10.22, 10.23, and 10.24 show the radiosurgical correlations of the various subtypes of parametrial infiltration.

Fig. 10.5 Deep endometriosis in lateral compartments. (**a**) Laparoscopic view before dissection: The right ureter split the lateral locations of deep pelvic endometriosis structures into two types, which are below the peritoneum. The ureter has an oblique orientation. Thus, some deep pelvic endometriosis (DPE) locations are above and below to the ureter (mediolateral parametrium), and other DPE locations are only below the ureter (the posterolateral parametrium or the sacrorectal septum). The star shows a right posterolateral DIE nodule. (**b**) Robotic surgery view after dissection showing the position of the left ureter (u) above an endometriotic nodule (star), which is in the left visceral fascia (i.e., the sacrorectal septum or the posterolateral parametrium) and under a second location (star) in the left proximal parametrium. *U* ureter, *vPF* visceral pelvic fascia, *V* vagina, *T* torus, *B* bladder, *R* rectum. (**c**) Schematic MR views. (1) Posterolateral compartment: USL distal/sacrorectal septum (posterolateral parametrium). (2) Mediolateral and anterolateral compartment: proximal (medio lateral) parametrium. (3) Mediolateral compartment: distal (medio lateral) parametrium. (**d**) Anatomy of the inferior hypogastric plexus within parametrial compartments. *Ur* ureter, *vPF* visceral pelvic fascia, *Pa* parametrium, *Apa* anterior parametrium, *T* torus, *US* uterosacral ligament

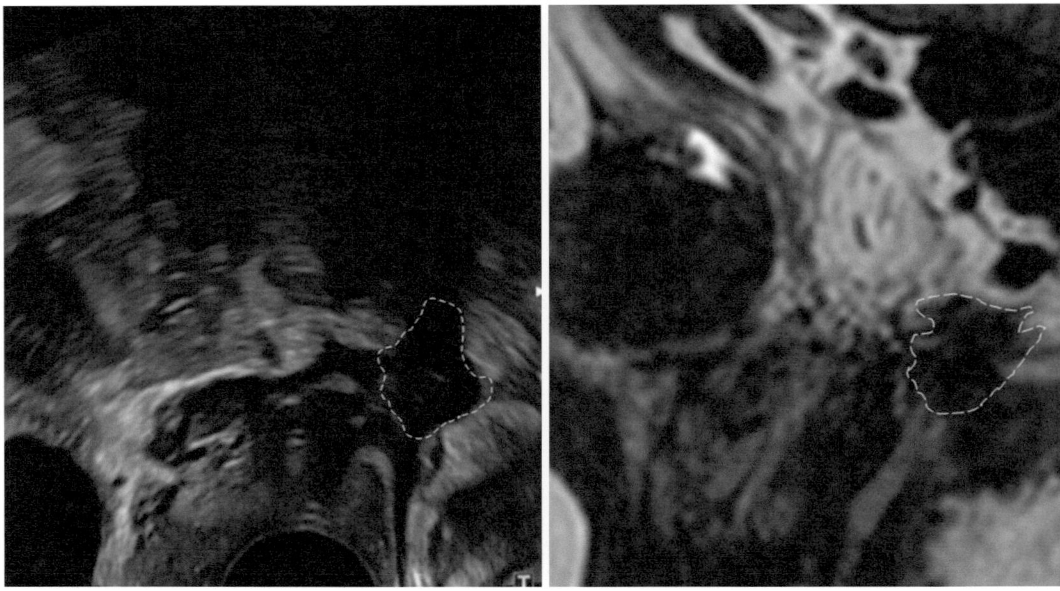

Fig. 10.6 Example of a fan-shaped lesion featuring the retraction of surrounding tissue located in the posterior and proximal paracervix on parasagittal TVUS and MR T2W slices

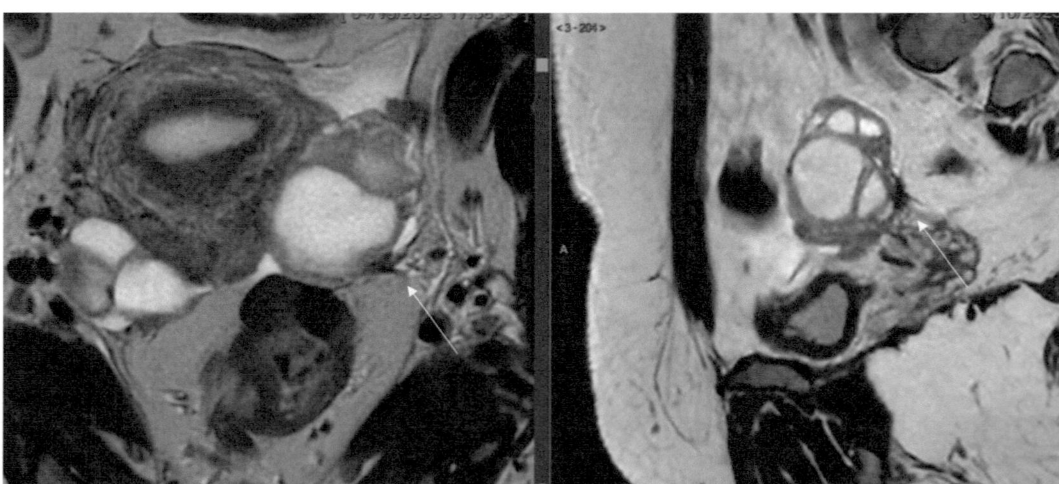

Fig. 10.7 Example of ovarian fossa involvement (or per-ovarian infiltration), which is visible on axial and parasagittal T2W sequences as a spiculated low-T2W nodule located below the ovary. This is not considered as parametrial infiltration

In conclusion, parametrium involvement in endometriosis is specific to its posterolateral location, involving the distal uterosacral ligament and visceral fascia or the sacrorecto-genital septum (SRGS). Thus, we distinguish between the mediolateral parametrium, the posterolateral parametrium, and, more recently, the anterolateral parametrium. The particularity of the posterolateral parametrium is its infraureteric location, where the hypogastric plexus is crossing. This latter plexus is the carrefour of the bladder and rectal innervation, explaining many digestive and pain symptoms in such patients. The surgical resection of the disease will lead to

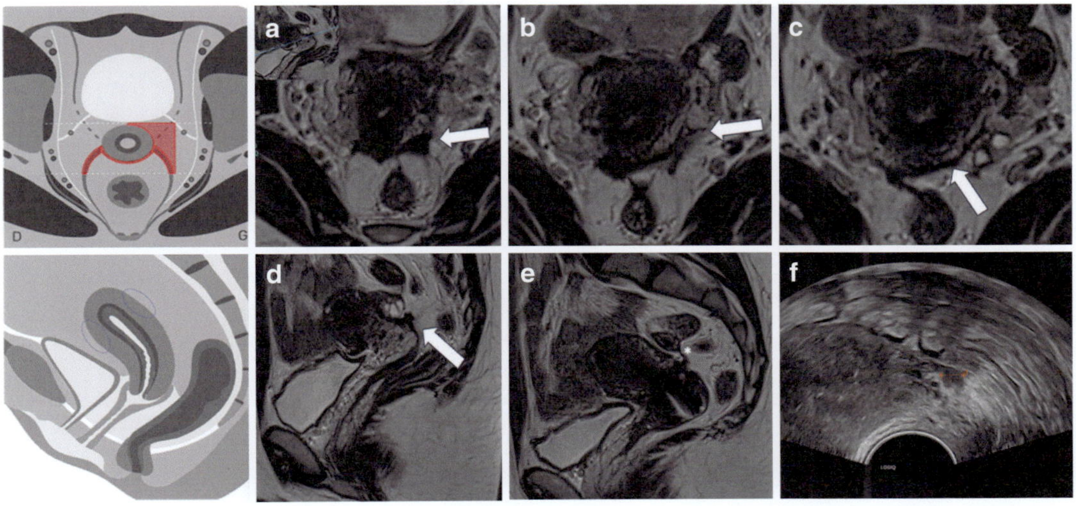

Fig. 10.8 Left mediolateral parametrial location. A low T2W signal infiltration (arrow) located mediolaterally to the uterus (**a**, **b**, **c**) with a supracentimetric nodule located under the left ovarian fossa (**d**) that is associated with low T2 signal infiltration between the uterus and the left ovary. This parametrial infiltration was proximal far from the ipsilateral ureter. On the right side was a thickened nodular uterosacral ligament (star) without parametrial infiltration (**e**). On ultrasonographic, the left medioparametrial proximal infiltration was detected as a low echoic nodule located laterally to the uterus (**f**)

voiding disorder—i.e., dysuria—in 20–35% of cases. The mediolateral parametrium can also be involved. The resection of such a disease also comes with a risk of bladder functional disorders. The management of patients with such a disease requires multidisciplinary expert centers because these locations are barely isolated and will need very different levels of expertise among those who make up the surgical teams, such as expert radiologists, procreation-assisted reproductive physicians, surgeons, psychologists, coordination nurses, sexologists, etc.

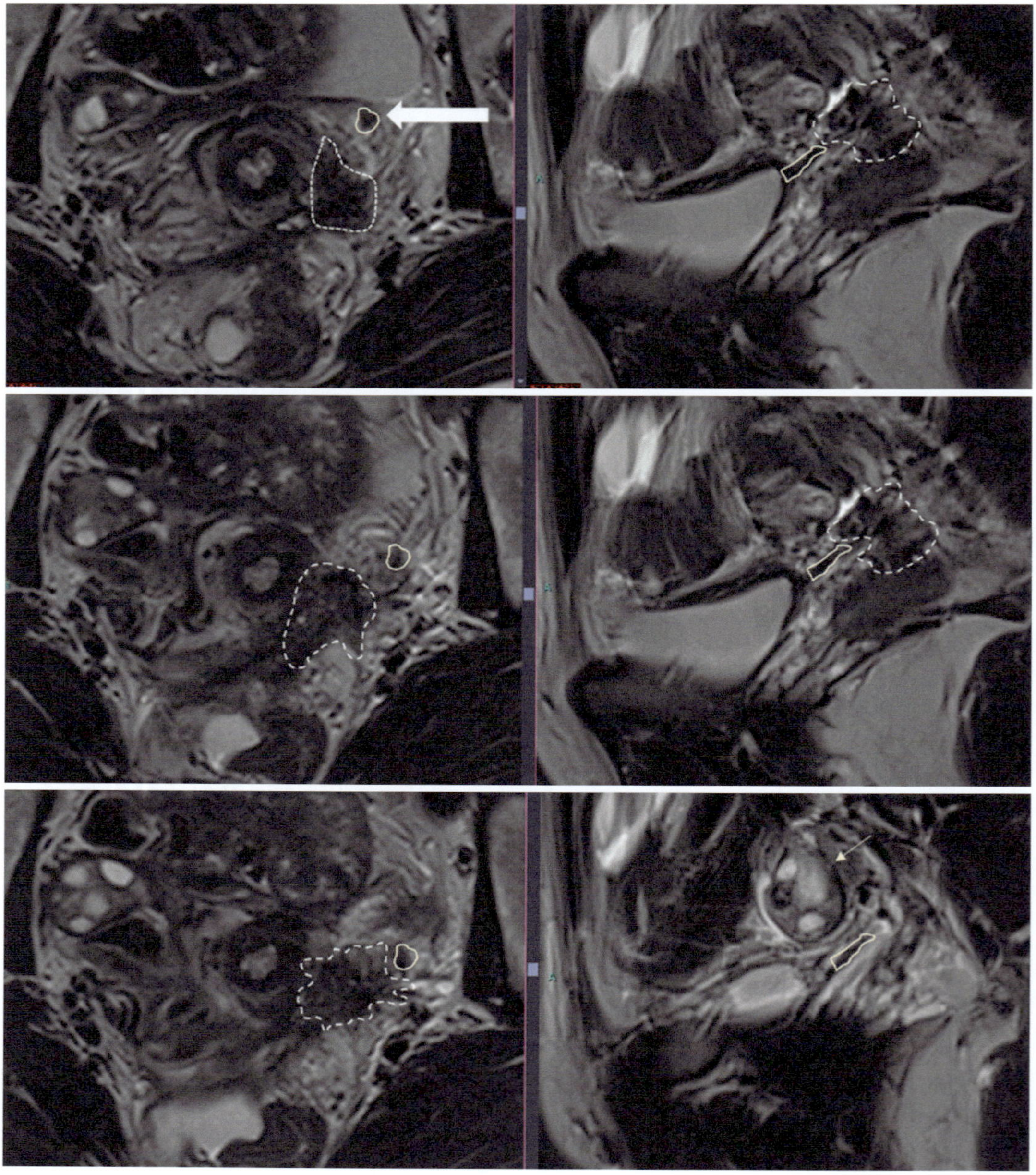

Fig. 10.9 Proximal left mediolateral parametrium. Dotted line: parametrial location; continuous line and thick arrow: ureter; thin arrow: ovary

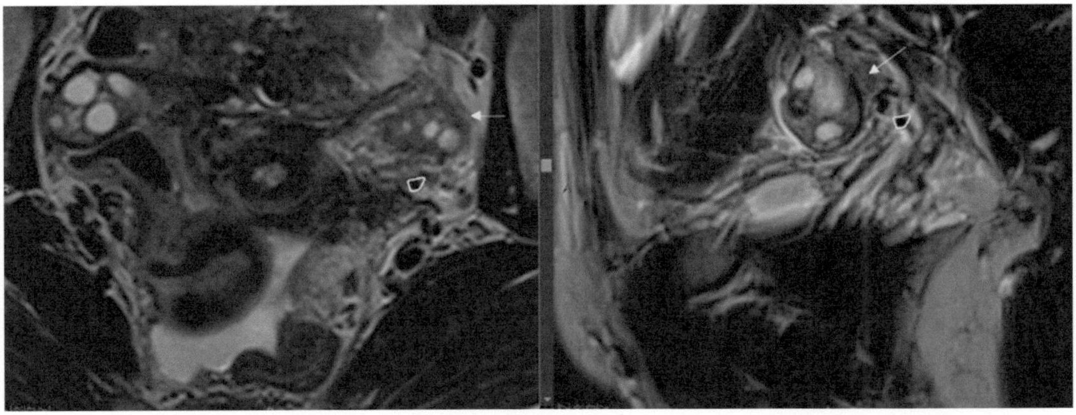

Fig. 10.9 (continued)

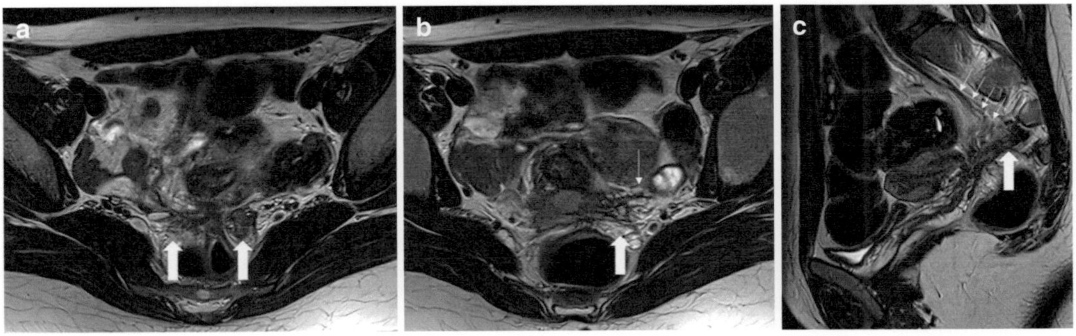

Fig. 10.10 Bilateral distal medio lateral parametrium. Thick arrow: DPE location on the parametrium; thin arrow: ureter. Bilateral parametrial infiltration (**a**) that extends on the left side to left adnexal (**b**) with an involvement of the ureter, which is visible crossing this infiltration in the parasagittal T2W plane (**c**)

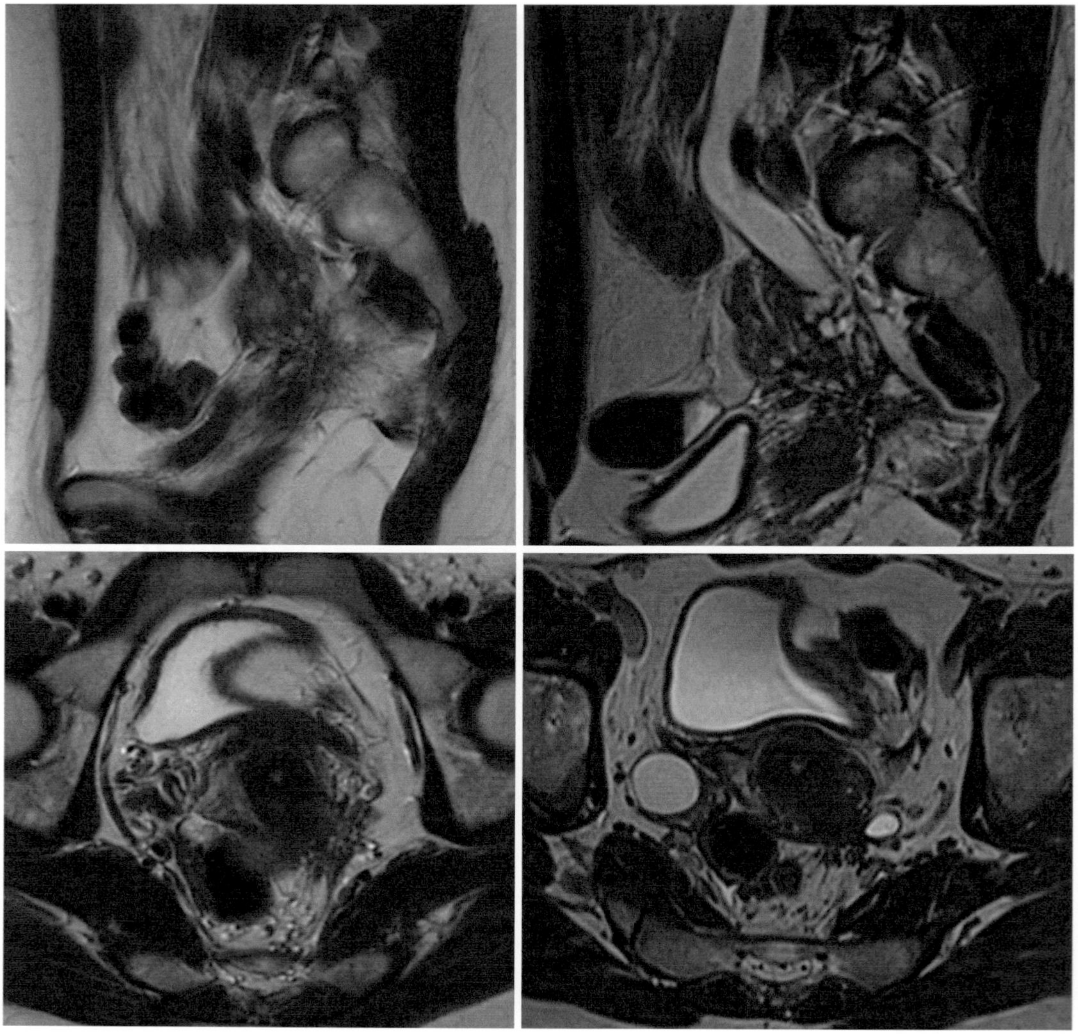

Fig. 10.11 Extrinsic disease involving left ureter

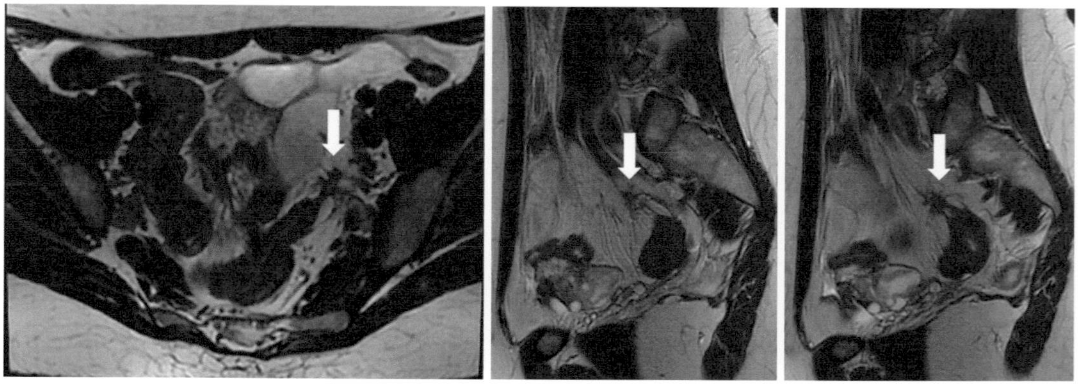

Fig. 10.12 Intrinsic disease ureteral involvement related to a deep location of endometriosis. A spiculated mass exists around the lumbar segment of the left ureter. Adjacent to this nodule are adherences with the sigmoid without a muscularis location

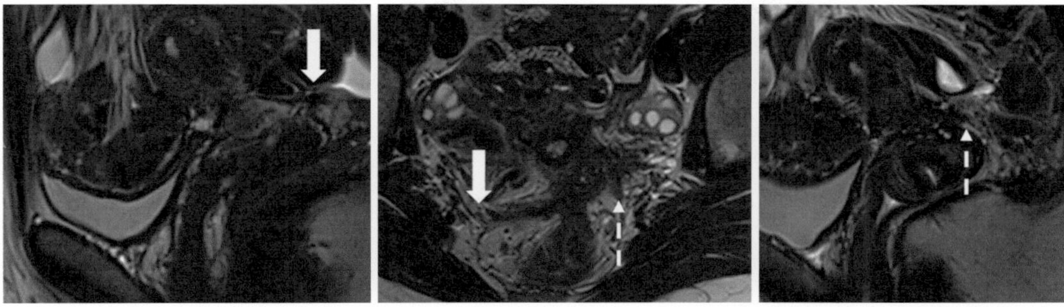

Fig. 10.13 Distal right USL.Plenty arrow: Right distal USL (posterolateral parametrium); dotted arrow: left mediolateral parametrial location

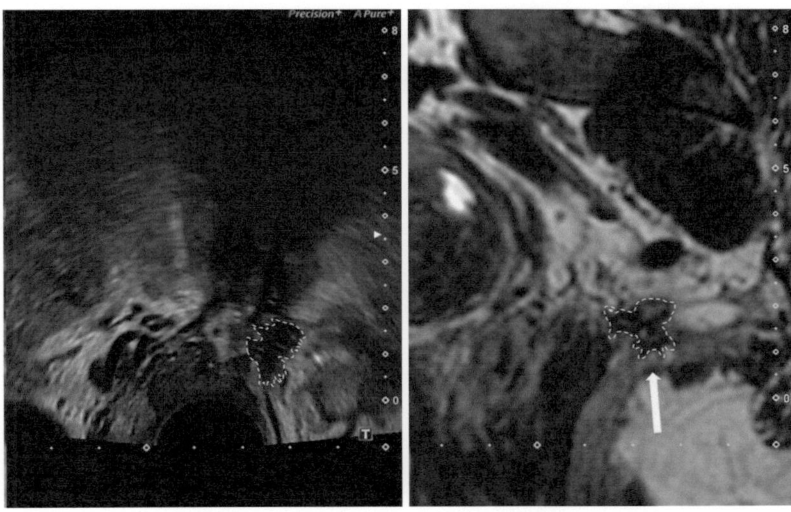

Fig. 10.14 Fusion US-MR image showing a focal involvement of the anterior part of the sacrorectal septum

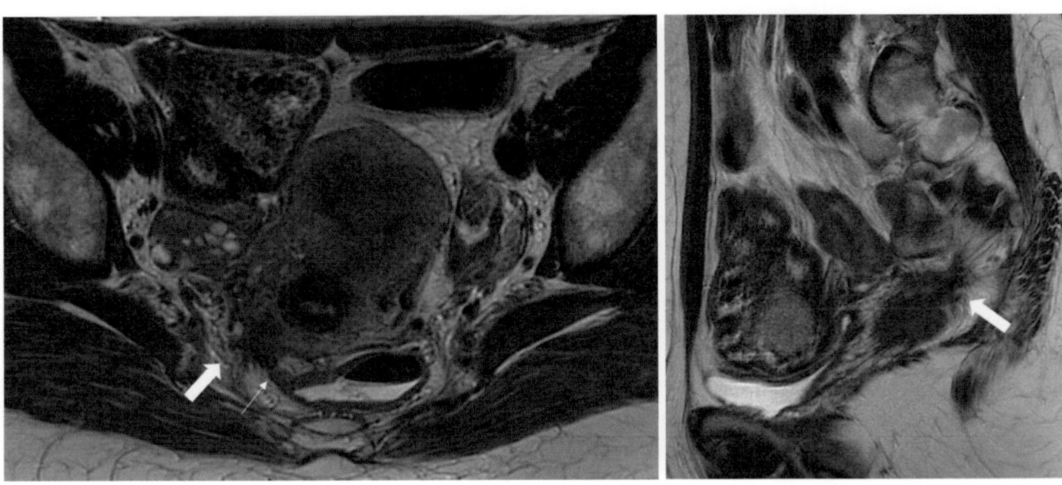

Fig. 10.15 Posterolateral parametrium: sacrorectal septum (Right) (thick arrow) associated with a mesorectal extension (thin arrow)

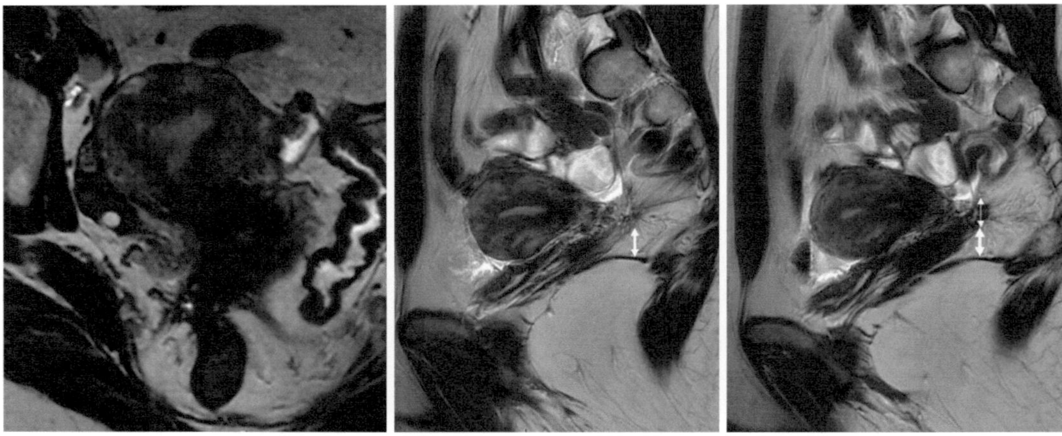

Fig. 10.16 Measurements for the evaluation of posterolateral parametrium (sacrorectal septum). DPE locations extend to the vagina, the rectum, and the uterosacral ligament proximal and distal to the sacrorectal septum. The vertical size of the nodule and its distance to the levator ani in a parasagittal plane are useful information to have before surgery

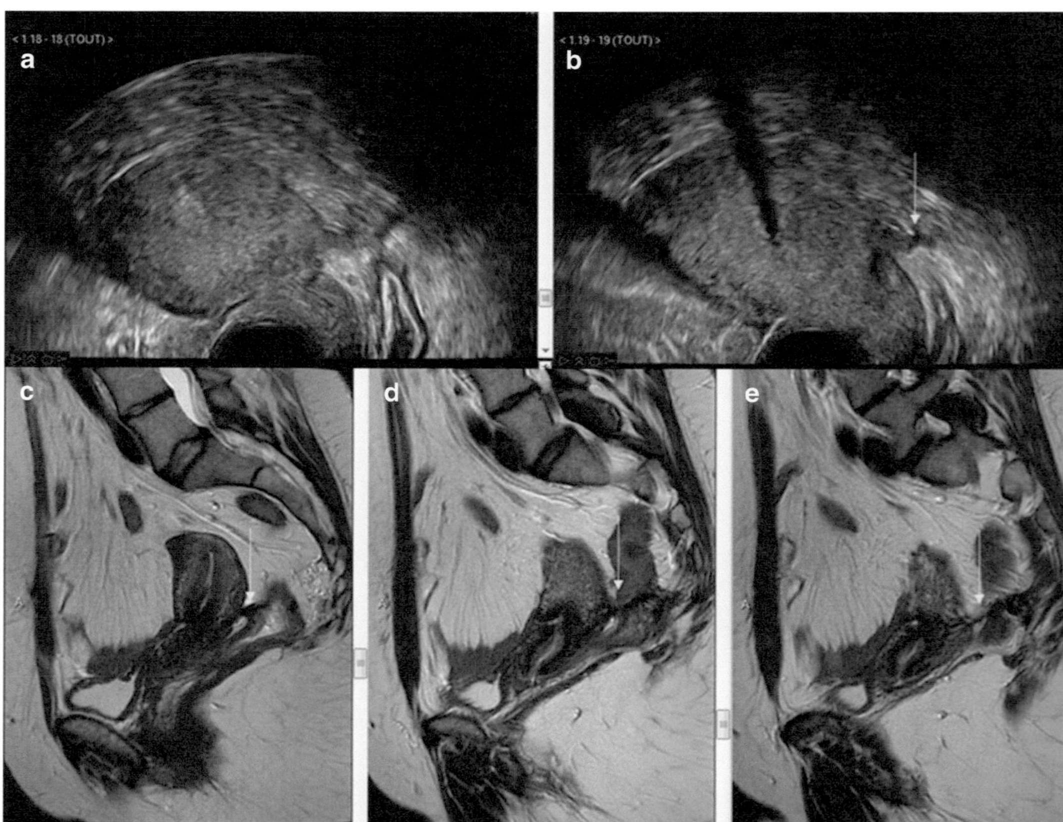

Fig. 10.17 Postoperative fibrosis after surgery for deep pelvic endometriosis. A 42-year-old with a personal history of pelvic surgery for deep pelvic endometriosis with colorectal resection referred for the suspicion of a recurrence of chronic pelvic pain on the right side. Ultrasonography (**a**, **b**) mode B: Nonspecific posterolateral hypoechoic infiltration. MRI (**c**, **d**, **e**) sagittal and parasagittal T2W sequence: smooth thickening on USL locations in its proximal and distal portion up to the pelvic wall appearing in very dark T2W signal

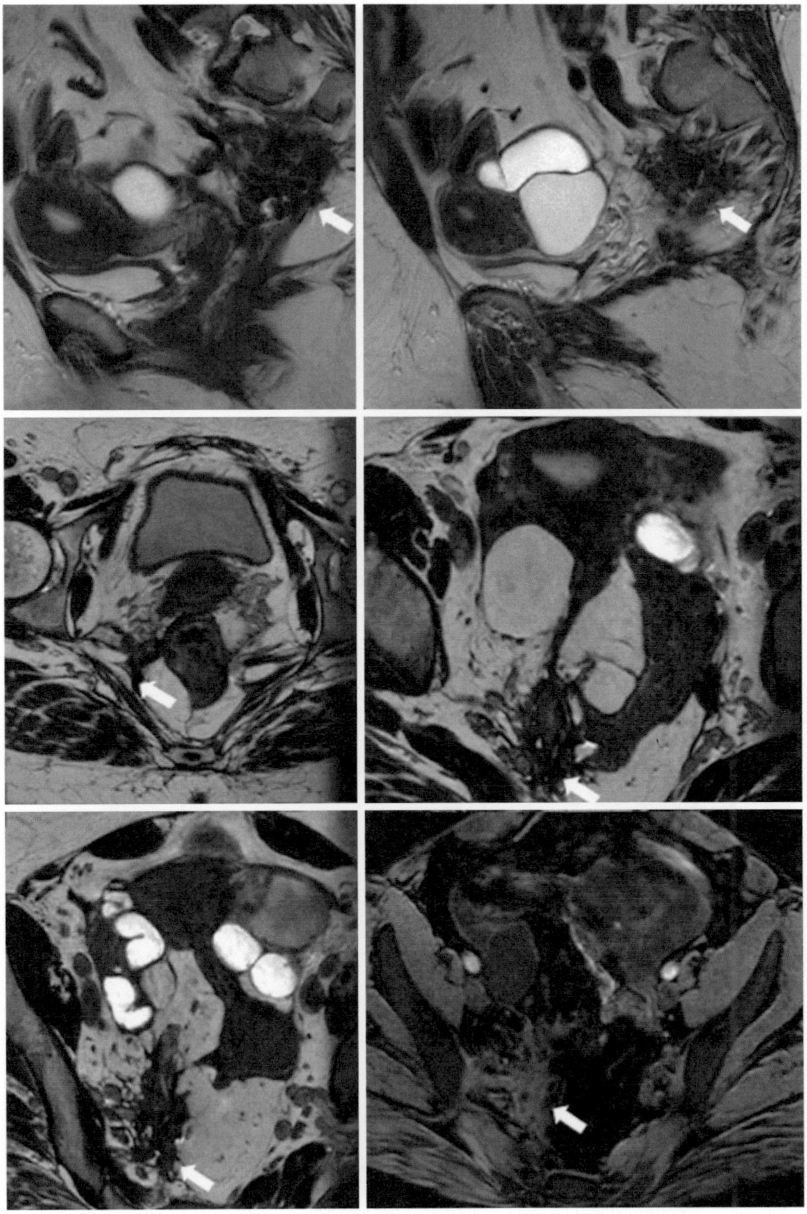

Fig. 10.18 Perirectal fibrosis and deep posterior pelvic desmoid tumor after surgery for deep pelvic endometriosis. A 36-year-old with a personal history of familial adenomatosis polypose with desmoid tumors and a personal history of sigmoid cancer treated via total coloprotectomy with ileo anal anastomosis who was referred for the suspicion of a recurrence of chronic pelvic pain on the right side

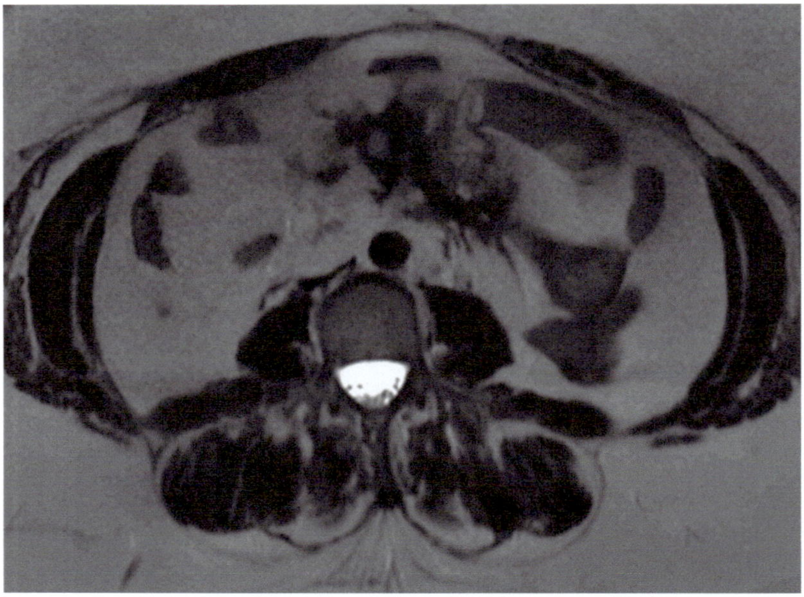

Fig. 10.18 (continued)

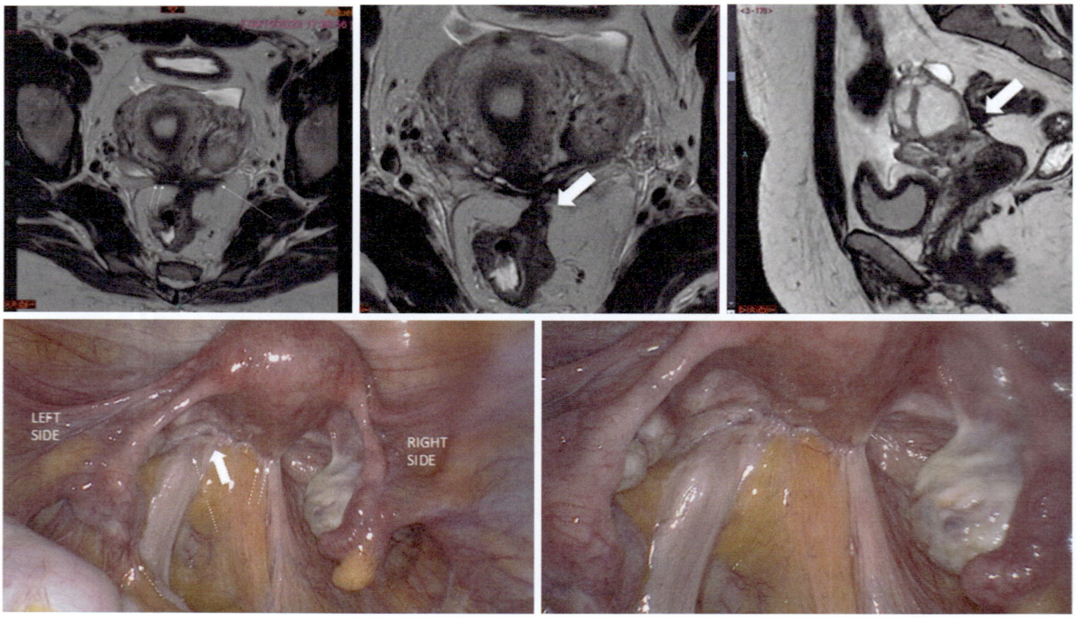

Fig. 10.19 Illustration of the importance of having an exhaustive description on MR imaging before surgery. MR imaging (Ax oblique T2W, Ax T2W, and sagT2W) showing a low T2W signal from the torus and both USLs associated with bilateral mediolateral parametrial proximal infiltration (thin arrows) and a centimetric location on the high rectum (thick arrows). The lateral infiltration is associated with a retraction of the left ovary and stays proximal far from both ureters. The laparoscopic view showing that the surgeon cannot see the presence and the potential depthless of the infiltration of lateral compartment. On the left side is a strong adherence between the proximal USL and the high rectum, as shown on MRI (thick arrow). On the right side is at least a location on the proximal USL ligament (double thin dashed arrow). The surgeon will have to perform a dissection to determine whether any parametrial involvement can be discovered below

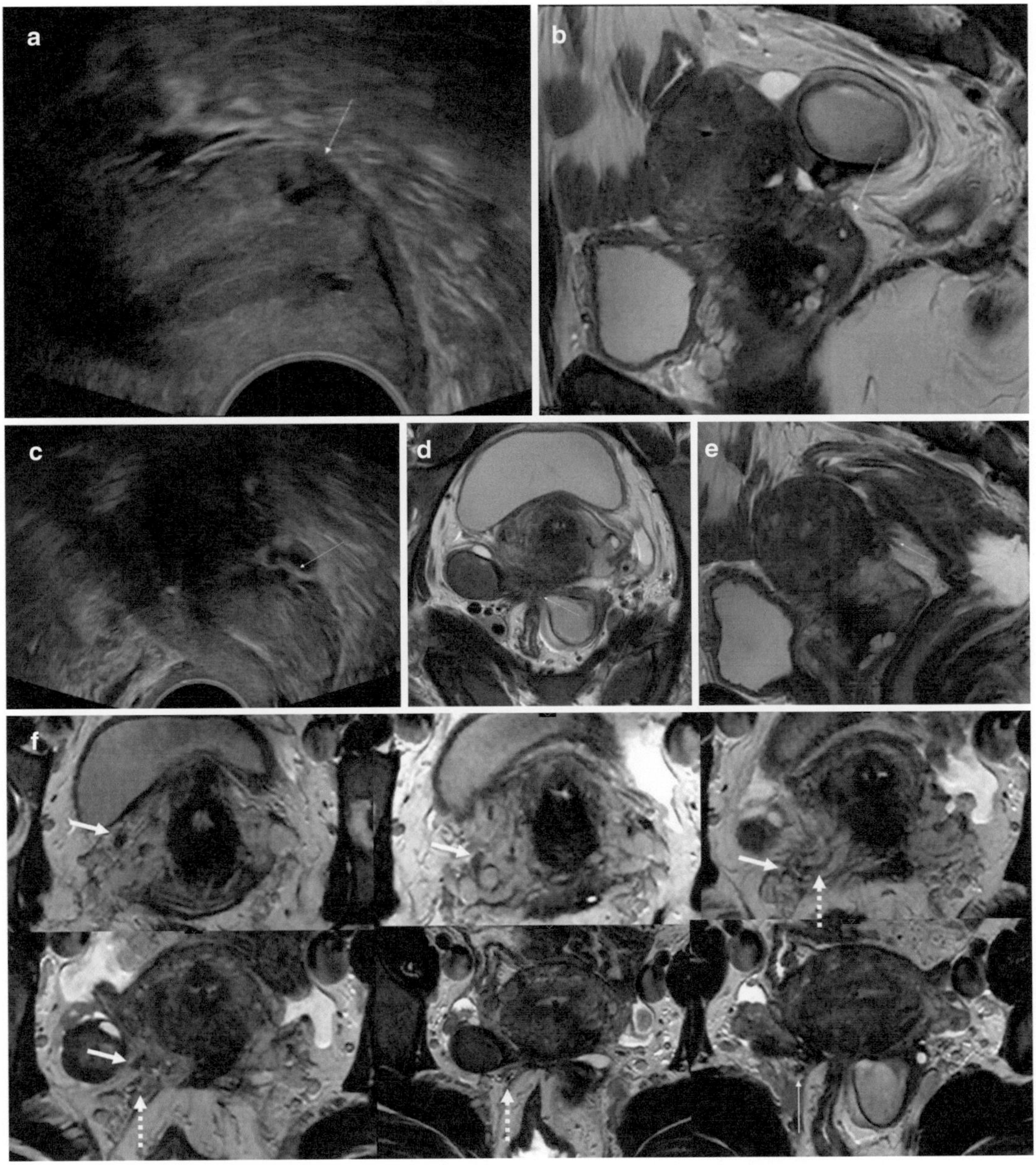

Fig. 10.20 Lateral supra ureteral parametrial location (mediolateral parametrium). Here the case of a 32-year-old woman, G3P1, suffered from chronic pelvic pain, including dysmenorrhea, dyspareunia, and dysuria. The radiologist described a left endometrioma associated with the deep pelvic endometriosis located on the torus; bilateral locations on the uterosacral ligament on their proximal segment, vagina (**a**, **b**), and mesosigmoid; and a centimetric sigmoid location, which extended to the right parametrium (**c**, **d**, **e**) without the involvement of the ureter or the uterin artery (**f**)—with a dPEI score rated at 4 (including three compartments: the mediocentral, right mediolateral, and posterocentral). The surgery consisted of a resection of the torus and both USLs, bilateral ureterlolysis, and a left mediolateral parametrial resection that confirmed a dPEI score at 4, confirmed at pathology. The operating time was 182 min. No complication occurred after surgery. The patient was hospitalized for 2 days after surgery without any postoperative dysfunction. (**a**) Ultrasonography and (**b**) sagT2W sequences. (**c**) Ultrasonography, (**d**) axial T2W sequence, and (**e**) sagital T2W sequence. (**f**) Axial oblique T2W sequence. (**g**) Radiosurgical correlation showing left mediolateral parametrial involvement (the radiological images have been inversed to easily correlate with the surgical view)

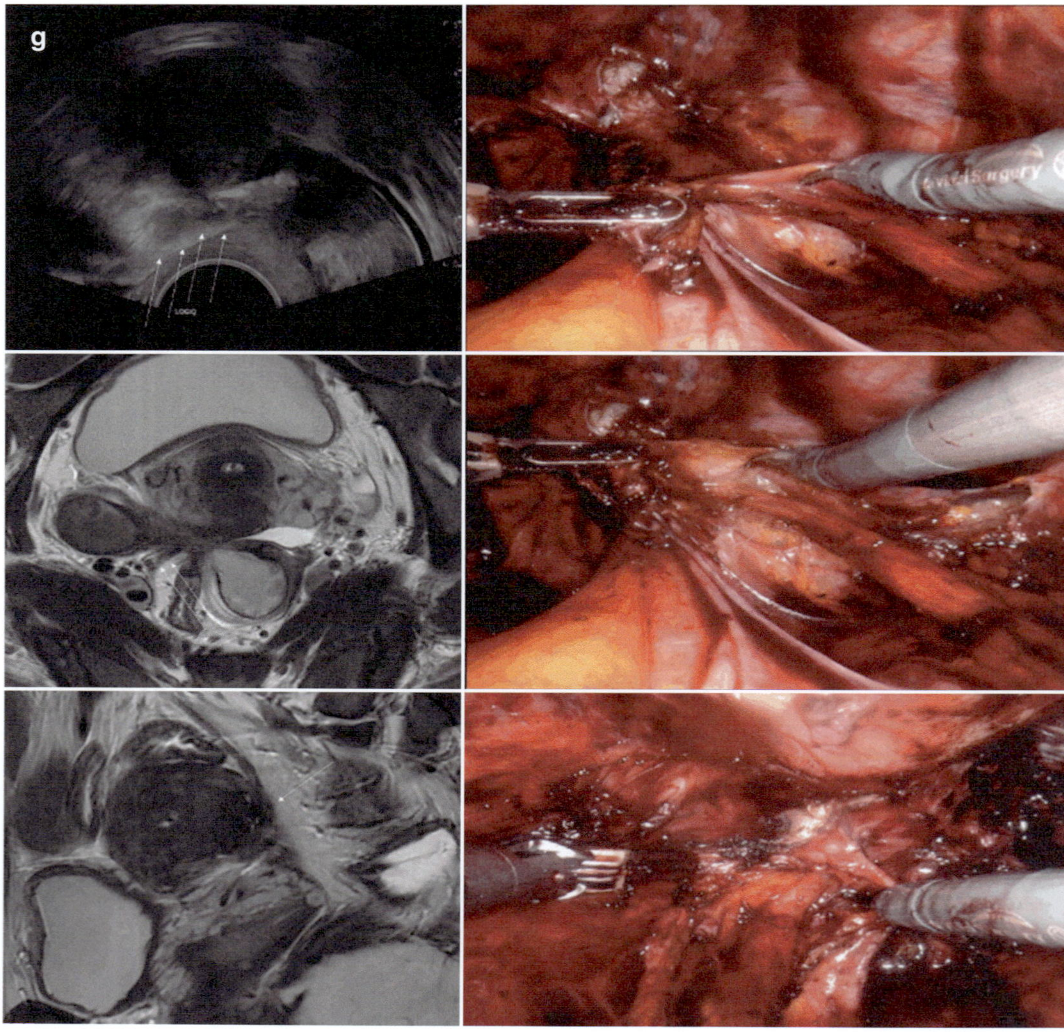

Fig. 10.20 (continued)

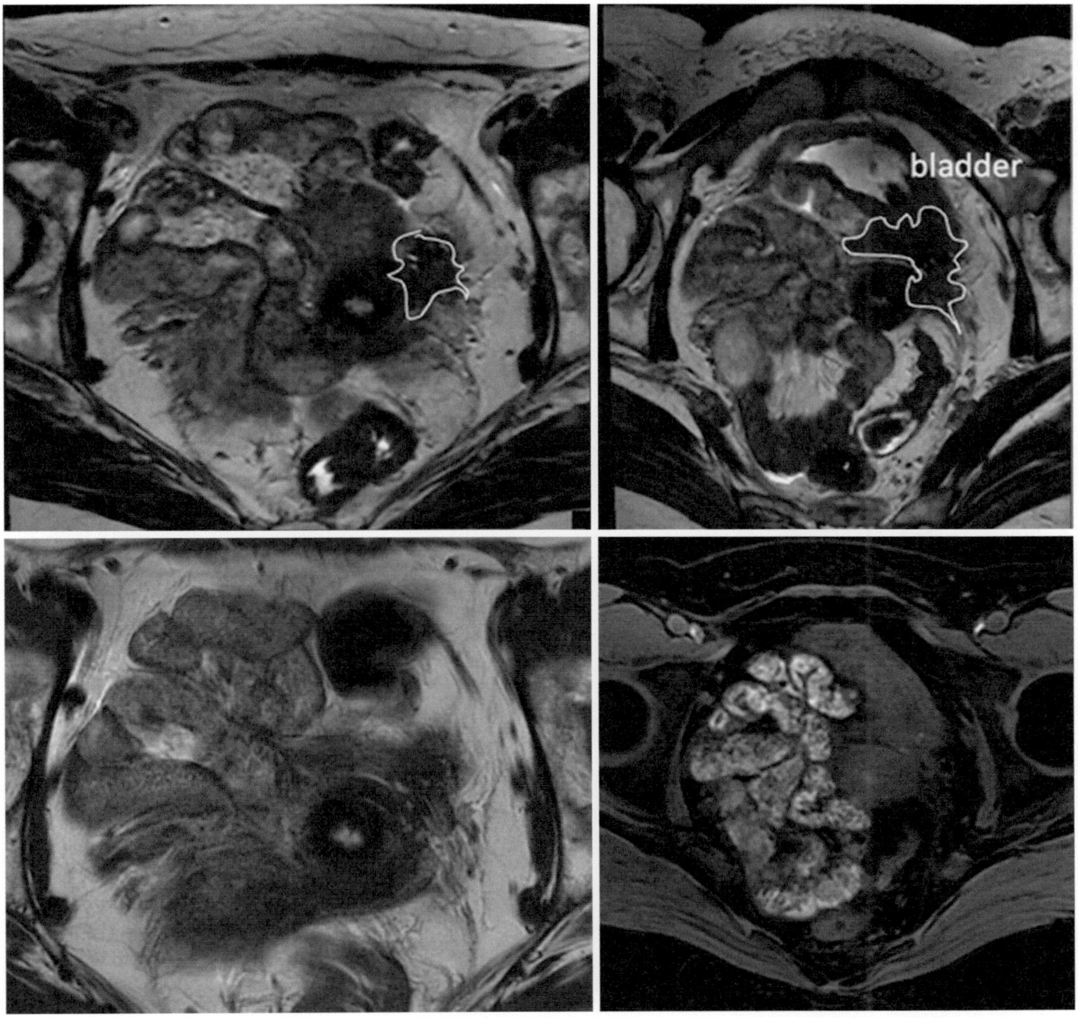

Fig. 10.21 Medio- and anterolateral parametrial location with ureteral and lateral bladder infiltration. Here the case of a 32-year-old woman, G3P1, suffered from chronic pelvic pain, including dysmenorrhea, dyspareunia, and dysuria. The radiologist described an endometrioma associated with a left ureteral dilatation caused by deep pelvic endometriosis centered on the left parametrium with the involvement of the uterin artery, ureter, and left lateral bladder wall and with a dPEI score of 5 (including four compartments—the mediocentral (external adenomyosis), left mediolateral, left anterolateral, and anterocentral (the bladder, including the trigone)—that are associated with a dilatation of the ureter). A JJ tube was placed before the MR examination to protect the left kidney. The surgery consisted of a resection of the left lateral parametrium after the ligation of the left uterine artery at its origin, the ureter, and the left lateral wall of the bladder. The reconstruction of the urinary tract was then performed via ureteral bladder reimplantation. The operating time was 250 min. No complication occurred after surgery. The patient was hospitalized for 6 days after surgery without any postoperative dysfunction

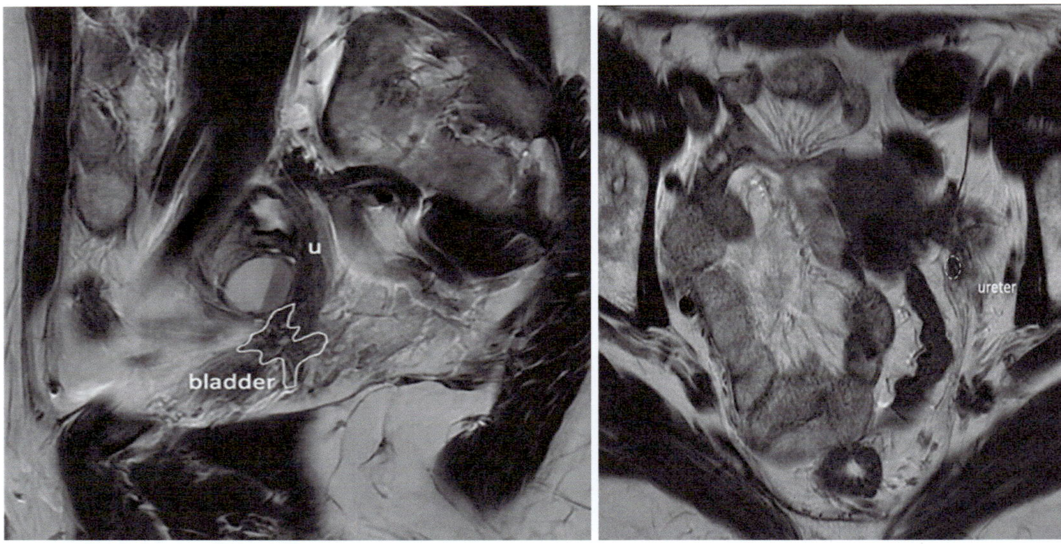

Fig. 10.21 (continued)

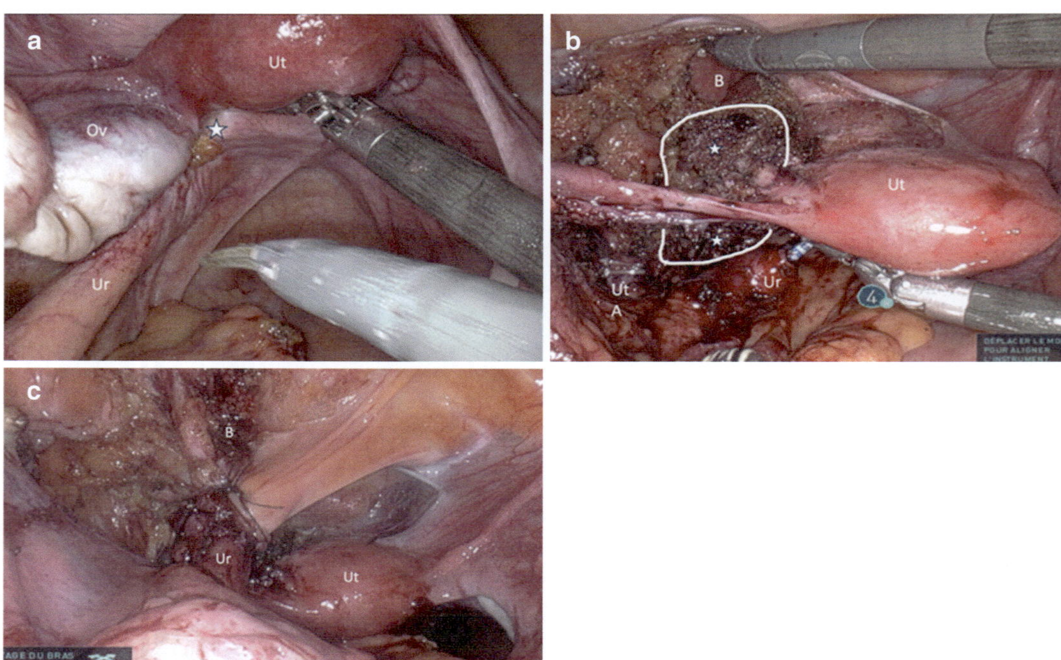

Fig. 10.22 Surgical correlation regarding the laparoscopic view of the pelvis: (**a**) Ureteral dilatation above the parametrial nodule (star) with attraction of the ovary. (**b**) Dissection of the parametrial nodule (star) after ligation and uterine artery sectioning, the section of the ureter, and bladder wall resection. (**c**) Urinary reconstruction via ureterovesical reimplantation and vesical suture. *Ut* uterus, *Ur* ureter, *Ut A* uterine artery, *B* bladder, *Star* voluminous left parametrial deep infiltrating endometriotic lesion (anterior + lateral + posterior parametrium)

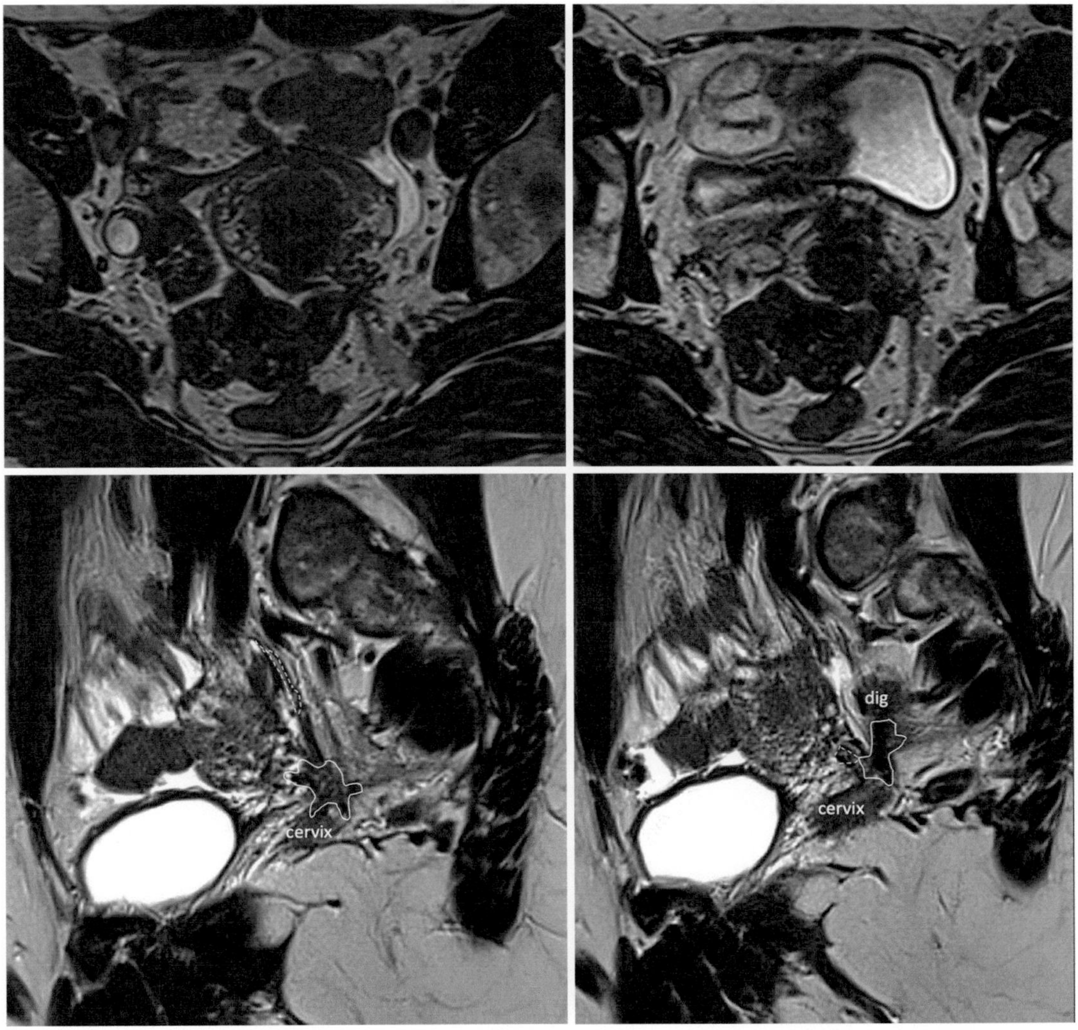

Fig. 10.23 Mediolateral and posterolateral parametrium. Here the case of a 45-year-old woman, G2P2, with a medical history featuring the resection of the torus and the USL and rectal shaving 4 years ago. She reported the recurrence of endometriotic symptoms with dysmenorrhea and intense dyspareunia and the failure of her medical treatments. The radiologist described a recurrent deep pelvic endometriotic nodule of the uterosacral ligaments on the distal left USL (without infiltration of the sacrorectal septum), including the left vPF and proximal left parametrium (white arrow in the MR imaging below), with a dPEI score of 4 (including three compartments: the mediocentral, left mediolateral, and left posterolateral + vaginal pouch). Rectal echoendoscopy found no rectum infiltration. The surgery consisted of a resection of the torus and both USLs, bilateral ureterolysis, a left vPF, and parametrium resection. The operating time was 205 min. She had initial dysuria with a bladder catheter for 3 days and normal miction. She was discharged on day 5 without any other complication and without late postoperative dysfunction

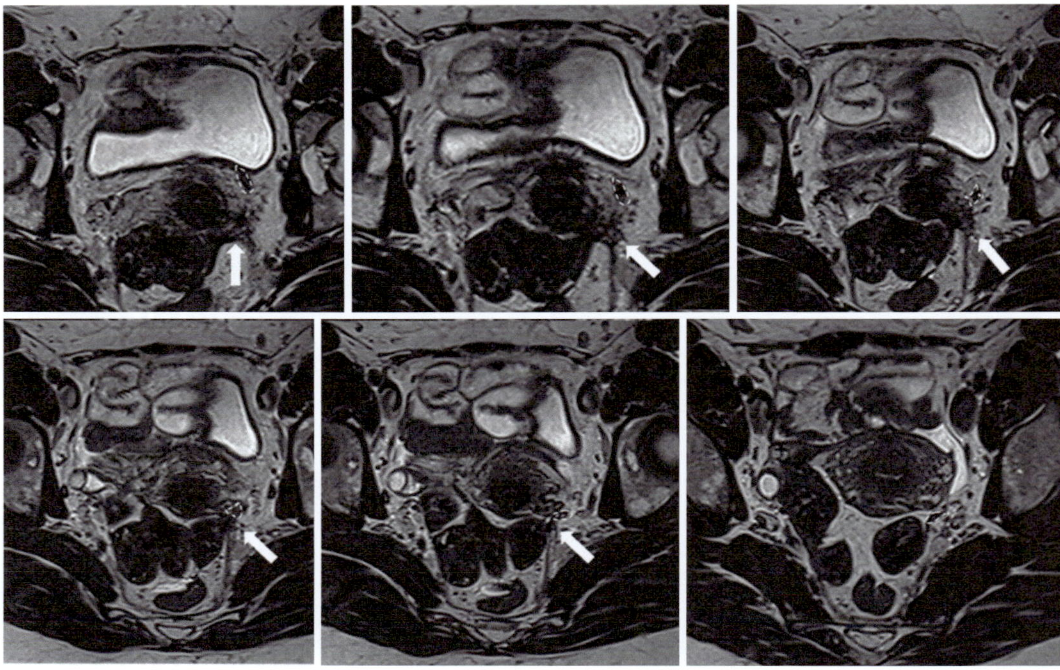

Fig. 10.23 (continued)

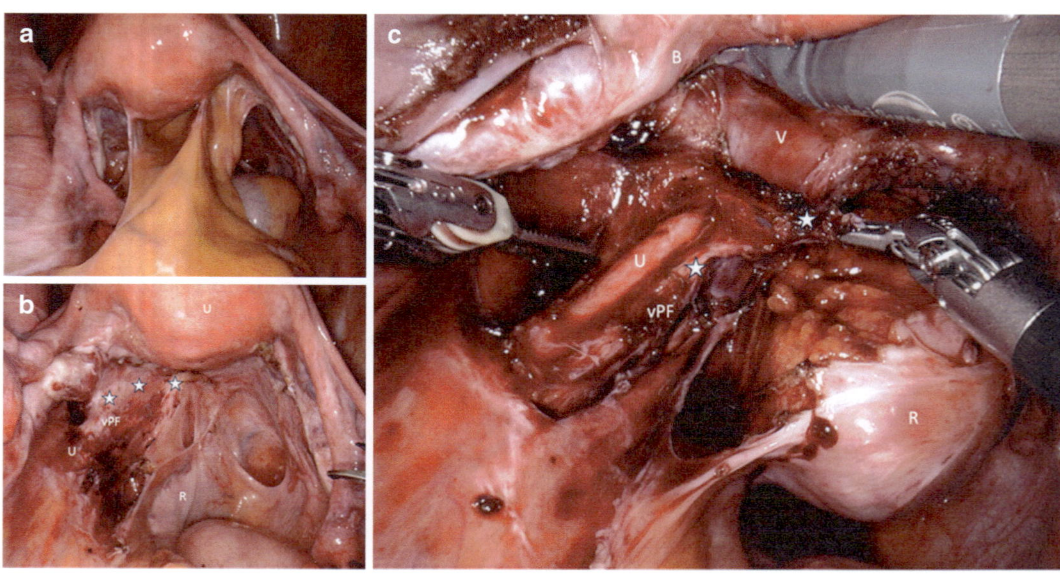

Fig. 10.24 Surgical correlation regarding the laparoscopic view of the pelvis: (**a**) Initial view with the adhesion of mesorectum and rectum. (**b**) After adhesiolysis, left USL and ovarian peritoneum are infiltrated by endometriosis (stars). (**c**) After rectal adhesiolysis, the left USL, parametrium, and vPF endometriosis (stars) are resected. *Ut* uterus, *Ur* ureter, *UtA* uterine artery, *B* bladder, *Star* left USL, parametrial, and vPF deep infiltrating endometriotic lesion, *vPF* visceral pelvis fascia, *AP* anterior parametrium (not involved)

References

1. Bazot M, Jarboui L, Ballester M, Touboul C, Thomassin-Naggara I, Daraï E. The value of MRI in assessing parametrial involvement in endometriosis. Hum Reprod. 2012;27(8):2352–8. https://doi.org/10.1093/humrep/des211.
2. Thomassin-Naggara I, Monroc M, Chauveau B, et al. Multicenter external validation of the deep pelvic endometriosis index magnetic resonance imaging score. JAMA Netw Open. 2023;6(5):e2311686. https://doi.org/10.1001/jamanetworkopen.2023.11686.
3. Ballester M, Santulli P, Bazot M, Coutant C, Rouzier R, Daraï E. Preoperative evaluation of posterior deep-infiltrating endometriosis demonstrates a relationship with urinary dysfunction and parametrial involvement. J Minim Invasive Gynecol. 2011;18(1):36–42. https://doi.org/10.1016/j.jmig.2010.08.692.
4. Touboul C, Fauconnier A, Zareski E, Bouhanna P, Daraï E. The lateral infraureteral parametrium: myth or reality? Am J Obstet Gynecol. 2008;199(3):242.e1–6. https://doi.org/10.1016/j.ajog.2008.04.003.
5. Höckel M, Horn L-C, Fritsch H. Association between the mesenchymal compartment of uterovaginal organogenesis and local tumour spread in stage IB-IIB cervical carcinoma: a prospective study. Lancet Oncol. 2005;6(10):751–6. https://doi.org/10.1016/S1470-2045(05)70324-7.
6. Ercoli A, Delmas V, Fanfani F, et al. Terminologia Anatomica versus unofficial descriptions and nomenclature of the fasciae and ligaments of the female pelvis: a dissection-based comparative study. Am J Obstet Gynecol. 2005;193(4):1565–73. https://doi.org/10.1016/j.ajog.2005.05.007.
7. Ceccaroni M, Clarizia R, Roviglione G. Nerve-sparing surgery for deep infiltrating endometriosis: laparoscopic eradication of deep infiltrating endometriosis with rectal and parametrial resection according to the Negrar method. J Minim Invasive Gynecol. 2020;27(2):263–4. https://doi.org/10.1016/j.jmig.2019.09.002.
8. Sanguin S, Roman H, Foulon A, Gondry J, Havet E, Klein C. Deep infiltrating endometriosis with sacral plexus involvement: improving knowledge through human cadaver dissection. J Gynecol Obstet Hum Reprod. 2021;50(8):102129. https://doi.org/10.1016/j.jogoh.2021.102129.
9. Ribeiro-Julio GS, Pereira JA, Ribeiro E, Gallo CM, Favorito LA. Anatomy of the lower hypogastric plexus applied to endometriosis: a narrative review. Int Braz J Urol. 2023;49(3):299–306. https://doi.org/10.1590/S1677-5538.IBJU.2022.9980.
10. Thomassin-Naggara I, Lamrabet S, Crestani A, et al. Magnetic resonance imaging classification of deep pelvic endometriosis: description and impact on surgical management. Hum Reprod. 2020;35(7):1589–600. https://doi.org/10.1093/humrep/deaa103.
11. De Cicco C, Schonman R, Craessaerts M, Van Cleynenbreugel B, Ussia A, Koninckx PR. Laparoscopic management of ureteral lesions in gynecology. Fertil Steril. 2009;92(4):1424–7. https://doi.org/10.1016/j.fertnstert.2008.08.021.
12. Yabuki Y, Sasaki H, Hatakeyama N, Murakami G. Discrepancies between classic anatomy and modern gynecologic surgery on pelvic connective tissue structure: harmonization of those concepts by collaborative cadaver dissection. Am J Obstet Gynecol. 2005;193(1):7–15. https://doi.org/10.1016/j.ajog.2005.02.108.
13. Rousset P, Florin M, Bharwani N, et al. Deep pelvic infiltrating endometriosis: MRI consensus lexicon and compartment-based approach from the ENDOVALIRM Group. Diagn Interv Imaging. 2023;104:95–112.
14. Guerriero S, Condous G, Rolla M, et al. Addendum to the consensus opinion from the international deep endometriosis analysis (IDEA) group: sonographic evaluation of the parametrium. Ultrasound Obstet Gynecol. 2024;64:275–80. https://doi.org/10.1002/uog.27558.
15. Mariani LL, Mancarella M, Novara L, Biglia N. Sonographic features of endometriosis infiltrating the lateral parametrium. J Gynecol Obstet Hum Reprod. 2021;50(7):102116. https://doi.org/10.1016/j.jogoh.2021.102116.
16. Guerriero S, Martinez L, Gomez I, et al. Diagnostic accuracy of transvaginal sonography for detecting parametrial involvement in women with deep endometriosis: systematic review and meta-analysis. Ultrasound Obstet Gynecol. 2021;58(5):669–76. https://doi.org/10.1002/uog.23754.

11 Lateral Deep Pelvic Endometriosis. Over Parietal Fascia: Nervous Locations

Luciana P. Chamié, Alice Brandão, and Izabela V. Pires Franco

11.1 Introduction

Neural endometriosis is a rare but underestimated entity. Because of its complexity and the medical community's lack of awareness about this type of endometriosis and pelvic neuroanatomy, it is considered one of the most difficult forms of deep endometriosis (DE) to detect and treat. Diagnosis is extremely difficult also because neuropathic pain is located distant to the pelvic site, in the lower back, in pudendal areas, in the buttocks, or in the lower extremities. All these pain locations are usually correlated with orthopedic and neurosurgical conditions, contributing to diagnosis delay and morbidity [1–4].

Neural endometriosis is defined by the compression, infiltration, distortion, and irritation of a pelvic nerve with or without neural entrapment, caused by DE or surrounding associated fibrosis [1–3].

Endometriosis can affect autonomic visceral innervation in the pelvis, which comprises the superior hypogastric plexus, hypogastric nerves, pelvic splanchnic nerves, and inferior hypogastric plexus or somatic innervation, which consists of sensory (afferent) and motor (efferent) nerves, such as the femoral nerve, obturator nerve, lumbosacral trunk, sciatic nerve, and pudendal nerve. The most frequently involved nerves are the hypogastric, inferior hypogastric plexus, sciatic, and obturator nerves [1–3, 5–7].

The pelvic sidewall and pelvic nerves are uncommon sites of endometriosis. However, it may be underestimated because a deeper comprehension of the anatomy and clinical findings of neural endometriosis is necessary to allow for the correct diagnosis. In a study conducted by Chiantera et al., the involvement of deep lateral tissues was detected in 40% of women with central lesions and in 72.7% of patients with hypogastric nerve involvement [1, 8–11].

Most often, pelvic nerves are affected by the contiguity of a large and infiltrative retrocervical and uterosacral lesion with parametrial and paracolpium extension. The theories proposed to explain extraperitoneal neural involvement are based on the lymphatic and vascular spread of endometrial-like cells associated with inflammation, angiogenesis, immunologic defects, and genetic predisposition [1, 8–10].

Neural endometriosis is one of the most challenging forms to manage. Clinical therapy is based on hormonal suppression, neuroleptics, pain management medication, and physiotherapy.

L. P. Chamié (✉)
Radiology, Chamié Imagem da Mulher,
São Paulo, São Paulo, Brazil
e-mail: luciana@chamie.com.br

A. Brandão
Radiology, Fonte Imagem,
Rio de Janeiro, Rio de Janeiro, Brazil

I. V. Pires Franco
Radiology, Clínica Izabela Pires Franco,
Belém, Pará, Brazil

I. Thomassin-Naggara (ed.), *Imaging of Endometriosis: A Comparative Guide of US, MRI and Surgery*, https://doi.org/10.1007/978-3-031-82750-1_11

Surgical treatment, whether resection or neurolysis with decompression, when indicated, must be performed by a highly skilled minimally invasive pelvic surgeon. The field of laparoscopic neurofunctional pelvic surgery has developed greatly in recent years, with the emergence of increasingly advanced techniques for neural preservation, such as the laparoscopic neuronavigation [1, 8, 12–17].

The aims of this chapter are to describe the anatomy and MRI findings of neural involvement in endometriosis through clinical cases and to discuss some clinical aspects that can highlight the diagnosis of neural involvement for the radiologist. Moreover, we included an MRI protocol consideration that can be employed to carry out an accurate diagnosis.

11.2 Clinical Aspects

Endometriosis can affect either autonomic visceral innervation in the pelvis or somatic innervation. In some patients, both innervations may be affected by the same DE lesion. The most frequently involved nerves are the hypogastric, inferior hypogastric plexus, sciatic, and obturator nerves [1–3, 5–7].

Clinical suspicious for nerve DE involvement is important because delayed diagnosis can foster clinical worsening, with difficult-to-manage symptoms that can become permanent, leading to sequelae and central sensitization [1, 18, 19].

The diagnosis of neural endometriosis requires a complete and detailed anamnesis, a targeted neurological and vaginal examination, and complementary tests, including a urodynamic test and an MRI of the pelvis [1, 2, 8].

Symptoms vary according to the nerve involved and the catamenial nature of the symptoms, and a comprehensive neurological examination can raise the suspicion of neural endometriosis. In chronic DE neural lesions, symptoms may occur in any phase of the menstrual cycle [1, 2, 12].

The dermatome affected is directly related to the sensory and motor dysfunction symptoms of somatic innervation. The dermatome is an area of the skin where all the sensory nerves come from a single nerve root. Therefore, an endometriosis lesion affecting the sciatic nerve may cause catamenial pain in the ipsilateral gluteal region and radiate to the lower extremity, with or without foot locomotor deficits. Obturator nerve involvement can cause weakness in thigh adduction and difficulty ambulating. A radiologist's knowledge of the dermatome distribution may contribute to their identifying and previewing somatic nerve involvement [1, 2, 12].

Clinical evaluation includes neurological and vaginal examinations, searching for hyperesthesia and hypoesthesia at the lumbosacral dermatomes and peripheral nerves and searching for motor deficits. The vaginal palpation of pudendal nerves and lower sacral nerve roots (S3, S4) can also be performed.

The visceral nervous system involvement can be the first clinical manifestation in patients with DE, especially complaints of bladder symptoms. The hypogastric nerves carry the sympathetic fibers that innervate the anal and internal urethral sphincters, rectum, and bladder, promoting the relaxation of the detrusor muscle and the contraction of the urethral sphincter and continence. The pelvic splanchnic nerves promote the contraction of the detrusor muscles and the innervation of the descending colon, sigmoid, and rectum, and the inferior hypogastric plexus carries nociceptive afferent signals from the pelvic viscera to the central nervous system. Therefore, patients may present increased catamenial bladder sensitivity, urinary urgency, and urgent incontinence or a decreased bladder capacity and compliance [1, 2, 12, 20].

The urodynamic test evaluates motor and sensitive urinary urgency, sphincter dysfunctions, and voiding difficulties. Nerve conduction studies and electromyography can be useful for some peripheral nerve evaluations [1, 2, 12, 21].

A specific clinical diagnosis is pudendal neuralgia. It induces pudendal pain, characterized by pain in the perineal and vulvar areas, and vulvodynia, typically worsened by sitting and relieved by standing and on toilet seat position [12]. Moreover, pudendal endometriosis can cause bladder disfunctions, retention in neurogenic lesion, hyperactivity or hypersensitivity in non-neurogenic lesions and rectal dysfunctions, such as rectal deviation and chronic constipation in neurogenic lesions and irritable colon in non-neurogenic lesions [2, 12]. Clinical examination is crucial in these cases, including the evaluation of the vulvar area for positive trigger points and the palpation of the pudendal nerve dorsomedial to the sciatic spine. A clinical examination of the perineum, anal canal, and rectum in some cases can demonstrate hyperalgesia, hypoesthesia, or allodynia in the S3 and S4 dermatomes. The evaluation of the postvoid residual volume and bladder wall thickness is important during a pelvic ultrasound [2, 12].

11.3 Diagnostic Imaging

MRI is considered the method of choice to evaluate neural involvement due to its high sensitivity and specificity in identifying neural involvement (ranging from 90.3% to 100% and 96.3% to 100%, respectively) [1].

MRI provides a comprehensive anatomical evaluation with high spatial and contrast resolution, as well as a large field of view that includes the pelvic sidewall and pelvic bone opening, perfect for the evaluation of neural involvement and preoperative planning. Furthermore, MRI offers increased accuracy compared to ultrasonography and computed tomography in identifying the exact location, type, and extension of the cause of the neuropathy or plexopathy [1, 2, 12, 21].

Even more, MRI can assist in the diagnosis of neural endometriosis in acute and chronic stages and demonstrates lesions in the vicinity or with infiltration into the peripheral nerves or plexus, Wallerian degeneration associated with axonal nerve injury, and the denervation of target muscles. In the acute phase, it can demonstrate nerve caliber and signal intensity changes, such as hyperintense signal and nerve thickening, as well as muscular edema related to the injured nerve. Chronic lesions present with fat muscle infiltration and atrophy [1, 3, 6, 8, 9].

Transvaginal sonography (TVUS) has a limited role in the diagnosis of neural endometriosis, requiring highly trained sonographers with extensive knowledge of advanced pelvic anatomy because most of the pelvic nerve fibers cannot be directly identified by TVUS. If neural endometriosis is suspected, MRI should always be performed to improve the identification of possible neural involvement [22, 23].

11.4 Considerations for a Dedicated MRI Protocol

The endometriosis MRI protocol has already been published and can vary according to the preferences of each institution. In the authors' opinion, the use of a specific protocol is essential to improve diagnostic accuracy. Patient preparation includes bowel preparation, 4 h of fasting, mild bladder distention, and the use of an anti-peristaltic agent. The protocol includes a coronal 3D T2-weighted isotropic sequence, sagittal and axial T2-weighted high-resolution sequences, and fast axial T1 and axial and sagittal T1 fat-suppressed sequences [1, 3].

In patients with potential neural involvement, pelvic MRI protocol should include dedicated sequences and MRI neurography to identify the affected nerve and the pattern of neural involvement. Using this protocol, the radiologist will be able to define the lesion's characteristics, location, nerve relationship (proximity or direct involvement), nerve damage, and chronicity. Altogether, it will allow better clinical counseling and surgical planning for a patient-centered approach [1, 3].

The MRI neurography protocol includes the following: (a) two-dimensional (2D) or three-dimensional (3D) high-resolution T1-weighted non-fat-suppressed images (T1WNFSIs), (b) 3D high-resolution coronal T2 isotropic non-fat-suppressed images, (c) a postcontrast coronal 3D high-resolution short tau inversion recovery (STIR) sequence, (d) diffusion-weighted imaging (DWI) sequences, (e) tractography diffusion tensor imaging (DTI), and (f) post-gadolinium isotropic T1 axial high-resolution fat-suppressed images (Fig. 11.1). This protocol maximizes the nerve signal intensity from the fat pelvic

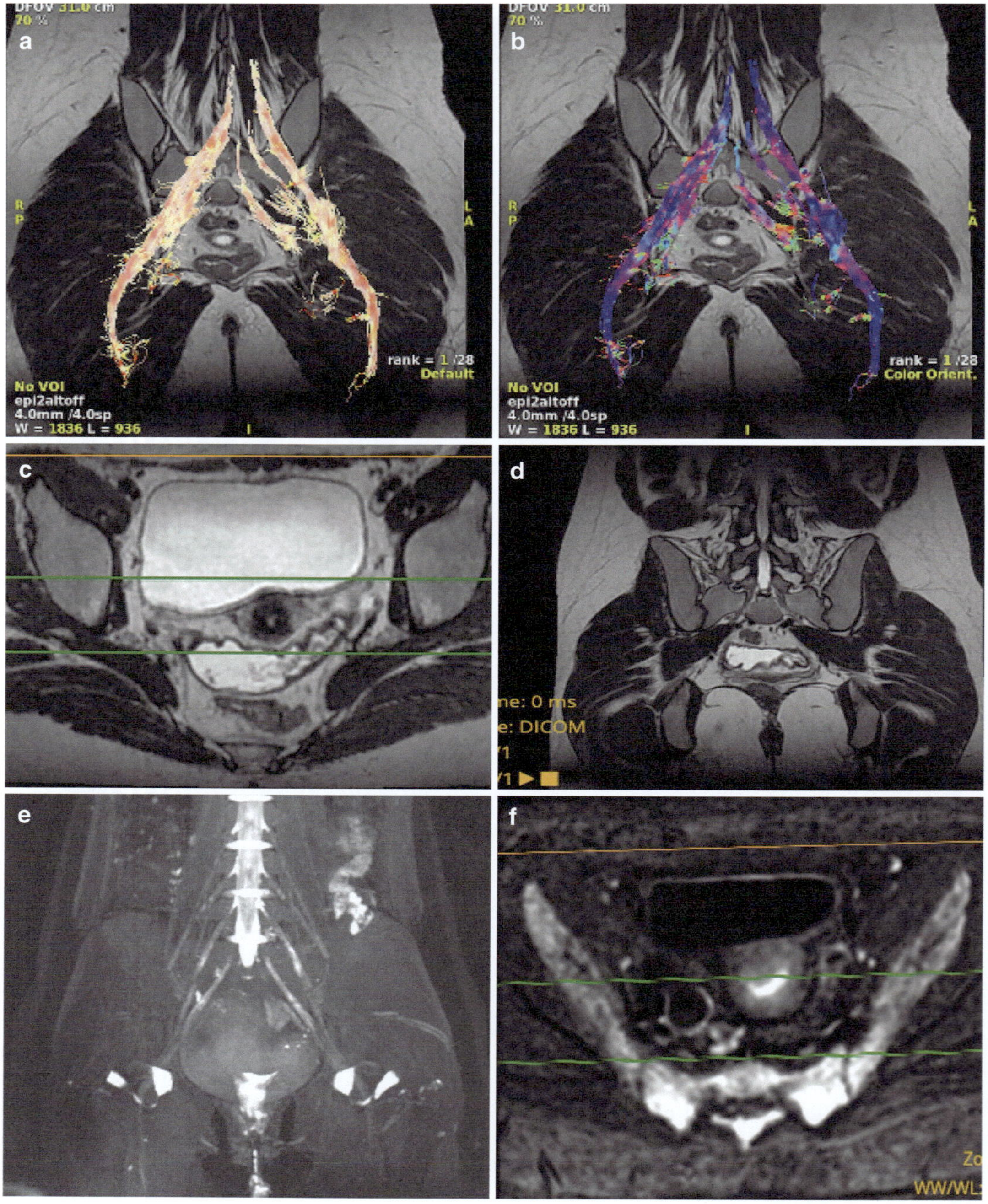

Fig. 11.1 Pelvic MRI tractography protocol: (**a**) and (**b**) tractography; (**c**) axial 3D T2WI (**d**) Coronal 3D T2WI (**e**) Coronal 3D T2WI STIR (**f**) DWI

background and suppresses vessels' signal intensity [1, 24–26].

The 2D and 3D high-resolution T1WNFSI and T2WNFSI sequences are crucial to identifying the nerves, improving the identification of the neural pathway in contrast to the hyperintense background of perineural tissue. A high-resolution 3D T2WI isotropic sequence enables multiplanar analysis, which can be critical for identifying the relationship of the endometriosis lesion with the nerve tissue [1, 24–26].

A 3D high-resolution T2W fat-suppressed short time inversion recovery (STIR) imaging sequence achieves an adequate and homogeneous fat suppression, allowing a proper differentiation because the hyperintense nerves are visualized against the hypointense background of the perineural fat. Because STIR is a fluid-sensitive sequence, nerve edema is well demonstrated, and it can be compared with the contralateral side. In addition, it enables an adequate signal suppression of the pelvic venous plexus, allowing better differentiation between nerves and vessels. Multiplanar imaging and 3D maximum-intensity projection MRI improve the identification of nerve pathways [1, 24–26].

A diffusion-weighted sequence provides a measure of the random movement of free water molecules in tissues (Brownian motion) and characterizes different tissue properties, such as orientational tissue organization. Unlike free-water diffusion, the movement of water molecules in biological tissues is restricted by interactions with cell membranes and macromolecules. In nerve tracts, the diffusion is anisotropic (directional), meaning water diffuses relatively freely along the long axis of the tract but is restricted by the myelin sheath in the short axis plane. Therefore, standard DWI does not provide data on the directionality of diffusion.

On the other hand, diffusion tensor imaging (DTI) estimates water diffusion in tissues in multiple directions (at least six) and diffusion-sensitizing gradients in a voxel, and it can be used to calculate fractional anisotropy (FA) maps and parameters on the basis of eigenvalues and mean diffusivity, which measure the integrity of nerves. Tractography provides a visual representation of the integrity of nerve bundles through postprocessing algorithms that link the direction of maximum diffusivity in adjacent voxels, which can allow the detection of neural alterations that could not be detected via conventional pelvic imaging protocols [1, 24–28].

Standard diffusion-weighted (DW) MRI and postcontrast 3D T1 high-resolution isotropic sequences are essential to evaluate associated findings like soft tissue and bone edema and inflammatory reaction, neural enhancement, and signs of muscle denervation and to identify associated pathologies that can have a similar clinical presentation.

11.5 Anatomic Background

11.5.1 Pelvic Connective Tissue, Muscles, and Bone Foramina: Anatomical Landmarks for Neural Identification

Comprehensive knowledge of pelvic neuroanatomy is crucial for diagnosing neural DE. Understanding neural endometriosis requires meticulous knowledge of the anatomy of the connective tissue of the pelvis and the bone foramina and their association with the nerves and the anatomical spaces of the pelvis [1, 18].

The connective tissue of the pelvis aims to connect, support, and bind other tissues. They are also important dissemination routes for DE and for surgical access. The functional organization of the pelvis is composed of dense connective tissue (the visceral ligaments and the parietal and visceral pelvic fasciae) and areas of loose connective tissue (the pelvic organs and abdominal walls). The retroperitoneal pelvic connective tissue is organized into three main groups of fasciae fused so that their intersections delimit the pelvic spaces and form the septa, which are filled with alveolar connective tissue, can be surgically cleaved, and, under physiological conditions, are virtual and collapsed depending on the amount of alveolar and fatty tissue they contain [5, 29].

These three groups are the parietal pelvic fascia (PPF), the visceral pelvic fascia (VPF), and the extraserosal pelvic fascia (EPF). The PPF surrounds the structures that delimit the pelvis (the levator ani, piriformis, obturator, and coccygeus muscles; the anterior surface of the sacrum and coccyx; and the hypogastric vessels and sacral roots). The PPF is divided into the obturator fascia; the pelvic superior fascia, which covers the levator ani and coccygeus muscles; and the piriformis fascia. The PPF is perforated by four bilateral foramina for the neurovascular bundles directed toward the legs and the gluteoperineal region. The VPF envelops the pelvic organs and attaches them to the pelvic sidewalls, creating the adventitious layer in each of them (Fig. 11.2). The EPF is the connective tissue between the PPF and the VPF, which supports the vascular and neural structures of the pelvis. The EPF consists of the parametrium, paracervix, lateral ligament of the rectum, superior vesical ligament, and presacral fascia [5, 18, 29].

Anatomical references for the lumbar plexus include the psoas, the anterosuperior iliac crest, and the obturator foramen. For the lumbosacral plexus, they include the piriformis muscle and the superior and inferior ischial foramina. The presacral fascia, the hypogastric fascia, and the ureter are the references for the hypogastric nerves; the nerve is located anteriorly to the presacral fascia, medially to the hypogastric fascia, and medially to the ureter [1–3].

11.5.2 MRI Features of Normal Pelvic Nerves and Neural Endometriosis

MRI can directly depict the somatic pelvic nerves. Nevertheless, imaging autonomic nerves remains challenging. Their small diameter and oblique path hamper differentiating them from adjacent structures. Knowledge of their anatomical topography enables their involvement to be inferred. However, through a dedicated imaging protocol for neural assessment, larger autonomic pelvic plexuses can be visualized [1, 25, 26].

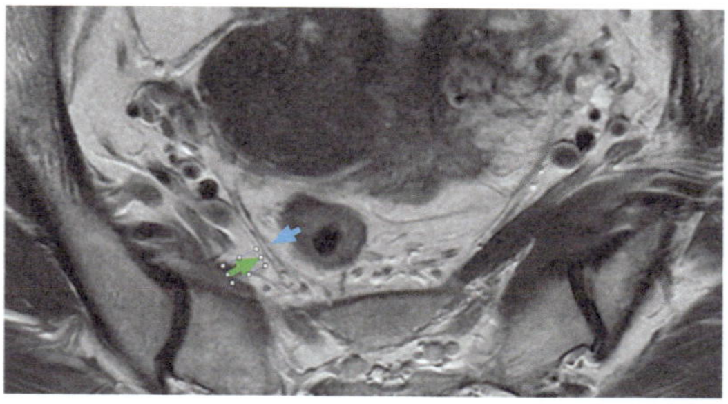

Fig. 11.2 Pelvic 2D T2W high-resolution MRI in the axial plane demonstrating the connective tissue structures. The parietal pelvic fascia is represented by the presacral fascia (green arrow), the visceral pelvic fascia is represented by the mesorectal fascia (blue arrow), and the extraserosal connective tissue is noted between the parietal and visceral fascia, where a visceral nerve is located

11.5.2.1 Normal Aspects of Somatic Nerves

Somatic nerves are straightforward to visualize via MRI. Normal nerves are isointense to slightly hyperintense to skeletal muscle on T2WI and isointense to skeletal muscle on T1WI. Somatic nerves have a smoother aspect compared to that of adjacent vessels and are slightly less hyperintense than vessels. Diffusion and STIR sequences suppress the vessels' signal intensity. Both the lumbar plexus and the lumbosacral plexus can be involved by DE, in most cases the lumbosacral [1].

11.5.2.2 MRI Findings of Neural Somatic Endometriosis

MRI findings include (a) solid spiculated nodules hypointense on T2WI, with or without cystic and hemorrhagic components; (b) cystic lesions resembling endometriomas (hypointense on T2WI and hyperintense on T1WI); and (c) complex cystic masses hyperintense on T2WI with septa and hematic content (Fig. 11.3). Associated findings include adjacent soft tissue edema and inflammatory reaction, demonstrated via post-contrast enhancement in acute stages and a diffuse increase in signal intensity on T2WI. Chronic stages can demonstrate signs of axonal nerve degeneration and denervated muscle, characterized by muscle atrophy and fatty infiltration into the target muscles of the affected nerve [1, 8, 30, 31].

Lumbar Plexus

The lumbar plexus is formed by the nerves from L1 to L4, along with the subcostal nerve (T12). From superior to inferior, the major branches of the lumbar plexus include the iliohypogastric nerve (L1), the ilioinguinal nerve (L1), the genitofemoral nerve (anterior L1-L2), the lateral femoral cutaneous nerve (L2-L3), the obturator nerve

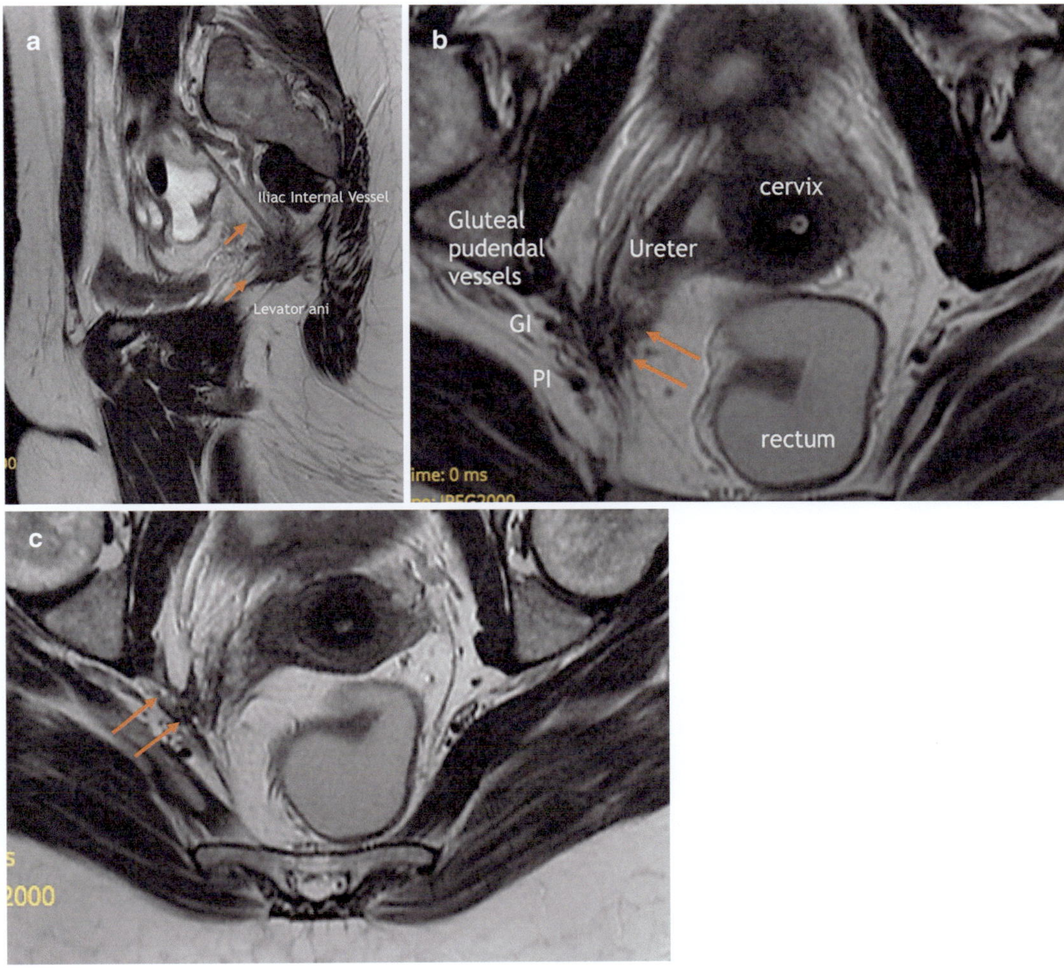

Fig. 11.3 DE solid spiculated nodule (arrows) hypointense on T2WI located at the pelvic floor and sciatic foramen. It retracts the inferior gluteal artery and vagina. Inferior hypogastric plexus involvement is also shown. Pelvic 2D T2 high-resolution MRI in sagittal plane (**a**) and axial plane (**b**, **c**). *GI* Glutea inferior, *PI* Pudenda Interna

(L2-L4), and the femoral nerve (L2-L4) [1, 25, 26]. Some branches of the lumbar plexus run into the pelvis and can be affected by endometriosis. Among them, the most important are the obturator and femoral nerves [1, 2, 5].

Obturator Nerve

The obturator nerve (ON) is a major peripheral nerve of the thigh. It is formed by fibers from the anterior divisions of L2, L3, and L4. The ON descends behind the psoas major, emerges from its medial border, runs laterally along the pelvic sidewall to the iliac external vessels, and leaves the pelvis through the obturator foramen into the obturator canal (Fig. 11.4). It is responsible for motor innervation to the adductor muscle of the hip and for sensory innervation to the skin on the medial thigh and knee. In cases where the obturator nerve is involved, the most common symptoms are catamenial pain and motor deficits in hip adduction and sensory disturbances in the medial thigh [1, 2, 21, 32].

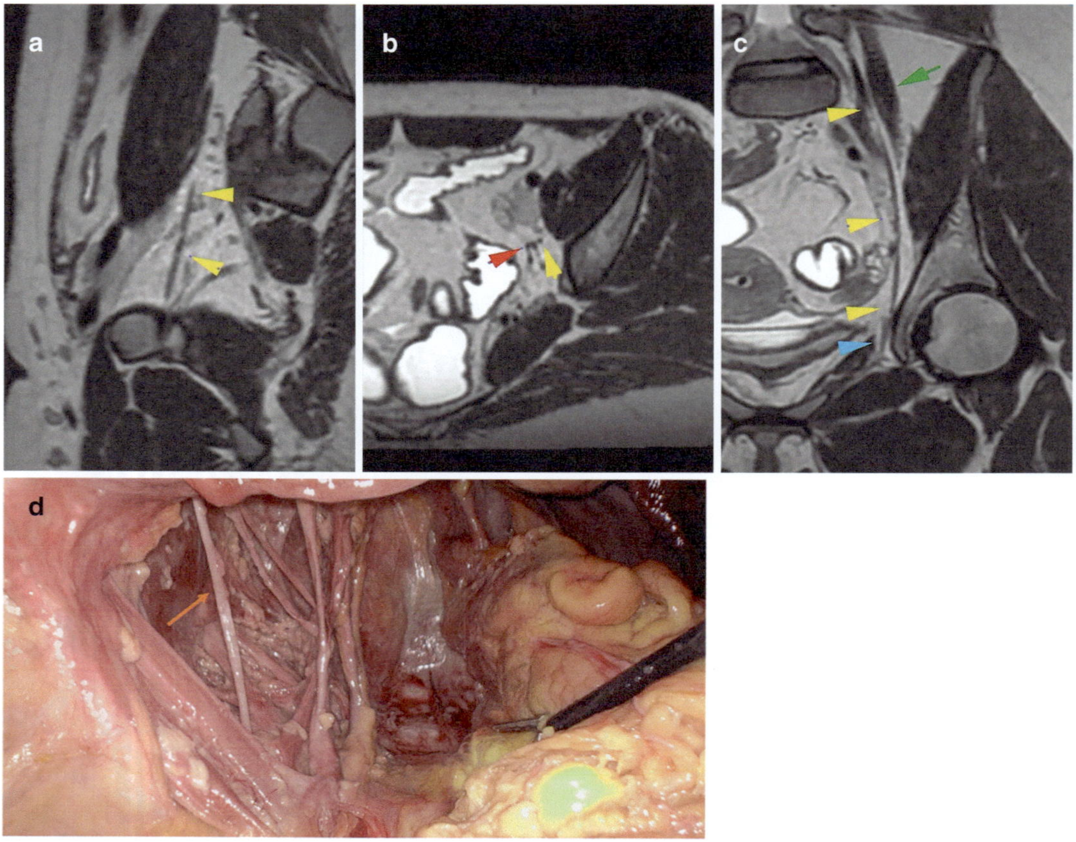

Fig. 11.4 Pelvic MRI demonstrating the obturator nerve (yellow arrows): sagittal (**a**), axial (**b**), and coronal (**c**). The path of the nerve is shown as medial to the psoas muscle in the pelvic retroperitoneum (green arrow) and with a descending path lateral to the obturator neurovascular bundle, a branch of the internal iliac (red arrow). Note its distal portion in the obturator foramen (blue arrow). Cadaver dissection of the ON (**d**). The ON is the most lateral, elongated structure (arrow on D). (Courtesy of Claudio Crispi, MD)

Obturator Nerve Endometriosis

Endometriosis lesions in the obturator fossa are rare, and only a few case reports appear in the literature. However, in the authors' experience, indirect ON involvement should be remembered because large endometriomas can cause compression on the nerve (Fig. 11.5). Signs of the denervation of the obturator muscle may be visible in the case of nerve damage (Fig. 11.6) [1, 3, 18, 21, 32].

Femoral Nerve

Femoral endometriosis is a rare condition that can cause catamenial episodes of cruralgia and partial motor and sensory loss in the femoral nerve territory. The femoral nerve is the largest nerve of the lumbar plexus. It forms from the dorsal divisions of the L2–L4 ventral rami. It is a lower limb motor and sensory nerve, controlling the primary hip flexor and knee-extension muscles. It also controls sensation over the anterior and medial thigh and the medial leg down to the hallux. It descends between the psoas and iliacus muscles until it leaves the pelvis under the inguinal ligament and divides into anterior and posterior branches (Fig. 11.7) [1].

Femoral Nerve Endometriosis

Endometriosis in the parietal colic gutter along the psoas and iliacus muscles can affect the femoral nerve before it exits the pelvis through the femoral canal, lateral to the femoral vessels

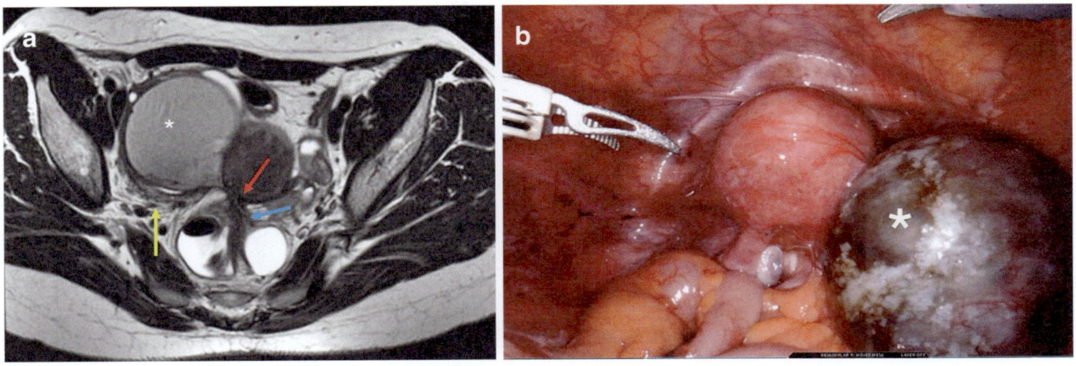

Fig. 11.5 Endometriosis in a 27-year-old woman with dysmenorrhea, deep dyspareunia, and pain that radiates to the lower right thigh. (**a**) Pelvic T2W MRI shows a right ovary endometrioma (*) compressing the right obturator nerve (yellow arrow), attached to a retrocervical (red arrow) and rectal lesion (blue arrow). (**b**) Laparoscopic view. Note the large endometrioma (*) compressing the lateral wall. (Courtesy of Thiers Soares, MD)

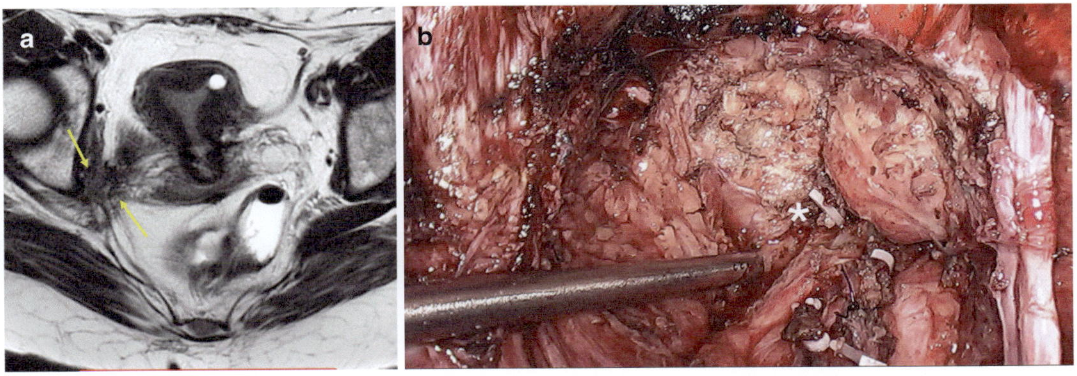

Fig. 11.6 Neural endometriosis in a 36-year-old woman with chronic pelvic pain that radiates to the lower right extremity and complaints of difficulty adducting the right leg associated with sensory changes in the ipsilateral limb. (**a**) Pelvic T2W MRI shows a DE lesion at the obturator fossa affecting the right obturator nerve and the lateral pelvic sidewall at the greater sciatic foramen (yellow arrows). (**b**) Laparoscopy demonstrating the nodule infiltrating the right ON (*). (Courtesy of Claudio Crispi, MD)

(Fig. 11.8). The extracavity portion of the femoral nerve is rarely affected by endometriosis. [1, 3].

Lumbosacral Plexus

The lumbosacral plexus is formed by the lumbosacral trunk, the ventral branches of the first to third sacral nerves, and part of the fourth. The anastomotic branch of L4 joins L5 to form the lumbosacral trunk. The lumbosacral trunk is near the medial margin of the psoas major muscle and runs inferiorly over the pelvic brim, joining with S1 and then successively with S2, S3, and S4 (Fig. 11.9). As anatomical landmarks, the superior gluteal vessels run between the lumbosacral trunk and S1. The lumbosacral trunk contributes to the formation of the sacral plexus, which gives rise to the superior and inferior gluteal nerves. It plays a crucial role in the function and stability of the gluteal muscles. The main branches of the sacral plexus are the sciatic nerve, the inferior and superior gluteal nerves, and the pudendal nerves [1, 2, 5].

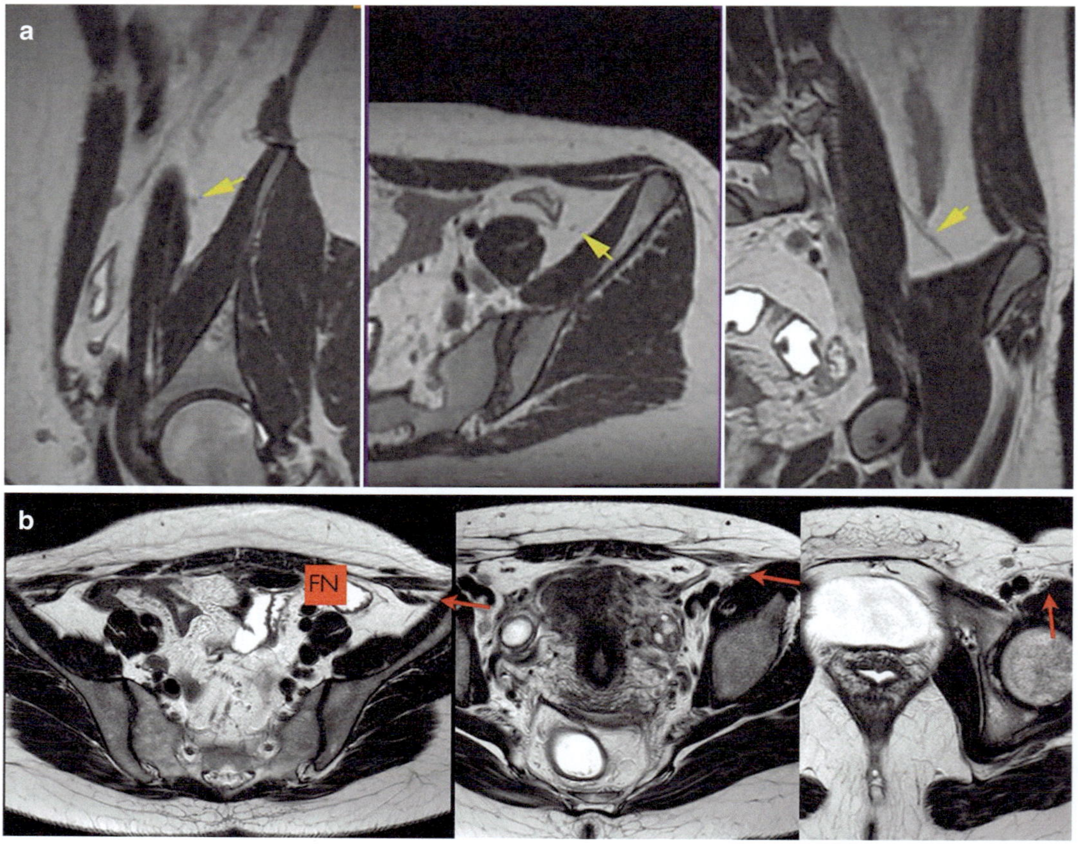

Fig. 11.7 Pelvic MRI demonstrating the femoral nerve. Pelvic 2D T2W high-resolution MRI: (**a**) Sagittal, axial, and coronal planes respectively demonstrating the femoral nerve (yellow arrows) in the pelvic retroperitoneum, between the psoas and iliacus muscles, before it exits the pelvis through the femoral canal, lateral to the femoral vessels. Injuries to the paretic colic gutter can affect this nerve. (**b**) Axial plane demostrating the extracavity portion of the nerve (red arrows). The nerve passes underneath the inguinal ligament to enter the femoral triangle. Within this triangle, the nerve is located lateral to the femoral vessels

Lumbosacral Plexus Endometriosis

Endometriosis can affect the lumbosacral plexus via the distortion or infiltration of their main branches: the sciatic, inferior and superior gluteal, and pudendal nerves. Large parametrial DE can infiltrate the continuum of the sacral plexus. Large lesions featuring the involvement of the lateral portion of the uterosacral ligament and rectovaginal space correlate with the involvement of sacral nerve roots S2, S3, and S4 (Fig. 11.10). Lesions infiltrating the ovarian fossae and cardinal ligaments can involve preferentially sacral nerve roots S1, S2, and S3 [1–3, 5, 14, 33].

Sciatic Nerve

The sciatic nerve is the thickest and longest nerve in the human body. It is composed of fibers from L4 and L5 coming from the lumbosacral plexus and fibers from S1, S2, and S3. These branches come together and converge in the posterior pelvic region to form the sciatic nerve, which leaves the pelvis through the suprapiriform hiatus of the greater ischial foramen (Fig. 11.11). It passes inferiorly to the piriformis muscle, accompanied by the pudendal nerve, the internal pudendal artery and vein, and the inferior gluteal neurovascular branch. The sciatic nerve then continues its

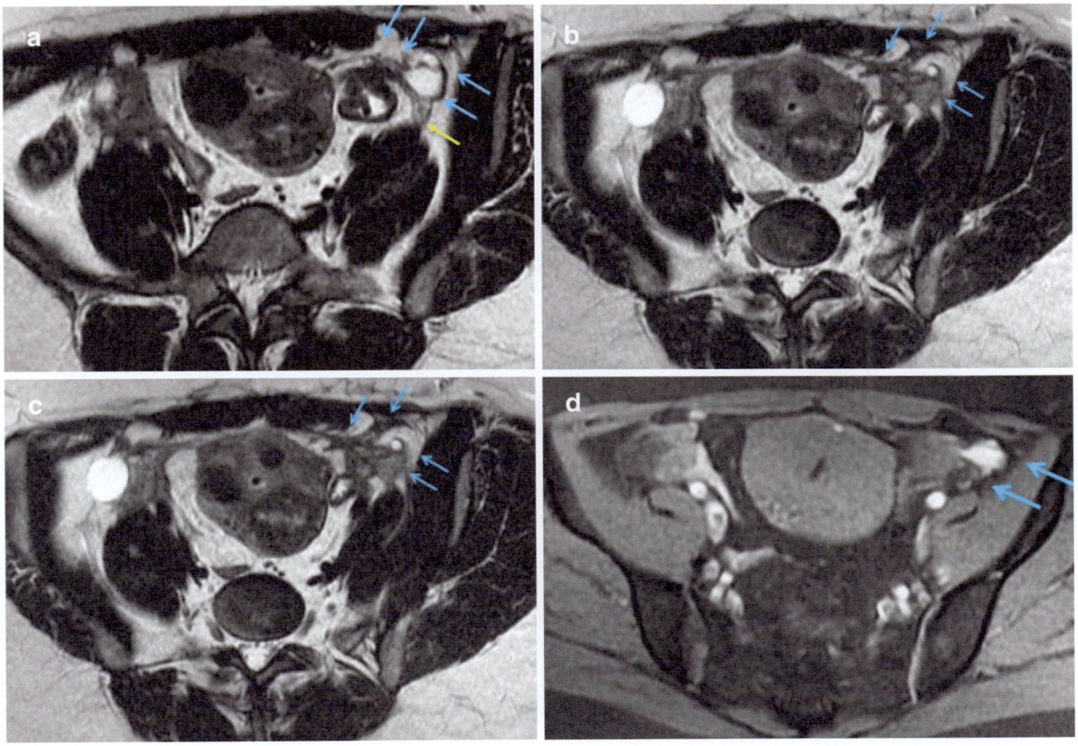

Fig. 11.8 Endometriosis in the parietal colic gutter (blue arrows). Note the DE hypointense plaque with blood in the left gutter (blue arrows). The ovary is positioned high. The plaque involves the ovary and infiltrates the retroperitoneum, adjacent to the psoas and iliac muscle and anterior to the femoral nerve (yellow arrows). (**a**, **b**, **c**) Axial T2WI and (**d**) axial T1WI with fat saturation

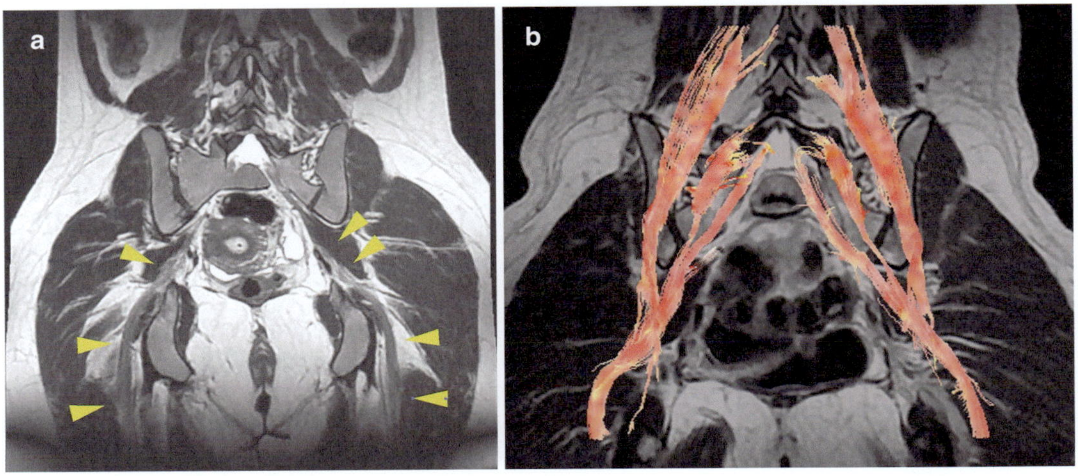

Fig. 11.9 MRI tractography shows the lumbosacral plexus. (**a**) 3D T2WI in the coronal plane showing the plexus and the sciatic nerves (yellow arrows). (**b**) Postprocessing tractography fused with 3D T2WI in the coronal plane. L4, L5, S1, and S2 are well delineated

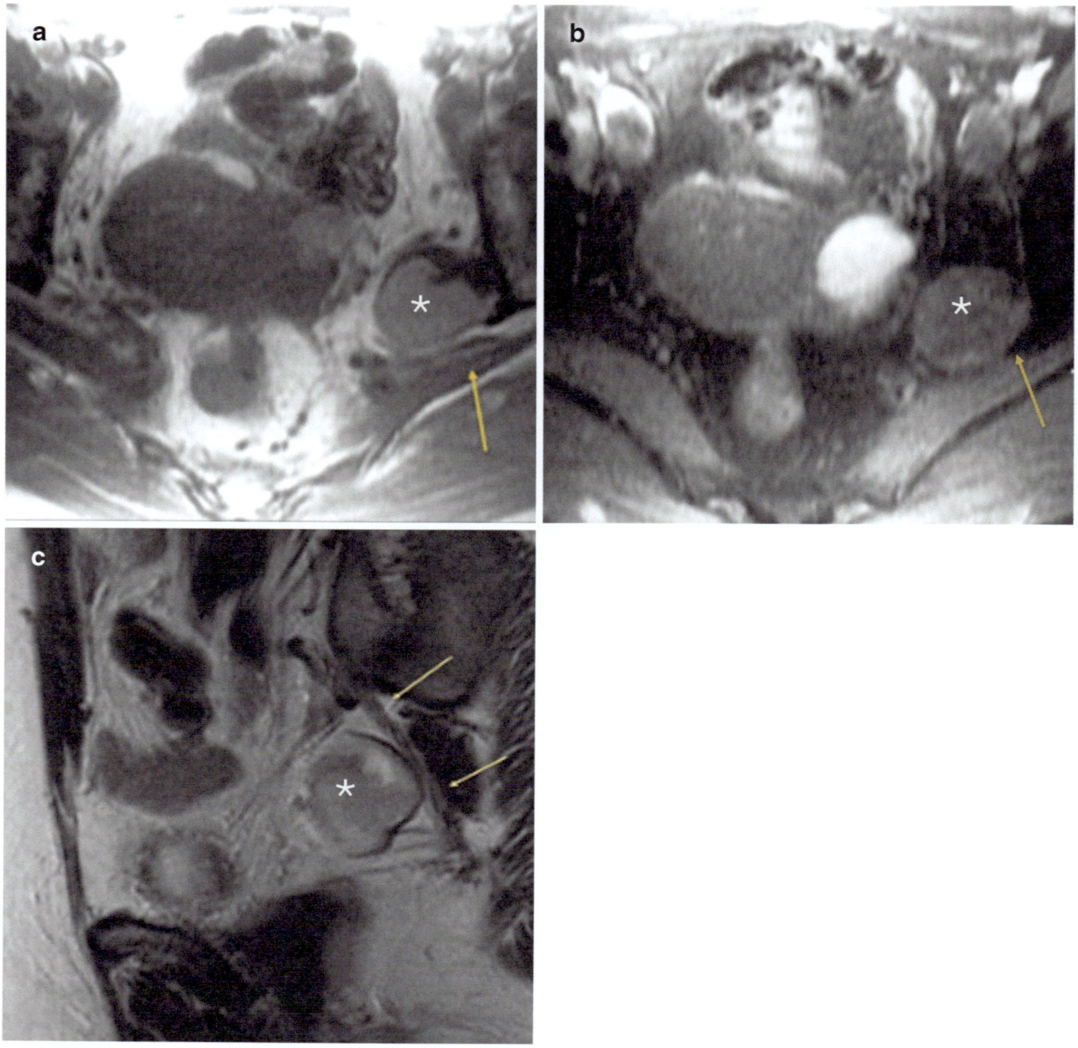

Fig. 11.10 Endometriosis in a 36-year-old infertile woman with dysmenorrhea and pain in the left gluteal region that radiates to the lower extremity. (**a**) Axial T2W MRI, (**b**) axial T1WFSI, and (**c**) sagittal T2W MRI shows an endometriotic cyst (*) displacing the lumbosacral plexus and the sciatic nerve (yellow arrows). Associated findings: endometrioma of the left ovary and retrocervical and intestinal DE

course through the posterior thigh and is divided, at the level of the knee, into its main branches, the common fibular and tibial nerves [1, 8, 9].

The sciatic nerve has sensitive branches to the upper gluteal region, posterolateral thigh, leg, ankle, and foot and motor branches to the hip extensors, abductors and rotators, knee flexors, and ankle and foot muscles [1, 8, 9, 14, 30].

Sciatic Nerve Endometriosis

The term *sciatica* refers to the compression or irritation of the sciatic nerve. It is characterized by pain in the ipsilateral gluteal region that radiates to the lower extremity. When related to endometriosis, initially, the pain is cyclical during the menstrual period, and, over time, it becomes continuous [1, 8, 9, 14, 30].

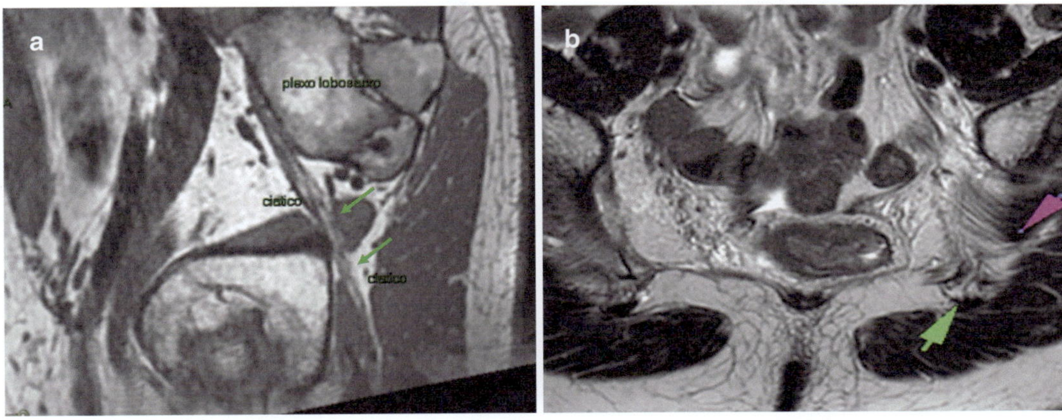

Fig. 11.11 Pelvic MRI demonstrating the sciatic nerve path (green arrows) through the greater ischial foramen (purple arrow): (**a**) sagittal oblique 3D T1W MRI and (**b**) coronal oblique T2W MRI

The sciatic nerve is the most affected peripheral nerve by DE. MRI findings of sciatic endometriosis include solid spiculated nodules hypointense on T2WI, cystic lesions like ovarian endometriomas, and complex cystic masses. MRI neurography demonstrates an endometriotic lesion centered at the sciatic notch. The sciatic nerve can demonstrate a marked and hyperintense signal on T2WI distal to the lesion, indicating axonal injury. In addition, atrophy and evidence of denervation can be found in the target muscles of the sciatic nerve and the distal lumbosacral plexus, most marked in the gluteal group and the quadratus femoris muscle [1, 3, 6, 8, 9].

Endometrioma-like cystic lesions are usually avascular and unilocular cysts with old hematic content, which is hyperintense on T1WFSI and hypointense on T2WI ("shading sign") in the path of the sciatic nerve. Usually, it has restricted diffusion due to thicker content and chronic bleeding. The differential diagnosis includes neurogenic benign tumors such as neurinoma and neurofibroma, which, differently from endometriosis lesions, show gadolinium enhancement and an intermediate signal on T2WI and T1WI [1, 3, 8, 9, 30].

Isolated sciatic endometriosis commonly affects the suprapiriform portion of the sciatic nerve. The endometriotic lesion grows inside the sciatic nerve and caudally broadens through the greater sciatic foramen. Symptoms are L5 and S1 sciatica and gluteal pain. Bladder dysfunctions and pudendal pain are absent in these cases. If surgical intervention is indicated, the intrafascicular neurolysis of the sciatic nerve with the resection of the damaged part of the nerve must be performed [1, 3, 8, 9, 31]. Depending on the location of the endometriotic nodule (before/after the greater sciatic foramen), different types of surgeries have to be performed (with possible transgluteal access).

Solid spiculated nodules at the posterolateral pelvic region and near the greater ischial foramen comprise a rare presentation of endometriosis affecting the sciatic and pudendal nerve (Figs. 11.12 and 11.13). These lesions are often infiltrative and can also affect the pelvic floor. Associated findings include adjacent muscle and bone edema and inflammatory reaction demonstrated by a diffuse increase in signal intensity on T2WI and postcontrast enhancement in acute stages. Muscle atrophy and fatty infiltration can be seen in chronic cases [1, 3, 8].

Pudendal Nerve

The pudendal nerve is one of the two main branches of the sacral plexus, along with the sciatic nerve. It originates in the pelvis, from the ventral rami of the S2 to S4 sacral roots, close to the upper edge of the sacrotuberous ligament and the ischiococcygeus muscle. It then runs inferi-

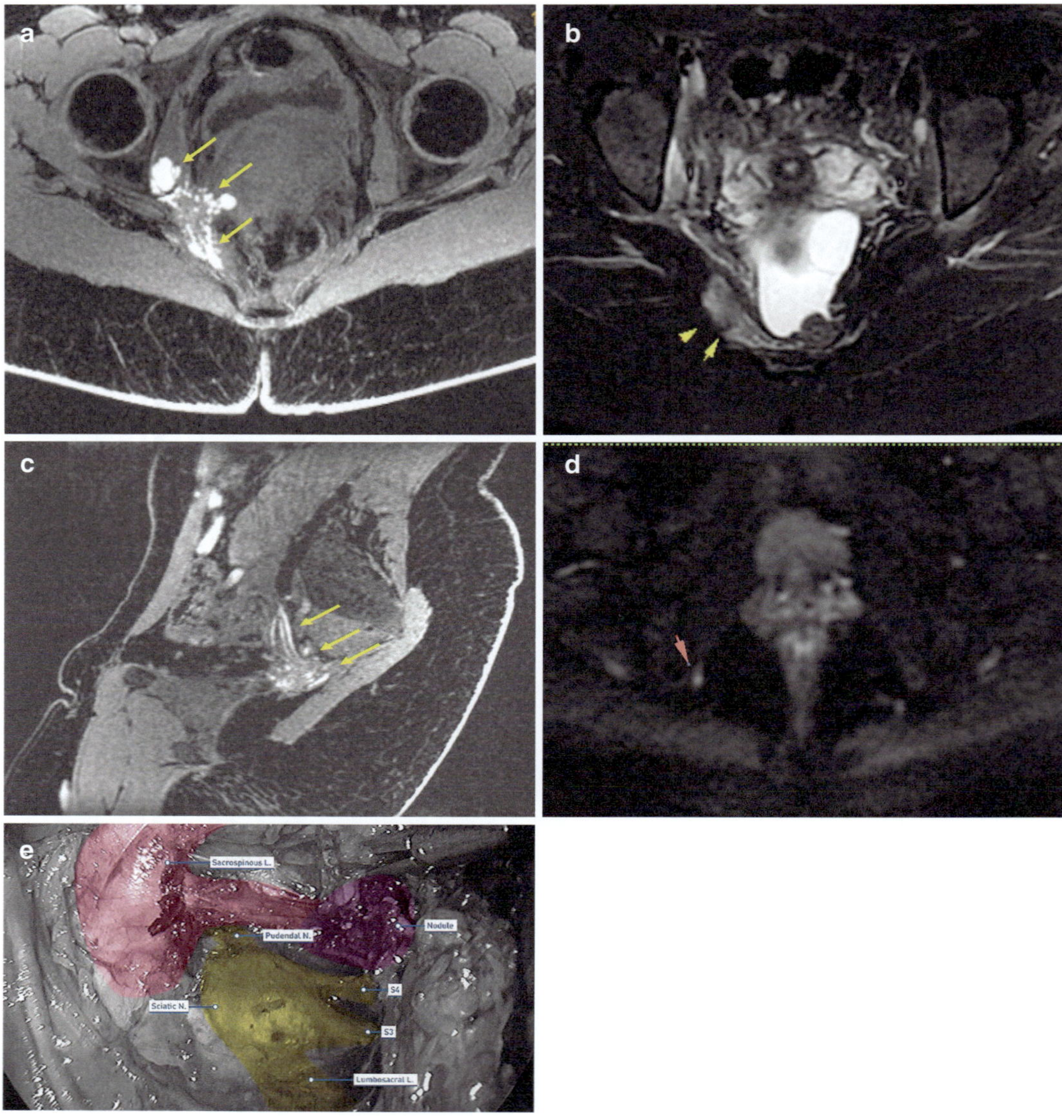

Fig. 11.12 DE lesion affecting the sciatic nerve (arrows in **a** and **c**) and the pudendal nerve (arrow in **d**). Blood is in the lesion, which causes nerve edema, better demonstrated with DWI. Note the associated edema in the right piriformis muscle seen on axial STIR (arrows in **b**). (**a** and **c**) 3D T1WFSI high-resolution sequence, (**b**) STIR axial sequence, (**d**) DWI in axial plane. Robotic surgery. (Courtesy of Claudio Crispi, MD)

orly and leaves the pelvis through the greater ischial foramen. After passing through the foramen, the nerve runs through the gluteal region, dorsally to the sacrospinous ligament, and medially to the internal pudendal vessels. Accompanied by the internal pudendal artery and vein, the pudendal nerve passes through the lesser ischial foramen and the pudendal canal (Alcock's canal) (Fig. 11.14). Toward the entrance to Alcock's canal, the pudendal nerve gives off the inferior rectal nerve, which innervates the external anal sphincter and the perianal skin. In the distal portion of the canal, the pudendal nerve bifurcates into two branches, the perineal nerve and the dorsal clitoral nerve [2, 3, 5].

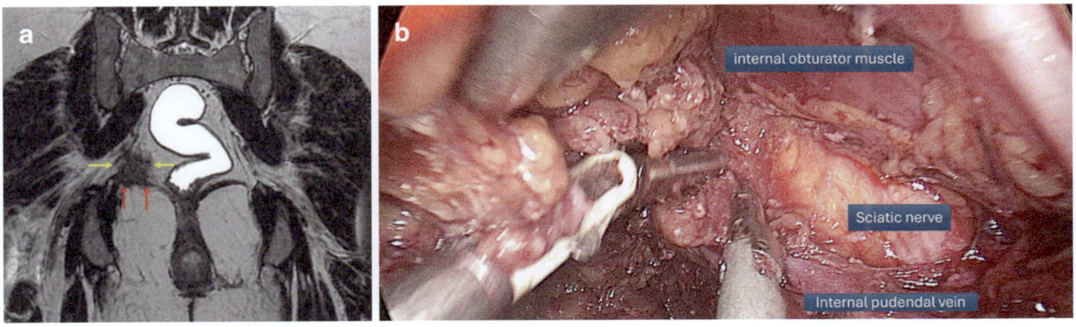

Fig. 11.13 (**a**) DE lesion involving the sciatic and pudendal nerves and the pelvic floor (yellow arrows) is well displayed in the 3D T2WI coronal sequence. The plaque retracts the S1, S2, and S3 nerves and retracts the levator ani muscle (red arrows), which shows signs of denervation. (**b**) Laparoscopic view of the pelvic cavity shown, with no signs of deep endometriosis. (Courtesy of Marco Aurelio Pinho de Oliveira, MD)

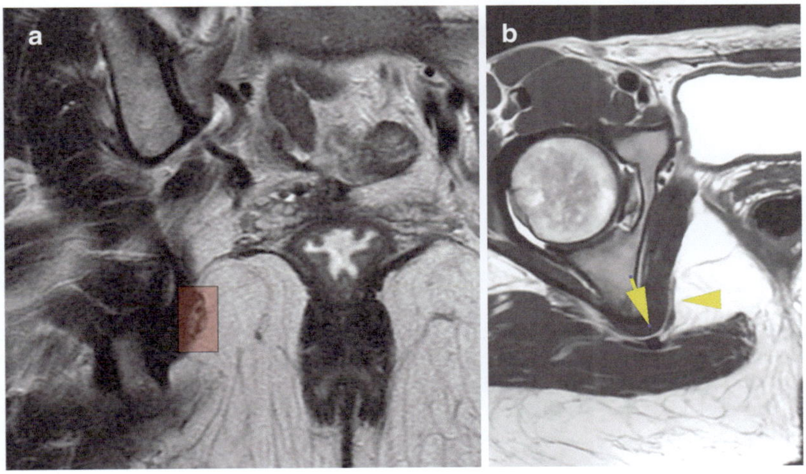

Fig. 11.14 Pelvic MRI demonstrating the pudendal nerve path in Alcock's canal: (**a**) coronal plane T2WI (rectangle) and (**b**) axial T2WI (arrows in Alcock's canal and the inferior sciatic foramen)

The pudendal nerve is the main nerve in the perineal region, with sympathetic sensory fibers for the external genital organs, the skin of the perineum, the lower gluteal region, and the motor fibers that control the levator ani muscle, and it is responsible for the continence and relaxing of the external urethral sphincter and external anal sphincter. It also has a potential modulating effect on bladder function and influences the function of the lower third of the vagina [1, 3, 5, 10].

Pudendal Nerve Endometriosis

Pudendal neuralgia induces pudendal pain and bladder and rectal disfunctions [2, 12]. Pudendal endometriosis can manifest due to an endometriotic lesion along the pelvic wall at the level of the endopelvic portion of the pudendal nerve between the sacrotuberous and sacrospinous ligaments or at Alcock's canal (Fig. 11.15 and 11.16) [1, 2, 6].

11.5.2.3 Normal Aspects of the Visceral Nerves and Plexus

The visceral nerves and plexus represent a challenge for MRI identification. However, Wisjmuller et al. were able to identify the superior and inferior hypogastric plexus and the hypogastric nerve in 70%, 70%, and 80% of their volunteers, respectively. To highlight their path, we included an anatomical reference such as bone or muscle structure and reinforced the concepts of the pelvic fascia and the autonomic nerves [6].

The superior hypogastric plexus (SHP) appears as a high-signal intensity small mesh-like structure

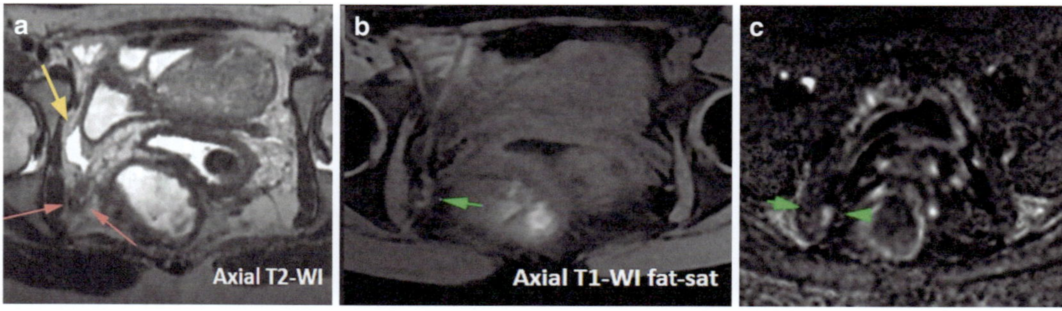

Fig. 11.15 Endometriosis in a 35-year-old woman with dysmenorrhea, dyspareunia, and perianal/perineal pain. (**a**) Axial T2W MRI shows DE of the right pelvic floor involving the pudendal nerve (pink arrows) that is associated with a peritoneal pocket (yellow arrow). (**b**) Axial T1WFSI shows hematic foci in the pudendal nerve (green arrow). (**c**) Synthetic DWI shows pudendal nerve edema (green arrows)

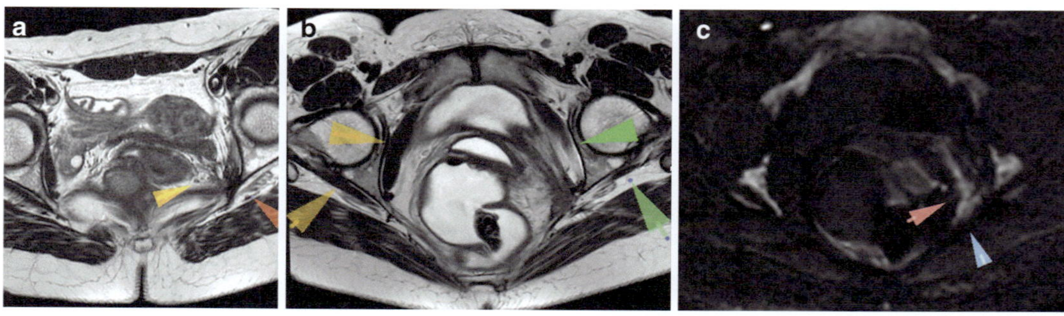

Fig. 11.16 Lesion in the small sciatic foramen and the pudendal canal involving the left pudendal nerve (head arrows in **a** and **c**). Note fat infiltration in the internal obturator and quadratus femoris muscle (green head arrows in **b compared to the normal appearance of the muscles shown by the yellow arrows**) and signs of denervation related to chronic nerve involvement. It also show neuropathy with pudendal nerve edema. (**a** and **b**) Axial T2WI and (**c**) DWI

located retroperitoneally at the level and in front of the sacral promontory and between the neural foramina (Fig. 11.17). The SHP is more straightforward to visualize than the inferior hypogastric plexus (IHP), probably because it has a relatively fixed presacral location and lacks surrounding confounding structures). The SHP receives sympathetic fibers from L3 and L4, parasympathetic from the pelvic splanchnic nerves (L3, L4), and both parasympathetic and sympathetic contributions from the aortic plexus. The main function is to carry innervation from the bowel (distal to the left colonic flexure) and pelvic visceral organs such as the vagina, uterus, cervix, fallopian tubes, rectum, and bladder; therefore, the dysfunction of this plexus can cause bowel, urinary, and reproductive dysfunction [1–3, 5, 29].

The SHP bifurcates at the level of aortic bifurcation and the sacral promontory into two hypogastric nerves (HNs), which have a lower path along the mesorectum, anteriorly to the presacral fascia, medially to the hypogastric fascia, and laterally to the mesorectal fascia, coursing bilaterally along the common iliac chains and pararectal fossa. The HNs appear as a linear structure posteromedial to the ureters and medial to the uterosacral ligament [1–3, 5, 29].

To better understand the location of the HNs in the pelvis, consider that it is involved by a fascia sheath common to the ureter, genital vessels and SHP in the retroperitoneal space deriving from the extensions of the renal fascia to their terminations in the pelvis (Figs. 11.18 and 11.19). Posterior to the rectum, this fascia fuses with the

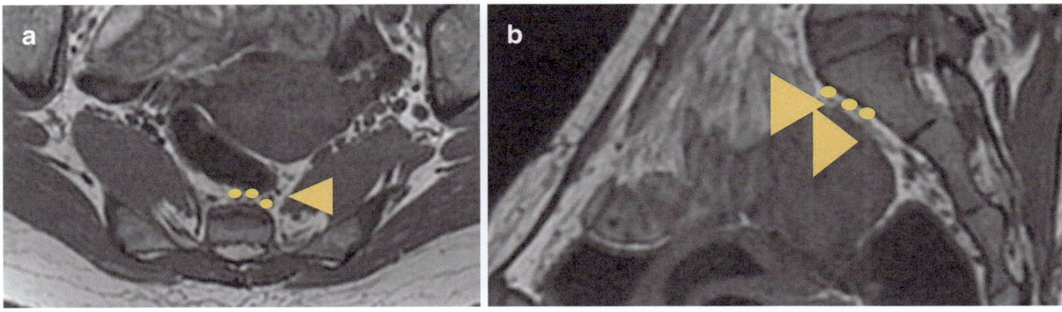

Fig. 11.17 Pelvic MRI shows the superior hypogastric plexus location (head arrows in **a**, **b**) anterior to the promontory and medial to the iliac vessels (circles in **a**) and ureters

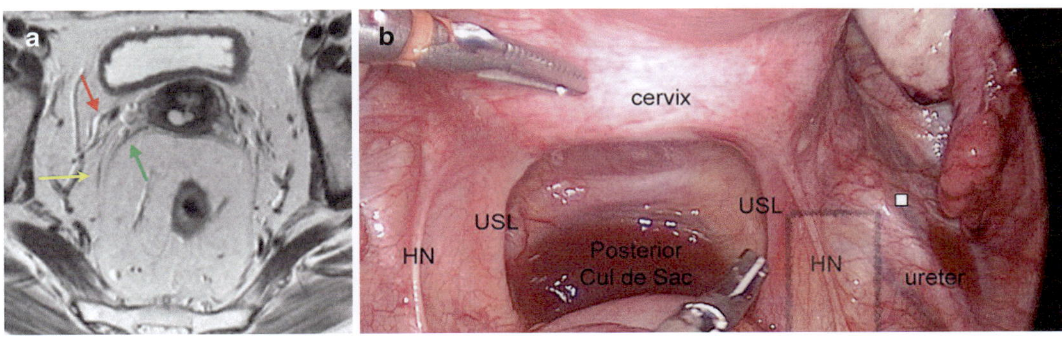

Fig. 11.18 (**a**) Pelvic MRI shows the hypogastric nerve location (yellow arrow) between the ureter (red arrow) and uterosacral ligament (green arrow). (**b**) The same view is shown from laparoscopy. (Courtesy of Marco Aurelio Pinho de Oliveira, MD)

mesorectal fascia at the level of the second to fourth sacral vertebrae. At this point the HNs will join the pelvic splanchnic nerves [3, 34].

The HNs divide into the bladder, uterine, and rectal bundles and join the pelvic splanchnic nerves to form the IHP at the level of the utero-sacral ligaments and the middle rectal vein. The IHP appears in axial, sagittal, and coronal sequences as a high-signal-intensity 3–4 cm mesh-like structure located retroperitoneally at the level of the upper third of the vagina. It has three main branches: the middle rectal plexus, the ureterovaginal plexus, and the bladder plexus [1, 25, 26].

The splanchnic nerves originate in the ventral S2-S4 sacral roots and cross the parametrium and the sacral hypogastric fascia, forming a mesh-work of smaller nerves not directly visualized on MRI. The splanchnic nerves anastomose with the hypogastric nerves (sympathetic system), forming the IHP, which is adjacent to the lateral part of the uterosacral ligament. These nerves provide parasympathetic innervation to the bladder and rectum, regulate urinary bladder emptying by controlling the internal urethral sphincter, enable rectal motility, and influence sexual functions like erection [1, 25, 26].

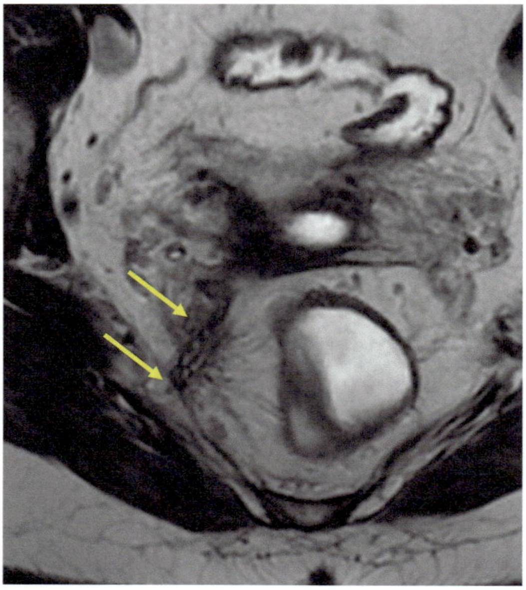

Fig. 11.19 Axial T2WI: a 4 cm right DE nodule involving the uterosacral ligament, mesorectum, and rectum (arrows). Note the lateral extension through the visceral and parietal fascia. The HNs are thickened and hypointense, as is the DE

11.5.2.4 Visceral Pelvic Nerve Endometriosis

The SHP has its location in the midline of the lower abdomen, and it is not a frequent site of endometriosis involvement [1–3, 5, 29]. Different from the SHP, the IHP and hypogastric nerve are common sites of pelvic endometriosis among cases of neurological involvement. Cases of parametrium infiltration pose a high risk of hypogastric nerve involvement, and in cases of paracolpium infiltration, the IHP is potentially at risk (Figs. 11.20, 11.21, 11.22 and 11.23) [2, 3, 5, 29].

Symptoms of splanchnic nerve involvement can vary from sexual dysfunction to chronic constipation and bladder retention. Because they are very thin structures, they are not usually directly identified on MRI. However, depending on the location of DE lesions, neural involvement may be inferred, especially if a strong clinical correlation exists [2, 6].

Fig. 11.20 Endometriosis in a 33-year-old woman with early onset dysmenorrhea, dyspareunia, and dyschezia for 15 years. (**a**) TVUS transversal view shows a parametrial and paracopium DE nodule (yellow arrows) deeply infiltrating the vaginal fornix (blue arrows) and extending to the pelvic floor (white arrows). (**b**) Axial T2W pelvic MRI shows a left parametrial endometriosis and a lateral wall endometriosis (yellow arrows) in the topography of the hypogastric fascia and the left hypogastric nerve, involved by the lesion, and it shows an ovarian endometrioma (*). (**c, d**) Sagittal T2W MRI shows parametrial endometriosis (yellow arrow) infiltrating the ureter, causing stenosis and upstream dilatation (blue arrows), with posterior extension to sacral roots S2, S3, and S4, represented by a thickening of the extra-foraminal portion of these sacral roots (red arrows). (**e**) Coronal T2W MRI shows parametrial nodule extending to the pelvic floor (yellow arrows), fatty atrophy of the left iliococcygeal muscle (signs of denervation—red arrows), and rectal endometriosis (blue arrow). The patient underwent surgery with a left nephrectomy and extensive resection of endometriosis. (**f**) Laparoscopy courtesy of Ricardo Quintairos, MD: Note that the photograph from surgery shows the DE lesion infiltrating the ureter, fascia, and hypogastric nerve (ureter: green, hypogastric nerve: orange, hypogastric fascia: purple, rectosigmoid: white)

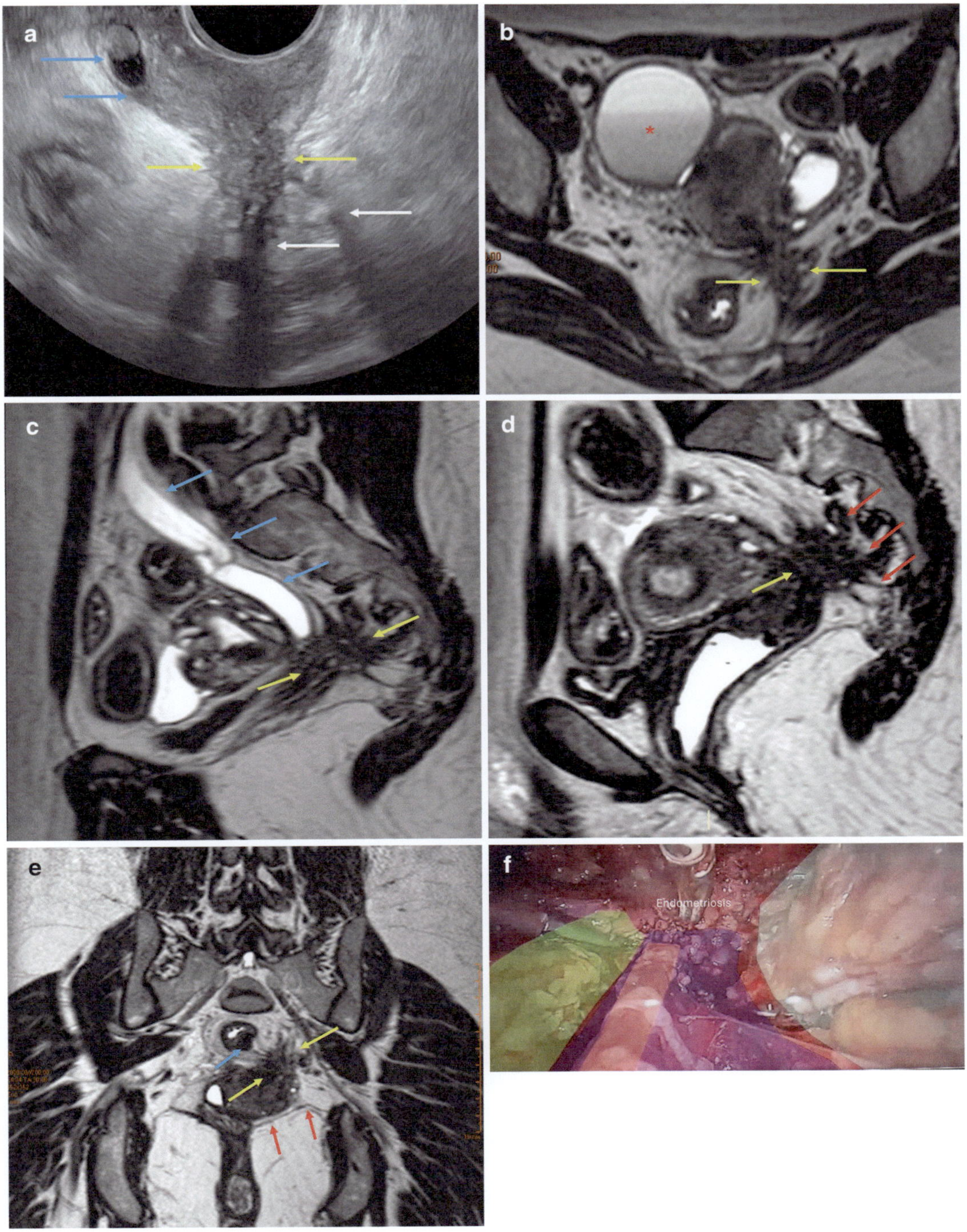
a
b
c
d
e
f
Endometriosis

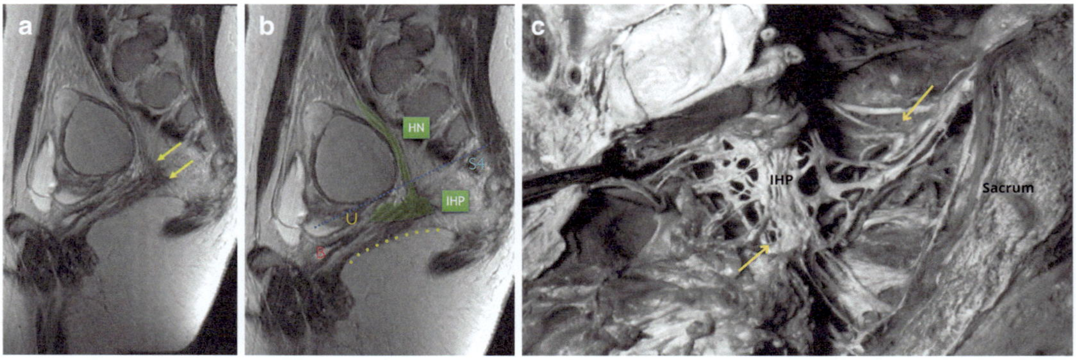

Fig. 11.21 DE involving the HNs and IHP: (**a**) Sagittal T2WI shows HN and IHP involvement (yellow arrows). (**b**) Note the relationship between the nerves and the ureter, bladder, levator ani, and piriform muscle. The location of the HNs (yellow arrows in a) is just below the junction of the ureter with the uterine artery, penetrated by multiple small vessels. (**c**) Anatomical dissection highlighting the inferior hypogastric plexus in a cadaveric specimen (yellow arrows). Reproduced with permission from Brown G. High-resolution MRI of the anatomy important in total mesorectal excision of the rectum. AJR Am J Roentgenol. 2004 Feb;182(2):431–9. https://doi.org/10.2214/ajr.182.2.1820431. PMID: 14736677

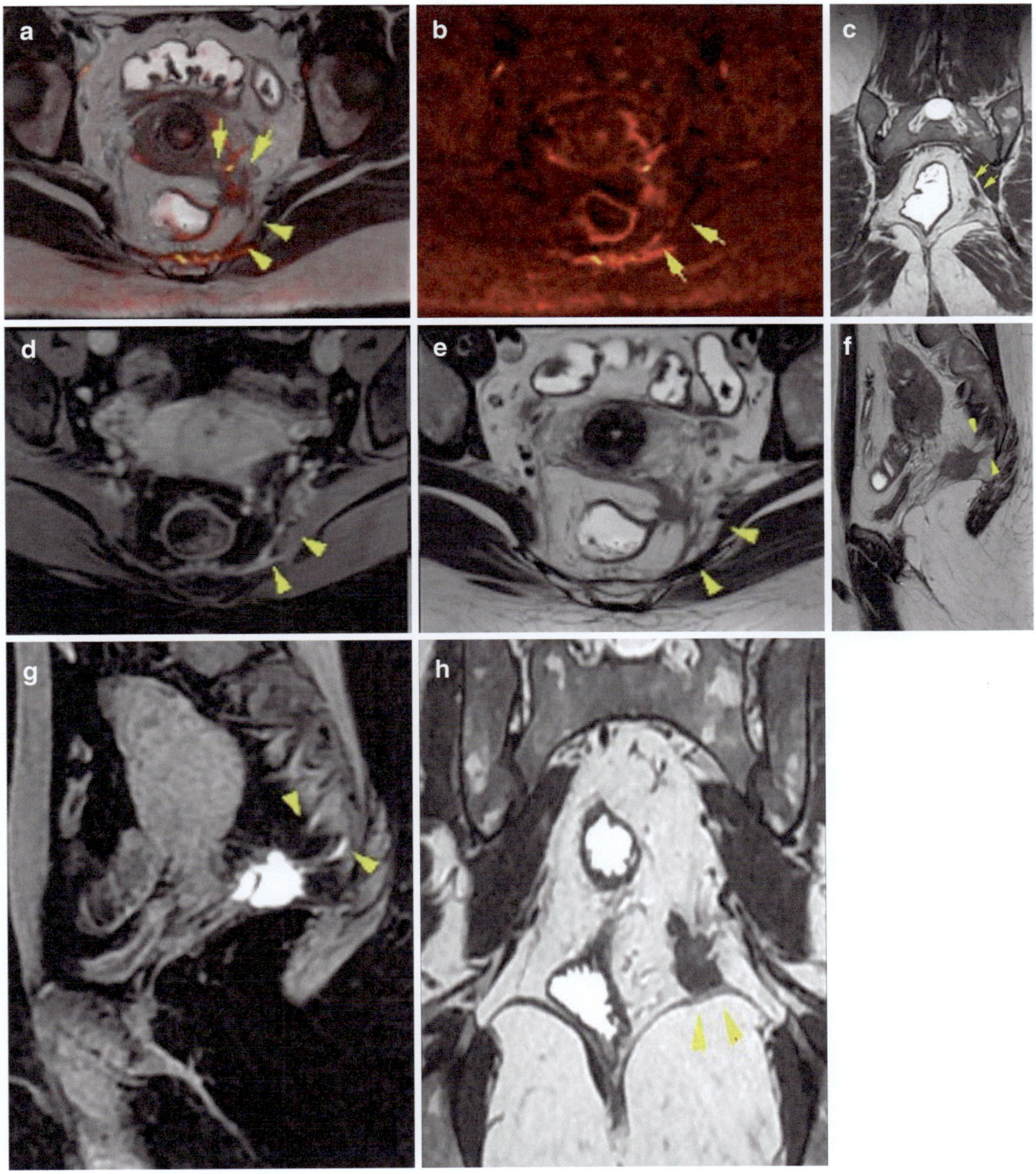

Fig. 11.22 Endometriosis in a 37-year-old woman with chronic pelvic pain, pain in the left gluteal region that radiates to the lower extremity, and bladder dysfunction. Pelvic MRI demonstrates a posterolateral DE nodule on the left (head arrows), involving the uterosacral ligament, mesorectum, lateral wall, and pelvic floor. It involves the hypogastric nerve and inferior hypogastric plexus laterally, goes beyond the mesorectal and hypogastric fascia, and extends to the inferior gluteal vessels and to the S3 and S4 roots in the lower third of the piriformis. These roots are thickened, with hematic foci, and have a hypersignal on T2 and enhancement, with an appearance similar to the rest of the endometriosis, suggestive of involvement and associated with signs of denervation in the levator muscle, which is characterized by muscle atrophy. Sciatic nerve with hypersignal, indicating edema, is also shown

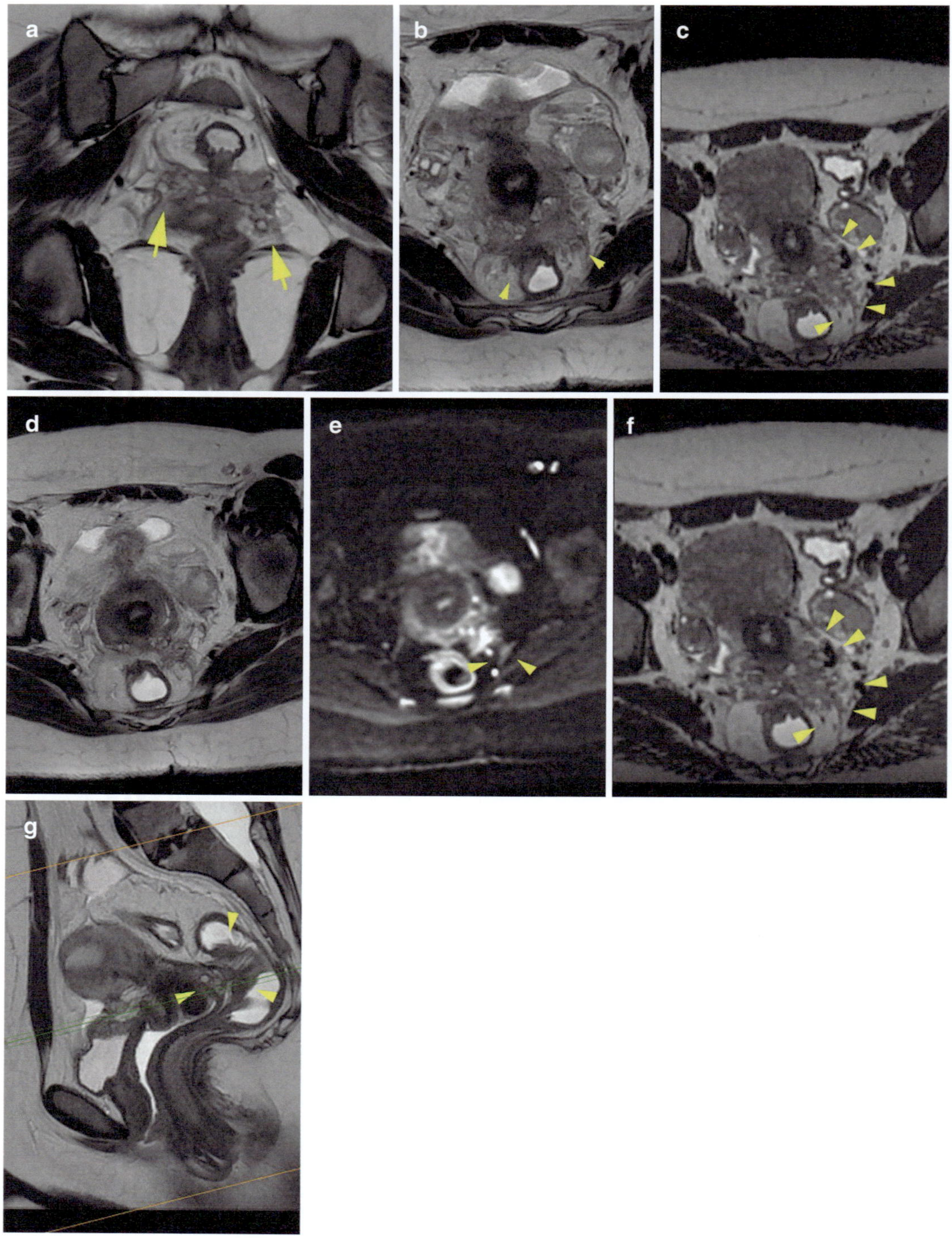

Fig. 11.23 Endometriosis in a 33-year-old woman with chronic pelvic pain that worsens during menstruation, pain in the anal area during menstruation, and dyschezia for 2 years. Along with dysuria, sensation of not emptying the bladder, and dyspareunia for 5 years. Pelvic MRI shows retrocervical endometriosis affecting the cervical insertion and the lateral portion of the uterosacral ligaments extending to the hypogastric/parietal fascia (head arrows in **a**, **b**, **c**, and **f**), close to sacral roots S3 and S4 (slightly thickened). Extension to the posterior parametrium and paracolpos, more evident on the left, is inseparable from the inferior hypogastric plexus, splanchnic nerves, and superficial uterine veins near the left pelvic floor, without evident muscular infiltration

11.6 Conclusion

Neural involvement in endometriosis represents a severe form of the disease, which is associated with incapacitating pain and with bladder, sexual, and intestinal dysfunction and which can lead to sequelae and central sensitization if left untreated. The key to obtaining an imaging diagnosis of neural endometriosis is the advanced knowledge of pelvic neuroanatomy. Despite being challenging, diagnosis is feasible in most cases and is crucial for appropriate treatment planning and patient counseling, impacting morbidity and avoiding sequelae. MRI is considered the imaging method of choice for evaluating neural endometriosis. Through a dedicated imaging protocol with high-resolution sequences, the main pelvic nerves involved in endometriosis can be identified. The most common imaging findings of somatic neural DE are solid spiculated nodules hypointense on T2WI, endometrioma-like cysts, and complex cystic masses. Visceral nervous DE has been observed mainly in cases featuring the lateral extension of retrocervical lesions in proximity to the hypogastric nerve and the inferior hypogastric plexus or posterolateral extension adjacent to the sacral roots.

References

1. Colak C, Chamie LP, Youngner J, Forney MC, Luna Russo MA, Gubbels A, et al. MRI features of pelvic nerve involvement in endometriosis. Radiographics. 2024;44(1):e230106.
2. Possover M. 22. Neuropelveology—the medicine of the pathologies of the pelvic nerves and plexuses. In: Saridoğan E, Kilic GS, Ertan K, editors. Minimally invasive surgery in gynecological practice [internet]. Berlin: De Gruyter; 2020. p. 247–54. https://doi.org/10.1515/9783110535204-022/html.
3. Brandão A. Atlas de endometriose profunda: correlação rm e laparoscopia. Rio de Janeiro: Revinter; 2014.
4. Ceccaroni M, Clarizia R, Alboni C, Ruffo G, Bruni F, Roviglione G, et al. Laparoscopic nerve-sparing transperitoneal approach for endometriosis infiltrating the pelvic wall and somatic nerves: anatomical considerations and surgical technique. Surg Radiol Anat. 2010;32(6):601–4.
5. Atlas de anatomia ginecológica laparoscópica. Não definido; 2019.
6. Wijsmuller AR, Giraudeau C, Leroy J, Kleinrensink GJ, Rociu E, Romagnolo LG, et al. A step towards stereotactic navigation during pelvic surgery: 3D nerve topography. Surg Endosc. 2018;32(8):3582–91.
7. Anaf V. Relationship between endometriotic foci and nerves in rectovaginal endometriotic nodules. Hum Reprod. 2000;15(8):1744–50.
8. Pham M, Sommer C, Wessig C, Monoranu CM, Pérez J, Stoll G, et al. Magnetic resonance neurography for the diagnosis of extrapelvic sciatic endometriosis. Fertil Steril. 2010;94(1):351.e11–4.
9. Moura Filho JP, Leão RV, Horvat N, Helito PVP, Amaral DT, Viana PCC, et al. What abdominal radiologists should know about extragenital endometriosis-associated neuropathy. Abdom Radiol. 2020;45(6):1818–28.
10. Niro J, Fournier M, Oberlin C, Le Tohic A, Panel P. Endometriotic lesions of the lower troncular nerves. Gynecol Obstet Fertil. 2014;42(10):702–5.
11. Diniz ALL, Resende JAD Jr, Andrade CMD Jr, Brandão AC, Gasparoni MP Jr, Favorito LA. Urological knowledge and tools applied to diagnosis and surgery in deep infiltrating endometriosis—a narrative review. Int Braz J Urol. 2023;49(5):564–79.
12. Possover M. Laparoscopic management of endopelvic etiologies of Pudendal pain in 134 consecutive patients. J Urol. 2009;181(4):1732–6.
13. Possover M, Schneider T, Henle KP. Laparoscopic therapy for endometriosis and vascular entrapment of sacral plexus. Fertil Steril. 2011;95(2):756–8.
14. Possover M. Laparoscopic management of neural pelvic pain in women secondary to pelvic surgery. Fertil Steril. 2009;91(6):2720–5.
15. Possover M, Rhiem K, Chiantera V. The "Laparoscopic Neuro-Navigation"—LANN: from a functional cartography of the pelvic autonomous neurosystem to a new field of laparoscopic surgery. Minim Invasive Ther Allied Technol. 2004;13(5–6):362–7.
16. Possover M, Baekelandt J, Kaufmann A, Chiantera V. Laparoscopic endopelvic sacral implantation of a Brindley controller for recovery of bladder function in a paralyzed patient. Spinal Cord. 2008;46(1):70–3.
17. Possover M. Five-year follow-up after laparoscopic large nerve resection for deep infiltrating sciatic nerve endometriosis. J Minim Invasive Gynecol. 2017;24(5):822–6.
18. Ceccaroni M, Clarizia R, Roviglione G, Ruffo G. Neuro-anatomy of the posterior parametrium and surgical considerations for a nerve-sparing approach in radical pelvic surgery. Surg Endosc. 2013;27(11):4386–94.
19. Possover M, Quakernack J, Chiantera V. The LANN technique to reduce postoperative functional morbidity in laparoscopic radical pelvic surgery. J Am Coll Surg. 2005;201(6):913–7.
20. Resende JAD Jr. DISFUNÇÕES do TRATO URINÁRIO inferior EM MULHERES com ENDOMETRIOSE PROFUNDA. 2016.

21. Waer P, Samson I, Sinnaeve F, Sciot R, Pans S. Perineural spread of endometriosis along the obturator nerve into the adductor thigh compartment. Jpn J Radiol. 2012;30(5):446–9.
22. Chamié LP, Ribeiro DMFR, Tiferes DA, Macedo Neto ACD, Serafini PC. Atypical sites of deeply infiltrative endometriosis: clinical characteristics and imaging findings. Radiographics. 2018;38(1):309–28.
23. Di Giovanni A, Casarella L, Coppola M, Falcone F, Iuzzolino D, Rasile M, et al. Ultrasound evaluation of retrocervical and parametrial deep endometriosis on the basis of surgical anatomic landmarks. J Minim Invasive Gynecol. 2022;29(10):1140–8.
24. Simon N, Kliot M. Diffusion weighted MRI and tractography for evaluating peripheral nerve degeneration and regeneration. Neural Regen Res. 2014;9(24):2122.
25. Brown G, Kirkham A, Williams GT, Bourne M, Radcliffe AG, Sayman J, et al. High-resolution MRI of the anatomy important in total mesorectal excision of the rectum. Am J Roentgenol. 2004;182(2):431–9.
26. De Paepe KN, Higgins DM, Ball I, Morgan VA, Barton DP, deSouza NM. Visualizing the autonomic and somatic innervation of the female pelvis with 3D MR neurography: a feasibility study. Acta Radiol. 2020;61(12):1668–76.
27. Brandão AC, Lehman CD, Partridge SC. Breast magnetic resonance imaging. Magn Reson Imaging Clin N Am. 2013;21(2):321–36.
28. Brandão AC, Silva AO. Diseases of the female pelvis. Magn Reson Imaging Clin N Am. 2013;21(2):447–69.
29. Ercoli A, Delmas V, Fanfani F, Gadonneix P, Ceccaroni M, Fagotti A, et al. Terminologia Anatomica versus unofficial descriptions and nomenclature of the fasciae and ligaments of the female pelvis: a dissection-based comparative study. Am J Obstet Gynecol. 2005;193(4):1565–73.
30. Yekeler E, Kumbasar B, Tunaci A, Barman A, Bengisu E, Yavuz E, et al. Cyclic sciatica caused by infiltrative endometriosis: MRI findings. Skeletal Radiol. 2004;33(3):165–8.
31. Possover M, Chiantera V. Isolated infiltrative endometriosis of the sciatic nerve: a report of three patients. Fertil Steril. 2007;87(2):417.e17–9.
32. Ekpo G, Senapati S, Advincula AP. Laparoscopic excision of endometriosis of the obturator nerve: a case report. J Minim Invasive Gynecol. 2007;14(6):764–6.
33. Possover M, Baekelandt J, Flaskamp C, Li D, Chiantera V. Laparoscopic neurolysis of the sacral plexus and the sciatic nerve for extensive endometriosis of the pelvic wall. Minim Invasive Neurosurg. 2007;50(1):33–6.
34. Kinugasa Y, Murakami G, Suzuki D, Sugihara K. Histological identification of fascial structures posterolateral to the rectum. Br J Surg. 2007;94(5):620–6.

12 Thoracic and Diaphragmatic Endometriosis

Aki Kido, Yuki Himoto, Toshihiro Ojima, and Tomoshi Tsuchiya

12.1 Introduction

Thoracic and diaphragmatic endometriosis are two of the most common sites of extrapelvic endometriosis, as are the abdominal wall and nerve, [1, 2]. The term *thoracic endometriosis* refers to the presence of endometriotic implants within the thoracic cavity: The lesions are on the diaphragmatic, parietal, and visceral pleura and within the lung parenchyma [3]. On the other hand, the term *diaphragmatic endometriosis* is used when endometriotic implants are encountered on the abdominal side (peritoneal surface) of the diaphragm [4].

The pathogenesis of endometriosis in this area is still discussed and debated. Because no theory has succeeded at comprehensively explaining all the clinical manifestations associated with the syndrome, the etiology is likely multifactorial [3]. The theories include the following: (a) The retrograde menstruation theory, which is also known as Sampson's theory, is largely accepted. Some of the menstrual blood flows backward thorough the fallopian tubes into the pelvic cavity. Then, the peritoneal fluid containing endometrial cells circulates within the peritoneal cavity from the pelvis through the right paracolic gutter toward the right hemidiaphragm. Right-side preference is due to the obstruction of flow by the falciform and phrenicocolic ligaments [5]. (b) The coelomic metaplasia theory is also thought to be a main etiology of the disease. Endometriosis arises via the metaplasia of mesothelial cells lining the pleural and peritoneal surfaces into the endometrial glands and stroma [6]. (c) The lymphatic and hematogenous dissemination theory, which may explain why bronchopulmonary endometrial lesions can occur on both sides. (d) On catamenial pneumothorax, the prostaglandin theory suggests that the rising levels of circulating prostaglandin F2α during menstruation might cause the constriction of bronchioles and blood vessels, which can lead to the rupture of alveoli within pre-existing subpleural blebs and bullae and ultimately to catamenial pneumothorax [3]. These locations are more frequently present on the right side than on the left side due to the peritoneal fluid movement. These locations justify to add a coronal and Sagittal T1W FS sequence in the MR protocol centered on the abdomen each time any symptom may suggest diaphragmatic locations. Some teams add systematically a fast

A. Kido (✉)
Department of Radiology, University of Toyama, Toyama, Japan

Y. Himoto
Department of Diagnostic Radiology and Nuclear Medicine, Kyoto University, Kyoto, Japan
e-mail: yhimoto@kuhp.kyoto-u.ac.jp

T. Ojima · T. Tsuchiya
Department of Thoracic Surgery, University of Toyama, Toyama, Japan
e-mail: ojitoshi@med.u-toyama.ac.jp; tsuchiya@med.u-toyama.ac.jp

I. Thomassin-Naggara (ed.), *Imaging of Endometriosis: A Comparative Guide of US, MRI and Surgery*, https://doi.org/10.1007/978-3-031-82750-1_12

coronalT1W Sequence with FS to screen these locations in any MR protocol to diagnose endometriosis. The description of these locations on the diaphragm is crucial before surgery, especially when hemorragic implants are located medially and posteriorly, as these locations are frequently missed at laparoscopy.

12.2 Thoracic Endometriosis and Thoracic Endometriosis Syndrome

Thoracic endometriosis includes endometrial implants in various thoracic locations, such as the airways, pleura, pericardium, and lung parenchyma, resulting in a variety of clinical and radiological manifestations collectively known as thoracic endometriosis syndrome (TES) [7]. TES encompasses four clinical entities: catamenial pneumothorax (CP) (80%), catamenial hemothorax (14%), catamenial hemoptysis (5%), and pulmonary nodules [3, 8]. The word *catamenial* is used to describe a clinical presentation that occurs in proximity to the menstrual period, typically spanning a duration of 24 h before and 72 h after the start of menstruation [9].

Thoracic endometriosis can be classified into two types: pleural and parenchymal [10]. As for pleural endometriosis, catamenial pneumothorax, or hemothorax, which affects predominantly the right side (in over 90% of cases), are the primary manifestations, typically presenting with symptoms of chest pain and dyspnea. Although rare, from the perspective of diagnostic medicine, catamenial pneumothorax must be considered as a differential diagnosis in premenopausal women with pneumothorax, especially if it occurs on the right side. In contrast, parenchymal endometriosis typically exhibits hemoptysis. Clinical complications commonly arise within 72 h of the onset of menstruation and tend to recur periodically [10]. Video-assisted thoracoscopic surgery (VATS) is considered the gold standard for the diagnosis and treatment of thoracic endometriosis. Computed tomography (CT) scans face challenges in detecting lesions, particularly smaller ones [11]. Endometrial glands are often not identified by hematoxylin–eosin (H&E) staining, so immunostaining is important.

12.2.1 Surgical Procedures

The gold standard for a definitive diagnosis of thoracic endometriosis is VATS [3]. Among patients with catamenial hemothorax, the main intraoperative findings were diaphragmatic lesions (38.8%); endometriosis of the visceral pleura (29.6%); discrete lesions, such as bullae, blebs, or scarring (23.1%); and no findings (8.5%) [12]. In VATS, diaphragmatic lesions manifest as red lesions, often co-occurring with numerous diaphragmatic apertures, fenestrations, perforations, and pores of varying dimensions, predominantly situated at the central tendon (Fig. 12.1) [13]. In those with diaphragmatic lesions, diaphragmatic perforation has been observed in 69% [12].

12.2.2 Treatment

As with pelvic endometriosis, hormonal therapy using antigonadotropic agents can help reduce endometriotic tissue. A high recurrence rate is known solely with hormonal therapy [14]. Therefore, surgical treatment can be combined with hormonal therapy, especially when considering the systemic nature of the disease [12, 14]. On the other hand, Korom et al. indicated that all surgical treatment options should be exhausted before considering hormonal treatment [12]. The surgery is generally performed in conjunction with the menstrual cycle, to facilitate the detection of blueberry spots representing endometriotic tissue [15]. When hormonal therapy precedes, the recognition of lesions can become more challenging. In the treatment using the VATS procedure, superficial endometriotic implants can be fulgurated by using bipolar diathermy, a CO_2 laser, an argon laser, or plasma energy, whereas deeper endometriotic implants should be excised via sharp dissection [3]. Diaphragmatic lesions or perforations are resected by using the endoscopic stapler device in cases where the resected surface is ultimately relatively small [3]. The use of syn-

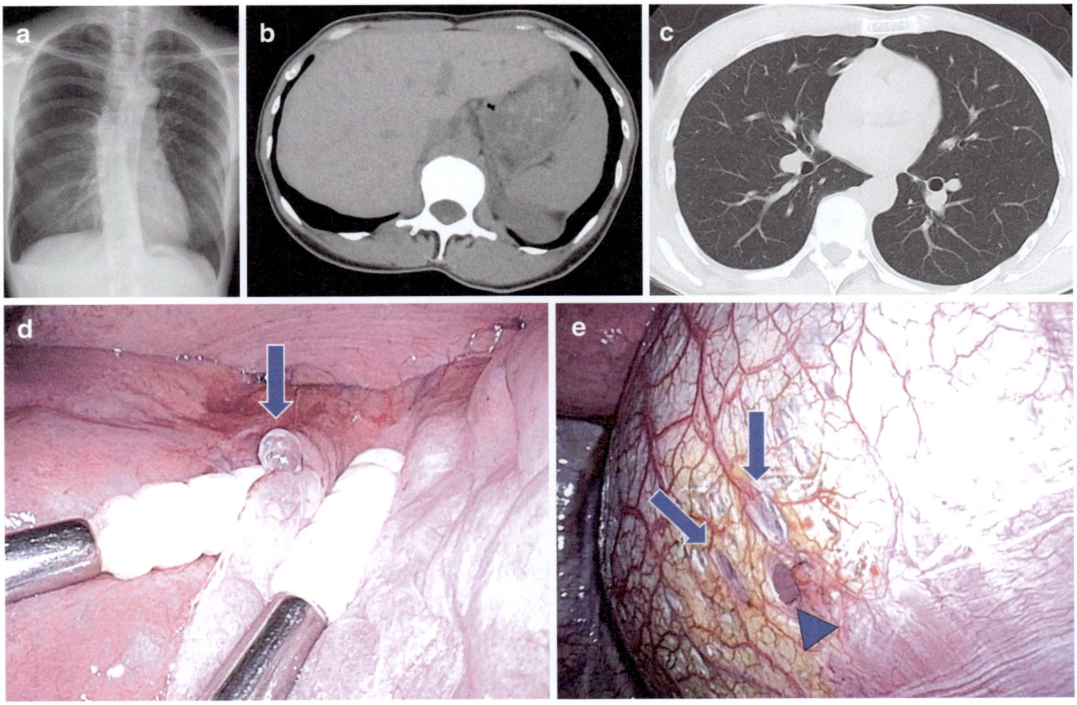

Fig. 12.1 A 47-year-old woman with repeated right chest pain since she was 30 years old. Sudden, severe chest pain occurred, and the patient arrived at the hospital. Chest X-ray showed right pneumothorax (**a**). Unenhanced CT could not detect any other abnormal findings before (**b**) or after drainage (**c**). VATS was performed, which revealed a small bulla in the right middle lobe (**d**, arrow) and several holes on the right diaphragm at the boundary between the central tendon and the muscular area (**e**, arrow and arrowhead). The surface of the liver was recognized from the hole (**e**, arrowhead). As a treatment, several endometriotic spots were resected and covered with polyglycolic acid sheets

thetic mesh is recommended to close larger diaphragmatic defects [16]. In cases with parenchymal endometriotic nodules or larger lesions, wedge resection with a stapling device or subsegmentectomy is considered [3]. Pleurodesis after VATS has been shown to decrease the recurrence of pneumothorax by 20–25% compared with those without pleurodesis [17].

12.2.3 Radiologic Findings

Pleural lesions are difficult to detect on CT imaging and magnetic resonance imaging (MRI), because if the lesions are tiny, then the report is very limited. The reported image finding of a pleural lesion is the same as that of a diaphragmatic lesion, as mentioned below, which is high signal intensity on fat-suppressed T1-weighted imaging (T1WI) [18, 19]. Pulmonary parenchymal endometriosis shows (cavitary) nodules, bullous changes, ground-glass opacities, consolidations, and linear opacities [20]. Those findings pathologically correspond to various stages of pulmonary hemorrhage. [20]. Another important role of CT in pneumothorax is to find other causes, including bulla, lymphangioleiomyomatosis (LAM), or Birt–Hogg–Dubé syndrome. LAM also affects young women (around 34 years old) and commonly manifests as exertional dyspnea and recurrent pneumothorax [21]. A differential diagnosis can be made via CT, which shows diffusely distributed thin-walled lung cysts [21]. Birt–Hogg–Dubé syndrome is a rare disease with multiple fibrofolliculomas as skin lesions observed in young women. It accompanies bullous emphysema, thin-walled cysts (80%), and pneumothorax [22].

12.3 Diaphragmatic Endometriosis

Diaphragmatic endometriosis is often found on the right side: 92.3% of the deep endometriosis (DE) patients in the report by Pagao F. et al. [23]. This tendency can be explained by the retrograde menstruation theory and the obstruction of the flow of peritoneal fluid by the falciform and phrenicocolic ligaments [5]. Cyclic right shoulder pain is often found in diaphragmatic endometriosis patients, in addition to dysmenorrhea and cyclic apnea. Also, diaphragmatic endometriosis has been associated with severe endometriosis—that is, rAFS III° or IV° in 78.4% of patients—and has resulted in a higher rate of infertility than those without diaphragmatic endometriosis [23].

12.3.1 Surgical Procedure

A routine evaluation of the abdominal side of the diaphragm is recommended in all patients undergoing laparoscopy for suspected pelvic endometriosis. Because the posterior right hemidiaphragm is the most common site for diaphragmatic endometrial implants, the optimal visualization of the diaphragm is achieved by positioning the patient in a steep reverse Trendelenburg position while gently pushing the liver caudally [3]. The laparoscopic findings of endometriotic implants are the same as those of the thoracic cavity, including being black, blue, or reddish-purple in appearance and sometimes accompanying liver adhesions [3]. In some cases, cutting the falciform ligament is required to carry out a complete evaluation of the right hemidiaphragm.

12.3.2 Treatment

The recommended therapeutic approach for lesions on the abdominal side of the diaphragm involves hydrodissection followed by excision, whereas superficial lesions may be treated with CO_2 laser vaporization [3]. Diaphragm lesions are resected from the thoracic side because obtaining a clear visual field from the abdominal side is difficult.

12.3.3 Radiological Findings

Because these lesions are tiny punctate foci, they is not easy to recognize on CT or magnetic resonance (MR) imaging. On MR imaging, they can be found as hyperintense nodules or plaques on T1-weighted images (Figs. 12.2 and 12.3) [24]. Rousset et al. evaluated the MR imaging findings of 23 surgically confirmed diaphragmatic endometriosis patients [25]. MRI showed a sensitivity of 78–83% at the patient level. At the lesion level, all the lesions were right sided, 72% were depicted as nodules, and 87.5% were located posteriorly to the vena cava [25]. In some patients, the differential diagnosis may be tricky with diaphragmatic hernia as some severe locations do a hole in the diaphragm that have to be measured before surgery (Fig. 12.4).

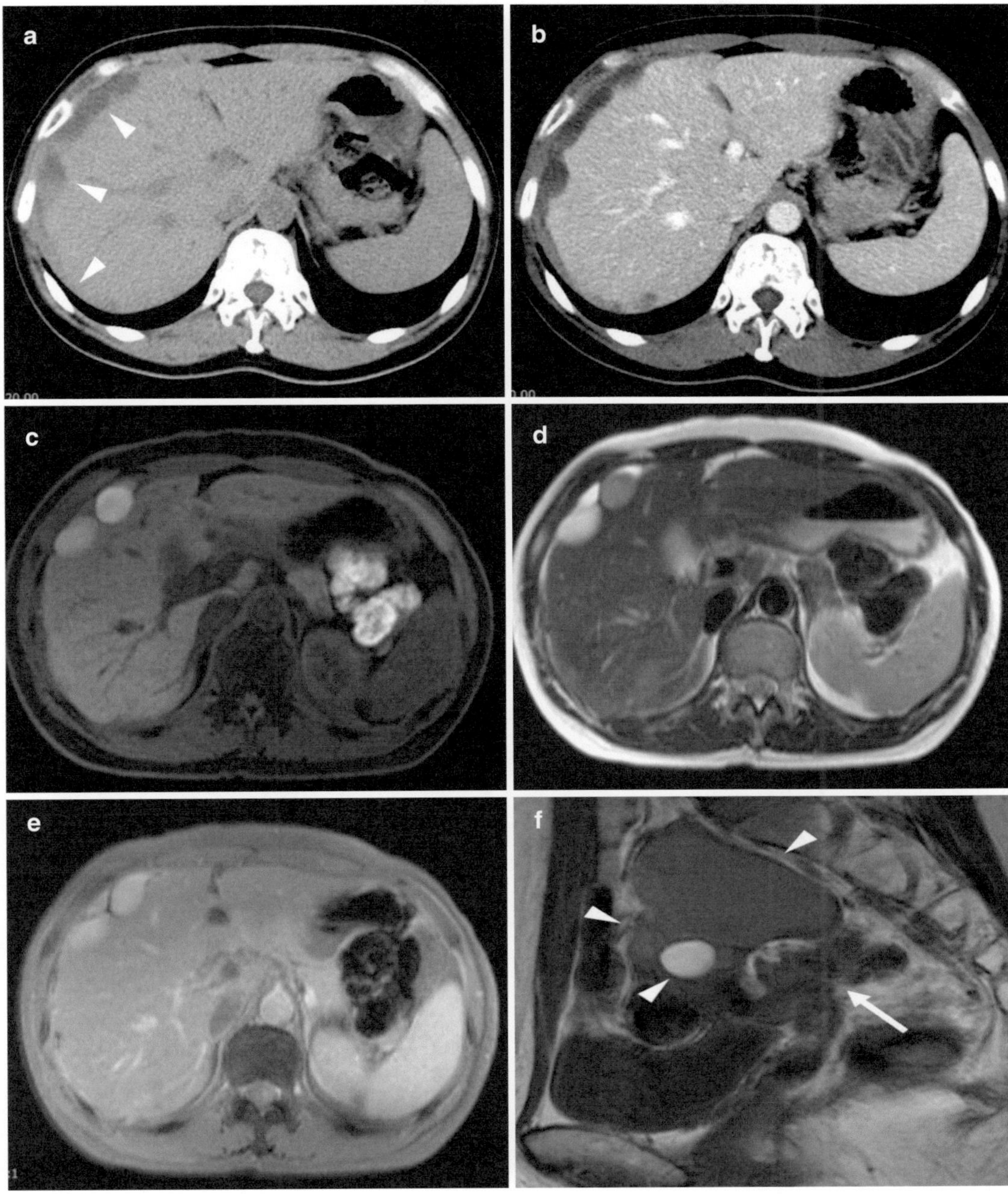

Fig. 12.2 A 44-year-old woman, after hysterectomy due to uterine fibroids. She had been experiencing periodic hypochondrial pain once a month for 2 years. Unenhanced CT (**a**) showed subdiaphragmatic lesions with fluid-fluid level (**a**, arrowheads) compressing the surface of the liver. The moderately high attenuation level was suspected to represent hemorrhage. Contrast-enhanced CT (**b**) depicted no enhanced parts within them. On unenhanced abdominal MRI, perihepatic lesions showed high signal intensity on fat-saturated T1-weighted images (**c**) and high signal intensity with shading on T2-weighted images (**d**, arrow), indicating hemorrhagic lesions. No enhanced parts appeared on contrast-enhanced T1-weighted images (**e**). Pelvic MRI (**f**, T1-weighted images; **g**, T2-weighted images) showed endometriotic cysts (arrowheads) accompanying strong adhesion among the endometriotic cysts, rectum, and vaginal stump (arrow). (**h**) After 3 months of hormonal therapy, multiple perihepatic lesions became unrecognizable on abdominal MRI (**h**, fat-saturated T1-weighted images)

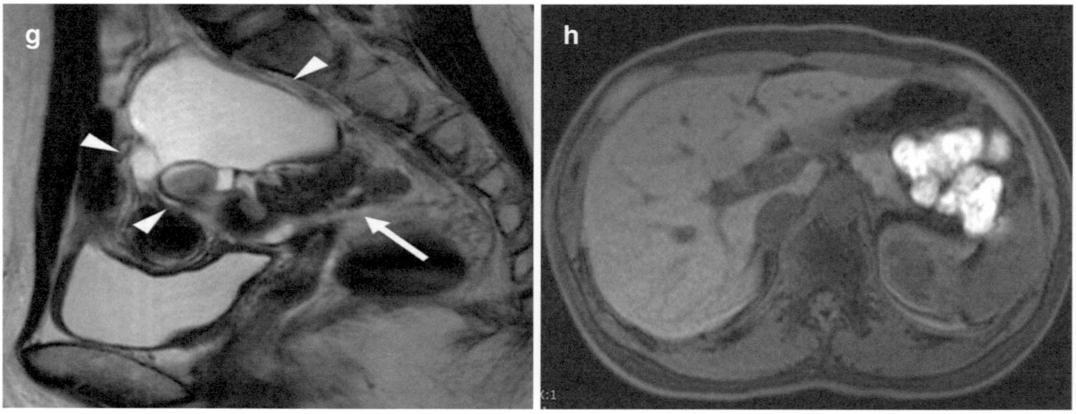

Fig. 12.2 (continued)

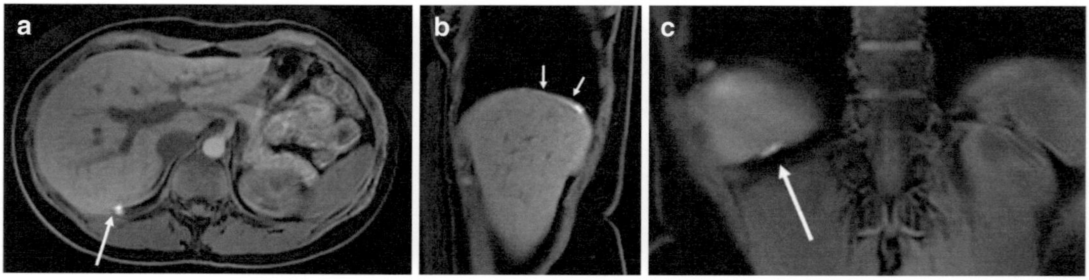

Fig. 12.3 A 37-year-old nulligravida woman, referred for the suspicion of recurrent endometriosis presenting with right hypochondrial pain associated with menstrual cycles. She had a history of pelvic endometriosis and resected torus, uterosacral ligaments, and vesicouterine cul-de-sac and the discoid resection of the rectum 10 years earlier. After that, she received a left salpingectomy for hydrosalpinx and a new digestive resection. On abdominal MRI performed on day 21 of the menstrual cycle, fat-saturated T1-weighted images (**a**, axial; **b**, sagittal; and **c**, coronal) showed multiple high-signal-intensity nodules and plaques located on the right posterior diaphragm (arrows), which indicate endometriotic lesions (Courtesy Isabelle Thomassin Nagggara)

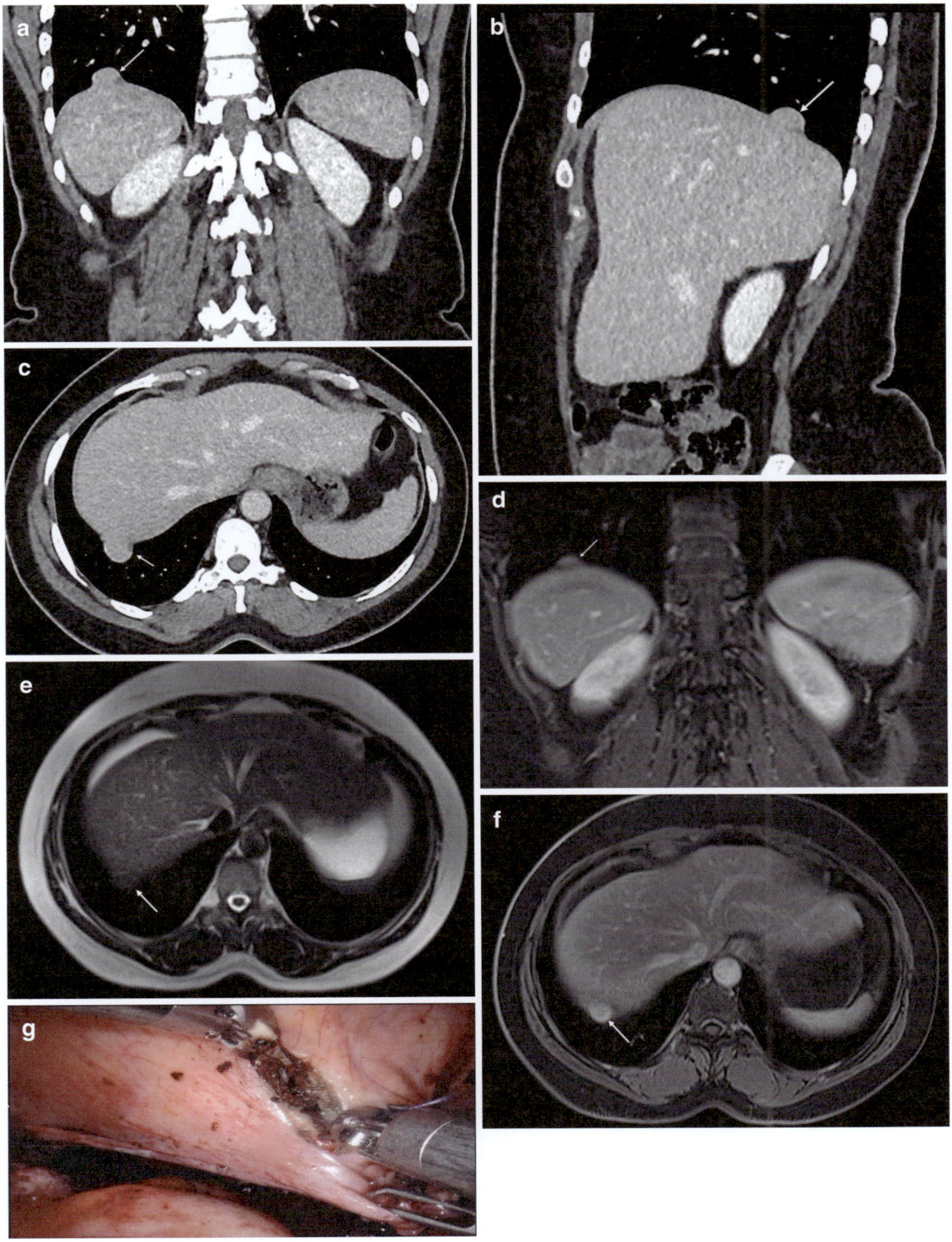

Fig. 12.4 A 49 year old women, referred in a context for severe endometriosis (mulitple digestive nodules and parametrial infiltration with ureter involvement) presenting with right hypochondrial pain associated menstrual cycles. A CT scan showed a diaphragmatic hernia (arrow) in coronal plane (**a**), sagital plan (**b**) and axial plane (**c**) located on the right diaphragm. A dedicated MRI showed that this lesion was not a hernia but a diaphragmatic nodule of endometriosis (arrow) in highT1W signal (**d** and **f**) and intermediate T2W signal (**e**). The surgery confirms this hypothesis of endometriotic location with a hole between thoracic and abdomnal cavities that was accessble and repared by the surgeon (courtesy Isabelle Thomassin Naggara and Cyril Touboul)

References

1. Andres MP, Arcoverde FVL, Souza CCC, Fernandes LFC, Abrao MS, Kho RM. Extrapelvic endometriosis: a systematic review. J Minim Invasive Gynecol. 2020;27:373–89.
2. Keckstein J, Saridogan E, Ulrich UA, Sillem M, Oppelt P, Schweppe KW, Krentel H, Janschek E, Exacoustos C, Malzoni M, Mueller M, Roman H, Condous G, Forman A, Jansen FW, Bokor A, Simedrea V, Hudelist G. The #Enzian classification: a comprehensive non-invasive and surgical description system for endometriosis. Acta Obstet Gynecol Scand. 2021;100:1165–75.
3. Nezhat C, Lindheim SR, Backhus L, Vu M, Vang N, Nezhat A, Nezhat C. Thoracic endometriosis syndrome: a review of diagnosis and management. JSLS. 2019;23:e2019.00029.
4. Vigueras Smith A, Cabrera R, Kondo W, Ferreira H. Diaphragmatic endometriosis minimally invasive treatment: a feasible and effective approach. J Obstet Gynaecol. 2021;41:176–86.
5. Vercellini P, Abbiati A, Vigano P, Somigliana ED, Daguati R, Meroni F, Crosignani PG. Asymmetry in distribution of diaphragmatic endometriotic lesions: evidence in favour of the menstrual reflux theory. Hum Reprod. 2007;22:2359–67.
6. Kovarik JL, Toll GD. Thoracic endometriosis with recurrent spontaneous pneumothorax. JAMA. 1966;196:595–7.
7. Hwang SM, Lee CW, Lee BS, Park JH. Clinical features of thoracic endometriosis: a single center analysis. Obstet Gynecol Sci. 2015;58:223–31.
8. Joseph J, Sahn SA. Thoracic endometriosis syndrome: new observations from an analysis of 110 cases. Am J Med. 1996;100:164–70.
9. Bobbio A, Canny E, Mansuet Lupo A, Lococo F, Legras A, Magdeleinat P, Regnard JF, Gompel A, Damotte D, Alifano M. Thoracic endometriosis syndrome other than pneumothorax: clinical and pathological findings. Ann Thorac Surg. 2017; 104:1865–71.
10. Honore GM. Extrapelvic endometriosis. Clin Obstet Gynecol. 1999;42:699–711.
11. Hirata T, Koga K, Osuga Y. Extra-pelvic endometriosis: a review. Reprod Med Biol. 2020;19:323–33.
12. Korom S, Canyurt H, Missbach A, Schneiter D, Kurrer MO, Haller U, Keller PJ, Furrer M, Weder W. Catamenial pneumothorax revisited: clinical approach and systematic review of the literature. J Thorac Cardiovasc Surg. 2004;128:502–8.
13. Chamie LP, Blasbalg R, Pereira RM, Warmbrand G, Serafini PC. Findings of pelvic endometriosis at transvaginal US, MR imaging, and laparoscopy. Radiographics. 2011;31:E77–100.
14. Velagapudi RK, Egan JP III. Thoracic endometriosis: a clinical review and update of current and evolving diagnostic and therapeutic techniques. Curr Pulmonol Rep. 2021;10:22–9.
15. Kuo PH, Wang HC, Liaw YS, Kuo SH. Bronchoscopic and angiographic findings in tracheobronchial endometriosis. Thorax. 1996;51:1060–1.
16. Sakamoto K, Ohmori T, Takei H. Catamenial pneumothorax caused by endometriosis in the visceral pleura. Ann Thorac Surg. 2003;76:290–1.
17. Light RW, O'Hara VS, Moritz TE, McElhinney AJ, Butz R, Haakenson CM, Read RC, Sassoon CS, Eastridge CE, Berger R, et al. Intrapleural tetracycline for the prevention of recurrent spontaneous pneumothorax. Results of a Department of Veterans Affairs Cooperative Study. JAMA. 1990;264:2224–30.
18. Marchiori E, Zanetti G, Rodrigues RS, Souza LS, Souza Junior AS, Francisco FA, Hochhegger B. Pleural endometriosis: findings on magnetic resonance imaging. J Bras Pneumol. 2012;38:797–802.
19. Rangunwala J, Sitta J, Vyas K, Roda M. Multimodality thoracoabdominal imaging findings in a rare case of thoracic endometriosis syndrome. Cureus. 2020;12:e6819.
20. Lee YR, Choi YW, Jeon SC, Paik SS, Kang JH. On the AJR viewbox. Pleuropulmonary endometriosis: CT-pathologic correlation. AJR Am J Roentgenol. 2006;186:1800–1.
21. Pallisa E, Sanz P, Roman A, Majo J, Andreu J, Caceres J. Lymphangioleiomyomatosis: pulmonary and abdominal findings with pathologic correlation. Radiographics. 2002;22:S185–98.
22. Seaman DM, Meyer CA, Gilman MD, McCormack FX. Diffuse cystic lung disease at high-resolution CT. AJR Am J Roentgenol. 2011;196:1305–11.
23. Pagano F, Schwander A, Vaineau C, Knabben L, Nirgianakis K, Imboden S, Mueller MD. True prevalence of diaphragmatic endometriosis and its association with severe endometriosis: a call for awareness and investigation. J Minim Invasive Gynecol. 2023;30:329–34.
24. Naem A, Andrikos A, Constantin AS, Khamou M, Andrikos D, Lagana AS, De Wilde RL, Krentel H. Diaphragmatic endometriosis—a single-center retrospective analysis of the patients' demographics, symptomatology, and long-term treatment outcomes. J Clin Med. 2023;12:6455.
25. Rousset P, Gregory J, Rousset-Jablonski C, Hugon-Rodin J, Regnard JF, Chapron C, Coste J, Golfier F, Revel MP. MR diagnosis of diaphragmatic endometriosis. Eur Radiol. 2016;26:3968–77.

Extrapelvic Location: Abdominal Wall Endometriosis. Diagnostic and Interventional Imaging

13

Léo Razakamanantsoa and Milan Najdawi

Abbreviations

AWE Abdominal wall endometriosis
CA Cryoablation
CNB Core needle biopsy
CO_2 Carbon dioxide
CT Computed tomography
DWI Diffusion-weighted imaging
FNA Fine-needle aspiration
GA General anesthesia
HIFU High-intensity focused ultrasound
IR Interventional radiology
MRI Magnetic resonance imaging
MW Microwave
NSAIDs Nonsteroidal anti-inflammatory drugs
RFA Radiofrequency
SUV Standard uptake value
US Ultrasound

L. Razakamanantsoa (✉)
Department of Specialized Radiology and Interventional Imaging, Tenon Hospital, Sorbonne University, Paris, France

Saint-Antoine Research Center (CRSA), INSERM, CNRS, Sorbonne University, Paris, France
e-mail: leo.razakamanantsoa@aphp.fr

M. Najdawi
Department of Specialized Radiology and Interventional Imaging, Tenon Hospital, Sorbonne University, Paris, France
e-mail: milan.najdawi@aphp.fr

Key Points

- AWE represents a unique and infrequent manifestation of endometriosis, occurring in 0.03% to 3% of individuals. This condition develops predominantly on surgical scars or, less commonly, arises spontaneously without any history of surgical procedures.
- The primary clinical feature of AWE is catamenial pain, which significantly impairs patients' quality of life.
- The diagnostic evaluation of AWE extensively relies on the use of ultrasound (US) and magnetic resonance imaging (MRI) enhanced with gadolinium contrast. These imaging modalities are crucial for determining the extent of the disease and for the strategic planning of surgical or interventional treatments.
- The initial approach to management typically involves surgical intervention and hormonal therapies aimed at symptom relief. However, these treatments have a variable recurrence rate of 5% to 40% over extended periods of observation.
- Emerging percutaneous minimally invasive treatments, such as cryoablation, show promise thanks to their safety and effectiveness. Nevertheless, the potential of cryoablation as a leading treatment option necessitates further validation through studies with larger participant groups and prolonged follow-up durations.

I. Thomassin-Naggara (ed.), *Imaging of Endometriosis: A Comparative Guide of US, MRI and Surgery*, https://doi.org/10.1007/978-3-031-82750-1_13

13.1 Introduction

Abdominal wall endometriosis (AWE), while uncommon, represents a distinct entity wherein endometrial-like tissue infiltrates the layers of the abdominal wall. This tissue retains its responsiveness to hormonal fluctuations, leading to a cyclical pattern of symptom exacerbation, often coinciding with the menstrual cycle [1]. Although the incidence of AWE is reported to be between 0.03% and 3.5%, typically manifesting within cesarean delivery scars, but not exclusively, the condition is believed to be significantly underrecognized [2]. This chapter provides an in-depth exploration of AWE, beginning with an overview of the abdominal wall's anatomy, delving into the underlying pathophysiology and clinical presentation, examining diagnostic strategies, reviewing conventional management strategies, and contemplating future trajectories in treatment and understanding.

13.2 Anatomy, Pathophysiology, and Clinical Presentation

13.2.1 Abdominal Wall Anatomy and Physiology

The abdominal wall is a complex structure made up of layers of muscles, connective tissues, and fasciae that enclose the abdominal cavity. This structure is demarcated superiorly by the xiphoid process and the costal margins, inferiorly by the pelvic bones—specifically the iliac crests and the pubic symphysis—and laterally by the vertebral column at the lumbar region [3]. Comprising distinct layers, the abdominal wall is a complex structure featuring the skin, subcutaneous fat, superficial and deep fasciae, and a trio of muscles—the external oblique, internal oblique, and transversus abdominis—followed by the transversalis fascia, preperitoneal fat, and finally the peritoneum (Fig. 13.1). Embedded within these layers are essential neurovascular components, including nerves, arteries, veins, and lymphatic vessels [4]. The abdominal muscles play critical roles in supporting the growth and enclosure of abdominal viscera, safeguarding internal organs, enabling trunk movements, and maintaining pressure within the abdominal and thoracic cavities [5].

13.2.2 Definition of Abdominal Wall Endometriosis

Endometriosis, characterized as a chronic neuro-inflammatory disorder, impacts an estimated 6–10% of women in their reproductive years. This condition is typified by the presence of endometrial-like tissue aberrantly located outside the uterine cavity [6]. The predominant manifestations of endometriosis are categorized into three main pelvic types: the superficial peritoneal, the ovarian (known as endometrioma), and the deep infiltrating forms of the disease. Yet the condition can also extend beyond the pelvic domain to involve the upper abdominal visceral structures, the diaphragm, the pleural surfaces, and even the central and peripheral nervous systems, with abdominal wall layers recognized as notable sites of disease [7]. AWE most frequently presents in the context of cesarean section scars, but not exclusively, around the umbilicus or within Nuck's canal [8–10] (Fig. 13.2). The pathology of AWE is such that it may pervade every stratum of the abdominal wall, ranging from superficial subcutaneous layers to the deep peritoneum, and may even encroach upon the visceral organs.

13.2.2.1 Etiology of Abdominal Wall Endometriosis

The etiology of AWE is generally considered to originate from the inadvertent transplantation of endometrial cells onto the abdominal fascia or subcutaneous tissue during surgeries—a process that is known as iatrogenic implantation and that leads to the occurrence of scar endometriosis in a time frame reported from 6 months up to 10 years [11]. These cells, under the influence of estrogen, become active and proliferate [12]. Nevertheless, the occurrences of spontaneous endometriosis in sites such as the umbilicus or Nuck's canal have given rise to an alternative theory suggesting the

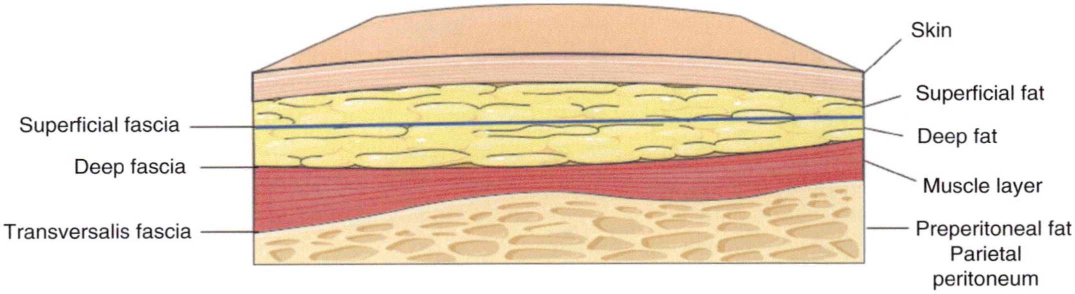

Fig. 13.1 Simplified drawing showing the different layers of the anterior abdominal wall

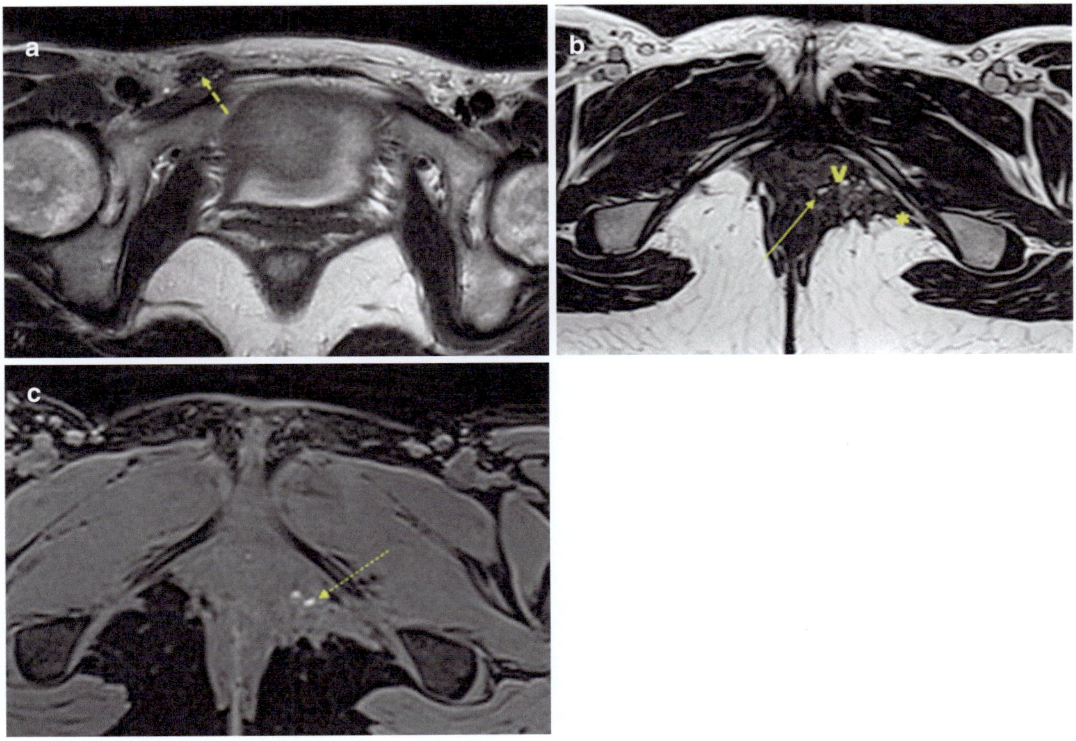

Fig. 13.2 (**a**) Axial T2-weighted MRI depicting a nodule (indicated by a yellow arrow), characterized by slight spiculation and a fibrous hypointense T2 signal interspersed with hyperintense T2 microcysts. Such features are indicative of endometriosis in Nuck's canal. This type of lesion is uncommon and can develop spontaneously without any previous surgical intervention, commonly presenting on the right side along the path of the round ligament. (**b**, **c**) Magnetic resonance imaging of pelvic endometriosis compromising the left ischiorectal fossa adjacent to the episiotomy scar. Within this T2-weighted imaging sequence (**b**), the lesion manifests as spiculated infiltration disrupting the adipose tissue of the left ischiorectal fossa, characterized by T2 hypointensity and the presence of microcysts (indicated by a solid arrow). The pathology extends into the left internal obturator muscle (highlighted by a star), particularly affecting Alcock's canal, and results in left-sided pudendal pain. The spread of the condition has been observed as nearing the vaginal wall (denoted as "v"). On the T1-weighted unenhanced imaging (**c**), hemorrhagic lesions are visible as areas of spontaneous T1 hyperintensity (marked with a dashed arrow), a hallmark feature of endometriotic invasion

migration of endometrial cells via the lymphatic route or along embryonic remnants within the umbilical fold, like the urachus and umbilical vessels [13]. The hypothesis of coelomic metaplasia has also been posited, wherein cells of similar embryonic origin to that of endometrial cells undergo transformation into endometrial-like tissue under certain unknown conditions, leading to endometriosis. Contributing factors may also include anomalies in immune response, the involvement of stem cells, and epigenetic modifications, all potentially playing a role in the pathogenesis of AWE [14].

13.2.2.2 Clinical Aspects of AWE

Typically, endometriosis is marked by cyclical pain that intensifies during the menstrual period, where this symptom predominantly manifests at the site of abdominal wall involvement [15]. Additional clinical manifestations may include changes in the skin such as hyperpigmentation or discoloration of scars, ecchymosis, spontaneous bleeding, or scar retraction (Fig. 13.3). A palpable mass correlating with the area of greatest discomfort is a common finding in the majority of patients [16]. Neurological symptoms are also notable features, where nerve irritation or entrapment leads to a host of sensations, such as spontaneous pain, a burning or stabbing feeling (akin to electric shocks), or tingling. These symptoms often stem from the involvement of the iliohypogastric, ilioinguinal, or genitofemoral nerves, reflecting the anatomical distribution of AWE.

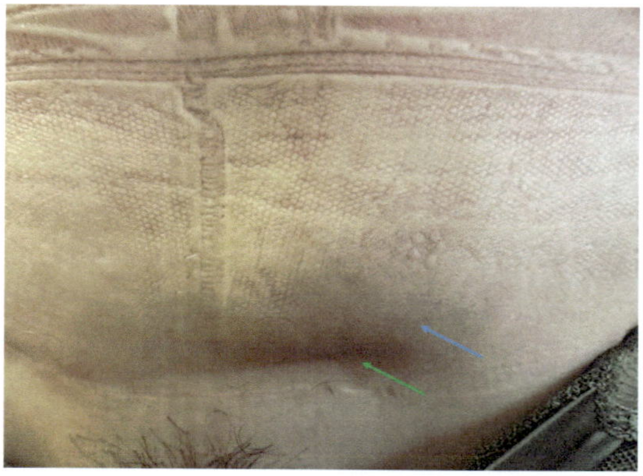

Fig. 13.3 Clinical presentation of a parietal endometriosis nodule. A 34-year-old female patient exhibits a painful palpable mass with cutaneous swelling (indicated by a blue arrow) along with skin retraction and color changes (indicated by a green arrow), corresponding to an underlying parietal endometriosis nodule

13.2.2.3 Differential Diagnosis of AWE

Nodules on the abdominal wall present a diagnostic challenge with a differential diagnosis that spans various etiologies, including traumatic causes like hematoma; infectious processes, such as abscesses or sebaceous cysts; and iatrogenic origins, including incisional hernia, suture granuloma, keloid formation, or retained surgical materials. The two primary conditions that necessitate differentiation from AWE are desmoid tumors and metastatic diseases of the abdominal wall. Desmoid tumors, unlike AWE, typically do not exhibit cyclical symptoms and are frequently located within the infraumbilical rectus sheath. However, the clinical and imaging characteristics of desmoid tumors may overlap with AWE, often necessitating pathologic evaluation for definitive diagnosis (Fig. 13.4) [17]. Conversely, abdominal wall metastases most commonly originate from colorectal, gastric cancers or result from iatrogenic seeding during laparoscopic procedures through trocar sites [18].

13.2.2.4 Malignant Potential of AWE

The potential for the malignant transformation of AWE is relatively low, occurring in approximately 1% of cases. Factors that may elevate the risk include advanced age, postmenopausal status, or the presence of a sizable tumor. When malignancy does arise within AWE, the predominant histological variant encountered is the notably aggressive clear cell carcinoma. Consequently, the management strategy for AWE often leans toward surgical or interventional procedures rather than follow-up, to mitigate the risk of such malignant progression regardless of its infrequency [19].

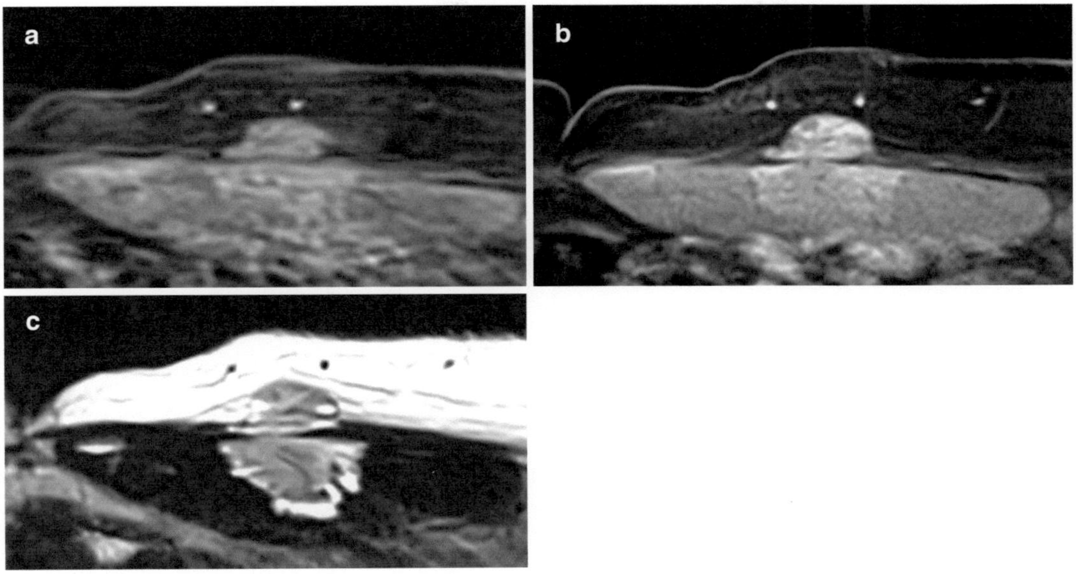

Fig. 13.4 The MRI features of a differential diagnosis for parietal endometriosis: desmoid tumor. A 17-year-old female patient with a left palpable subcutaneous nodule. (A) MRI in axial plane, T1 Dixon unenhanced water sequence, displaying an iso-intense T1 mass relative to the muscle. (B) Axial plane, T1 Dixon sequence after contrast, demonstrating the heterogeneous contrast enhancement of the mass embedded within the left rectus muscle and fat. (C) Axial cut, T2 sequence, showing a heterogeneously hyperintense T2 mass

13.3 Diagnostic Management

Beyond the scope of clinical symptomatic guidance, diagnostic imaging plays a pivotal role in the evaluation of abdominal wall endometriosis. It is essential not only for ascertaining the diagnosis but also for devising an appropriate surgical or interventional radiology strategy, ensuring a comprehensive treatment response, and excluding differential diagnoses, particularly those of a malignant nature.

13.3.1 Ultrasonography

Sonography is frequently the initial imaging modality employed by clinicians to explore the symptomatic correlation with the palpable tumorous lesion, favored due to its accessibility, affordability, and nonionizing nature and due to the convenience of bedside execution in the outpatient setting. Characteristic imaging findings typically depict a lesion within the subcutaneous tissue or residing within the stratified layers of the abdominal wall. These lesions often exhibit a hypoechoic and heterogeneous echotexture with variable internal echogenicity. Certain lesions may present with cystic alterations, areas of increased echogenicity, or calcifications. Doppler ultrasonography may further delineate these findings, occasionally revealing lesions with increased vascularity that is indicative of low-flow vascular patterns (Fig. 13.5) [15]. Elastography, an advanced technique, can improve the diagnostic accuracy of the detection of AWE by measuring changes in the firmness caused by the nodule [20]. However, using ultrasound comes with some downsides. It can be less clear for patients who are obese or have nodules that are located deep within the body. The process can be uncomfortable because it involves pressing down on the nodule to get a better view. Also, the results can vary depending on the skill and experience of the person performing the ultrasound.

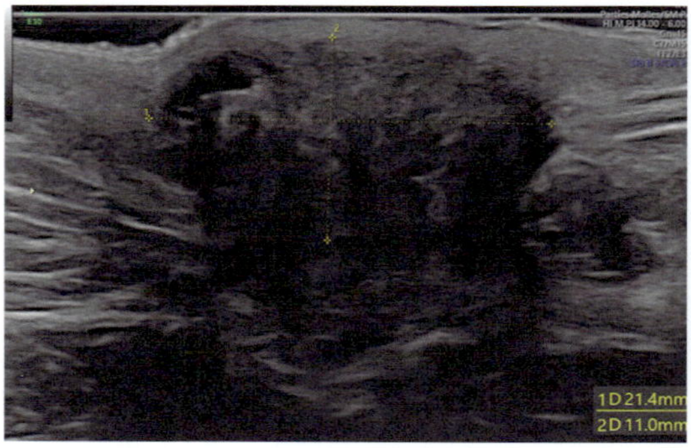

Fig. 13.5 Ultrasonographic characteristics of an abdominal wall endometriosis nodule. This nodule, displayed with its two transverse dimensions, is hypoechoic and heterogeneous. Skin invasion, which is readily detectable via ultrasound, would be indicated by hypoechoic spiculation extending into the skin layer, although it is not observed in this case. The firmness of the nodule can vary. The nodule may also contain cystic spaces (indicated by a white star), and tenderness upon probe pressure is a common feature

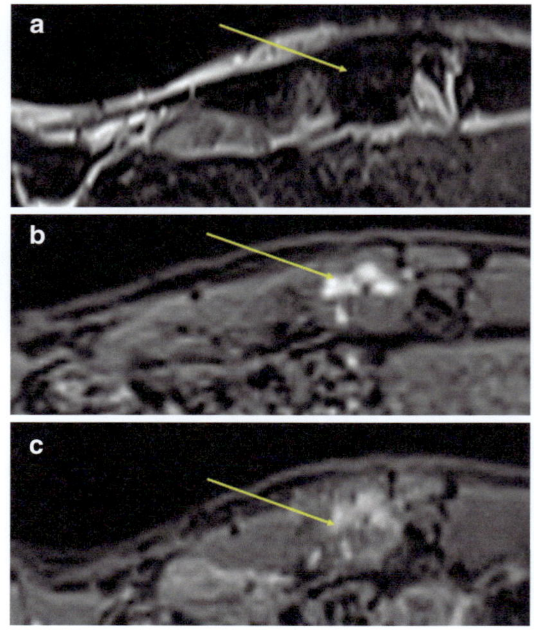

Fig. 13.6 Typical MRI appearance of a parietal endometriosis nodule in a 42-year-old female patient experiencing pain with a palpable nodule in the right rectus abdominis muscle (yellow arrow). (**a**) Axial MRI slice, T2-weighted image showing a nodule embedded within the right rectus muscle, with a circumscribed hypointense T2 signal. (**b**) Axial MRI slice, T1-weighted Dixon unenhanced water sequence, revealing pockets of spontaneous hyperintense T1 signal indicative of endometriotic tissue. (**c**) Axial MRI slice, T1-weighted Dixon contrast-enhanced water sequence exhibiting the heterogeneous enhancement of the mass

13.3.2 Magnetic Resonance Imaging

Magnetic resonance imaging (MRI) has emerged as an indispensable diagnostic adjunct in the management of endometriosis, particularly for providing definitive diagnoses, optimizing surgical interventions, and monitoring post-treatment outcomes in patients. Its efficacy in detecting extrapelvic endometrial implants, delineating their precise anatomical distribution within the abdominal wall strata, and assessing the extent of infiltration has been well documented. The conventional imaging protocol mandates the acquisition of T2-weighted and T1-weighted fat-suppressed sequences in no fewer than two orthogonal planes [21]. The use of contrast-enhanced imaging is advocated to enhance the diagnostic sensitivity for AWE, thereby facilitating accurate lesion characterization and aiding in preoperative planning [22]. MRI phenotypically characterizes AWE as either a homogeneously solid mass or a composite mass with solid and cystic components, which may pervade the abdominal wall from the subcutaneous layer to the serosal peritoneum. The lesions typically exhibit low-to-intermediate signal intensity on T2-weighted sequences, occasionally punctuated by microcystic structures and, at times, raising fluid–fluid levels. T1-weighted fat-suppressed sequences without contrast material can demonstrate a hyperintense signal consistent with endometriotic tissue, characterized by high signal intensities within the cystic or tumorous components (Fig. 13.6) [23]. Contrast-enhanced T1-weighted imaging further delineates the lesions, which may present with either well-defined or indistinct margins. Magnetic susceptibility sequences are valuable in identifying the blooming artifact indicative of methemoglobin and hemosiderin deposition [24]. Additionally, diffusion-weighted imaging (DWI) may prove beneficial in the detection of abdominal wall nodules, albeit with variable sensitivity contingent on the phase of the menstrual cycle [25]. Moreover, MRI serves various roles by facilitating the exclusion of differential diagnoses, staging coexisting pelvic endometriosis or adenomyosis, and enabling ovarian follicular assessment pertinent to fertility evaluation [1].

13.3.3 Computed Tomography (CT) Imaging

In the diagnostic approach to abdominal wall endometriosis, CT scan utilization is relatively infrequent, primarily due to concerns over radiation exposure in patients of childbearing age. When employed, CT imaging typically reveals nonspecific features, such as a solid mass enhancing within the abdominal wall, primarily serving to preoperatively delineate the disease's extent [15]. A particular diagnostic characteristic, termed *the Gorgon sign*, has been identified by some researchers as indicative of abdominal wall endometriosis. This sign is characterized by linear infiltration extending into the surrounding subcutaneous fat from a central nodule, mirroring histopathological patterns seen in deep pelvic endometriosis (DPE)—marked by histiocytic infiltration, fibrosis due to chronic hemorrhage, and minimal gland presence [26].

13.3.4 Positron Emission Tomography-Computed Tomography (PET-CT)

The application of positron emission tomography-computed tomography (PET-CT) in this context is limited, attributed to the low metabolic activity of the endometriosis cells and concerns over radiation [16]. Despite these limitations, PET-CT can still identify nonspecific markers such as fibrosis and inflammation through fluorodeoxyglucose (FDG) uptake with variable intensity. The measurement of 18F-FDG standard uptake value (SUV) on PET-CT scans may assist in distinguishing between endometriosis and potential malignant transformations, such as clear cell carcinoma development [27].

13.3.5 Fine-Needle Aspiration Cytology (FNAC) and Core Needle Biopsy (CNB)

Fine-needle aspiration cytology (FNAC) is a straightforward, minimally invasive technique that can be utilized preoperatively to detect epithelial cells, stromal cells with a spindle morphology, and macrophages containing hemosiderin. Despite its simplicity, the cytological representation of endometriosis via FNAC may vary significantly due to hormonal fluctuations, potentially presenting a broad range of cellular morphologies. Such variability increases the risk of misdiagnosing endometriotic lesions as malignant neoplasms [28]. The technical challenges associated with ultrasound-guided fine-needle aspiration (FNA)—such as the influence of patient body composition and the presence of substantial adipose or scar tissue, along with its low sensitivity and dependency on the operator's skill—further complicate its diagnostic reliability. To circumvent these limitations, some experts advocate for the routine use of ultrasound-guided core needle biopsy prior to treating abdominal wall nodules, aiming to eliminate the possibility of malignancy (Fig. 13.7). Nonetheless, a universal guideline for preoperative biopsy has not been established, because surgical intervention frequently facilitates a definitive diagnosis of abdominal wall endometriosis. The emergence of percutaneous procedures as a diagnostic tool has only recently gained attention, suggesting a shift toward more-direct methods of confirming the presence of endometriosis [29].

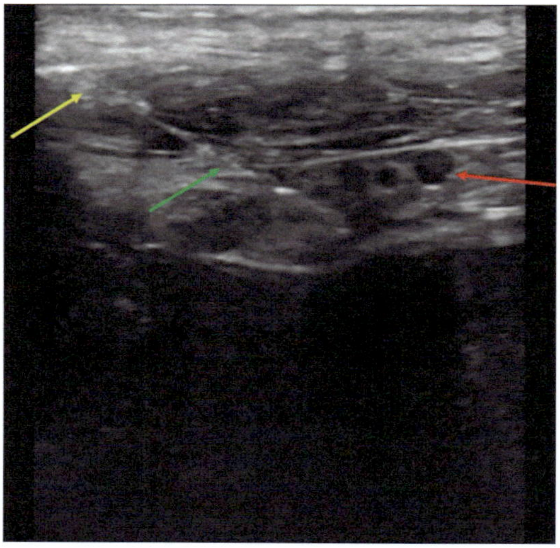

Fig. 13.7 Illustration of a percutaneous biopsy of a suspected intramuscular parietal endometriosis nodule. Biopsy can be conducted in uncertain cases to rule out differential diagnoses. The procedure is performed under ultrasound guidance (sagittal section) along the needle's path by using a coaxial system (yellow arrow). The deployment of the biopsy window is indicated (green arrow). Continuously monitoring the needle movement via ultrasound is necessary to avoid the at-risk inferior epigastric vascular bundle (red arrow)

13.4 Current Management and Surgical and Interventional Imaging Techniques

In this section, we present a comprehensive overview of common therapeutic strategies in AWE management, highlighting their efficacy, limitations, and associated challenges.

13.4.1 Drug Treatment

The initial line of treatment usually involves hormonal therapies alongside nonsteroidal anti-inflammatory drugs (NSAIDs) aimed at symptom alleviation. Despite these interventions, complete symptom relief is not guaranteed, where many patients experience persistent pain and symptom recurrence upon treatment discontinuation. The literature reveals modest outcomes with the use of oral progesterone and gonadotropin-releasing hormone analogs, noting a high rate of symptom resurgence after treatment and the necessity to discontinue these therapies when the patient desires pregnancy [30].

13.4.2 Surgical Treatment

Surgical excision stands out as the conventional method for AWE treatment for the complete removal of nodules. Recurrence rates after surgery exhibit a broad spectrum, documented between <5% and 39.1% at the 60-month follow-up mark [31, 32]. Surgical strategy emphasizes the importance of extensive nodule excision, maintaining a clear margin of at least 1 cm, to both effectively remove the mass and achieve a definitive histological diagnosis of parietal endometriosis [33]. The challenge escalates when addressing large or deeply situated nodules, necessitating elaborate surgical procedures that might include extensive resection and innovative reconstructive techniques, such as muscle flaps and mesh parietal repair. These measures are critical in averting recurrence and managing parietal defects [30]. Therefore, some minimally invasive treatments have been developed to optimize the efficacy of treatment while reducing morbidity.

13.4.3 Percutaneous Minimally Invasive Therapies

Amid the quest for less-invasive options, several emerging treatments have garnered attention.

13.4.3.1 Ultrasound-Guided Ethanol Sclerotherapy

Ultrasound-guided ethanol sclerotherapy, for instance, has shown promise in managing AWE but comes with its own set of risks, including the possibility of causing difficult-to-repair muscle necrosis and potential peritoneal damage in cases where endometriosis foci extend into the intraperitoneal area [34].

13.4.3.2 High-Intensity Focused Ultrasound (HIFU)

High-intensity focused ultrasound (HIFU) ablation represents a breakthrough in noninvasive treatment, leveraging the last decade's advances in solid tumor therapy [35]. This method employs a piezoelectric transducer to concentrate high-energy pulses on the target area while sparing surrounding tissues [36]. Despite its appeal, HIFU ablation has been associated with adverse effects, such as skin thermalgia, tenderness, orange-peel skin appearance, and hematuria [37].

13.4.3.3 Radiofrequency Ablation (RFA)

Thermal-based radiofrequency has been tested in AWE, but only one case report study exists, leading to an efficacy that needs to be confirmed by conducting larger, prospective studies [38].

13.4.3.4 Microwave (MW)

Microwave (MW) ablation had promising results in a recent study that reported significant pain relief in patients. However, this technique is not without its drawbacks, including risks of skin thermalgia and infection [39].

13.4.3.5 Cryoablation (CA)

Cryoablation emerges as one of the most innovative and rapidly growing techniques in the field of AWE treatment. Its increasing worldwide application prompts a closer examination of its underlying principles, technical nuances, and potential as a viable treatment option. In the subsequent section of this chapter, we will explore the foundational principles and technical considerations of using cryoablation as an illustrative example of a percutaneous minimally invasive approach for treating abdominal wall endometriosis (AWE).

Cryoablation Principles

Cryoablation is based on using intense cold, which can be rapidly generated either by depressurizing a gas within a needle (the Joule–Thomson effect) or by directly circulating a liquid gas through a needle [40]. This concentrated cold at the needle's tip leads to the formation of a variably sized ice ball, with temperatures within the ice ball varying depending on the distance from the needle. For instance, a 0 °C isotherm is situated at the periphery of the ice ball, while the needle tip can reach temperatures as low as −170 °C at maximum power. One notable advantage of cryoablation is the real-time visibility of this ice ball when using both ultrasound and CT scans. The volume of the ice ball closely corresponds to the actual ablation zone, improving the prediction and control of the treated area, which is less easy to visualize when using heat-based technologies. Another benefit is the preservation of collagenous fibrous structures, contributing to favorable aesthetic outcomes and sparing the supportive tissue [41]. Cell death occurs directly below −40 °C through the formation of intracellular ice crystals and direct membrane damage. Cell death can also happen above this temperature through various biological mechanisms. Indirect cell death results from intracellular dehydration due to changes in osmolality caused by extracellular ice formation. Ischemic phenomena occur due to local vasoconstriction and platelet activation secondary to vascular endothelial damage, leading to localized microthrombosis [42]. Additionally, reversible cellular damage initiates an apoptotic cascade that culminates in cell death. Finally, the release of intact antigens triggers significant immune responses.

Technical Setup

An advanced interventional radiology suite ensures optimal conditions for performing this procedure comfortably and safely (Fig. 13.8). Given its low complication rate and minimally invasive nature, outpatient facilities are ideally suited for this technique. The procedure is carried out under sedation supplemented with local anesthesia or under general anesthesia (GA). An interventional CT scanner is essential for treating deep nodules to monitor the risk to the digestive tract as the formation of the ice causes a posterior acoustic shadow that obstructs ultrasound visualization. The setup for cryoablation equipment (such as generators and gases) varies depending on the specific machine used, each

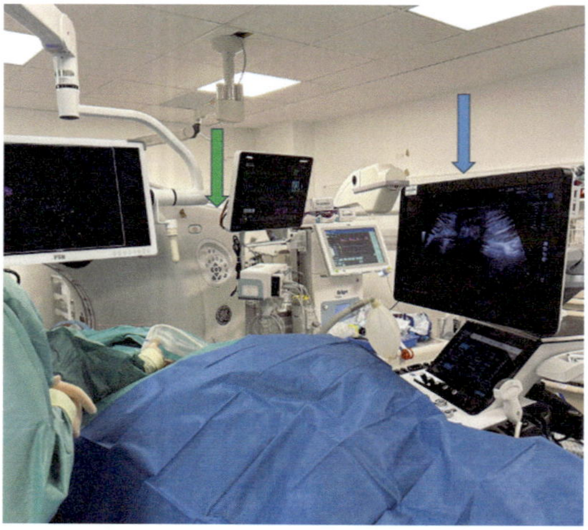

Fig. 13.8 Illustrative photo depicting the technical setup for the procedure conducted in an interventional radiology suite. Ideally, it is equipped with dual-guidance capabilities: ultrasound for the real-time positional analysis of the instruments (indicated by a blue arrow) and CT scan for monitoring protective techniques such as carbon dioxide dissection (indicated by a green arrow)

offering its own set of advantages and disadvantages. Moreover, CO_2 bottles equipped with regulators and appropriate filters are essential for carbodissection techniques.

Preoperative Consultation

A preoperative consultation with an interventional radiologist is mandatory. It involves reviewing the pre-existing MRI (eliminating differential diagnoses, searching for secondary locations, regional extension, at-risk structures) to better plan the intervention and provide personalized information to the patient about the procedure and its associated risks.

Main Anatomical Structures at Risk

The Skin

Contact between the ice ball and the skin poses a risk of causing cutaneous burns, ranging from first- to third-degree burns. This complication is easily predictable and almost always preventable by using appropriate techniques. The skin plane is easily identifiable on ultrasound with a high-frequency superficial probe. It consists of two primary layers: the epidermis (the most superficial hyperechogenic line, which is nonmeasurable) and the dermis (approximately 1 mm thick, uniformly hypoechogenic). Deeper lies the hypodermis, which corresponds to the subcutaneous fat layer. Hydrodissection techniques are most effective in preventing this complication by distancing the ice ball from the dermis. External skin warming, such as by using a sterile glove filled with warm water applied to the skin, is often performed (Fig. 13.9). Ultrasound monitoring can be conducted through the glove. Skin massages stimulate microcirculation and promote cold dissipation. Skin frostbite may be observed intraoperatively as white, indurated skin. In such cases, blisters may appear as early as postoperative day 1. This complication is rare and typically occurs when the operator deliberately decides to treat cutaneous endometriosis involvement.

The Digestive Tract

The risk of digestive tract involvement is parietal necrosis complicated by digestive fistula. Evocative symptoms often occur within the first few days following the procedure, manifesting as abdominal pain corresponding to the ablation zone in the 10 days following the procedure, complicated by localized peritonitis. This potentially serious complication can theoretically lead to surgical resection. This risk can be monitored and controlled only with intraoperative CT scanning because ultrasound cannot explore the deeper half of the ice ball. Additionally, carbodissection techniques, often used to control this risk, can be performed only with CT guidance because ultrasound cannot explore beyond a gas interface (Fig. 13.10). Preintervention planning must systematically include risk management, and an adapted platform with interventional CT is essential for managing deep parietal nodules.

The Nerves

Nerves are particularly sensitive to cold. Nerve stun occurs at temperatures as low as 5 °C and can be intentionally used for analgesic effect in cases of treatment under local anesthesia alone (in this case, power escalation must be very gradual). Nerve lesions become irreversible below

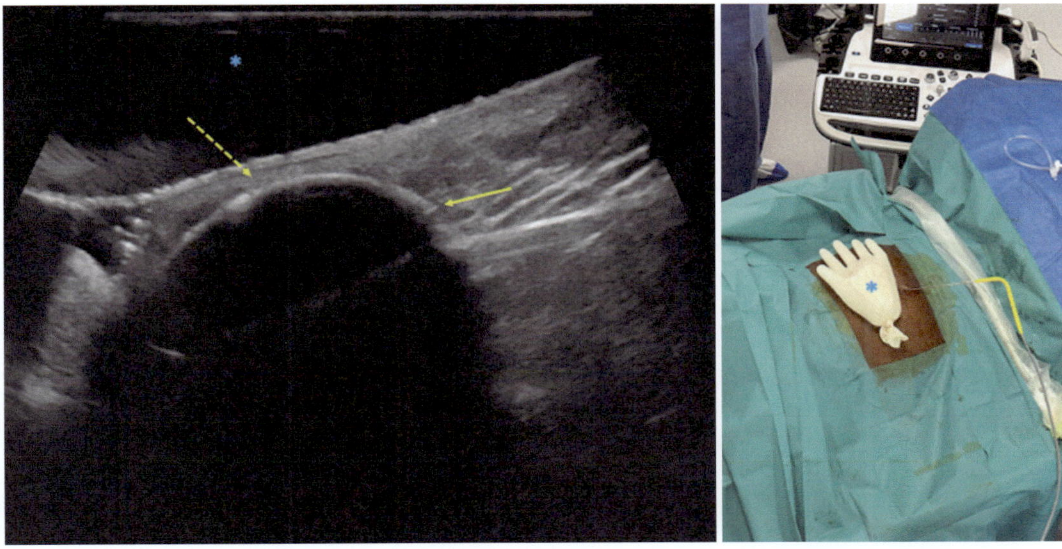

Fig. 13.9 Real-time cryoablation procedure under ultrasound guidance. The image is a sagittal section. The ice ball control (solid yellow arrow) can be easily performed under ultrasound. Normal cutaneous structures are also identified (dotted yellow arrow). A glove filled with saline solution is placed on the skin to protect it by providing warmth (blue star), and it also facilitates the monitoring of the ablation area due to its sonographic transparency

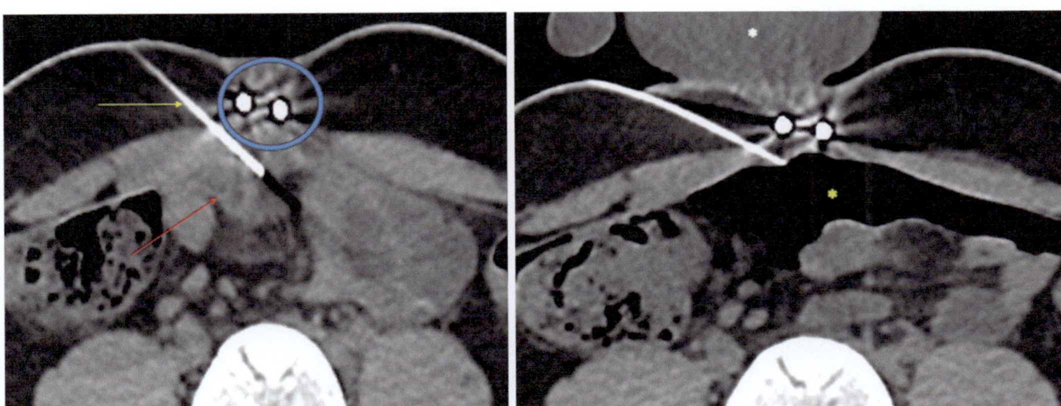

Fig. 13.10 Illustration of carbodissection during a parietal cryoablation procedure to protect intra-abdominal structures. After positioning the cryoprobes under ultrasound, a control CT scan is carried out to set up carbodissection, which moves the small bowel loops away from the anterior abdominal wall (cryoprobes circled in blue). The nearest small bowel loop is indicated by a red arrow. Here, two cryoprobes are used to create an ice ball that is wider than it is thick, ensuring treatment coverage over the nodule's entire width at lower cryoablation powers, thus minimizing the risk of cutaneous burns. A carbodissection needle (yellow arrow) is positioned in the peritoneal cavity, right behind the anterior abdominal wall. Following the confirmation of its placement outside of mesenteric vessels (the absence of blood reflux), CO_2 insufflation is carried out, constituting the carbodissection. After the carbodissection (yellow star), the small bowel loops have been displaced from the wall, facilitating safe ice ball formation with minimal digestive risk. The small bowel loop previously in immediate contact with the peritoneum beneath the nodule is now illustrated as being well clear of the ablation zone. A sterile glove (white star) filled with warm saline is placed on the skin, and cutaneous hydrodissection is performed under ultrasound to further reduce the risk of skin burns

−20 °C. The anterior abdominal wall has the advantage of not being traversed by nerve trunks, unlike the inguinal region.

The Bladder

Lower lesions of the anterior abdominal wall may be near the bladder. Perioperative bladder emptying (intermittent catheterization or indwelling catheterization) usually prevents this risk.

The Uterus

Some median and infiltrating anterior parietal lesions may be continuous with an external adenomyosis of the uterus. Treating parietal endometriosis also treats these contiguous external adenomyosis areas and could improve efficacy, as recently demonstrated [43].

Step-By-Step Procedure for Percutaneous Cryoablation of AWE

The procedural protocol for percutaneous cryoablation in the management of parietal endometriosis is simplified and delineated as follows (Fig. 13.11):

1. Commence with a meticulous review of the preoperative preparatory measures, encompassing a thorough examination of the patient's recent radiological imaging, the verification of the informed consent duly signed by the patient, and a comprehensive analysis of the biological data.
2. Position the patient in a prone posture within the sanctum of the interventional radiology suite, ensuring optimal access and comfort for the ensuing procedure.
3. Initiate anesthetic conditioning, which encompasses the establishment of monitoring parameters and venous access for perfusion. A critical decision is made at this juncture between employing general anesthesia (GA) or opting for anesthetic sedation (AS), based on specific requirements and the complexity of the procedure.

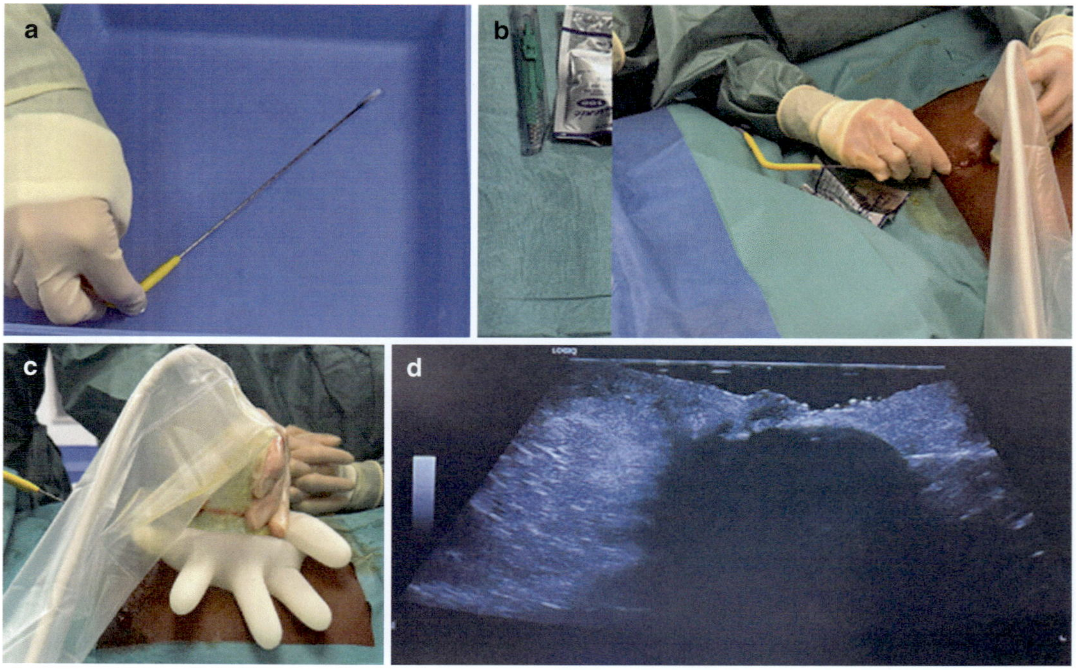

Fig. 13.11 Sequential phases of simplified cryoablation. (**a**) The preliminary assessment of the cryoprobe, which is used to verify the correct formation of the ice ball at the needle tip prior to insertion into the patient. (**b**) The deployment of the cryoablation needle into the lesion under ultrasonic guidance. (**c**) The real-time monitoring of the needle's position utilizing the acoustic shadowing of the thermoprotective warm glove. (**d**) Ultrasonographic visualization in real-time demonstrating the deep formation of the ice ball and the implementation of thermoprotective measures to prevent cutaneous burns

4. Execute a rigorous disinfection protocol at the operative site, followed by the strategic placement of sterile operating fields to maintain an aseptic environment throughout the intervention.
5. Utilize ultrasonography, employing a sterilely covered ultrasound probe, to precisely localize the nodule within the abdominal wall, ensuring accuracy in the intervention's target.
6. Administer local anesthesia in the vicinity of the nodule by employing xylocaine to mitigate discomfort and facilitate a pain-free procedural experience for the patient.
7. Conduct a preliminary assessment of the cryoprobe to verify the formation of the ice ball at its tip, preparing the device for optimal performance during the cryoablation process.
8. Carefully insert the cryoprobe adjacently or directly into the lesion, where deciding on one or the other is influenced by the number of cryoprobes utilized. Continuous ultrasonography monitoring is imperative throughout this phase to circumvent any potential harm to vital structures.
9. In instances necessitating further precaution, proceed to insert a slender needle either subcutaneously or into the peritoneal cavity. This measure is prepared to facilitate carbon dioxide dissection or liquid dissection as thermoprotective strategies during the cryoablation.
10. Initiate the cryoablation by activating the freezing and thawing cycle, meticulously monitoring the process to ensure the ablation of the targeted endometriotic tissue.
11. Prior to concluding the procedure, undertake a final assessment through ultrasonography and computed tomography (CT) scans to ascertain the absence of any complications, thereby ensuring safety and success.

Techniques: Depending on the Location of AWE

The Anterior Abdominal Wall

Two of the main areas to control risk are the skin and the digestive tract. For the skin, skin-protection techniques, such as those described above (hydrodissection, external warming, and skin massage), are typically employed. For the digestive tract, both hydrodissection and carbodissection techniques can be used. Fluid that is directly injected into the abdominal cavity tends to follow the slope and not remain in place between the anterior peritoneum and the small intestine or colon where it would be protected. Therefore, hydrodissection within the virtual space between the transversalis fascia (the deep fascia of the rectus muscle) and the peritoneum is preferred. Carbodissection, on the other hand, is ideal in the abdominal cavity, remaining readily in place between the anterior peritoneum and the digestive tract. Notably, because gas is a better thermal insulator than water, a thinner layer of gas is sufficient to achieve the desired thermal isolation.

The Inguinal Region

The specificity of this location concerns large nodules (> 2 cm) that may be in immediate proximity to the skin (risk of burns) but especially to the femoral nerves. The risk–benefit balance is systematically considered to minimize the risk of nerve complications. Anatomically, an inguinal nodule lies along the path of the round ligament and inevitably involves the sensitive genital branches of the ilioinguinal and genitofemoral nerves. However, postoperative anesthesia applied to the ipsilateral labia majora is not systematic, likely due to extensive sensory nerve interconnection in this region near the midline. Furthermore, because the innervation is primarily associated with the pudendal nerve, located deeply in the pelvic cavity, patients need not worry about any impact on orgasm.

Follow-Ups After the Procedure

Cryoablation generally leads to a strong local inflammatory reaction in the days following the procedure. The peak of inflammation typically occurs between postoperative days 3 and 5. Transient bodily changes related to this inflammation (edema, redness, and warmth) may be clinically impressive for the patient, and clear information on this point is important to alleviate any concerns. The discomfort is generally mild, and its duration depends primarily on the size of the ice ball created. According to empirical experience, it can range from 10 days to a month. Oral anti-inflammatory treatment may be administered in the early days of recovery, along with mild-to-moderate analgesics. No scar care is necessary, because the skin incision required for needle insertion is only 5 mm wide, ideally concealed in the pubic hair area, and typically heals within 72 h after the procedure. Serous drainage can delay the healing of needle-entry points due to edematous infiltration, and the patient should be informed of this possibility. Parietal pain from the nodule should no longer reappear following the intervention, indicating its effectiveness. Recurrences are possible but rare, often associated with nodules not identified in the initial assessment and therefore left untreated. Occasionally, cutaneous anesthesia or paresthesia over 1 or 2 cm^2 may occur adjacent to the ablation zone, particularly when treating superficial nodules. Sensory recovery is possible but may be lengthy and uncertain.

Following cryoablation, the nodule becomes fibrous and tends to decrease in size. If it was palpable before the intervention, patients should be informed that it may still be palpable afterward. The crucial point is that it will no longer be painful. Occasionally, patients may start to feel the fibrous scar nodule after losing weight (with the resumption of physical activity following the relief of abdominal pain), which they did not palpate before, due to a thicker adipose layer.

Follow-up MRI can be performed, but currently, no specific guidelines on radiological follow-up are available (Fig. 13.12).

13.5 Future Directions

Despite the considerable progress made in delineating the complex pathophysiology of endometriosis, an urgent and unmet need for extensive future research aimed at deepening our understanding of abdominal wall endometriosis (AWE) remains. Specifically, the prevalence and underlying biological mechanisms that drive the manifestation of extrapelvic endometriosis must be elucidated, particularly those cases that emerge on the abdominal wall in the absence of prior surgical history. This exploration is crucial for identifying potential etiological factors unique to AWE and understanding its development pathways.

In the clinical domain, a more detailed and focused approach is required to identify specific and reliable clinical indicators of AWE. This endeavor is essential not only for enhancing diagnostic accuracy but also for evaluating the broader implications of AWE on patients' quality of life. Such assessments are key to understanding the full spectrum of the disease's impact on daily activities, mental health, and overall well-being. Establishing dedicated tertiary centers of excellence for endometriosis and streamlining patient referral processes could play pivotal roles in achieving higher diagnostic accuracy. This structured approach would facilitate early and accurate diagnoses, allowing for timely intervention and the convening of multidisciplinary teams. These teams, comprising specialists from diverse medical backgrounds, would collaborate to customize treatment plans that are both effective and mindful of minimizing patient morbidity.

The evolving preferences among patients, particularly those leaning toward reducing their intake of hormonal therapies and favoring minimally invasive procedures, indicate a significant shift toward alternative therapeutic strategies. This shift underscores the growing importance of developing and refining interventional treatments that can provide relief and positive outcomes for patients seeking less-invasive options. While surgical interventions remain a critical option, reserved for intractable cases or those not amenable to other treatments, the exploration and incorporation of innovative interventional techniques, such as cryoablation or high-intensity focused ultrasound, present promising avenues. However, the relative novelty of these techniques has left a significant gap in long-term, prospective data comparing their efficacy and outcomes to traditional surgical methods.

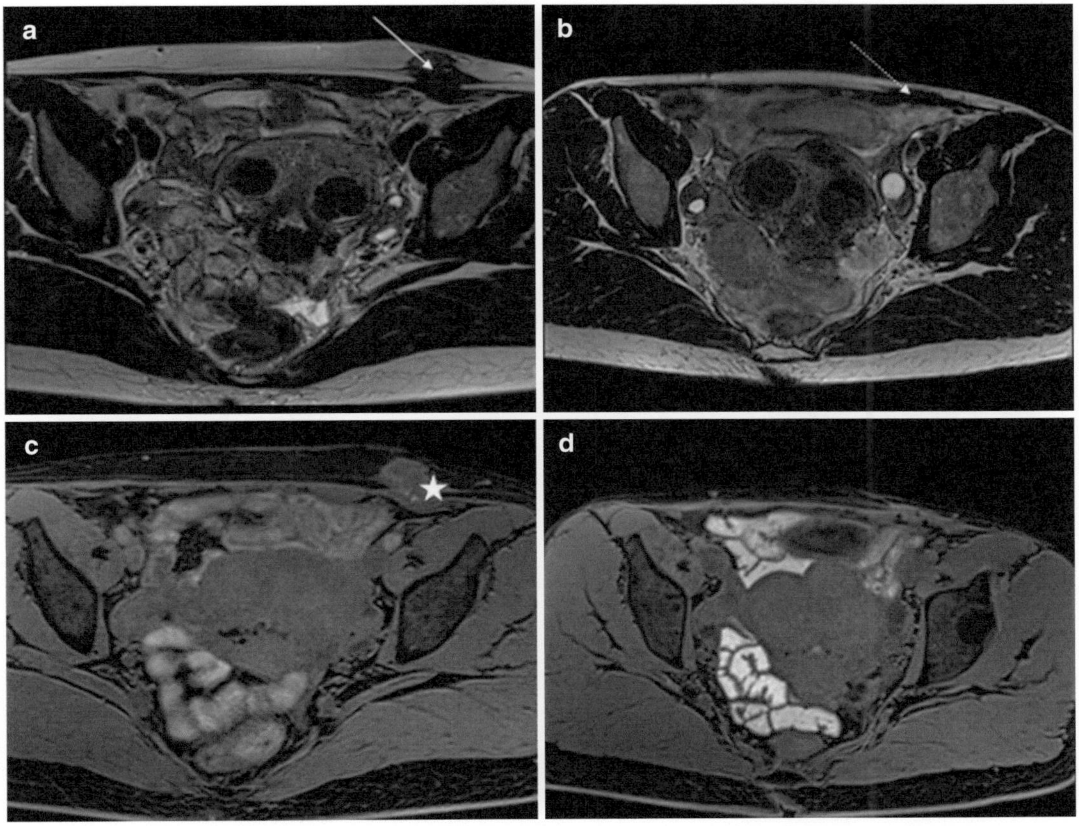

Fig. 13.12 A 37-year-old patient undergoing cryoablation for a parietal endometriosis nodule on the left abdominal wall. (**a**) Axial T2-weighted MRI slice demonstrating the nodule in isointense infiltration through the fat and the left rectus abdominis muscle (white arrow). (**b**) Axial T2-weighted MRI slice taken 12 months after treatment revealing nodule regression with a fibrous scar in linear T2 hypointensity (white dotted arrow). (**c**) Axial T1-weighted water sequence without contrast pretreatment displaying the initial endometriotic spots (white star). (**d**) Axial T1-weighted water sequence without contrast 12 months following treatment illustrating the nodule's regression

This gap highlights the critical need for establishing comprehensive registries and conducting in-depth evaluations to thoroughly assess these emerging modalities. Such research should include rigorous comparisons to established surgical interventions, thereby providing a clearer understanding of their relative benefits and limitations. Additionally, the integration of these techniques raises important questions about the role and feasibility of histological analysis in the context of percutaneous treatments. Unlike traditional surgical approaches, which allow the excision of tissue that can be sent for pathological examination to confirm diagnoses and rule out malignancy, many percutaneous techniques do not afford the same opportunity for post-treatment histological evaluation.

Lastly, the economic implications of adopting new and innovative treatments for AWE cannot be overlooked. Comprehensive medico-economic studies are urgently needed to evaluate the cost-effectiveness of various treatment modalities. Such studies are essential for ensuring that patients receive the most effective treatments, ones that not only address the physical manifestations of the disease but also do so in a manner that is financially sustainable and delivers the best possible outcomes for morbidity reduction and quality-of-life improvement. Through meticulous and targeted research efforts, the medical community can advance toward a more nuanced understanding and management of abdominal wall endometriosis, ultimately benefiting patients across the globe.

References

1. Horton JD, Dezee KJ, Ahnfeldt EP, Wagner M. Abdominal wall endometriosis: a surgeon's perspective and review of 445 cases. Am J Surg. 2008;196:207–12. https://doi.org/10.1016/j.amjsurg.2007.07.035.
2. Benedetto C, Cacozza D, de Sousa CD, Coloma Cruz A, Tessmann Zomer M, Cosma S, et al. Abdominal wall endometriosis: report of 83 cases. Int J Gynecol Obstet. 2022;159:530–6. https://doi.org/10.1002/ijgo.14167.
3. Flament JB. Functional anatomy of the abdominal wall. Chirurg. 2006;77:401–7. https://doi.org/10.1007/s00104-006-1184-5.
4. Flynn W, Vickerton P. Anatomy, abdomen and pelvis: abdominal wall. In: StatPearls. Treasure Island, FL: StatPearls Publishing; 2024.
5. Read JW, Ibrahim N, Jacombs ASW, Elstner KE, Saunders J, Rodriguez-Acevedo O. Imaging insights into abdominal wall function. Front Surg. 2022;9:799277.
6. Zondervan KT, Becker CM, Missmer SA. Endometriosis. N Engl J Med. 2020;382:1244–56. https://doi.org/10.1056/NEJMra1810764.
7. Andres MP, Arcoverde FVL, Souza CCC, Fernandes LFC, Abrão MS, Kho RM. Extrapelvic endometriosis: a systematic review. J Minim Invasive Gynecol. 2020;27:373–89. https://doi.org/10.1016/j.jmig.2019.10.004.
8. Zhang P, Sun Y, Zhang C, Yang Y, Zhang L, Wang N, et al. Cesarean scar endometriosis: presentation of 198 cases and literature review. BMC Womens Health. 2019;19:14. https://doi.org/10.1186/s12905-019-0711-8.
9. Dridi D, Chiaffarino F, Parazzini F, Donati A, Buggio L, Brambilla M, et al. Umbilical endometriosis: a systematic literature review and pathogenic theory proposal. J Clin Med. 2022;11:995. https://doi.org/10.3390/jcm11040995.
10. Prodromidou A, Pandraklakis A, Rodolakis A, Thomakos N. Endometriosis of the canal of Nuck: a systematic review of the literature. Diagnostics. 2020;11:3. https://doi.org/10.3390/diagnostics11010003.
11. Koger KE, Shatney CH, Hodge K, McClenathan JH. Surgical scar endometrioma. Surg Gynecol Obstet. 1993;177:243–6.
12. Sasson IE, Taylor HS. Stem cells and the pathogenesis of endometriosis. Ann N Y Acad Sci. 2008;1127:106–15. https://doi.org/10.1196/annals.1434.014.
13. Nellihela L, Al-Adnani M, Kufeji D. Primary umbilical endometriosis in an adolescent girl: unsuspected pathology. Eur J Pediatr Surg Rep. 2020;8:e10–3. https://doi.org/10.1055/s-0039-1700987.
14. Petrosellini C, Abdalla S, Oke T. The many guises of endometriosis: giant abdominal wall endometriosis masquerading as an incisional hernia. Int J Fertil Steril. 2018;11:321–5. https://doi.org/10.22074/ijfs.2018.5126.
15. Hensen J-HJ, Van Breda Vriesman AC, Puylaert JBCM. Abdominal wall endometriosis: clinical presentation and imaging features with emphasis on Sonography. Am J Roentgenol. 2006;186:616–20. https://doi.org/10.2214/AJR.04.1619.
16. Carsote M, Terzea DC, Valea A, Gheorghisan-Galateanu A-A. Abdominal wall endometriosis (a narrative review). Int J Med Sci. 2020;17:536–42. https://doi.org/10.7150/ijms.38679.
17. Cărăuleanu A, Popovici RM, Costea CF, Mogoş RA, Scripcariu DV, Florea ID, et al. Abdominal wall endometriosis versus desmoid tumor—a challenging differential diagnosis. Rom J Morphol Embryol. 2020;61:45–50. https://doi.org/10.47162/RJME.61.1.05.
18. Rouhani P, Fletcher CDM, Devesa SS, Toro JR. Cutaneous soft tissue sarcoma incidence patterns in the U.S.: an analysis of 12,114 cases. Cancer. 2008;113:616–27. https://doi.org/10.1002/cncr.23571.
19. Bahall V, Barry LD, Rampersad A. Clear cell carcinoma arising from abdominal wall endometriosis—a report on two cases and literature review. World J Surg Oncol. 2022;20:86. https://doi.org/10.1186/s12957-022-02553-x.
20. Wozniak S, Czuczwar P, Szkodziak P, Wozniakowska E, Milart P, Paszkowski M, et al. Elastography improves the accuracy of ultrasound in the preoperative assessment of abdominal wall endometriosis. Ultraschall Med. 2015;36:623–9. https://doi.org/10.1055/s-0034-1398834.
21. Busard MPH, Mijatovic V, van Kuijk C, Hompes PGA, van Waesberghe JHTM. Appearance of abdominal wall endometriosis on MR imaging. Eur Radiol. 2010;20:1267–76. https://doi.org/10.1007/s00330-009-1658-1.
22. Onbas O, Kantarci M, Alper F, Kumtepe Y, Durur I, Ingec M, et al. Nodular endometriosis: dynamic MR imaging. Abdom Imaging. 2007;32:451–6. https://doi.org/10.1007/s00261-006-9038-7.
23. Arkoudis N-A, Moschovaki-Zeiger O, Prountzos S, Spiliopoulos S, Kelekis N. Caesarean-section scar endometriosis (CSSE): clinical and imaging fundamentals of an underestimated entity. Clin Radiol. 2023;78:644–54. https://doi.org/10.1016/j.crad.2023.05.020.
24. Chu W. EP20.05: magnetic resonance imaging of abdominal wall endometriosis clinically and sonographically mimicking a tumour. Ultrasound Obstet Gynecol. 2018;52:272. https://doi.org/10.1002/uog.20073.

25. Genç B, Solak A, Sahin N, Genç M, Oğul H, Sivrikoz ON, et al. Diffusion-weighted imaging in the evaluation of hormonal cyclic changes in abdominal wall endometriomas. Clin Radiol. 2014;69:130–6. https://doi.org/10.1016/j.crad.2013.08.015.
26. Yarmish G, Sala E, Goldman D, Lakhman Y, Soslow R, Hricak H, et al. Abdominal wall endometriosis: differentiation from other masses using CT features. Abdom Radiol. 2017;42:1517–23. https://doi.org/10.1007/s00261-016-0998-y.
27. Balogova S, Daraï E, Noskovicova L, Lukac L, Talbot J-N, Montravers F. Interference of known or suspected endometriosis in reporting FDG PET/CT performed in another indication. Clin Nucl Med. 2022;47:305. https://doi.org/10.1097/RLU.0000000000004049.
28. Ail DA, Joshi AR, Manzoor I, Patil S, Kulkarni M. Fine-needle aspiration cytology of abdominal wall endometriosis: a meaningful adjunct to diagnosis. Oman Med J. 2018;33:72–5. https://doi.org/10.5001/omj.2018.14.
29. Reategui C, Grubbs D, Abdominal wall endometriomas. Should the approach vary based on its relationship to the fascia? A case report and review of the literature. Int J Surg Case Rep. 2021;78:62–6. https://doi.org/10.1016/j.ijscr.2020.11.143.
30. Bektaş H, Bilsel Y, Sari YS, Ersöz F, Koç O, Deniz M, et al. Abdominal wall endometrioma; a 10-year experience and brief review of the literature. J Surg Res. 2010;164:e77–81. https://doi.org/10.1016/j.jss.2010.07.043.
31. Kim SJ, Choi SH, Won S, Shim S, Lee N, Kim M, et al. Cumulative recurrence rate and risk factors for recurrent abdominal wall endometriosis after surgical treatment in a single institution. Yonsei Med J. 2022;63:446. https://doi.org/10.3349/ymj.2022.63.5.446.
32. Ferjaoui MA, Arfaoui R, Khedhri S, Abdessamia K, Hannechi MA, Hajjami K, et al. Abdominal wall endometriosis: a challenging iatrogenic disease. Int J Surg Case Rep. 2021;88:106507. https://doi.org/10.1016/j.ijscr.2021.106507.
33. Sumathy S, Mangalakanthi J, Purushothaman K, Sharma D, Remadevi C, Sreedhar S. Symptomatology and surgical perspective of scar endometriosis: a case series of 16 women. J Obstet Gynaecol India. 2017;67:218–23. https://doi.org/10.1007/s13224-016-0945-4.
34. Bozkurt M, Çil AS, Bozkurt DK. Intramuscular Abdominal Wall endometriosis treated by ultrasound-guided ethanol injection. Clin Med Res. 2014;12:160–5. https://doi.org/10.3121/cmr.2013.1183.
35. Orsi F, Arnone P, Chen W, Zhang L. High intensity focused ultrasound ablation: a new therapeutic option for solid tumors. J Cancer Res Ther. 2010;6:414–20. https://doi.org/10.4103/0973-1482.77064.
36. Bachu VS, Kedda J, Suk I, Green JJ, Tyler B. High-intensity focused ultrasound: a review of mechanisms and clinical applications. Ann Biomed Eng. 2021;49:1975–91. https://doi.org/10.1007/s10439-021-02833-9.
37. Wang S, Li B-H, Wang J-J, Guo Y-S, Cheng J-M, Ye H, et al. The safety of echo contrast-enhanced ultrasound in high-intensity focused ultrasound ablation for abdominal wall endometriosis: a retrospective study. Quant Imaging Med Surg. 2021;11:1751–62. https://doi.org/10.21037/qims-20-622.
38. Carrafiello G, Fontana F, Pellegrino C, Mangini M, Cabrini L, Mariani D, et al. Radiofrequency ablation of abdominal wall endometrioma. Cardiovasc Intervent Radiol. 2009;32:1300–3. https://doi.org/10.1007/s00270-008-9500-8.
39. Liu Y, Wen W, Qian L, Xu R. Safety and efficacy of microwave ablation for abdominal wall endometriosis: a retrospective study. Front Surg. 2023;10:1100381. https://doi.org/10.3389/fsurg.2023.1100381.
40. Erinjeri JP, Clark TWI. Cryoablation: mechanism of action and devices. J Vasc Interv Radiol. 2010;21:S187–91. https://doi.org/10.1016/j.jvir.2009.12.403.
41. Yakkala C, Chiang CL, Kandalaft L, Denys A, Duran R. Cryoablation and immunotherapy: An Enthralling Synergy to Confront the Tumors. Front Immunol. 2019;10:2283.
42. Pusceddu C, Paliogiannis P, Nigri G, Fancellu A. Cryoablation in the management of breast cancer: evidence to date. Breast Cancer. 2019;11:283–92. https://doi.org/10.2147/BCTT.S197406.
43. Marcelin C, Brun J-L, Caprais J, Molina-Andreo I, Jambon E, Le Bras Y, et al. Percutaneous cryoablation of symptomatic uterine adenomyomas: initial experience. J Gynecol Obstet Hum Reprod. 2024;53:102727. https://doi.org/10.1016/j.jogoh.2024.102727.

Part III

Technique and Reporting of the Different Imaging Techniques and Classifications

Techniques and Reporting of the Different Imaging Techniques and Classifications: Ultrasonography

14

Thierry Van den Bosch, Celine Bafort, and Dominique Van Schoubroeck

14.1 Introduction

Ultrasonography in patients with suspected endometriosis is a dynamic and interactive examination combining detailed imaging of the pelvis with organ mobility evaluation, site-specific pain assessment, patient's visual feedback, and patient information.

The reason for referral is often pain, from among dyspareunia, dysmenorrhea, dyschezia, dysuria, lower abdominal pain, or more-diffuse pain symptoms. The aims of an endometriosis scan are not only to detect endometriosis but also to objectivate and report other possible reasons for the pain (e.g., introital pain at the start of the vaginal scan, site-specific tenderness over the bladder trigonum, pelvic inflammatory disease, or postoperative adhesions).

Phenotypically, three types of endometriosis lesions can be distinguished: superficial/peritoneal endometriosis, deep endometriosis, and ovarian endometriotic cysts (endometriomas) [1]. Ultrasonography is the first-line imaging technique in the detection of deep endometriotic lesions and endometriomas [2]. Superficial endometriosis often remains undetected on ultrasonography. However, because ultrasonography is a dynamic exam, site-specific tenderness and reduced organ mobility are indirect signs of superficial endometriosis [3, 4].

Patients undergoing an endometriosis scan often have high expectations. In patients in whom one or more selectively painful deep endometriosis nodules are diagnosed, a proper sonographic mapping of the deep endometriosis will allow a targeted surgical removal of the lesions [5]. In those cases, the prognosis of the surgery in terms of pain symptoms is good. However, in patients for whom no endometriosis can be visualized on ultrasonography, the management is more complex. Therefore, the patient may be disappointed after the completion of a negative scan. Women with complex/centralized pelvic pain need a long-term multidisciplinary approach even if endometriosis is present.

The examination must be performed in a calm and relaxing environment. The examiner must take time to explain the aim of the scan and encourage the patient to report when they feel some discomfort or pain.

The scan is performed gently, avoiding excessive or brisk pressure with the probe. Elicited pain can cause secondary uterine cramping or

T. Van den Bosch (✉) · C. Bafort
Department of Obstetrics and Gynecology, University Hospital Leuven, Leuven, Belgium

Department of Development and Regeneration, KU Leuven, Leuven, Belgium
e-mail: thierry.vandenbosch@uzleuven.be; celine.bafort@uzleuven.be

D. Van Schoubroeck
Department of Obstetrics and Gynecology, University Hospital Leuven, Leuven, Belgium
e-mail: dominique.vanschoubroeck@uzleuven.be

I. Thomassin-Naggara (ed.), *Imaging of Endometriosis: A Comparative Guide of US, MRI and Surgery*, https://doi.org/10.1007/978-3-031-82750-1_14

more-generalized pelvic or abdominal pain, precluding further examination. This should be considered in the context of combining an endometriosis scan with other tests (e.g., hysterosalpingosonography or hysteroscopy) when a one-stop setting is being contemplated.

According to the IDEA consensus [6], four items should be addressed during the sonographic examination in women with a clinical suspicion of deep endometriosis: (1) an evaluation of the uterus and adnexa (including the evaluation of direct and indirect signs of adenomyosis); (2) an evaluation of "soft markers," including site-specific tenderness and ovarian mobility; (3) an assessment of the organ sliding in the anterior and posterior compartment ("sliding sign") [7]; and (4) the detection of deep endometriosis nodules in the anterior, posterior, and lateral compartments. Figure 14.1 shows a schematic overview of the anterior and posterior locations of deep endometriosis [6].

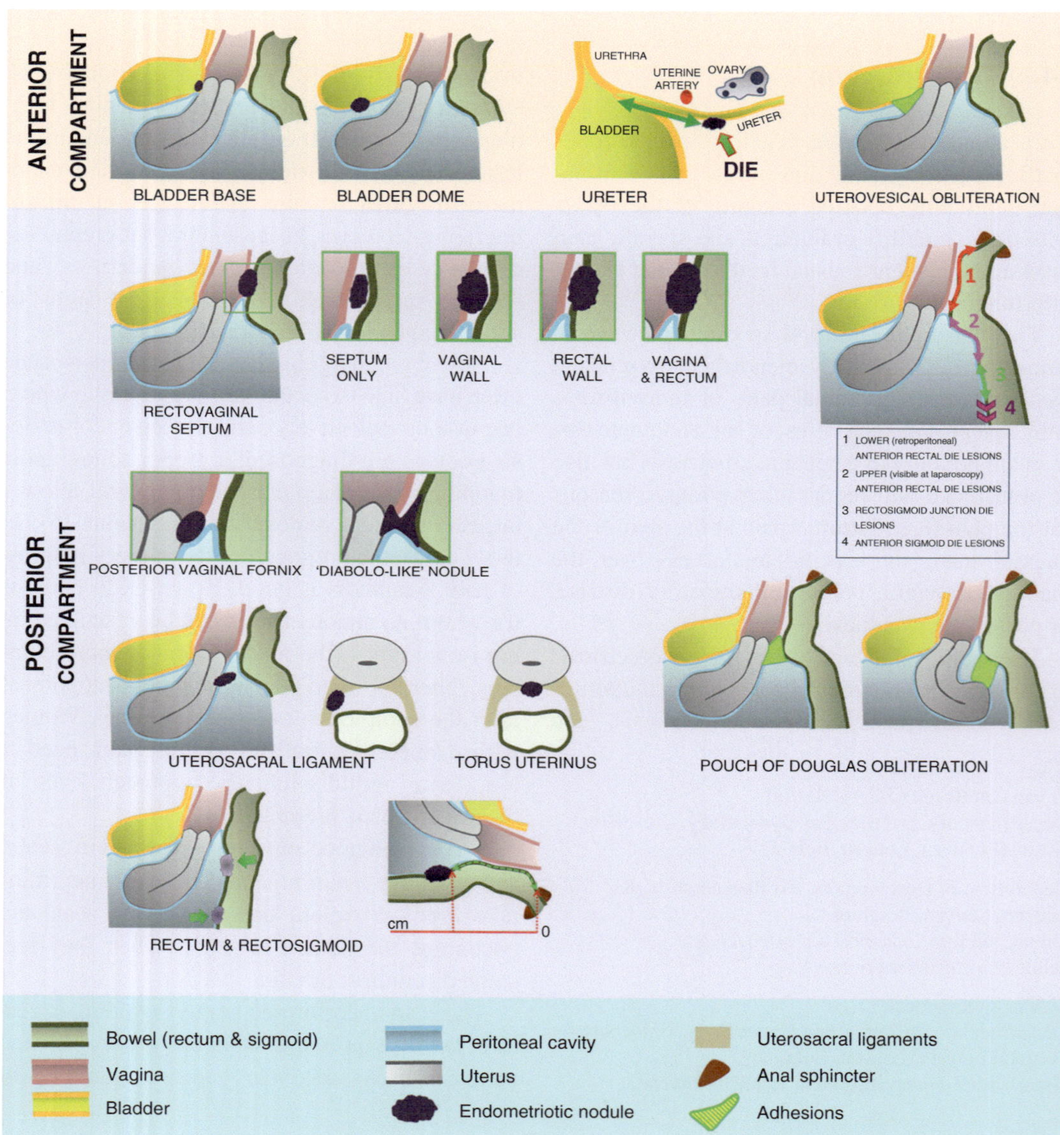

Fig. 14.1 Schematic overview of anterior and posterior locations of deep endometriosis. (From https://doi.org/10.1002/uog.15955 [6])

Endometriosis ultrasonography is usually performed via transvaginal scanning. To optimize superficial tissue image quality in the assessment of the vaginal wall, rectovaginal septum, and pouch of Douglas, creating a gel interface in the probe cover above the top of the probe (the stand-off technique) is advisable.

Sufficient gel should be applied onto the probe cover to optimize the sliding of the probe. In patients with introital pain and/or pelvic floor hypertonia, the introital application of lidocaine gel some minutes before the examination may be helpful. Explaining the sonographic images while slowly inserting the probe and allowing the necessary time for the pelvic floor to relax will improve the patient's confidence and cooperation.

An endometriosis nodule is a hypoechogenic, poorly vascularized solid lesion, sometimes irregular or ill-defined. At elastography, the nodule is typically relatively hard. An endometriotic implant is often, but not invariably, selectively painful when some pressure is applied with the probe. Therefore, especially for small lesions, good communication between the patient and the examiner is crucial. The patient will guide the ultrasound examiner toward the lesion. This is known as *tenderness-guided sonography* and is key in optimal endometriosis sonography [8].

14.2 Anterior Compartment

In the anterior compartment, the bladder wall, the vesicouterine pouch, and the insertion of the round ligaments are evaluated. Some bladder filling will optimize the sonographic image quality, but a full or overly full bladder will restrict the proper evaluation of anterior sliding and of anterior and posterior compartment lesions.

The landmarks of the bladder trigone are the urethral ostium and both ureteral ostia. To visualize the urethra, the probe must be pointed toward the anterior wall of the vagina. The urethra is situated between the vaginal wall and the symphysis pubis, and it can be followed toward its origin in the bladder. From there, both ureters are identified laterally and cranially of the urethral ostium. The terminal part of the ureter runs through the bladder wall and is visible as a hypoechogenic tubular structure tangentially ending in the bladder. To visualize the left ureter, the probe is slowly moved laterally to the left while the probe is slightly turned anticlockwise; for the right ureter, the probe is slowly moved to the right while the probe is slightly turned clockwise.

The organ sliding between the bladder and the uterus is evaluated by gently moving the probe into the anterior fornix and pushing the uterus or via deep palpation on the suprapubic region with the examiner's free hand. In the event of the partial or total obliteration of the vesicouterine pouch, the sliding sign will be negative. A negative sliding sign suggests adhesions. These may be due to endometriosis, pelvic infection, or postoperative sequalae (e.g., after cesarean section).

The bladder wall is scrutinized for endometriotic implants in the trigonum, the bladder base, the bladder dome, and the retroperitoneal part of the bladder—the latter rarely being involved. An endometriotic nodule presents as a hypoechogenic, somewhat irregular mass in the bladder serosa and muscularis, sometimes invading the bladder mucosa. Besides its size and the level of involvement of the bladder wall, reporting the exact location of the lesion using the landmarks of the trigonum is also crucial. To detect/exclude hydroureteronephrosis, a transabdominal ultrasound needs to be performed. Figure 14.2 schematically shows the landmarks in the anterior compartment.

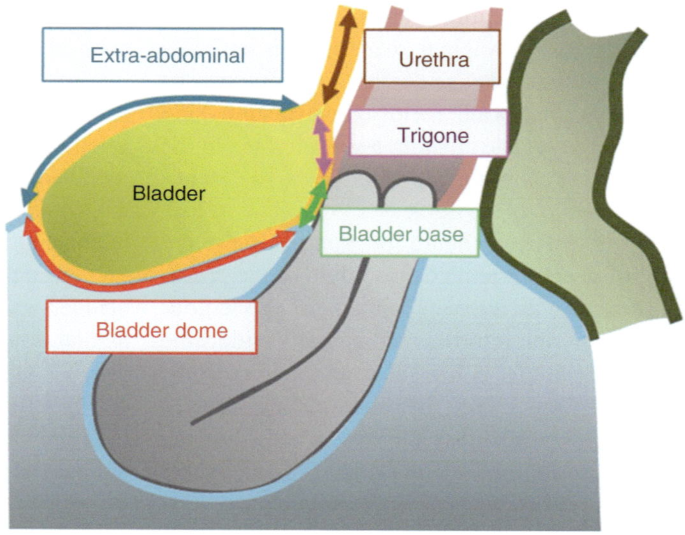

Fig. 14.2 Schematic overview of the landmarks in the anterior compartment. (From https://doi.org/10.1002/uog.15955 [6])

14.3 Posterior Compartment

The posterior compartment comprises the posterior vaginal wall up to the posterior fornix, the rectovaginal septum, the rectal- and rectosigmoid wall, the uterosacral ligaments, the retrocervical area (including the torus uteri), and the pouch of Douglas.

Starting a sonographic examination via the evaluation of the rectovaginal wall may be advisable. Starting from the introitus, the more hypoechogenic vaginal wall is followed up to the posterior fornix. To optimize image quality, the instillation of an excess of gel into the probe cover may be considered to obtain an acoustic window. This "standoff" technique improves the detection of small vaginal wall endometriosis lesions. The rectovaginal septum is the linear echogenic tissue underneath the vaginal wall. The underlying rectal muscularis is a hypoechogenic band that can be followed from the anal sphincter up to the rectosigmoid portion of the bowel. The typical three rectovaginal "hypoechogenic-hyperechogenic-hypoechogenic" layers are easily visible up to the caudal fold of the pouch of Douglas.

Once the pouch of Douglas has been reached, the rectum runs slightly dorsally. At this point the rectal wall often makes a U-shaped dorsal fold, where visualizing the continuity of the rectal muscularis can be more difficult.

The upper rectal- and rectosigmoid wall is visible as an alternation of hyperechogenic and hypoechogenic stripes: starting from the echogenic serosa, the hypoechogenic muscularis externa and interna (in between, a fine echogenic line is often visible), the hyperechogenic submucosa, and finally the hypoechogenic muscularis mucosae, the hyperechogenic intestinal mucosa, and the bowel lumen. Reporting whether the inner muscularis and the submucosa are involved is important for surgeons.

If an endometriotic lesion is visualized in the bowel wall, the lesion size, location, and depth of wall involvement need to be reported. Because such visualization may be relevant for (surgical) management, a three-dimensional (3D) acquisition might be convenient to obtain a proper transverse section of the affected bowel segment and allow a reliable estimation of the affected bowel circumference.

A nonobliterated posterior compartment may contain some anechogenic fluid in the pouch of Douglas, allowing the evaluation of the peritoneal surface for the presence of tiny (superficial endometriosis) lesions and adhesions.

The uterosacral ligaments (USL) are hyperechogenic bandlike structures originating from the torus at the upper posterior part of the cervix and running laterally toward the sacrum. The orientation of the uterosacral ligaments is rather horizontal unless the cervix is pushed cranially with a probe. The uterosacral ligaments are assessed on transverse section. When using 3D acquisition starting from the midsagittal position, the USL will appear on the B-plane (transverse section).

The posterior compartment may be partially or totally obliterated. In the latter case, organ sliding between the posterior uterine wall and the rectosigmoid wall will be completely absent.

Figure 14.3 schematically shows the landmarks in the posterior compartment.

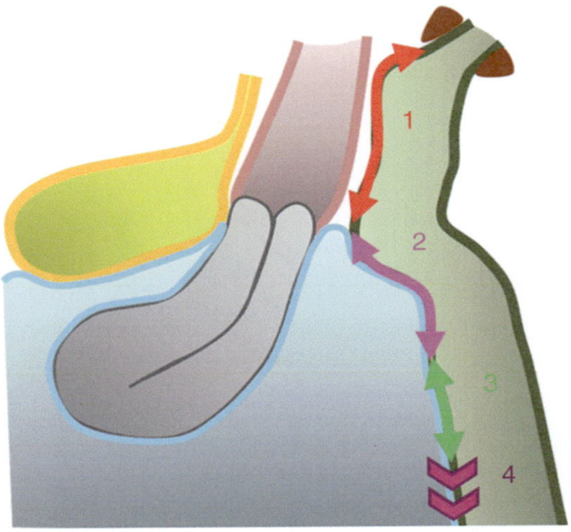

Fig. 14.3 Schematic overview of the landmarks in the posterior compartment. (From https://doi.org/10.1002/uog.15955 [6])

14.4 Lateral Compartments

The evaluation of the lateral compartments starts at the ureters. Each ureter is followed up cranially from the bladder ostium toward the overcrossing of the uterine artery and further over the lateral pelvic wall. In the case of endometriotic implants in the proximity of the ureter, the deviation from and infiltration into the ureter wall should be scrutinized [9].

Other landmarks of the lateral compartment include the iliac vessels, the pelvic side walls, the highly echogenic anterior face of the sacrum, and the presacral nerve roots running ventrolaterally from the sacrum. Figures 14.4, 14.5 and 14.6 shows the schematic overview of the female pelvic structures with the identification of the lateral parametrial area.

Fig. 14.4 Schematic drawing of female pelvic structures featuring the identification of parametrial areas in a transverse pelvic section. (From https://doi.org/10.1002/uog.27558 [9])

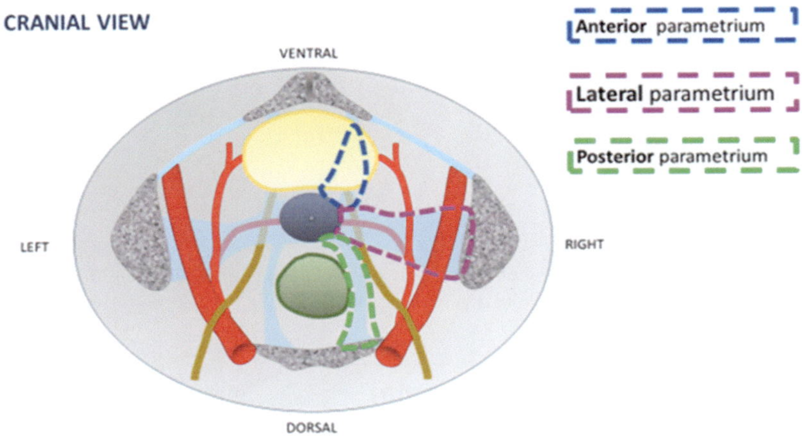

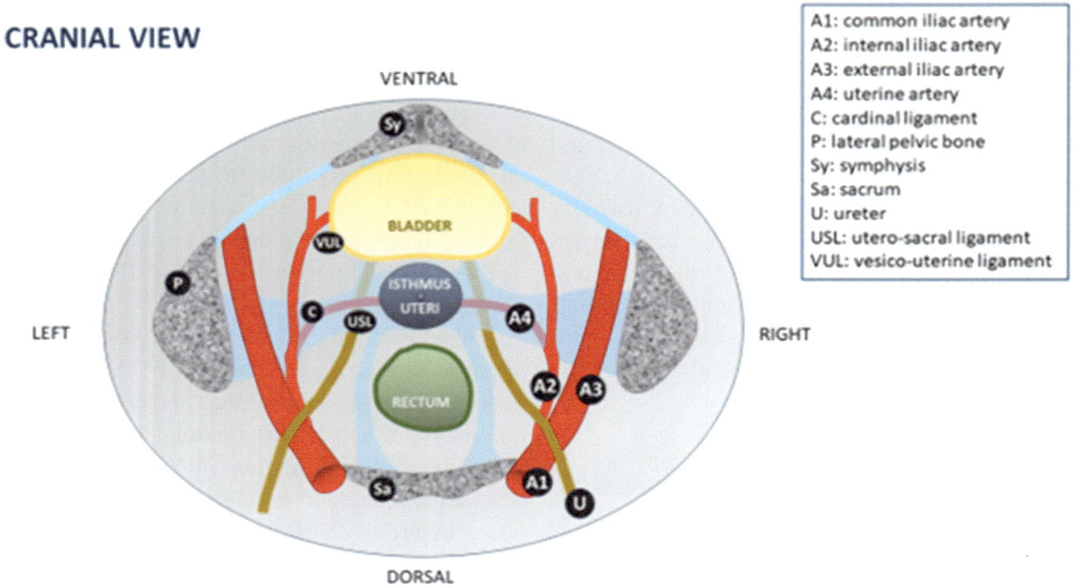

Fig. 14.5 Schematic drawing of female pelvic parametrial ligament in a transversal pelvic section. (From https://doi.org/10.1002/uog.27558 [9])

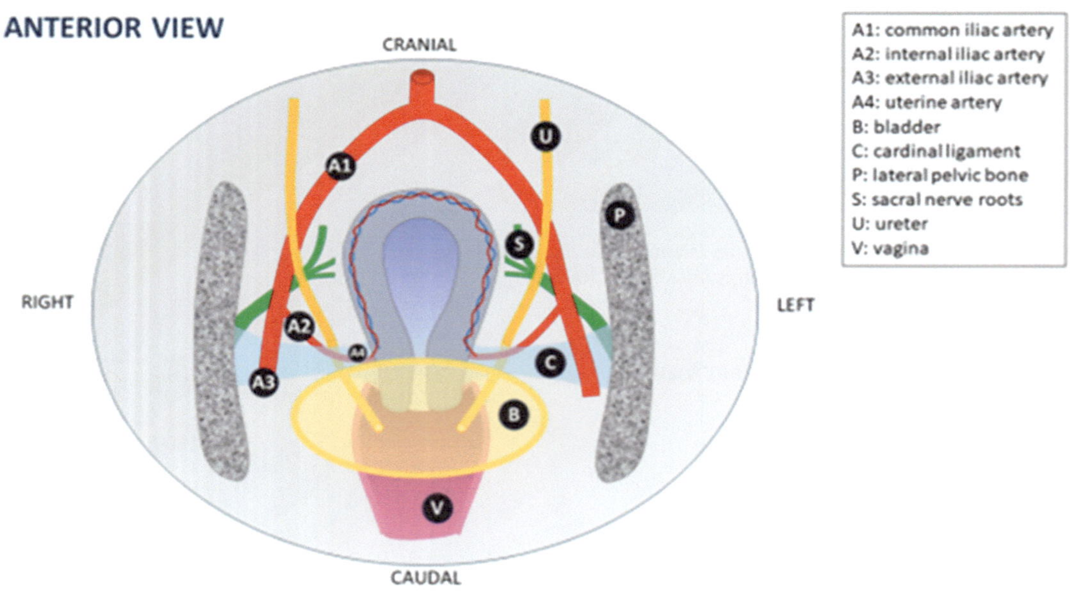

Fig. 14.6 Schematic drawing of female pelvic structures featuring the identification of the lateral parametrial area in a coronal section. (From https://doi.org/10.1002/uog.27558 [9])

14.5 Ovaries (Endometrioma)

The ovaries are evaluated for the presence or absence of cystic endometriosis, typically defined in a premenopausal woman as the presence of a cystic lesion with one to four locules with ground-glass content, without solid parts [10]. The sliding of the ovary to the pelvic sidewall, the uterus, the uterosacral ligaments, or the bowel wall is to be evaluated with gentle pressure with the vaginal probe or with the abdominal free hand of the examiner.

14.6 Uterus (Direct and Indirect Signs of Adenomyosis)

Due to endometriosis or adhesions in the posterior compartment, the fundus uteri may be pulled backward significantly, resulting in steep fundal retroflexion as visible in sagittal section: The uterine position is then reported as an "ear sign" or a "question mark sign."

Pelvic nodules are often associated with adenomyosis, especially adenomyosis affecting the external myometrium (e.g., focal adenomyosis of the outer myometrium).

Besides the evaluation of site-specific tenderness over the uterus, direct and indirect signs of adenomyosis should be searched for. Direct signs of adenomyosis reflect the presence of ectopic endometrial tissue in the myometrium and include subendometrial echogenic lines and buds, myometrial echogenic islands, and myometrial cysts. Indirect signs of adenomyosis are features secondary to the ectopic myometrial tissue and include an asymmetric myometrium, a globular uterus, an irregular or interrupted junctional zone, fan-shaped shadowing, and translesional vascularity.

14.7 Other Locations (Abdominal Wall Endometriosis)

Abdominal wall endometriosis is seen mainly after abdominal surgery (e.g., cesarean section). On clinical examination, the pain can be pointed at with one finger, and a small hard nodule can be palpated. Contracting the abdominal wall muscles may increase selective tenderness. At abdominal ultrasound, preferably with a linear probe, an irregular, hypoechogenic, and nonvascularized nodule is seen.

14.8 Conclusion

Endometriosis requires taking a holistic multidisciplinary team approach, ultrasound examination being part of it. Ultrasonography is essential in the diagnostic workup of patients with pelvic pain. It enables a detailed evaluation confirming or excluding the presence of endometrioma(s) and endometriotic nodules and allows preoperative mapping in those planned for surgery.

References

1. Zondervan KT, Becker CM, Missmer SA. Endometriosis. N Engl J Med. 2020;382(13):1244–56.
2. Piketty M, Chopin N, Dousset B, Millischer-Bellaische AE, Roseau G, Leconte M, et al. Preoperative work-up for patients with deeply infiltrating endometriosis: transvaginal ultrasonography must definitely be the first-line imaging examination. Hum Reprod. 2009;24(3):602–7.
3. Van Den Bosch T, Van Schoubroeck D. Ultrasound diagnosis of endometriosis and adenomyosis: state of the art. Best Pract Res Clin Obstet Gynaecol. 2018;51:16–24.
4. Okaro E, Condous G, Khalid A, Timmerman D, Ameye L, Van Huffel S, et al. The use of ultrasound-based "soft markers" for the prediction of pelvic pathology in women with chronic pelvic pain—can we reduce the need for laparoscopy? BJOG. 2006;113:251.
5. Menakaya U, Reid S, Lu C, Bassem G, Infante F, Condous G. Performance of ultrasound-based endometriosis staging system (UBESS) for predicting level of complexity of laparoscopic surgery for endometriosis. Ultrasound Obstet Gynecol. 2016;48(6):786–95.
6. Guerriero S, Condous G, Van Den Bosch T, Valentin L, Leone FPG, Van Schoubroeck D, et al. Systematic approach to sonographic evaluation of the pelvis in women with suspected endometriosis, including terms, definitions and measurements: a consensus opinion from the international deep endometriosis analysis (IDEA) group. Ultrasound Obstet Gynecol. 2016;48(3):318–32.
7. Reid S, Lu C, Casikar I, Reid G, Abbott J, Cario G, et al. Prediction of pouch of Douglas obliteration in women with suspected endometriosis using a new real-time dynamic transvaginal ultrasound technique: the sliding sign. Ultrasound Obstet Gynecol. 2013;41(6):685–91.
8. Guerriero S, Ajossa S, Gerada M, Virgilio B, Angioni S, Melis GB. Diagnostic value of transvaginal "tenderness-guided" ultrasonography for the prediction of location of deep endometriosis. Hum Reprod. 2008;23(11):2452–7.
9. Guerriero S, Condous G, Rolla M, Hudelist G, Ferrero S, Alcazar JL, et al. Addendum to the consensus opinion from the international deep endometriosis analysis (IDEA) group: sonographic evaluation of the parametrium. Ultrasound Obstet Gynecol. 2024;64:275.
10. Van Holsbeke C, Van Calster B, Guerriero S, Savelli L, Paladini D, Lissoni AA, et al. Endometriomas: their ultrasound characteristics. Ultrasound Obstet Gynecol. 2010;35(6):730–40.

15 Techniques and Reporting of the Imaging Techniques and Classifications: MR Imaging

Isabelle Thomassin-Naggara, Rana Al Rouhban, and Lucia Manganaro

15.1 Introduction

"Optimised communication between patients and the imaging team is an essential component of providing patient-centered and value-based care" [1], as underlined by European Society of Radiology. Imaging reporting is a crucial tool for communication. Moreover, communication with the clinician who referred the patient for the examination needs to be thorough; communication with the patient is another key issue, especially for patients with severe endometriosis [2]. Endometriosis is a benign disease that may, however, require very complex surgery with potentially long-term impacts on the quality of life of the patient. Thus, particularly in endometriosis, communication with the patient should be thorough because they will be involved in determining the type of surgery. Thus, MR reporting must be detailed and understood by the patient, and a recent publication underlined the usefulness of using imaging classifications in endometriosis [2] for three main goals:

1. To correctly plan the surgery given that some locations may be difficult to remove and must be treated by an expert surgeon, such as deep endometriotic disease, which may involve different pelvic organs, such as urinary or digestive organs, and may thus require coordination among different surgical specialties in a same operation room
2. To help guide the patient to a tertiary center, with expertise in cases of severe endometriosis disease requiring a multidisciplinary team, including an expert radiologist, a fertility physician, a pain specialist, and an expert surgeon, for endometriosis and supportive care
3. To correctly inform the patient about the surgery by giving them practical information on operating time, hospital stay, and/or the risk of de novo dysuria

Among the several MR classifications proposed [3, 4], the dPEI score was the first MR score to be correlated with operating time, hospital stay, and postoperative complications [5]. Moreover, this score was validated in a large mul-

The original version of the chapter has been revised. A correction to this chapter can be found at https://doi.org/10.1007/978-3-031-82750-1_17

I. Thomassin-Naggara (✉)
Imageries Radiologiques et Interventionnelles Spécialisées (IRIS), Tenon Hospital, AP-HP, Sorbonne Université, Paris, France
e-mail: isabelle.thomassin@aphp.fr

R. Al Rouhban
Centre Intercommunal de Creteil, Créteil, France
e-mail: Rana.Alrouhban@chicreteil.fr

L. Manganaro
Department of Radiological, Oncological and Pathological Sciences, Sapienza University "of Rome, Rome, Italy
e-mail: veronica.celli@uniroma1.it

I. Thomassin-Naggara (ed.), *Imaging of Endometriosis: A Comparative Guide of US, MRI and Surgery*, https://doi.org/10.1007/978-3-031-82750-1_15

ticentric cohort on 605 patients, confirming high reproducibility and high accuracy, which helps clinicians to correctly inform the patient on these elements [6]. Finally, many publications have revealed the role of structured reporting in improving the communication of diagnostic radiology findings [7]. In this chapter, we will present a structured report proposed by the Société d'Imagerie de la Femme (SIFEM) and the European Society of Urogenital Radiology.

15.2 MR Technique

The pelvic MR protocol is based on the recommendations of the European Society of Urogenital Radiology [8]. Regarding the preparation of the patient, a consensus was reached on the necessity of fasting (for 3–6 h) and belt strapping. An antiperistaltic agent is useful to limit movement artifacts and a half-empty bladder to not compress the posterior region of the pelvis.

Bowel enema preparation is crucial to optimize the quality of MR examination. This allows digestive distension and artifacts due to gas to be avoided. In addition, this improves the analysis of the rectosigmoid wall to depict any endometriotic location in the muscularis. This limits the value of rectal/vaginal opacification, which remains under debate. In fact, even if rectal/opacification enhances the detection of rectal/locations, the distension of these cavities obscures certain subtle deep endometriotic locations in the uterosacral ligaments (USLs). Rectal opacification should be performed in the case of inefficient bowel preparation (Fig. 15.1). Vaginal opacification can be useful before surgery to have a good evaluation a nodule in the posterior vaginal pouch. If systematically used, the radiologist should limit the amount of jelly (10-20cc). Another option is to perform gadolinium injection, which may improve the diagnostic performance of vaginal locations. The other indications of gadolinium injection are atypical adnexal endometriosis, the suspicion of a nodule in the abdominal wall, a suspicion of nerve injuries or an equivocal location on the bladder wall.

Regarding the acquisition MR protocol, magnet fields of 1.5 T or 3.0 T are equally recommended. The protocol needs to minimally include T2-weighted (T2W) images in different planes—the sagittal two-dimensional (2D) and axial 2D planes—and thin slices for 2D T2W images as part of the plan for the USLs. The alternative is to perform 3D T2W acquisition, which has the advantage of allowing a multiplanar analysis, which improves diagnostic performance [9]. Moreover, a 3D T1-weighted (T1W) Dixon sequence must be performed to recognize endometriotic fluid and hemorrhagic implants.

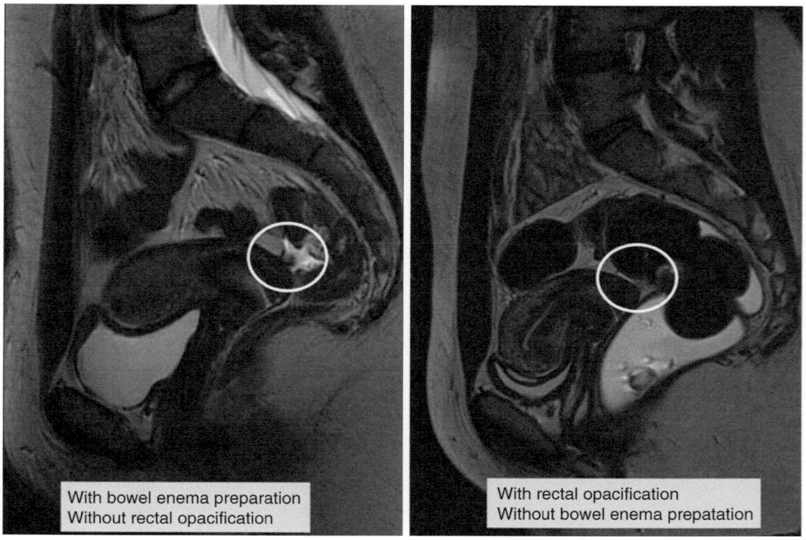

Fig. 15.1 MR technique

15.3 MR Reporting

15.3.1 General Considerations

As with any imaging report, different clinical elements should be mentioned, such as patient age, gestity, parity (the number of cesareans), the day of the menstrual cycle, and the indications for which symptoms the patient was referred in the context of a clinical suspicion of endometriosis: chronic pelvic pain associated with dysmenorrhea (EVA), deep dyspareunia, menstrual pain with urination and defecation, or scapular pain (side) during menstruation or infertility. This section should also mention whether the patient has any history of pelvic surgery or pelvic infection that may mimic deep pelvic endometriosis. Hormonal treatment and desire for pregnancy are also important details to report. In addition to the MR protocol and information on patient preparation, the technical quality of the examination should be stated: good/satisfactory/poor (motion artifacts or poor digestive preparation). Anatomic considerations should also be included, such as a description of the uterus (the size, the location, and laterodeviation), endometrial thickness, the presence of fibroids and internal adenomyosis, the position of the ovaries, whether ovarian parenchyma is visible, and the presence of hydrosalpinx with water or hemorrhagic signal.

15.3.2 Specific Description of Endometriotic Disease (Table 15.1)

15.3.2.1 Adnexal Endometriosis

The description of any endometrioma, defined as an ovarian cyst with high or very high T1W signal with SI equal or higher thant fat on non fat sat T1W sequence, must include the number, size, side, bilaterality, and presence of normal ovarian parenchyma. If a solid component is suspected on a T2W sequence, a gadolinium injection with a dynamic contrast sequence should be performed.

If the hemorrhagic cyst is smaller than 10 mm, it will be described as an ovarian implant (the side, the number, the size, whether it is central or peripheral, and whether it is typical). The presence or absence of endometriotic hematosalpinx is also part of an adnexal endometriosis description, for which the side (right or left) and the diameter should be mentioned.

15.3.2.2 Superficial Endometriosis

The presence of peritoneal pseudocysts with purely cystic or hemorrhagic signal, the presence of pelvic adhesions, and the presence or absence of peritoneal effusion should be mentioned. The complete obliteration of the Douglas pouch with suspended fluid in low abundance, highlighting pelvic adhesions, is also key information to report Moreover a periovoarian infiltration can be present medially and possibly associated with kissing ovaries. Finally, location in vesico uterin pouch without infiltration of the uterus or bladder is also considered as a superficial nodule.

15.3.2.3 Deeply Infiltrating Endometriosis

The description of deeply infiltrating endometriosis (DIE) in the dPEI reporting system is conducted through compartmental analysis, which involves dividing the pelvis into its anterior, medial, posterior regions and into its central and lateral compartments. In the following, we will use this classification to delineate the various locations within nine pelvic compartments and an additional extrapelvic compartment. A compartimental analysis is recommended with a division defining two horizontal lines with an anterior line passing anterior to the cervix or vagina and a posterior line passing anterior to the rectum and two vertical lines passing from back to front by the USL and the underlying mesorectal fascia, the lateral border of the uterine cervix or vagina, and the lateral wall of the bladder

Mediocentral Compartment This compartment encompasses the torus uterinum, proximal uterosacral ligaments (USLs), posterior vaginal pouch, rectovaginal septum, mesorectum and (if present) external anterior/posterior myometrial infiltration. The identification of endometriotic lesions within each of these structures, including

Table 15.1 Lexicon

Adnexal lesions	
Endometrioma	MR features: O-RADS descriptors Content is hypointense on T2WI and hyperintense on T1WI higher or equal to fat on non fat sat T1W sequence No internal enhancement No wall enhancement Size, unique/multiple, uni/bilateral, ipsilateral normal ovarian parenchyma, contralateral normal ovary (Size and number of follicules) If internal enhancement, atypical endometrioma that needs to be characterized with DW and DCE and rated with O-RADS MR score
Hematosalpinx	Dilated fallopian tubes with intraluminal hyperintense signal on fat suppressed T1W images. The low T2W signal intensity (T2 shading) frequently associated with endometriomas is not typically seen
Superficial endometriosis	
Peritoneal cystic lesion Endometriotic spot	Peritoneal cyst or bright T1W spot located on ovarian fossa, mesosalpinx, Douglas pouch, parietal peritoneum Uterin serosal plaques
Adhesions	Uterin deviation Uterin Z shape (in case of posterior adhesions) Periovarian infiltration Kissing ovaries (adhesions in ovarian fossa) Douglas symphysis
Deep pelvic endometriosis	
Medial locations	
Torus, proximal	Transversal orientation Positive diagnosis if: - Nodular (defined as if nodule is present in two planes). - Retraction (spiculate defined as irregularity present in two planes, distortion of the shape, surrounding fat infiltration) - Presence of hemorrhagic implant(s) whatever the thickening. Uncertain diagnosis (dashed circle) if: - Irregular or pseudonodular (present in only one plane). - Regular fibrotic thickening
Vagina	Nodule or thickening of the posterior vaginal wall. O'clock position. Length, thickness (double-headed arrows), transverse axis, and circumference by degree
Rectovaginal septum and anterior mesorectum	Nodule or mass located or extended between the vagina and the rectum, below the peritoneal pouch of Douglas reflexion. Length, transverse axis, thickness and distance to the anal verge.
Myometrial infiltration (anterior or posterior)	Nodular fibrotic extrinsic infiltration of the myometrium with ill defined borders § hemorrhagic cystic area. Length (double-headed arrows). Two level of extension in depth: - Moderate (limited to the subserosal external myometrium). - Severe (up to the junctional zone or more). Distance from the endometrium.

(continued)

Table 15.1 (continued)

Mediolateral parametrium	Irregular and/or retractile fibrotic infiltration +/- hemorrhagic cystic area of vascular and adipocellular tissue of lateral or posterolateral cervical (arrows) or vaginal regions, between the anterior and posterior lines.
Ureter	Fibrotic infiltration with abolition of the peri ureteric cellular and fat signal at the entry of the ureter in the parameter or more posteriorly at the level where it ran behind the posterior leaf of the broad ligament. +/- Ureteral dilatation. Involvement circumference (= or <360°). Length of involved ureter. Distance from ureterovesical junction.
Uterine artery	Fibrotic infiltration surrounding the uterine artery (serpiginous flow void) (arrows) with abolition of the peri artery cellular and fat signal
Pelvic wall, external iliac and/or obturator vessels, nerves	Fibrotic infiltration of external iliac and obturator vessels (dashed circles) and obturator muscles, up to the pelvic wall/obturator muscle Involvement of obturator nerve
Posterior locations	
Rectum and rectosigmoid junction	Thickening or mass of the rectosigmoid wall. Location within the rectosigmoid, considering the distance between the anal verge and the middle point of the rectal lesion, as follows: Lower rectum (0–5 cm) Middle rectum (5–10 cm) Upper rectum (10–15 cm) Recto-sigmoid junction (>15 cm). Distance to the anal verge and the lower point of the lesion. O'clock position. The length, transverse axis and the thickness. Circumference (by degree or by dividing the rectal wall into eight radii). Submucosal edema.
Posterolateral parametrium (Distal USL, Sacrorectal septum) infra ureteral parametrium	Positive diagnosis if: fibrotic nodular infiltration within the lateral pelvic compartment, behind the posterior horizontal line passing anteriorly to the rectum, either unilaterally or bilaterally, with loss of the normal appearance of the retro- and subperitoneal pararectal space located outside the mesorectal fascia. The USL represents the roof of the sacrorectal septum, therefore, an endometriotic deposit that infiltrates underneath and outside the USL into the pararectal space invades the sacrorectal septum. Diagnostic criteria of distal USL location are the same than proximal USL
Sacral roots, sciatic nerve, internal iliac vessels and pelvic wall	Fibrotic infiltration of sacral roots, sciatic nerve, internal iliac vessels, and pelvic wall, often in continuity with the infiltration of the sacro-recto-genital septum.

(continued)

Table 15.1 (continued)

Anterior locations	
Bladder	Nodule or mass involving the muscularis layer. Lateralization of the lesion: median, right sided, or left-sided. Three different locations within the bladder wall: Anterior dome. At the level of vesicouterine pouch. Bladder base. Size in the three planes. Distance to ureteral orifice.
Proximal Round ligaments	"Proximal" correspond to intrapelvic third of round ligament. Fibrotic nodular thickening (generally > 1cm) § hemorrhagic cystic area (arrows) Often associated with external adenomyosis. Size.
Distal round ligaments	Distal" correspond to the intrapelvic two thirds of round ligament, up to the deep orifice and/or into the inguinal canal. Fibrotic nodular thickening (generally > 1cm) § hemorrhagic cystic area (arrows). Size.
Extra pelvic locations	
Cecum-ileum-appendix	Fibrotic nodular infiltration of the caecum and ileum (+/- ileum distension) including distance to the ileocecal valve or appendicular wall (+/- appendix distension), with size of lesion.
Sigmoid colon	Lesion located above the rectosigmoid junction, indicating the proximal or distal part of the sigmoid. Size and number of lesions. Length, thickness and circumference +/- upstream distension.
Abdominal wall	Fibrotic nodular infiltration +/- hemorrhagic cystic area of the rectus muscles and/or lateral muscles, or subcutaneous fat tissue with size, percentage of muscular infiltration, relationship with the muscle fasciae and distance to the skin. Umbilical nodule
Inguinal regions	Nodular fibrotic infiltration +/- hemorrhagic cystic area of the terminal extra pelvic part of the round ligament at the level of the superficial orifice of inguinal canal or in the labia majora.

Orange: central compartments; blue: lateral compartments; and green: extrapelvic compartments their measurements in mm along two orthogonal axes, should be reported.

Posterocentral Compartment In the posterocentral compartment, lesions on the low/medium/high rectum or rectosigmoid junction wall lesions should be specified, detailing their height, axial diameter, and anteroposterior thickness of each lesion in mm; their distance to the anal margin in cm; and the degree of circumference involvement. The presence of submucosal edema is also pertinent information. Single or multiple lesions of the rectosigmoid wall may be present, necessitating a detailed description of each lesion.

Anterocentral Compartment In the anterocentral compartment, the involvement of the proximal intrapelvic third of the left or right round ligament should be delineated, including the nature of its involvement (nodular thickening and hemorrhagic spots), its size, and its relation to adjacent external anterior adenomyosis.

Bladder lesions should be categorized according to three locations in the bladder wall: the anterior two-thirds of the dome, the posterior third of the dome at the level of the vesicouterine pouch, and the bladder base. The description should encompass the lesion's dimensions in three planes, lateralization (median, right sided or left sided), and its distance to the right/left ureteral meatus.

Left and Right Mediolateral Compartments Reporting DIE in this compartment entails a description of the involvement of the mediolateral parametrium (supra ureteral parametrium), the ureter, the uterine artery, and the pelvic wall, including the external iliac vessels, obturator vessels, and obturator muscles. Mediolateral parametrium corresponds to vascular and adipose tissue of the lateral or posterolateral cervical or vaginal regions. This typically arises from a nodular lesion (over 1 cm) in the proximal uterosacral ligament extending downwards and outwards or from a lesion in the inferior and posterior broad ligament.This description should specify the type of involvement (fibrotic infiltration) and the side; for the ureter, the description should include not only these data points but also the involvement circumference (= or < 360°), length of the involved ureter, and distance from the ureterovesical junction.

Left and Right Posterolateral Compartments For the left and right posterolateral compartments, descriptions should include the involvement of the posterolateral parametrium, behind the posterior horizontal line passing anteriorly to the rectum, either unilaterally or bilaterally, with loss of the normal appearance of the retro- and subperitoneal pararectal space located outside the mesorectal fascia. The distal USL represents the roof of the sacrorectal septum, therefore, an endometriotic deposit that infiltrates underneath and outside the USL into the pararectal space invades the sacrorectal septum.

- Distal uterosacral ligaments, specifying the type of involvement (nodulari, spiculate, and/or the presence of hemorrhagic implants), and any uncertain diagnoses (pseudonodular, retractile, or fibrotic regular thickening).
- Additionally, details on the involvement of the sacrorectal septum, including its laterality, height, and distance or extension to the iliococcygeus muscle of the levator ani, should be provided. Infiltration into the sacral roots, the sciatic nerve, the internal iliac vessels, and/or the pelvic wall should also be documented.

Left and Right Anterolateral Compartments Regarding the left and right anterolateral compartments, lesions of the distal intrapelvic two-thirds of the round ligament up to the deep orifice and/or into the inguinal canal should be described. Information on the size of the lesion and the presence or absence of hemorrhagic implants should be included in the report. Anterolateral parametrium correspond to perivesical space which should be particularaly described in case of infiltration of the proximal protion of the ureter.

Extrapelvic Compartment Each lesion should be individually documented.

Caecum and ileum: Fibrotic nodular infiltration into the caecum and ileum, including the distance from the ileocecal valve or appendicular wall, along with the lesion's size, should be noted.

Sigmoid colon: Lesions above the rectosigmoid junction should be specified by indicating their location in the proximal or distal part of the sigmoid. The size and number of lesions, as well as the length, thickness, circumference, and upstream distension, should be noted.

Abdominal wall: Fibrotic nodular infiltration, with or without hemorrhagic cystic areas, into the rectus muscles, lateral muscles, or subcutaneous fat tissue should be described in detail by including the size, percentage of muscular infiltration, relationship with the muscle fasciae, and distance to the umbilical nodule.

Inguinal regions: Nodular fibrotic infiltration, with or without hemorrhagic cystic areas, in the terminal extrapelvic part of the round ligament at the superficial orifice of the inguinal canal or in the labia majora should be included in the report.

15.4 MR Classifications

Several published MR classifications that describe endometriosis have had several objectives: (1) to standardize MR report, (2) to evaluate the severity of the disease, (3) to predict the impact of the disease on fertility, and (4) to preoperatively inform patients of the risk of complications. Historically, the first and the most widely used one is a classification proposed by the American Society for Reproductive Medicine (ASRM). This classification is a surgical one that includes a description of superficial and adnexal endometriotic disease but lacks a description of most deep endometriotic nodules, especially the nodules nonvisible on laparoscopy.

Thus, a second classification, one based on surgical findings, was proposed, named ENZIAN classification, which was recently modified and became the #ENZIAN classification. This classification is based on the identification of three types of lesions, depending on their location. The lesions are labeled "A" when in the vagina–rectovaginal space, labeled "B" in the uterosacral ligaments, and labels "C" in the rectum sigmoid colon. For all these locations, a measurement must be performed to categorize the lesion: category 1 (<1 cm), category 2 (2–3 cm), and category 3 (>3 cm). In addition, the presence of adenomyosis (FA), bladder nodules (FBs), an extension to the ureters (FU), and intestinal involvement (the coecum and ileum) (FI) should be specified. The severity of lesions in compartments A and C are correlated with operating time, hospital stay, and the presence of postoperative complications [5]. Unfortunately, the assessment of the lesions located in the B compartments has a huge reproducibility problem. A prospective multicenter study (the cENZIAN study) showed very poor reproducibility for theses lesions, which are the most frequent locations using ENZIAN for the ratings of preoperative MR studies [10]. In fact, in clinical practice, performing a measurement on the USLs is complex because the orientation of the USLs varies considerably among patients. Thus, intra and inter-reproducibility assessment is poor [5].

Because of this limitation, a dedicated classification created from MR images has been developed. Because MR imaging allows the description of lesions that are not visible at surgery, it meets an urgent need. In addition, to improve reproducibility, the PCI model inspired the development of a new classification, named dPEI classification. This classification is based on the description of nine pelvic compartments and one extrapelvic compartment. The nine compartments are the three classical ones in the center of the pelvic (anterior, medial, posterior) and these compartments are separated from the lateral ones by the visceral fascia. Thus, six other compartments exist: the anterolateral, mediolateral, and posterolateral compartments on both sides [11] (Fig. 15.2). This classification was developed and validated first at one center [5] and then at multiple centers [6]. A dPEI value is calculated by adding the number of compartments where the disease is detected and adding additional points

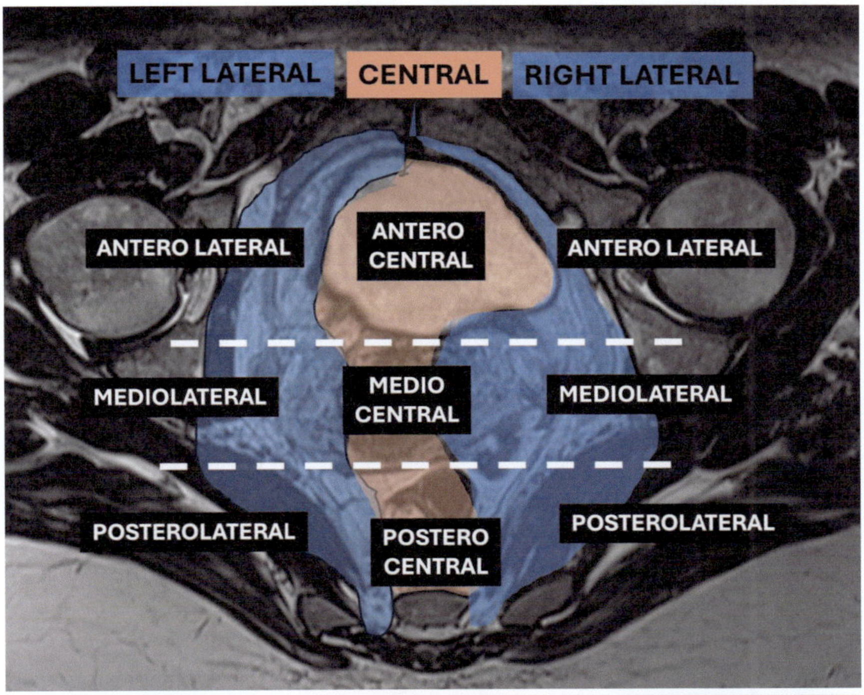

Right anterolateral	Anterocentral	Left anterolateral
Anterolateral parametrium Distal round ligament	Bladder Proximal round ligament	Anterolateral parametrium Distal round ligament
Right mediolateral	**Mediocentral**	**Left mediolateral**
Mediolateral parametrium Ureter – Uterine artery Pelvic wall (Muscle, Nerve, Vessels)	Torus and proximal USL External myometrial infiltration Vagina Rectovaginal septum Mesorectum	Mediolateral parametrium Ureter – Uterine artery Pelvic wall (Muscle, Nerve, Vessels)
Right posterolateral	**Posterocentral**	**Left posterolateral**
Posterolateral parametrium (=infraureteral) 1) Distal USL 2) Sacro rectal septum Pelvic wall (Muscle, Nerve, Vessels)	Rectum Rectosigmoid junction	Posterolateral parametrium (=infraureteral) 1) Distal USL 2) Sacro rectal septum Pelvic wall (Muscle, Nerve, Vessels)
Extra pelvic		
Caecum, ileum appendix, Sigmoid colon, Abdominal wall, inguinal regions, ureter at the level of common iliac artery		

Fig. 15.2 Deep Pelvic Endometriosis Index

in the event of vaginal pouch location, lombar ureteral distension, bladder basis location, or a location detected on the pelvic wall. This overall score predicts operating time and hospital stay with a linear correlation between the score and these features (Fig. 15.3). Moreover, this classification helps to define three levels of risk for postoperative complications, where the low-risk group (score 1–2) is only at a 3.3% risk of postoperative complications, the intermediate group (score 3–4) is at a 5.5% risk, and the high-risk group (score 5 and more) is at a 10.2% risk. Both publications show that the highest scores are associated with the presence of lateral locations, which clearly define the level of difficulty in surgeries and the risk of nerve injuries that are responsible mainly for these postoperative complications, such as de novo dysuria. Using dPEI also allows for predicting postoperative complications, which is crucial to discuss with patients before deciding on a surgery. The use of such classifications is an important tool to communicate with patients and helps in shared decision-making.

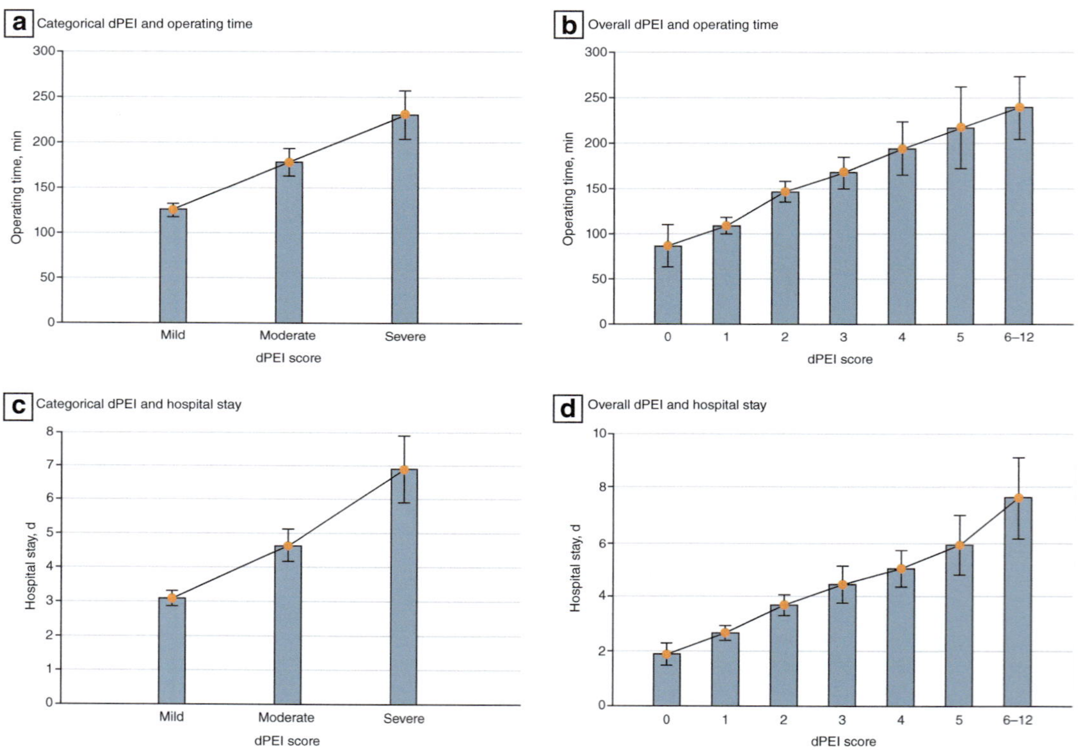

Fig. 15.3 Prediction of operating time and hospital stay with dPEI. (Source: Thomassin-Naggara et al. [6])

15.5 Key Images and Drawings

In the introduction, we underlined the importance of communication, especially during multidisciplinary team (MDT) sessions with clinicians. In endometriosis, this is particularly important because it illustrates the findings with key images to guide the surgeon on how to approach lesions that will not be visible before they open the peritoneum. The radiologist should select key images and insert arrows to explain the findings.

In addition, an easy way to improve communication with patients is to use drawings. The terms used in a MR report are complex and difficult to understand. Drawings may help the surgeon to explain the surgery and may help in shared decision-making with the patient.

Example 1 Example of Standardized Report: Adnexal Endometriosis

Clinical Information

A 31-year-old patient, GP0, presenting with pelvic pain and dysuria, referred for the suspicion of endometriosis

No previous medical or surgical history

Technique

Bowel preparation (4 h of fasting, enema, and injection of 1 mL of glucagon)

T2-weighted images in sagittal plane, and axial plane, 3D cube T2-weighted images, and 3D T1-DIXON weighted images were also obtained on the pelvis

Results

The uterus is normal in shape and in size, anteflexed, displaced to the right, measuring 79 × 23 × 47 mm

The myometrium is homogeneous without myomas or signs of adenomysis

The endometrium measures 6 mm in thickness, without an intracavitary lesion

The cervix is unremarkable

The ovaries are in proximity, both attracted to the midline with adherence to the posterior uterine wall: "Kissing ovaries"

No visible tubal abnormality

Adnexal Endometriosis

Right endometrioma measuring 43 mm (CC) × 34 mm (AP) × 21 mm (T)

The right normal ovarian parenchyma is compressed, measuring 7 mm in thickness with a few follicles (around four)

Left endometrioma of 71 mm (CC) × 61 mm (AP) × 69 mm (T)

The left normal ovarian parenchyma is compressed, measuring 8 mm in thickness with a few follicles (around five)

Superficial Peritoneal Endometriosis

Millimetric implant of the right fallopian tube

Deep Endometriosis

Mediocentral compartment: small nodular lesion of the torus between the converging ovaries, measuring 5 × 4 mm, without adjacent myometrial infiltration

Posterocentral compartment: no involvement of the rectal wall

Anterocentral compartment: no bladder involvement

No involvement of the proximal round ligaments

Lateral compartments: no extension to the parametria or lateral pelvic side wall

Extrapelvic compartment: no detectable abnormalities in the region of the ileocecal junction.

No visible abnormalities on the anterior abdominal wall (including the umbilicus).

No dilatation of the pyelocaliceal cavities

No peritoneal fluid

Conclusion

Bilateral endometriomas

No visible superficial endometriosis

Deep pelvic endometriosis involving the mediocentral compartment

dPEI score 1 (mild risk) with only the mediocentral compartment affected

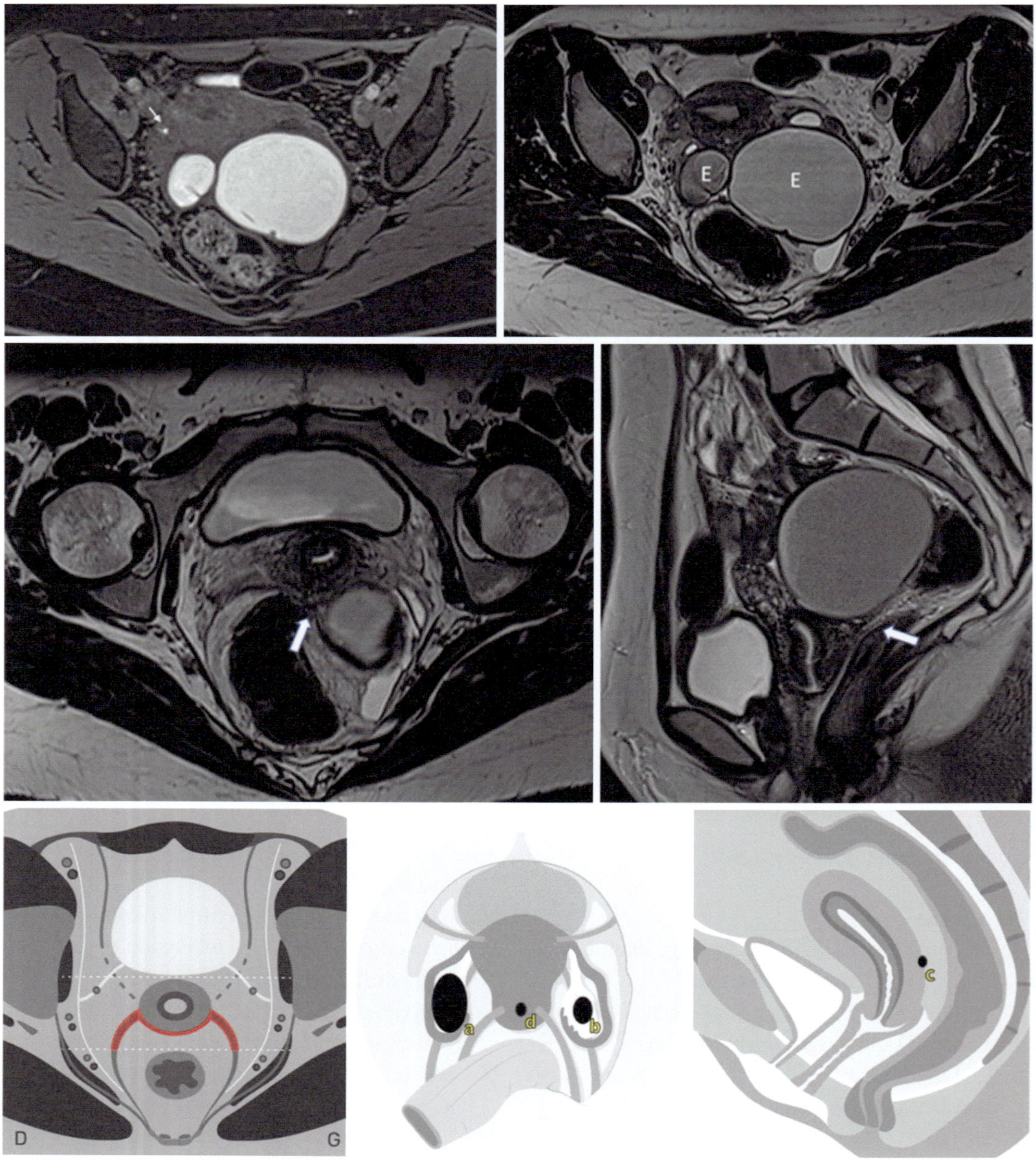

Key images (**a**) Axial T1W sequence, (**b**) axial T2W sequence, (**c**) axial T2W sequence, (**d**) sagittal T2W sequence drawings

Example 2 Example of Standardized Report: Mild Deep Pelvic Endometriotic Disease (dPEI score)

Clinical Information

A 36-year-old patient, known to have fibroids, presenting with dyspareunia, referred for fibroids cartography and the suspicion of endometriosis

Technique

Bowel preparation (4 h of fasting, enema, and injection of 1 mL of glucagon)

T2-weighted images in sagittal plane and axial plane, 3D cube T2-weighted images, and 3D T1-DIXON weighted images were also obtained on the pelvis

Results

The uterus is normal in shape, retroflexed, median in position, measuring 98 × 83 × 89 mm

The myometrium shows many fibroids (more than 10), all displaying low signal on T2 sequences, of which

- A FIGO6 left posterior fibroid, measuring 46 × 29 mm
- A FIGO4 left anterior fibroid, measuring 31 × 36 mm
- A FIGO6 left posterior fundic fibroid, measuring 31 × 30 mm

Diffuse deep internal adenomyosis

The endometrium measures 3 mm in thickness, without an intracavitary lesion

The cervix is unremarkable

The ovaries are attracted to the posterior wall of the uterus ("kissing ovaries"), measuring 4.4 cm² for the right ovary and 2.4 cm² for the left one, each showing very few follicles

There is no adnexal mass, no visible tubal abnormality

Adnexal Endometriosis

There is no detectable endometriotic implant or cyst.

Deep Endometriosis

Mediocentral compartment: nodular thickening of the torus and proximal uterosacral ligaments, measuring 22 mm (T) × 10 mm (AP) × 13 mm (CC)

Posterocentral compartment: no rectal involvement

Anterocentral compartment: no involvement of the bladder or round ligaments

Lateral compartments: no parametrial involvement or lateral pelvic side wall

Extrapelvic compartment: no detectable abnormalities in the region of the ileocecal junction and no visible abnormalities on the anterior abdominal wall (including the umbilicus)

No dilatation of the pyelocaliceal cavities

Conclusion

Multiple uterine fibroids

Deep diffuse symmetrical adenomyosis

No adnexal endometriosis

No visible superficial endometriosis

Deep pelvic endometriosis involving the torus uterinum and proximal uterosacral ligaments

dPEI score 1 (mild risk) with only one compartment affected

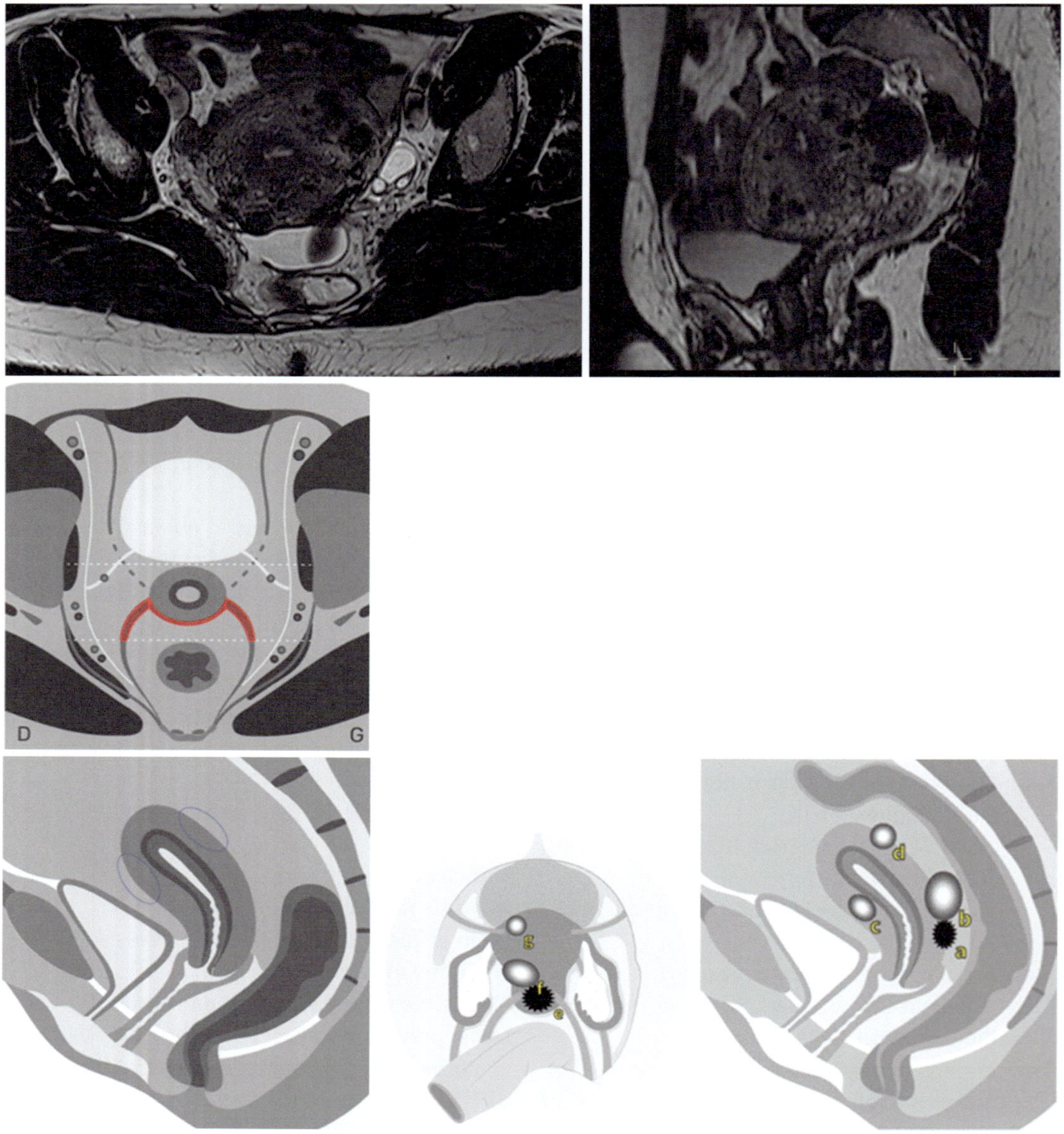

Key images (**a**) Axial T2W sequence, (**b**) sagittal T2W sequence and drawings

Example 3 Example of Standardized Report: Mild Disease (dPEI Score 1)

Clinical Information

A 32-year-old patient G2P0, presenting with pelvic chronic pain, dysmenorrhea, and dyspareunia, referred for the suspicion of deep pelvic endometriosis

Technique

Bowel preparation (4 h of fasting, enema (normacol), and injection of 1 mL of glucagon)

T2-weighted images in sagittal plane and axial plane, 3D cube T2-weighted images, and 3D T1-weighted images with and without fat saturation were also obtained on the pelvis

Results

The uterus is normal in shape, anteverted and anteflexed, median in position, measuring 99 × 41 × 51 mm

The myometrium is homogeneous without myomas or signs of adenomysis

The endometrium measures 6 mm in thickness, without an intracavitary lesion

The cervix is unremarkable

The ovaries are normal in position and in size with normal follicular count

No adnexal mass and no visible tubal abnormality

Adnexal Endometriosis

No detectable endometriotic implant or cyst.

Deep Endometriosis

Mediocentral compartment: a nodular spiculated thickening of the torus and right proximal uterosacral ligament measuring 4 mm in thickness and extending to 8 mm with hemorrhagic implant on T1

Posterocentral compartment: no rectal involvement

Anterocentral compartment: no involvement of the bladder or round ligaments

Lateral compartments: no parametrial involvement or lateral pelvic side wall locations

Extrapelvic compartment: no detectable abnormalities in the region of the ileocecal recess and no visible abnormalities on the anterior abdominal wall (including the umbilicus)

No dilatation of the pyelocaliceal cavities

Conclusion

Deep pelvic endometriosis involving the torus uterinum and proximal uterosacral ligaments

DPEI score 1 (mild risk) with only one compartment affected

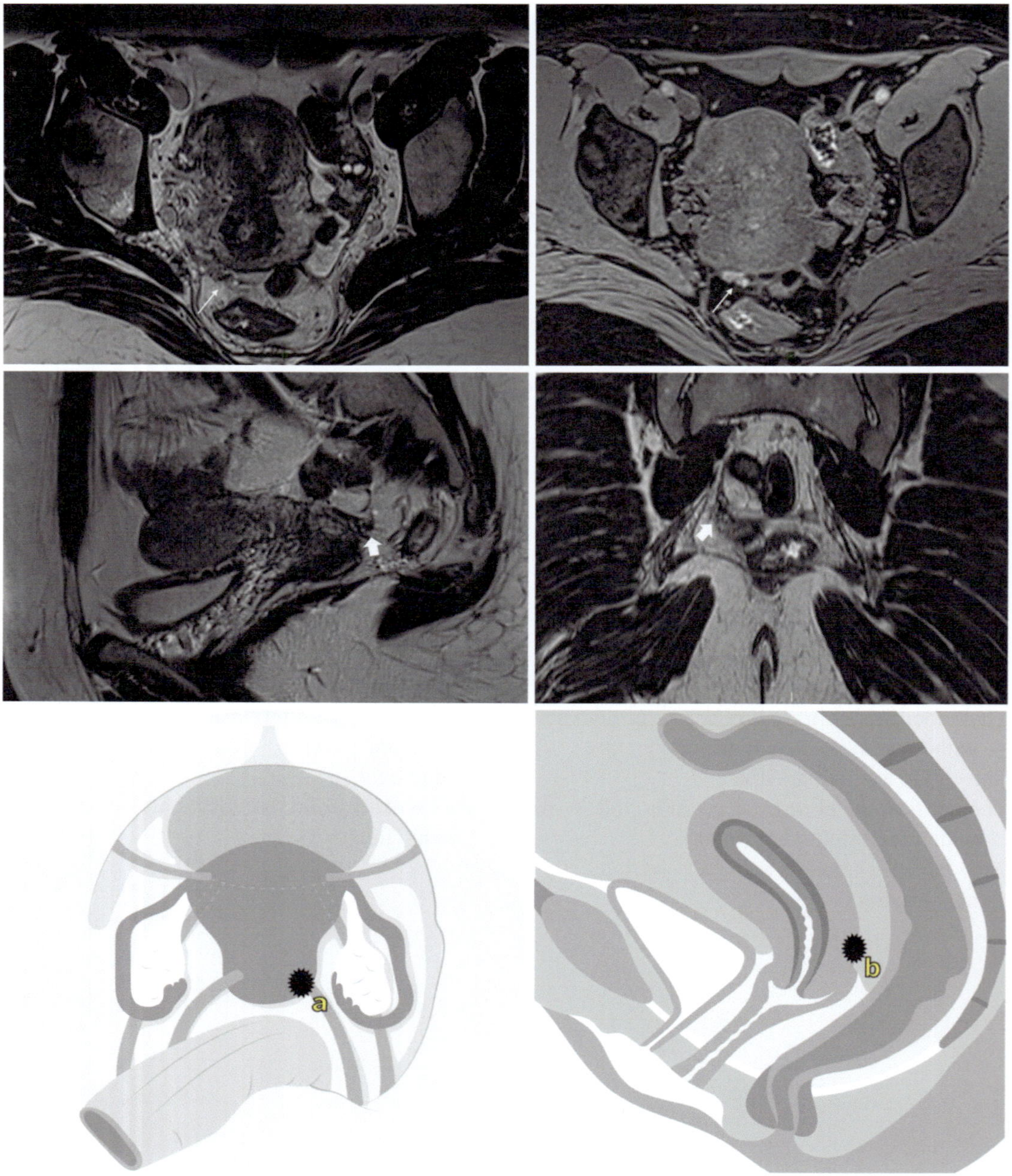

Key images (**a**) Axial T2W, (**b**) axial T1W sequence, (**c**) sagittal T2W, and (**d**) coronal T2W and drawings

Example 4 Example of Standardized Report: Mild Disease (dPEI Score 2)

Clinical Information

A 37-year-old patient, nulliparous, without contraception (stopped Optimizette medication 9 months ago), seen on cycle day 22, with a history of endometriosis without imaging, minimally symptomatic today referred for a Assisted Medical Procreation assessment

Technique

Bowel preparation (4 h of fasting, enema (normacol), and injection of 1 mL of glucagon)

T2-weighted images in sagittal plane and axial plane, 3D cube T2-weighted images, and 3D T1-DIXON weighted images were also obtained on the pelvis

Results

The uterus has regular contours, anteverted, anteflexed, median, normal in size—measuring 85 × 42 × 53 mm

The myometrium displays normal signal intensity without evidence of internal adenomyosis or myoma

The endometrium measures 16 mm, compatible with an endometrium of secretory phase without intracavitary anomalies

The cervix is unremarkable

The ovaries are in anatomical position:

- The right ovary measures 5 cm², with normal follicular count and a 13 mm corpus luteum associated with mild ovarian edema, without endometrioma or ovarian implant
- The left ovary measures 5 cm², with normal follicular count, without endometrioma or ovarian implant

No visible tubal anomalies

Adnexal Endometriosis

No endometrioma or hematosalpinx

Superficial Endometriosis

No superficial peritoneal implants

No peritoneal inclusion cysts

Small peritoneal effusion

Deep Endometriosis

Mediocentral compartment: asymmetric thickening of the proximal left uterosacral ligament (USL) of 3 mm, extending posterolaterally

No involvement of the torus, vagina, or rectovaginal septum

No external isthmic adenomyosis

Posterocentral compartment: thin adhesions of the Douglas pouch, without rectosigmoid involvement

Anterocentral compartment: no involvement of the bladder, vesicouterine pouch, or round ligaments

Lateral compartments: irregular nodule measuring 16 mm × 11 mm in the left sacrorectogenital fascia with endometriotic implants, located 3 mm from the lateral pelvic wall

Some adhesions extending to the posterior pelvic wall

No involvement of the parametria

Extrapelvic compartment: no detectable abnormalities in the region of the ileocecal recess and no visible abnormalities on the anterior abdominal wall (including the umbilicus)

No dilatation of the pyelocaliceal cavities

Conclusion

No adnexal endometriosis

No visible superficial endometriosis

Deep pelvic endometriosis with active implants featuring the involvement of the left proximal and distal uterosacral ligament extending to the ipsilateral sacrorectogenital fascia associated with endometriotic active implants

dPEI 2 (mild risk) with mediocentral involvement (proximal left USL) and posterolateral involvement (left sacrorectogenital fascia).

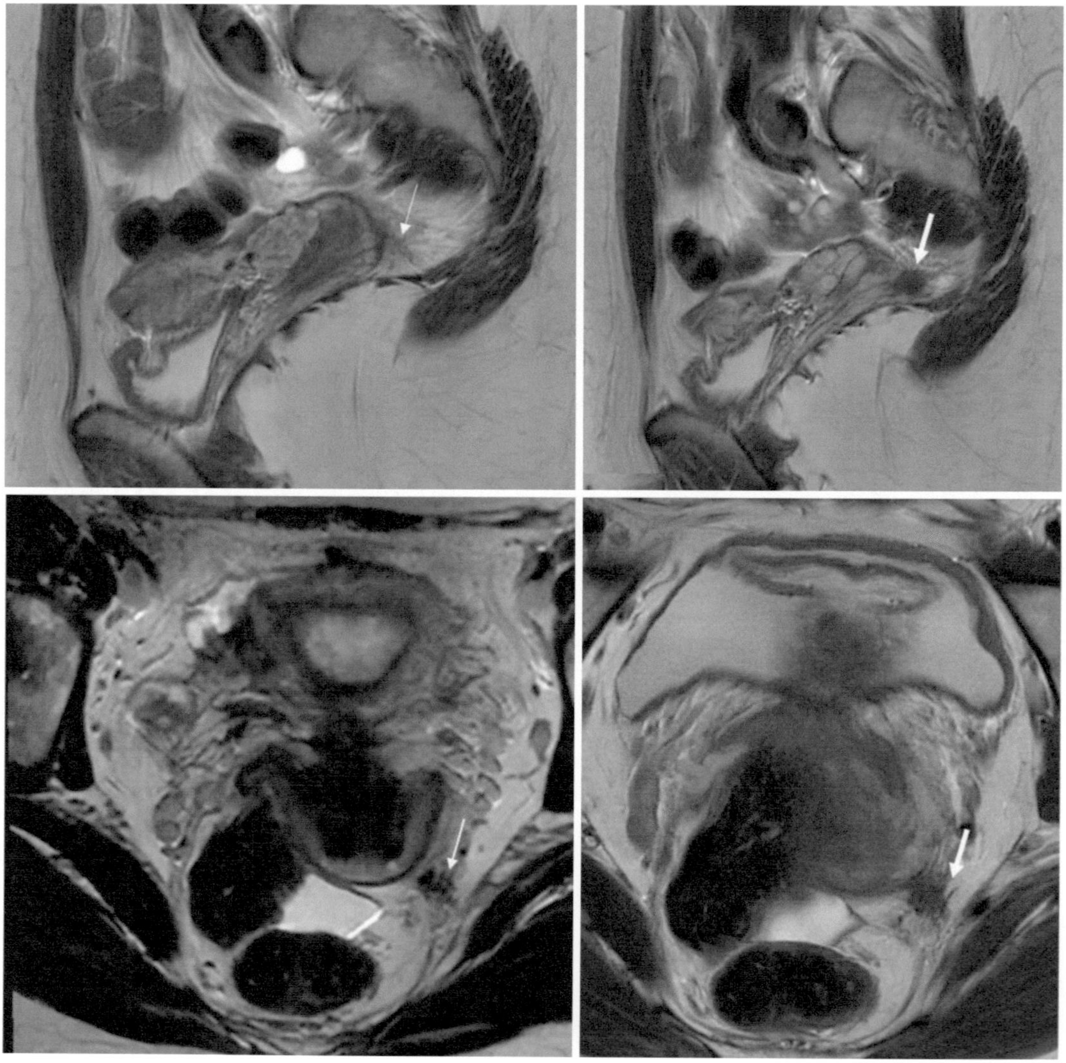

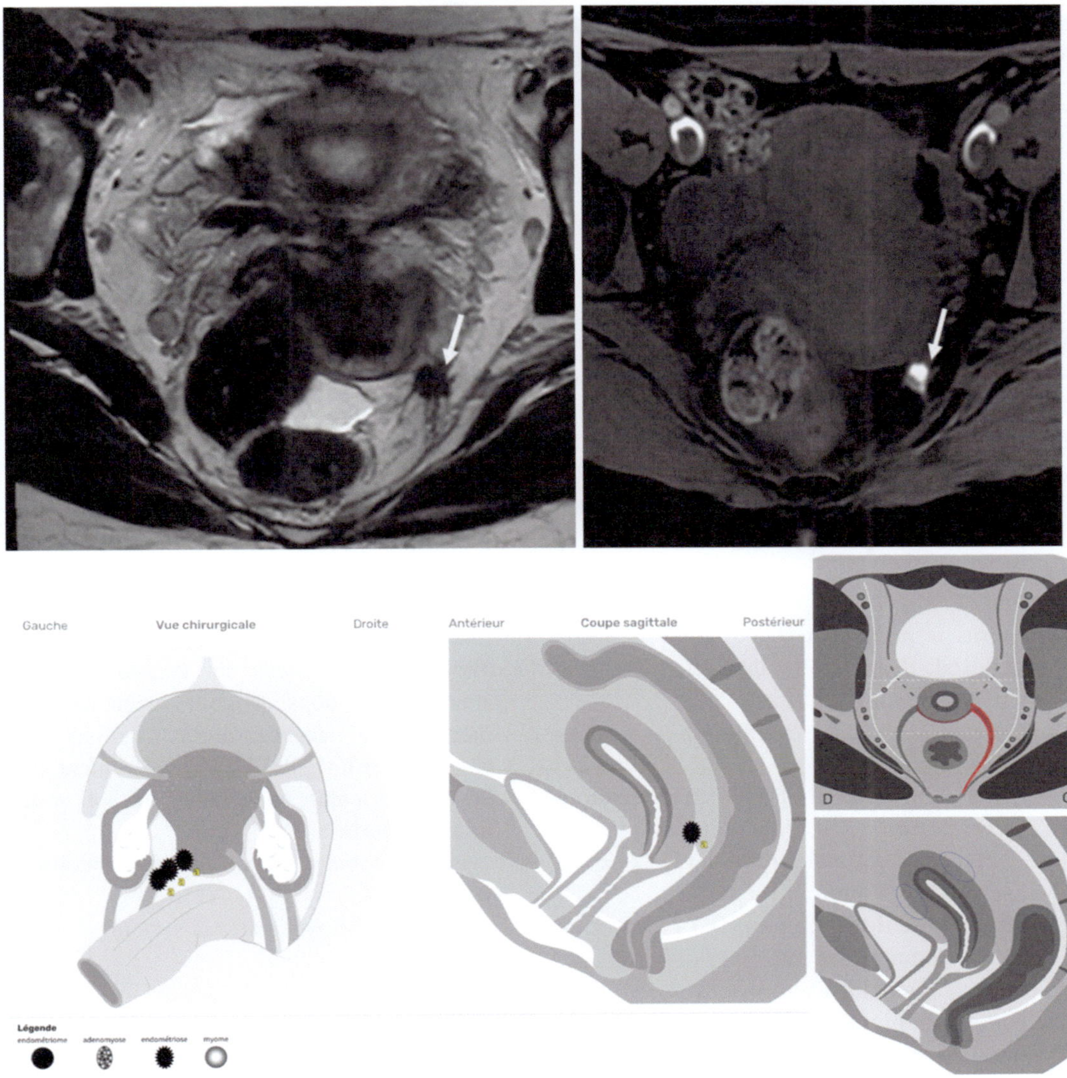

Key images (**a**, **b**) Sagittal T2W sequence, (**c**–**e**) axial oblique T2W sequence, and (**f**) axial T1W and drawings

Example 5 Example of Standardized Report: Moderate Disease (dPEI Score 3)

Clinical Information

A 43-year-old patient, nulligravida, under hormonal treatment (Dienogest) presenting with chronic pelvic pain referred for the suspicion of endometriosis

No previous surgical history

Technique

Bowel preparation (4 h of fasting, enema (normacol), and injection of 1 mL of glucagon)

T2-weighted images in sagittal plane and axial plane, 3D T2-weighted images, and 3D T1-DIXON weighted images were also obtained on the pelvis.

Results

The uterus is normal in shape, anteverted and anteflexed, displaced to the left, measuring 88 × 59 × 63 mm

The myometrium shows several fibroids displaying low signal on T2:

- Anterior corporal FIGO 5 measuring 25 × 19 mm
- Left posterior fundic corporal FIGO 4 measuring 15 × 9 mm
- Right posterior corporal FIGO 4 measuring 11 × 10 mm

No detectable internal adenomyosis

The endometrium measures 3 mm in thickness, without an intracavitary lesion

The cervix is unremarkable

The right ovary is not visualized

The left ovary is in normal position and measures 1.5 cm²

No adnexal mass and no visible tubal abnormality

Adnexal Endometriosis

No detectable endometriotic implant or cyst

Deep Endometriosis

Mediocentral compartment: endometriosic nodular lesion of the torus and proximal uterosacral ligaments, with high signal intensity spots on T1, measuring approximately 17 × 10 mm, associated with external posterior corporal adenomyosis and adhesion to the sigmoid colon at the rectosigmoid junction without the involvement of its wall

No vaginal involvement

Posterocentral compartment: no rectal wall involvement

Anterocentral compartment: probable bladder involvement at the level of vesicouterine pouch

Nodular lesion of the proximal left round ligament measuring 6 mm

Lateral compartments: no parametrial or sacrorectogenital fascia or lateral pelvic wall involvement

Extrapelvic compartment: the distension of the small bowel loops, without visible involvement at the ileocecal recess sigmoid dolichocolon with sigmoid wall involvement over 26 mm in length adjacent to the left round ligament nodule

No visible anomaly on the anterior abdominal wall

No dilation of the pyelocaliceal system

Conclusion

No adnexal endometriosis

No superficial endometriosis visible

Deep pelvic endometriosis involving the mediocentral compartment (the torus and proximal uterosacral ligaments) with external posterior corporal adenomyosis, the anterocentral compartment (the bladder and proximal left round ligament), and an extrapelvic (sigmoid) compartment

dPEI score 3 (moderate risk) with DE in mediocentral, anterocentral, and extrapelvic compartments

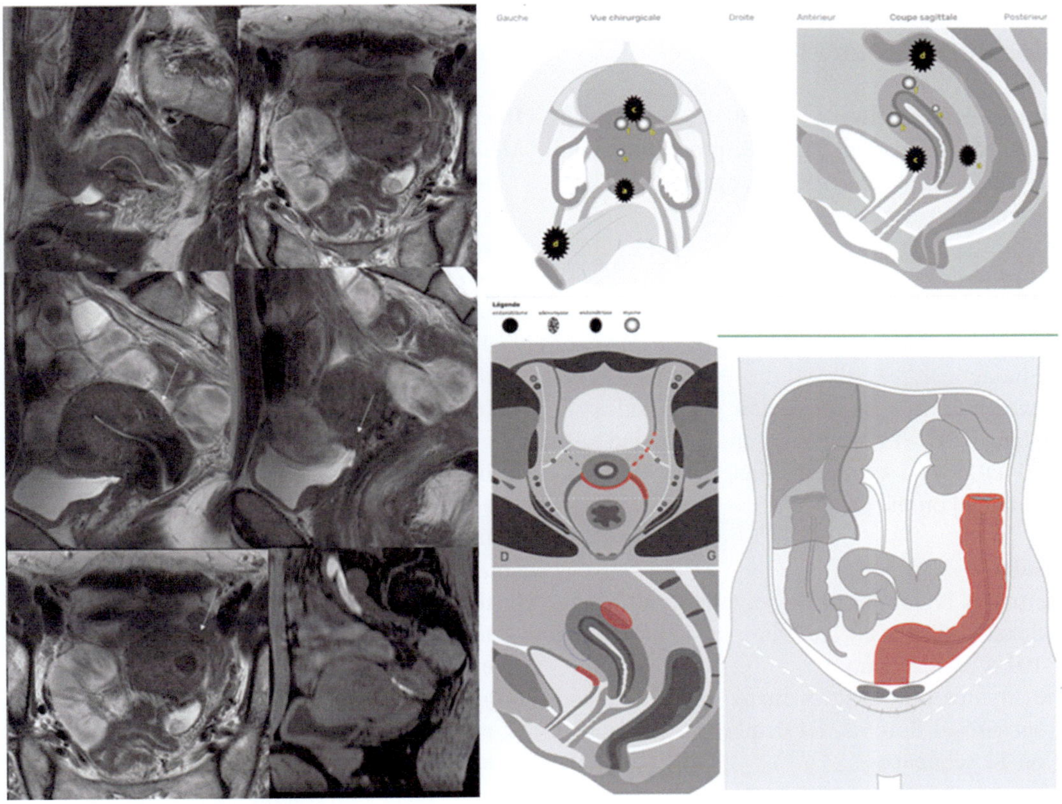

Key images (**a**) Sagittal T2W, (**b**) coronal T2W, (**c**, **d**) sagittal T2W, (**e**) axial oblique T2W, (**f**) sagittal T1W and drawings

Example 6 Example of Standardized Report: Moderate Disease (dPEI Score 4)

Clinical Information

A 40-year-old patient, G10P2, presenting with dysmenorrhea, dyspareunia, cycle related dysuria, and dyschezia

Technique

Bowel preparation (4 h of fasting, enema (normacol), and injection of 1 mL of glucagon)

T2-weighted images in sagittal plane and axial plane, 3D T2-weighted images, and 3D T1-DIXON weighted images were also obtained on the pelvis

Results

The uterus is normal in shape, anteverted, retroflexed, displaced to the left, measuring 101 × 58 × 73 mm

The myometrium shows many interstitial and subserosal fibroids, all displaying low signal on T2 sequences

Diffuse deep internal adenomyosis

Anterior isthmic cesarian section scar

The endometrium measures 5 mm of thickness, without an intracavitary lesion

The cervix is unremarkable

The ovaries are attracted to the posterior uterine wall

The right ovary measures 4.5 cm² and contains a corpus luteum of 12 mm

The left ovary measures 3.4 cm² and contains three antral follicles

There is no adnexal mass, no visible tubal abnormality

Adnexal Endometriosis

No detectable endometriotic implant or cyst

Deep Endometriosis

Mediocentral compartment: nodular lesion of the torus and proximal uterosacral ligaments measuring 16 × 10 mm, associated to adjacent external adenomyosis

Posterocentral compartment: extension to the upper rectum, with rectal wall thickening at 14 cm from the anus, measuring 8 mm in thickness, extending to 16 mm in height, involving 96° of the circumference

Anterocentral compartment: no bladder involvement

The involvement of the proximal left round ligament

Lateral compartments: the bilateral extension of the lesion to the parametria without the involvement of sacrorectogenital fascia or lateral pelvic wall

Extrapelvic compartment: no detectable abnormalities in the region of the ileocecal junction and no visible abnormalities on the anterior abdominal wall (including the umbilicus)

No dilatation of the pyelocaliceal cavities

No peritoneal fluid

Conclusion

Multiple uterine fibroids and deep diffuse symmetrical adenomyosis

No adnexal endometriosis

No visible superficial endometriosis

Deep pelvic endometriosis involving the mediocentral and posterocentral compartments and both mediolateral compartments

dPEI score 4 (moderate risk)

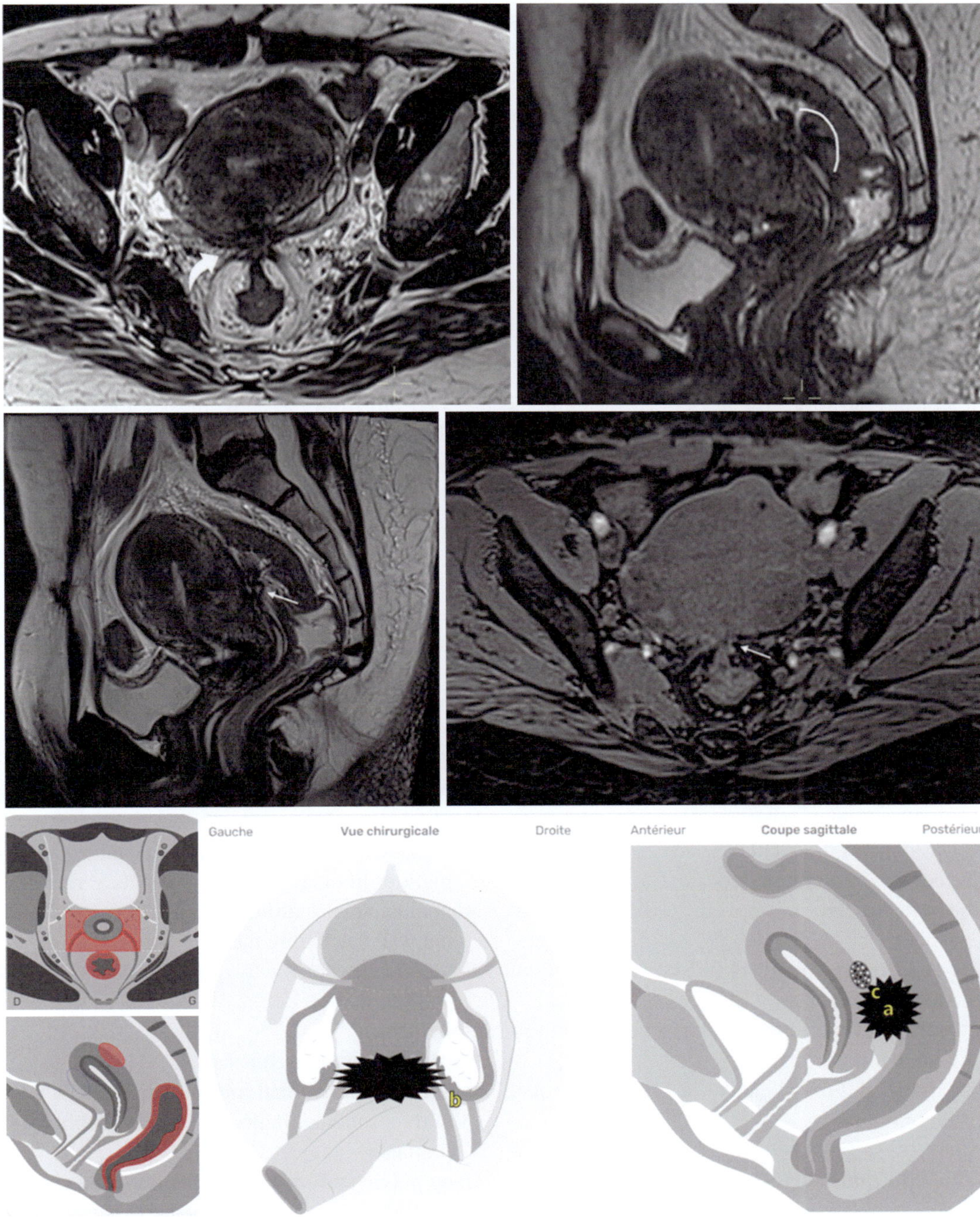

Key images (**a**) Axial T2W, (**b**, **c**) sagittal T2W, (**d**) axial T1W with fat saturation (axT1WFS) and drawings

Example 7 Example of Standardized Report: Severe Recurrent Postoperative Disease (dPEI 6)

Clinical Information

A 37-year-old patient, G1P1, who was referred for the suspicion of recurrent endometriosis in the context of infertility and who had a history of deep pelvic endometriosis surgically treated 3 years ago via the resection of the torus and rectal shaving

Technique

Bowel preparation (4 h of fasting, enema (normacol), and injection of 1 mL of glucagon)

T2-weighted images in sagittal plane and axial plane, 3D cube T2-weighted images, and 3D T1-weighted images with and without fat saturation were also obtained on the pelvis

Results

The uterus is normal in shape, anteverted, retroflexed, displaced to the left, measuring 83 × 35 × 49 mm

The myometrium is homogeneous without myomas or signs of adenomyosis

The endometrium measures 2 mm in thickness, without an intracavitary lesion

The cervix is unremarkable

The ovaries are normal in position and in aspect

The right ovary measures 3.2 cm² with normal follicular count

The left ovary measures 3.3 cm² with normal follicular count

No adnexal mass and no visible tubal abnormality

Adnexal Endometriosis

No detectable cyst

Endometriotic implant of the left ovary measuring 5 mm

Superficial Peritoneal Endometriosis

Right subdiaphragmatic and subhepatic abdominal endometriotic peritoneal implants measuring 5 and 8 mm, respectively

Deep Endometriosis Involving Many Compartments

Mediocentral compartment: nodular lesion of the torus and proximal uterosacral ligaments measuring 24 × 16 × 16 mm, associated with adjacent external adenomyosis

Posterocentral compartment: extension to the upper rectum, with rectal wall thickening at 12.7 cm from the anus, measuring 10 mm in thickness, extending to 17 mm in height, involving 78° of the rectal circumference

Anterocentral compartment: nodular lesion in the vesicouterine pouch measuring 16 mm (CC) × 13 mm (T) × 9 mm (AP) laterally on the left, invading the serosa of the bladder wall at the level of the dome at 16 mm above the left ureterovesical junction

The involvement of the left proximal round ligament, measuring 11 mm in thickness

Lateral compartments: the extension of the lesion to the parametria bilaterally and to the right sacrorectogenital fascia without extension to the ureter

No dilatation of the pyelocaliceal cavities

Extrapelvic compartment: no detectable abnormalities in the region of the ileocecal recess

No visible abnormalities on the anterior abdominal wall (including the umbilicus)

No pelvic effusion

Conclusion

No adnexal endometriosis

Superficial peritoneal implants in the abdomen with subdiaphragmatic and subhepatic implants

Deep pelvic endometriosis involving the anterocentral, mediocentral, posterocentral, and mediolateral, compartments.

dPEI score 6 (severe)

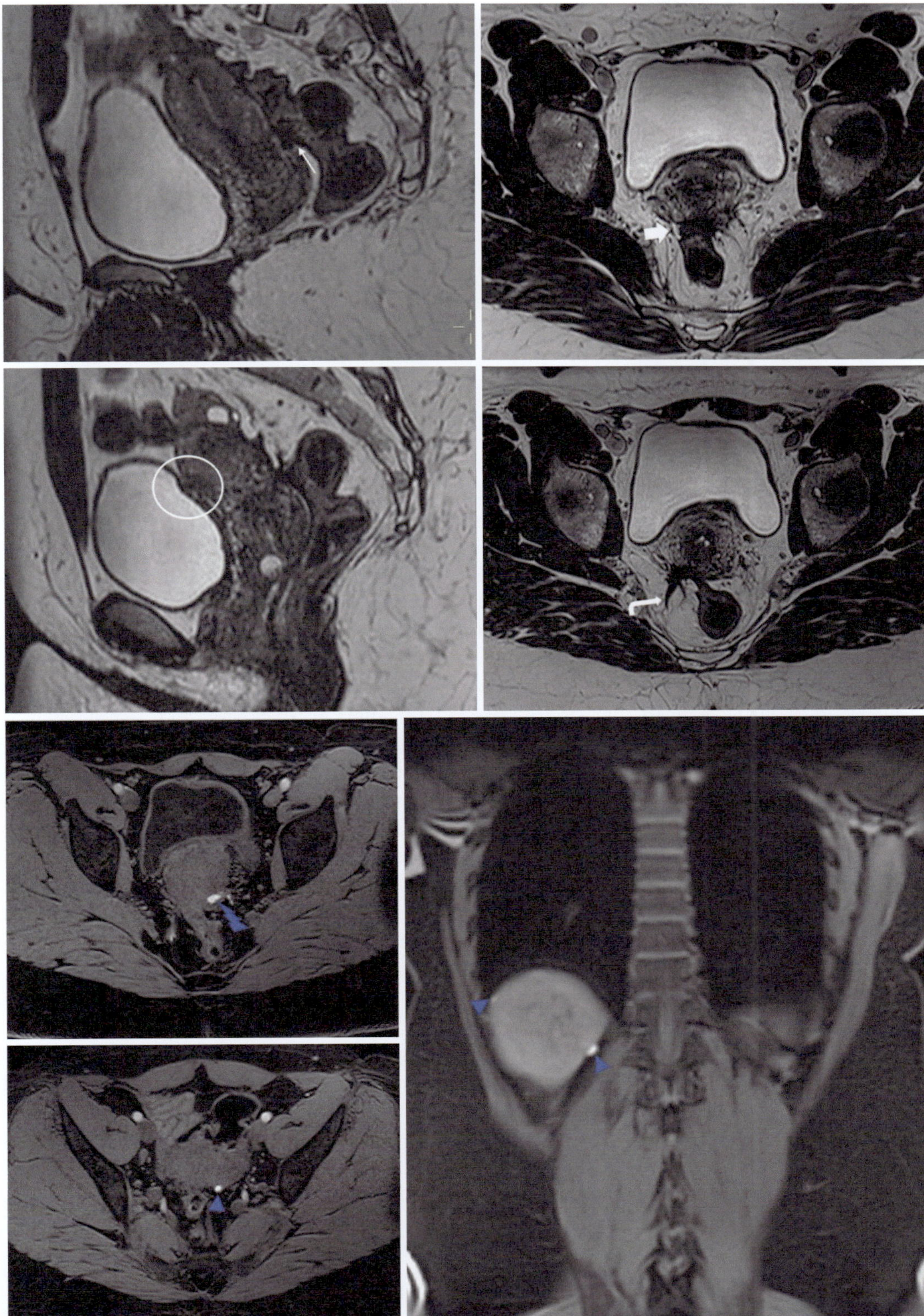

Key images (**a**, **b**) Sagittal T2W, (**c**, **d**) axial T2W, (**e**, **f**) axial T1W, and (**g**) coronal T1W and drawings

Standardized Reporting from ESUR

Clinical Information

[<>] years old patient, Gravidity [<>]

Parity [<>], day [<>] of the cycle, (number of cesarean sections) referred for clinical suspicion of endometriosis: chronic pelvic pain and/or dysmenorrhea (EVA), and/or deep dyspareunia, and/or dysuria/dyschezia during menstruation, and/or menstrual scapular pain (side)/infertility

No history of pelvic surgery or pelvic infection

Hormonal treatment: Desire for pregnancy.

Referring Physician: Dr. [<>]

Technique

Performed on 1.5/3.0 T machine

Bowel preparation (fasting, enema (type of enema), and administration of antispasmodic agents (type))

T2-weighted images of the pelvis were obtained in sagittal plane, axial plane, and coronal plane, 3D cube/space T2-weighted images/ thin slice T2-weighted images obtained in oblique plane in the axis of the uterosacral ligaments. 3DT1-weighted images of the pelvis.

+/– Vaginal opacification

Image quality: satisfactory/degraded by motion artifacts

Findings

The uterus is normal in size and shape, anteverted/retroverted, anteflexed/retroflexed, displaced to right/left, measuring [<>] × [<>] × [<>]mm

The myometrium displays normal signal intensity

Absence/presence of fibroids (description with FIGO type)

Absence/presence of internal adenomyosis: diffuse or focal thickening of junctional zone, with/without cystic foci. The endometrium is normal measuring [<>] in thickness

Focal endometrial lesion is detected (description)/No detectable intracavitary anomaly

The cervix is unremarkable/abnormal (abnormality description) cesarean-section scar [<>]

The ovaries are normal in size and show presence of multiple/few small follicles. No adnexal mass lesion is detected/adnexal mass (description)

Right/left hydrosalpinx measured at [<>], with fluid or hemorrhagic signal

Absence/presence of free fluid in the pelvis

Adnexal Endometriosis

Endometriomas/endometriotic implants (side, number, size, central or peripheral, typical or not)

Endometriotic hematosalpinx right/left measured at [<>]

Normal ovarian parenchyma (size)

Superficial Endometriosis:

Implants, adhesions

Deep Endometriosis

Mid-central compartment: Torus/proximal USL/ posterior vaginal fornix/rectovaginal septum/ anterior/posterior external adenomyosis measuring [<>]mm

Posterocentral compartment: Rectum/rectosigmoid over [<>] mm in length at [<>] cm from the anal margin. This involvement measures [<>]mm in thickness and concerns [<>] degrees of the circumference

Single or multiple

Anterocentral compartment: Bladder (dome/ base/trigone at [<>] mm from the right/left ureteral meatus)

Lateral compartments: Over visceral fascia: Right/left mediolateral parametrium/distal right/left USL/right/left posterolateral parametrium/anterolateral parametrium

Over parietal fascia: Right/left pelvic sidewall/ ischial notch/levator muscles/sacral roots

Extrapelvic compartment: Ileocecal-appendiceal junction/sigmoid colon/Anterior abdominal wall

Complete obliteration of the pouch of Douglas with loculated fluid, highlighting pelvic adhesions

Conclusion

Adnexal endometriosis: Endometrioma (right/ left ovarian endometrioma of … mm, hematosalpinx)

Superficial peritoneal endometriosis (implants, adhesions)

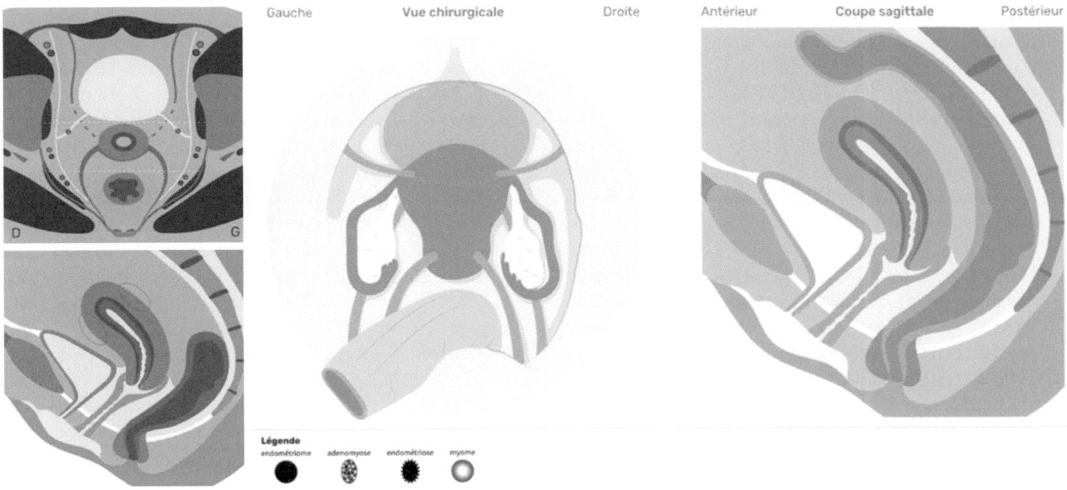

Examples of drawings including axial and sagittal sections and surgical views. These drawings are useful at the end of the MRI report to improve patient understanding (Source: Keydiag)

Deep pelvic endometriosis involving torus, uterosacral ligaments, vagina, and rectosigmoid over × mm with Douglas's symphysis, mediolateral/posterolateral parametrium, and anterolateral involving vesicouterine pouch, bladder, and round ligaments.

dPEI score XX mild, moderate, severe with [<>] compartments involved

Images and Drawings

15.5.1 Specific Situation: Postoperative Recurrence

After resection, the endometrioma recurrence rate ranges between 6% and 30%, corresponding to either a recurrence of a previously removed endometrioma or a newly developed endometrioma in the ipsilateral ovary or contralateral ovary [12]. On MRI, recurrent endometrioma is easy to detect because it displays the same characteristics and signal as those of a native endometrioma. This is not the case for deep endometriosis recurrence, however, which may have MRI features similar to those of native deep endometriosis (DE) or which may appear as a solid infiltrative nodule located on a posthysterectomy vaginal vault. These signs are not specific in a postoperative context and may correspond only to postoperative fibrosis unless they are associated with a high-signal glandular focus on T2-weighted images or bright "spots" on fat-suppressed T1-weighted images. Thus, on postoperative follow-up MRI, deep endometriosis recurrence should not be declared on the basis of the sole sign of an irregular or nodular thickening of the region of the torus or the USLs unless it is associated with consistent clinical symptoms.

Acknowledgements All drawings were realized with "keydiag" software.

References

1. Rockall AG, Justich C, Helbich T, Vilgrain V. Patient communication in radiology: moving up the agenda. Eur J Radiol. 2022;155:110464. https://doi.org/10.1016/j.ejrad.2022.110464.
2. Thomassin-Naggara I, Rousset P, Touboul C, Razakamanantsoa L, Manganaro L. Reasons why it is time to change imaging guidelines on endometriosis. Eur Radiol. 2024;34:6175. https://doi.org/10.1007/s00330-024-10595-w.
3. Keckstein J, Saridogan E, Ulrich UA, et al. The #Enzian classification: a comprehensive non-invasive and surgical description system for endometriosis. Acta Obstet Gynecol Scand. 2021;100(7):1165–75. https://doi.org/10.1111/aogs.14099.

4. Bazot M, Daraï E, Benagiano GP, et al. ENDO_STAGE magnetic resonance imaging: classification to screen endometriosis. J Clin Med. 2022;11(9):2443. https://doi.org/10.3390/jcm11092443.
5. Thomassin-Naggara I, Lamrabet S, Crestani A, et al. Magnetic resonance imaging classification of deep pelvic endometriosis: description and impact on surgical management. Hum Reprod. 2020;35(7):1589–600. https://doi.org/10.1093/humrep/deaa103.
6. Thomassin-Naggara I, Monroc M, Chauveau B, et al. Multicenter external validation of the deep pelvic endometriosis index magnetic resonance imaging score. JAMA Netw Open. 2023;6(5):e2311686. https://doi.org/10.1001/jamanetworkopen.2023.11686.
7. Schwartz LH, Panicek DM, Berk AR, Li Y, Hricak H. Improving communication of diagnostic radiology findings through structured reporting. Radiology. 2011;260(1):174–81. https://doi.org/10.1148/radiol.11101913.
8. Bazot M, Bharwani N, Huchon C, et al. European Society of Urogenital Radiology (ESUR) guidelines: MR imaging of pelvic endometriosis. Eur Radiol. 2017;27(7):2765–75. https://doi.org/10.1007/s00330-016-4673-z.
9. Bazot M, Beldjord S, Jarboui L, Ferrier C, Bendifallah S, Daraï E. Value of 3D MRI and vaginal opacification for the diagnosis of vaginal endometriosis. Front Surg. 2020;7:614989. https://doi.org/10.3389/fsurg.2020.614989.
10. Enzelsberger S-H, Oppelt P, Nirgianakis K, et al. Preoperative application of the Enzian classification for endometriosis (the cEnzian study): a prospective international multicenter study. BJOG. 2022;129:2052. https://doi.org/10.1111/1471-0528.17235.
11. Rousset P, Florin M, Bharwani N, et al. Deep pelvic infiltrating endometriosis: MRI consensus lexicon and compartment-based approach from the ENDOVALIRM group. Diagn Interv Imaging. 2023;104:95.
12. Guerra A, Daraï E, Osório F, et al. Imaging of postoperative endometriosis. Diagn Interv Imaging. 2019;100:607. https://doi.org/10.1016/j.diii.2018.11.003.

16 Technique and Reporting of the Imaging Techniques and Classifications: Laparoscopic Surgery

Adrien Crestani, Benjamin Merlot, and Horace Roman

16.1 Introduction

In 1860, Rokitansky described endometriosis as the presence of a polypoid peritoneal lesion resembling an endometrium [1]. This first macroscopic and microscopic description was a milestone in our understanding of the pathology of endometriosis. Although our knowledge on this topic has progressed through our understanding of genetic, epigenetic, and metabolomic mechanisms [2], the phenotypic evaluation of endometriosis remains a complex issue. Indeed, the visual description of the disease, in addition to being considered the gold standard of diagnosis [2], must enable us to associate the pathology with certain symptoms [3] or even to understand whether it is evolving [4]. However, no consensus has yet been reached on how to explore, describe, and report these lesions.

Moreover, although surgery has been shown to reduce pain, improve patients' quality of life, and improve postoperative fertility [2, 5], the exploration at the beginning of the procedure will inform the choice of surgical technique and will condition the postoperative follow-up and subsequent care of the patient.

Therefore, the first objective of the surgery should be a complete, exhaustive, and standardized description of all endometriosis lesions, with images and/or videos if possible. The surgeon should take care to use a validated common lexicon: the Terminologia Anatomica. The second objective of the surgical report is to describe in detail all the procedures and techniques performed during the operation and any events or complications that may have resulted.

In 2021, a lexicon for endometriosis was validated by the scientific societies of endometriosis; it standardizes the terms used by practitioners and surgeons in particular [6]. It describes not only the disease and its various forms but also the anatomical spaces, procedures, and techniques used. This standardization of practices should enable clinicians to speak a common language to optimize postoperative management and better inform patients.

16.2 Standardization of Surgical Reporting

In 2016, a Consensus on Recording Deep Endometriosis Surgery (CORDES) statement was published in *Human Reproduction* in two

A. Crestani (✉) · B. Merlot
Franco-European Multidisciplinary Endometriosis Institute (IFEMEndo), Clinique Tivoli-Ducos, Bordeaux, France

H. Roman
Franco-European Multidisciplinary Endometriosis Institute (IFEMEndo), Clinique Tivoli-Ducos, Bordeaux, France

Department of Gynecology and Obstetrics, Aarhus University Hospital, Aarhus, Denmark

I. Thomassin-Naggara (ed.), *Imaging of Endometriosis: A Comparative Guide of US, MRI and Surgery*, https://doi.org/10.1007/978-3-031-82750-1_16

parts [7]. In the first one, the authors proposed a deep endometriosis surgical sheet (DESS) for the standardized reporting of surgery for DE. It was essentially based on the World Endometriosis Research Foundation Endometriosis Phenome and Biobanking Harmonisation Project [8], which brought together 54 clinical, academic, and industry leaders in endometriosis research and management worldwide and developed a standard recommended form and a minimum required form to collect data on the surgical phenotype of endometriosis. The DESS is shown in Table 16.1. In the second part, the authors presented a consensus for the standardization of reporting surgical trials in patients with DE (see Table 16.2).

In 2021, the Enhancing the Quality and Transparency of Health Research (EQUATOR) Network (https://www.equator-network.org/) published nearly 500 reporting guidelines. The CONSORT-NPT guideline concerns randomized controlled trials on nonpharmacological treatments [9], the most recent STROCSS guideline for observational study in surgery [10], the PROCESS guideline for surgical case series [11], and the SCARE guideline for surgical case reports [12]. Yet none of these guidelines has provided a standardized surgical report method.

Table 16.1 Standardized reporting of surgical treatment for deep endometriosis, by Vanhie A et al.

Category	Details
Preoperative information	Record essential preoperative information: • Essential clinical covariates • Menstrual history and current hormonal treatment • Previous endometriosis surgery • Pre-operative imaging results • Use of prophylactic drugs • Indications and decision on type of surgery
Staging and description	Record detailed description and staging of endometriosis: • Staging—ASRM and EFI (optional: ENZIAN) • Extent of peritoneal/superficial endometriosis • Number, size and exact localization of each lesion • Extent of ovarian endometriosis • Number, size and localization of endometrioma(s) • Extent of deep endometriosis • Number, size and exact localization of each lesion • For bowel DE, – Depth of infiltration in intestinal wall – Circumferential involvement – Distance to anal verge • For urological DE: – Depth of infiltration in bladder and ureter – Presence of hydro-ureteronephrosis • Extent of adhesions
Surgical procedures	Record detailed description of surgical procedures performed: • Clear description of surgical procedures performed (standardized terminology) • Record surgical risk factors for negative outcomes
Postoperative information	Record essential post-operative information: • Operation times, length of hospital stay, and postoperative management • Detailed description of the abdomen after surgery • Detailed histological report • Intra- and postoperative complications

ASRM American Society for Reproductive Medicine, *EFI* endometriosis fertility index, *DE* deep endometriosis, *WERF-EPHectEPQ* World Endometriosis Research Foundation Phenomeand, Biobanking Harmonisation Project, *EPQ* Endometriosis Patient Questionnaire, NRS numerical rating scale, *QoL* qualityoflife, *PRO* patient reported outcome, *BFLUTS* Bristol Female Lower Urinary Tract Scale, *ICIQ* International, Consultationon Incontinence Modular Questionnaire, *FLUTS* Female Lower Urinary Tract Symptoms, *GIQLI* Gastrointestinal Quality of life Index, *KESS* Knowles-Eccersley-Scott Symptom questionnaire, *FIQLI* Fecal Incontinence Quality of Lifescale. *BMI* body mass index *PRO* patient-reported outcome *QoR* quality of recovery

Table 16.2 Standardized reporting of surgical trials for DE, by Vanhie A et al.

Category	Details
Methods	Report methods according to international standards: • CONSORT • STROBE • PRISMA
Participants	Record WERF-EPHect EPQ for all patients and report detailed description of the population studied: • Age, BMI, and ethnicity • Medication and substance use • Medical history and treatment • Menstrual history • Previous use of hormonal treatment • Previous diagnosis of endometriosis • Previous therapeutic surgery • Obstetrical history • Family history of endometriosis Report detailed description of pre-operative workup: • Details on imaging techniques used • Detailed description of results—preoperative endometriosis mapping
Interventions	Report details on indications for surgery: • Pain symptoms without infertility • Pain symptoms with infertility • Infertility without pain symptoms • No infertility or pain symptoms • Asymptomatic hydroureteronephrosis Report details on decisions on type/technique of surgery: • Pre- or intraoperative decision • Decision criteria/treatment algorithm Report interventions using the DESS: • Description endometriosis at start of surgery • Staging of endometriosis—ASRM + EFI (+ENZIAN) • Standardized description of all surgical procedures • Description of abdomen at end of surgery Report detailed histological results: • Histologic confirmation of endometriosis + histologic type/pattern • Largest diameter of each lesion • Depth of invasion (in bowel, bladder, ureter, or other area) for each lesion • *Bowel specimens*: • Presence of lymphatic dissemination • Median length of the resected bowel segments (in cm) • Number + location of positive section margins

(continued)

Table 16.2 (continued)

Category	Details
Results	Report details on all primary outcomes: *Pain*: • Daily ratings with 11-point NRS • Separate ratings for: dyspareunia, dysmenorrhea, chronic pelvic pain, dyschezia and mictalgia • Record and report concomitant use of other drugs/analgesics/therapies • Address cyclicity—menstrual diary *QoL*: • EHP-30 Assessment at baseline (minimum 1) + follow up (minimum 1) *Fertility*: • Report cumulative pregnancy rate • Report details on mode of conception • Report details on post-operative hormonal treatment (secondary prevention) *Recurrence*: • Report cumulative suspected and proven recurrence rate *Complications*: • Report all complications + management + outcome in absolute numbers • Classify complications according to the Clavien–Dindo system • Report comprehensive complication index (CCI)
Secondary outcomes	Report details on secondary outcomes: *Sexual function*: • Define method used for assessment of sexual (dys)function • Assessment at baseline (minimum 1) + follow-up (minimum 1) • *Suggested PRO's*: • FSFI = Female sexual function index • MFSQ = McCoy Female Sexuality Questionnaire • GSSI = Global Sexual Satisfaction Index *Urinary function*: • Define the method used for assessment of urinary (dys)function • Recommended use of PRO combined with urodynamics • Assessment at baseline (minimum 1) + follow-up (minimum 1) • Suggested PRO: BFLUTS (=ICIQ-FLUTS) Bowel function: • Define the method used for assessment of bowel (dys)function • Assessment at baseline (minimum 1) + follow up (minimum 1) • *Suggested PRO's*: • General GI symptoms—GIQLI • Constipation—KESS • Incontinence—FIQLI • Classification of feces—Bristol stool chart
Tertiary outcomes	Optionally, report details on tertiary outcomes: Cost-effectiveness Recovery—QoR-40 or CARE Patient centeredness—ENDOCARE questionnaire

WERF-EPHectEPQ World Endometriosis Research Foundation Phenome and Biobanking Harmonisation Project, *EPQ* Endometriosis, Patient Questionnaire, *NRS* numerical rating scale, *QoL* quality of life, *PRO* patient reported outcome, *BFLUTS* Bristol Female Lower Urinary Tract Scale, *ICIQ* International Consultation on Incontinence Modular Questionnaire, *FLUTS* Female Lower Urinary Tract Symptoms, *GIQLI* Gastrointestinal Quality of life Index, *KESS* Knowles-Eccersley-Scott Symptom questionnaire, *FIQLI* Fecal Incontinence Quality of Life scale, *BMI* body mass index, *PRO* patient-reported outcome, *QoR* quality of recovery

Most recently, Zhang et al. developed a standardized checklist of items applicable to all types of surgery. The Surgical Technique Reporting Checklist and Standards (SUPER) guideline aims to define reporting standards for surgical technique on the basis of the models of standardization like Strengthening the Reporting of Observational Studies in Epidemiology (STROBE).

Yet by looking through even the most recent publications, the scientific community's compliance with these recommendations is obviously low. Inspired by these models, we propose a standardized surgical report containing 24 items.

16.2.1 Surgical Indications

The aim of surgical indications are to contextualize the surgery so that the indications for surgery and the objectives set with the patient prior to surgery are clear.

1. *Patient's history and disease, clinical examination, imaging, and preoperative radiological classifications*

An oriented description of the medical history of the patient and clinical examination are mandatory. The surgeon should summarize the imaging reports on the basis of different international standard classifications (see Chaps. 13 and 14).

2. *Rationale: symptoms, medical treatments, and fertility*

Three main clinical situations may be more or less associated with the rationale for surgery: infertility, pain resistance to a well-conducted multimodal treatment, and endometriosis lesions endangering an organ (hydronephrosis, occlusion, etc.). The involvement of each of these situations must be specified.

3. *Objectives*

In line with the rationale, the objectives of the surgery must be clearly defined in the context of the abovementioned elements (pain, infertility, etc.).

4. *Planned procedures and/or techniques and the surgical route*

This item should clearly list the proposed procedures and therefore whether a colorectal/urological/thoracic surgeon and/or robot-assisted laparoscopy are needed.

5. Eventual inclusion in a research protocol needs also to be specified

16.2.2 Presurgical Preparation

6. *Names of surgeons and staff, date, and operating time*
7. *Preoperative drugs: bowel preparation, residue-free diet, and premedication*

For colorectal surgery, preoperative bowel preparation measures have been shown to have a positive impact on reducing the rate of postoperative complications [13]. In a recent meta-analysis of nine studies, dietary rehabilitation combined or not with physical activity before colorectal surgery reduced hospital stay by 2 days [14]. Some surgeons may propose a residue-free diet to reduce the volume of the colon and therefore improve the surgical view, even in cases of endometriosis not involving the bowel. The most recent Cochrane review has demonstrated the benefits of bowel preparation combined with antibiotic prophylaxis, particularly in preventing surgical site infections and postoperative fistulae [15].

8. *Equipment required: bladder catheterization, uterine manipulator, tubal permeability test, and types of energy*

A foley catheter is systematically introduced to empty the bladder to expose the pelvic organs and avoid injuries while introducing the suprapubic trocar into the abdomen. The use of a uterine manipulator and the type of energy should be listed.

9. *Anesthesia/analgesia*

Laparoscopy is performed under general anesthesia. The injection of an analgesic at the trocar sites prior to incision and intraperitoneal instillation at the end of the procedure improves postoperative recovery [16, 17].

10. *Operating position: supine position, Trendelenburg, and compression point management*

For pelvic surgery, the patient is positioned supine, with their hands at their sides in the Trendelenburg position. In this way, the small intestines are forced upward and backward by gravity. For diaphragm endometriosis surgery, excision should, in our opinion, not be concomitant with pelvic surgery. To have comfortable access to the hepatophrenic area, the patient is positioned in the left lateral decubitus position, with a log under the scapula to open up the angle between the diaphragmatic dome and the liver as much as possible and with the trocars positioned under the twelfth rib [18–20].

11. *Asepsis and type of drape*

16.2.3 Exploration

12. *Laparoscopic entry technique and security tests if needed*

The optic trocar can be introduced directly via a contending trocar, into which the optic is inserted; by inserting a needle with a safety valve to create the pneumoperitoneum, enabling the optic trocar to be inserted without visual control; or via a direct incision into the aponeurosis (open). A recent Cochrane meta-analysis that evaluated the benefits and risks of different laparoscopic entry techniques in gynecological and nongynecological surgeries concluded that evidence was insufficient to support the use of one laparoscopic entry technique over another. Researchers noted an advantage of direct trocar entry over Veress needle entry for failed entry [21].

13. *Topographical description of lesions*

Becker et al. proposed nine “zones” for documenting the phenotype of the disease (see Table 16.3) [8]. In our experience, the exploration of the abdominal cavity should follow the surgical position of the patient. A description of the diaphragm should therefore be the first step because it is performed in the 0° decubitus position. If the suspicion of diaphragm endometriosis is high, using a proclive position will improve visibility.

The patient is then placed in a supine position, 10° to 30°, and the small bowel is explored, along with the appendix and the colon. Deep and superficial endometriosis should be described using the Terminologia Anatomica [22], which is used in Becker’s checklist. A detailed description of the lesion in superficial, ovarian, and deep endometriosis is required, including the number, size, and exact location of each lesion (superficial or deep); the presence of endometriomas and/or hydrosalpinxes; and the extent of adhesions.

For bowel endometriosis, the localization and number of intestinal DE lesions (multifocality), the depth of intestinal DE lesions in the intestinal wall, the length and the width of the lesions, and the distance between colorectal lesions and the anal verge should be documented [23, 24]. For urological endometriosis, the localization and number of urinary tract DE lesions, the depth of infiltration into the bladder wall, intrinsic/extrinsic ureteral endometriosis, and the presence of hydroureteronephrosis should be documented [25, 26]. Other sites outside the abdominopelvic area, including the umbilicus, scars, etc., should not be forgotten. Finally, peritoneal fluids should be applied or a peritoneal biopsy performed even if the exploration is negative for endometriosis [8].

14. *Preintervention assessment of tubal functionality*
15. *Imaging and surgical classifications*

Numerous endometriosis scores and classifications have been published. These are intended to standardize lesion description, assess the severity of the disease, evaluate the complexity of the procedures performed, and estimate the risk of postoperative complications and the likelihood of postoperative pregnancy.

Most classifications (except dPEI scores) have been established on the basis of surgical findings. Many of them have failed to describe lateral locations that are deep under the peritoneum and thus not visible on laparoscopy. This is n why imaging findings should be mentioned at the beginning of any surgical report. As described in the previous

Table 16.3 Suggested zones for surgical video and photographic documentation, by Becker et al.

Zone	Boundaries	Contents
I	Bilateral: round ligaments Posterior: uterus Midline anterior abdominal cavity limited by the round ligaments bilaterally and the uterus posteriorly	Midline anterior abdominal peritoneum Anterior surface of the broad ligaments Bladder dome Internal ring and inferior epigastric vessels
II	Anterior: bladder peritoneum Bilateral: broad ligaments and adnexae Caudal: torus uterinus	Uterus
III	Anterior: torus uterinus Bilateral: uterosacral ligaments Posterior: sacral pelvic brim	Pouch of Douglas/posterior cul-de-sac Rectovaginal septum Sigmoid colon Presacral peritoneum
IV	Anterior: right round ligament Medial: right broad ligament and adnexa	Right lateral peritoneum Anterior surface of right broad ligament
V	Medial: uterus and right uterosacral ligament Anterior: right fallopian tube Lateral: right infundibulopelvic ligament	Fallopian tube and ovary Mesovarium Posterior surface of the broad ligament Ovarian fossa Vessels and ureter
VI	Anterior: right round ligament Medial: right broad ligament and adnexa	Left lateral peritoneum Anterior surface of left broad ligament
VII	Medial: uterus and left uterosacral ligament Anterior: left fallopian tube Lateral: left infundibulopelvic ligament	Fallopian tube and ovary Mesovarium Posterior surface of the broad ligament Ovarian fossa Vessels and ureter
VIII	Not applicable	Other abdominopelvic areas including: • Adipose tissue • Bowel • Ureter • Anterior abdominal wall • Diaphragm • Other
IX	Not applicable	Other sites outside the abdominopelvic area: • Umbilicus • Scars • Chest • Other

chapters, the modified ASRM classification is outdated, and its predictive value concerns only the natural conception. Using the #Enzian classification is recommended in both preoperative and intraoperative situations because it helps to plan not only the duration of the operating time [27–29] but also the rate of postoperative complications [30].

The dPEI score is an MRI score whose result is directly proportional to the operative time, hospital stay, and probability of severe complications [31]. This information is therefore crucial to the global organization of care. The Endometriosis Fertility Index score [32] is based on clinical criteria such as the patient's age, the duration of infertility, the presence of pregnancy, the physical criteria of tubal functionality, and, finally, the lesion volume of endometriosis as estimated by the AFSR score. This score is therefore not a means of estimating lesion severity or the risk of surgical complications.

16.2.4 Surgical Procedures

16. *Surgical approach to the lesions*

Obviously, the approach to mild, localized and superficial lesions varies greatly depending on the surgical approach taken for severe, multifocal lesions. Determining the approach to severe endometriosis lesions is often the most complex phase. The surgeon systematically begins the operation by freeing the colosigmoid angle [33, 34], which often adheres to the abdominal wall, to increase the mobility of the left colon. Bilateral ureterolysis is mandatory, as is determining where the hypogastric nerves are located, posteriorly and medially, in relation to the ureters.These steps can be facilitated via ovarian and/or uterine suspension with transcutaneous threads or with a uterine manipulator and vaginal/rectal probes.

17. Description of the surgical procedure

In this section, the surgeon must limit their personal interpretation by using anatomical landmarks, adjacent structures and organs, spaces, fossae, etc. In the CORDES statement by Vanhie et al. [7], the authors defined the procedures for bowel and urinary tract endometriosis. These items are also used in the international terminology proposed by Tomassetti et al. [6].

16.2.4.1 Colorectal Endometriosis

For colorectal endometriosis, the surgeon frees the lesion from its lateral adhesions by opening the pararectal fossae and the Okabayashi space [35], separating the nerves and ureter laterally from the rectum medially [36]. Anteriorly, the surgeon separates the nodule from its uterovaginal attachments.

For shaving or partial-thickness excision, the lesion infiltrates the muscularis propria. In the case of deep muscular excision, the surgeon may repair the site of the excision by suturing the defect. The two criteria for choosing the right procedure are the depth of muscular invasion and the surface area of the rectal wall—therefore, the width and length of the nodule [34, 37, 38].

For a full-thickness excision, the lesion extends through the entire thickness of the muscularis and possibly the mucosa. The surgeon resects a patch of rectal wall. In most cases, this resection is performed by using a circular stapler inserted through the patient's anus; in other cases, the defect is sutured with absorbable thread. Therefore, rectosigmoid stenosis constitutes a first obstacle, which the surgeon will investigate via interrogation (subocclusive syndrome) and imaging [39].

The second criterion for the feasibility of circular transrectal stapling is the affected surface area of the rectum. The surgeon must ensure the complete shaving of the budding portion of the digestive lesion to reduce its thickness. The aim is to allow as much of the rectal surface as possible to enter the circular stapling forceps. Discs over five centimeters in diameter can thus be removed [40]. If the excision is not complete and conditions are favorable, the surgeon may consider a second full-thickness resection on the basis of the same principle [41], aiming to avoid segmental resection, which is known to be associated with a higher risk of fistula, low anterior rectal resection syndrome [42], and stenosis than discoid resection is [43].

16.2.4.2 Ureteral Endometriosis

Ureterolysis is the first surgical step in the management of ureteral endometriosis (UE). It is defined as follows by Vanhie et al. [7]: "Restoration of the normal mobility and anatomical position of the ureter through the resection of adhesions and the selective dissection of the ureter from a lesion, either mechanically or with diathermy, laser or any other energy source." It begins in a healthy zone, generally below the crossing with the iliac artery, allowing an easier and safer approach to the ureter, before progressing step by step toward the uterosacral ligament, thus freeing the ureter. This dissection can be performed by using cold scissors, a CO_2 laser, electrocoagulation, or an ultrasonic scalpel; having good knowledge of the diffusion of the energy used is essential for the procedure to run smoothly. Ureterolysis must preserve ureteral vascularization as much as possible. In numerous cases [44–46], when the ureter is merely surrounded (extrinsic ureteral endometriosis) but not infiltrated by the disease (intrinsic ureteral endometriosis), ureterolysis may be the only therapeutic procedure. The preoperative placement of a JJ catheter may facilitate the surgical procedure, or it may be necessary during the operation depending on the findings or possible

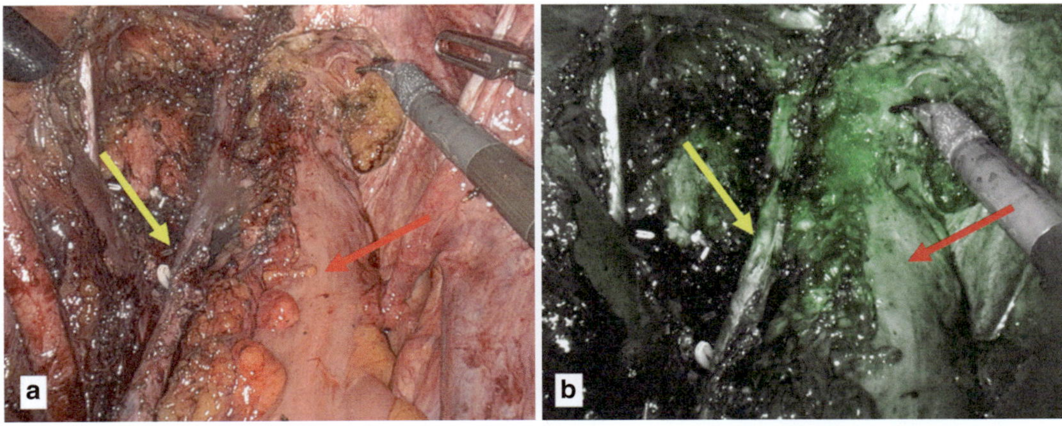

Fig. 16.1 Use of indocyanine green to evaluate left ureter (yellow arrow) and sigmoid (red arrow) perfusion

complications (wounds and extensive devascularization). To optimize the results of conservative management, several teams have reported the use of indocyanine green in endometriosis surgery and have reported other pathologies requiring a ureterolysis step (Fig. 16.1). Raimondo et al. recently described the intravenous use of indocyanine green to assess the residual perfusion of the ureters and thus to indicate whether a JJ catheter should be inserted [47] .

When simple ureterolysis is not sufficient, the gynecological surgeon, assisted by a urological surgeon, may have to perform a ureteral resection followed by ureteroureteral anastomosis in 6%, ureteroneocystostomy after ureteral resection in 21%, and nephrectomy in 0.45% of patients [45]. To the best of our knowledge, no minimum length is required for reimplantation, but whatever technique is used, the urological surgeon will begin by detaching the anterior surface of the bladder to mobilize it in the direction of the lesion and reduce tension on the anastomosis. In some cases, the bladder is lateralized and fixed to the psoas.

16.2.4.3 Bladder Endometriosis

As for colorectal lesions, bladder lesions can be excised through a partial-thickness or a full-thickness excision [7]. Bladder endometriosis comes in two types: solitary nodules of the bladder dome and anterior adenomyosis lesions that anteriorly invade the bladder. The radiological report must explicitly specify which type of lesion is being described because the surgical approach, risks, and side effects of each type differ. The former are the easiest to deal with. The surgeon frees the bladder from its anterior and lateral attachments by opening the prevesical space of Retzius and then the paravesical fossae. The nodule is then contoured to preserve as much of the healthy surface as possible. Suturing is then performed in two planes: the mucosal and the muscular.

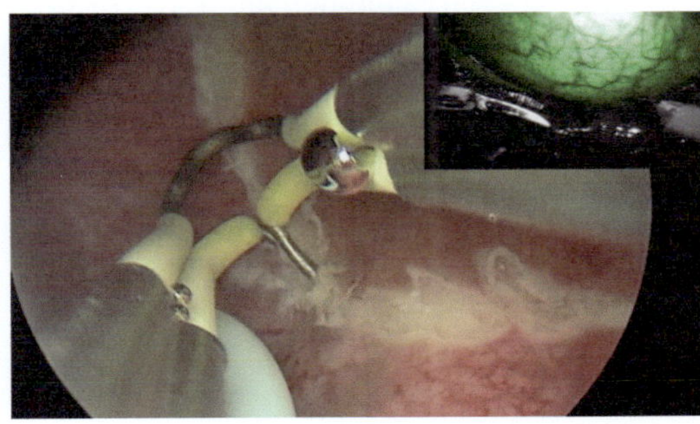

Fig. 16.2 Simultaneous cystoscopic and laparoscopic (robot assisted) view for a lesion of the bladder trigone

The latter are more complex due to the risk of trigonal invasion and their relationship with the ureters. In this case, preoperative imaging should determine the distance to the ureters. If the distance is less than 1 cm, concomitant reimplantation may be indicated. In any case, these lesions require preoperative JJ catheterization, during which the actual distance between the meatus and the lesion can be assessed. The use of a double surgical approach, both laparoscopic and cystoscopic (Fig. 16.2), enables us to control both the resection and suturing procedures [48–50].

16.2.4.4 Parametrial Endometriosis

According to the Terminologia Anatomica, the term *parametrium* should refer to the cranial portion (above the ureter) of the cardinal ligament (unofficial term), and the term *paracervix* should refer to the caudal portion (below the ureter) of the same ligament.

The radiologist's perspective is necessarily different from the surgeon's, as in laparoscopy, the uterus is anteverted and lateralized by the uterine manipulator, the peritoneum is open, and often the ovary and its infundibulum are tensioned by the assistant or suspended by a transcutaneous thread.

The involvement of the lateral compartments exposes the patient to the surgical risk of sectioning or the neuropraxia of the sympathetic and parasympathetic nerve fibers to the pelvis.

The identification and dissection of the hypogastric nerves (Fig. 16.3) is one of the standardized steps in the surgical approach to rectal and sacral nerve root lesions [51]. If the surgeon is able to fully visualize the sacral plexus (Fig. 16.4), they should clip and section several vessels of the internal iliac arterial and veinous networks because these vessels completely cover the sacral roots and are interposed between nerves and the endoscope.

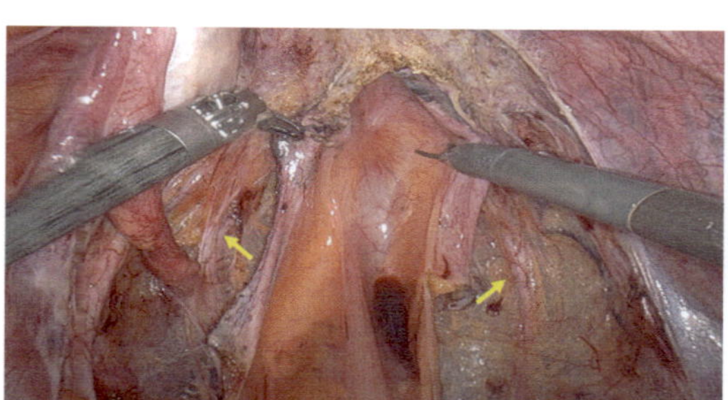

Fig. 16.3 Left and right hypogastric nerves

18. End-of-Procedure Control Procedures

The perfusion of the rectum and/or the ureters can be estimated with an infrared module in the camera and indocyanine green perfusion (see Fig. 16.1). It could reduce the rate of leakage [52]. For the evaluation of colorectal anastomosis, the surgeon inserts a foley catheter into the rectum and injects air while the abdominal cavity is filled with saline solution (bubble test). The tubal permeability test is also mandatory if fertility is an issue. Blue dye or indocyanine green can be used.

16.2.5 Postoperative Considerations

19. *The completeness of the resection is a fundamental information*

At the end of the procedure, the surgeon must describe the abdominal cavity and document any lesions left in place, with images and/or videos if possible, because the completeness of the surgical excision has been correlated with higher recurrence rates [53].

20. *Intraoperative complications*

Intraoperative complications have to be documented.

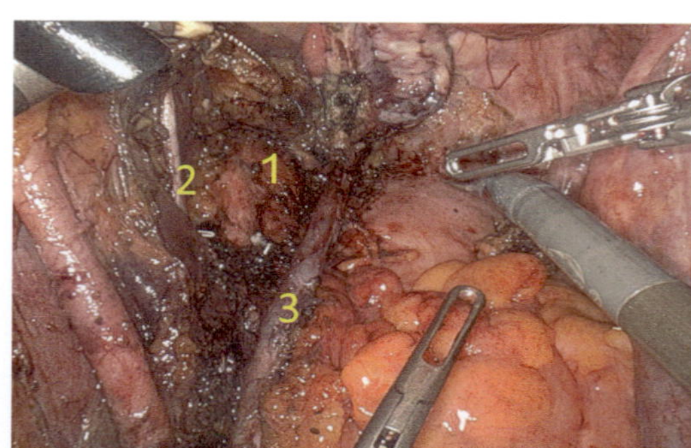

Fig. 16.4 Intraoperative view: a left endometriosis nodule on contact with the sciatic nerve (1) was resected, and numerous clips can be seen between the obturator nerve (2) and the ureter (3)

21. *Operation time, the length of hospital stay, and postoperative management*

The operation time, the length of hospital stay, and postoperative management details have to be specified.

The definition of the operation time should be explicit: door to door, narcosis, skin to skin, etc. Each is defined in the CORDES [7]. Any specific recommendations on immediate and long-term postoperative management should also be detailed.

References

1. Karl Freiherr von Rokitansky (1804–1878). Embryo Project Encyclopedia [Internet]. https://embryo.asu.edu/pages/karl-freiherr-von-rokitansky-1804-1878. Accessed 24 Jul 2024.
2. Giudice LC. Endometriosis. N Engl J Med. 2010;362(25):2389–98.
3. Vercellini P, Fedele L, Aimi G, Pietropaolo G, Consonni D, Crosignani PG. Association between endometriosis stage, lesion type, patient characteristics and severity of pelvic pain symptoms: a multivariate analysis of over 1000 patients. Hum Reprod. 2007;22(1):266–71.
4. Netter A, d'Avout-Fourdinier P, Agostini A, Chanavaz-Lacheray I, Lampika M, Farella M, et al. Progression of deep infiltrating rectosigmoid endometriotic nodules. Hum Reprod. 2019;34(11):2144–52.
5. Becker CM, Bokor A, Heikinheimo O, Horne A, Jansen F, Kiesel L, et al. ESHRE guideline: endometriosis†. Hum Reprod Open. 2022;2022(2):hoac009.
6. Tomassetti C, Johnson NP, Petrozza J, Abrao MS, Einarsson JI, Horne AW, et al. An international terminology for endometriosis, 2021. J Minim Invasive Gynecol. 2021;28(11):1849–59.
7. Vanhie A, Meuleman C, Tomassetti C, Timmerman D, D'Hoore A, Wolthuis A, et al. Consensus on recording deep endometriosis surgery: the CORDES statement. Hum Reprod. 2016;31:1219.
8. Becker CM, Laufer MR, Stratton P, Hummelshoj L, Missmer SA, Zondervan KT, et al. World endometriosis research foundation endometriosis phenome and biobanking harmonisation project: I. Surgical phenotype data collection in endometriosis research. Fertil Steril. 2014;102(5):1213–22.
9. Boutron I, Moher D, Altman DG, Schulz KF, Ravaud P, for the CONSORT Group. Extending the CONSORT statement to randomized trials of nonpharmacologic treatment: explanation and elaboration. Ann Intern Med. 2008;148(4):295.
10. Rashid R, Sohrabi C, Kerwan A, Franchi T, Mathew G, Nicola M, et al. The STROCSS 2024 guideline: strengthening the reporting of cohort, cross-sectional, and case-control studies in surgery. Int J Surg. 2024;110(6):3151–65.
11. Agha RA, Sohrabi C, Mathew G, Franchi T, Kerwan A, O'Neill N, et al. The PROCESS 2020 guideline: updating consensus preferred reporting of CasESeries in surgery (PROCESS) guidelines. Int J Surg. 2020;84:231–5.
12. Sohrabi C, Mathew G, Maria N, Kerwan A, Franchi T, Agha RA, et al. The SCARE 2023 guideline: updating consensus surgical CAse REport (SCARE) guidelines. Int J Surg. 2023;109(5):1136–40.
13. Crestani A, Merlot B, Goualard PH, Grigoriadis G, Chanavaz Lacheray I, Dennis T, et al. Bowel endometriosis: surgical customization is demanding. Best Pract Res Clin Obstet Gynaecol. 2024;94:102495.
14. Gillis C, Buhler K, Bresee L, Carli F, Gramlich L, Culos-Reed N, et al. Effects of nutritional Prehabilitation, with and without exercise, on outcomes of patients who undergo colorectal surgery: a systematic review and meta-analysis. Gastroenterology. 2018;155(2):391–410.e4.
15. Willis MA, Toews I, Soltau SL, Kalff JC, Meerpohl JJ, Vilz TO. Preoperative combined mechanical and oral antibiotic bowel preparation for preventing complications in elective colorectal surgery. Cochrane Database Syst Rev. 2023;2(2):CD014909. https://www.cochranelibrary.com/cdsr/doi/10.1002/14651858.CD014909.pub2/full. Accessed 2 Jan 2024.
16. Saccardi C, Gizzo S, Vitagliano A, Noventa M, Micaglio M, Parotto M, et al. Peri-incisional and intraperitoneal ropivacaine administration: a new effective tool in pain control after laparoscopic surgery in gynecology: a randomized controlled clinical trial. Surg Endosc. 2016;30(12):5310–8.
17. Daghmouri MA, Chaouch MA, Deniau B, Benayoun L, Krimi B, Gouader A, et al. Efficacy and safety of intraperitoneal ropivacaine in pain management following laparoscopic digestive surgery: a systematic review and meta-analysis of RCTs. Medicine (Baltimore). 2024;103(29):e38856.
18. Roman H, Dennis T, Grigoriadis G, Merlot B. Robotic management of diaphragmatic endometriosis in 10 steps. J Minim Invasive Gynecol. 2022;29(6):707–8.
19. Bourdel N, Fava V, Budianu MA, Chauvet P, Canis M, Chadeyras JB. Laparoscopic resection of diaphragmatic endometriosis in 10 steps. J Minim Invasive Gynecol. 2019;26(7):1224–5.
20. Moawad G, Youssef Y, Ayoubi JM, Feki A, De Ziegler D, Roman H. Diaphragmatic endometriosis: robotic approaches and techniques. Fertil Steril. 2022;118(6):1194–5.
21. Ahmad G, Baker J, Finnerty J, Phillips K, Watson A. Laparoscopic entry techniques. Cochrane Database Syst Rev. 2019;1(1):CD006583.
22. Takeda S. Anatomical terminology/Terminologia Anatomica: a melting pot for creating a universal language of anatomy. Anat Sci Int. 2024;99:331.
23. Roman H, Bubenheim M, Huet E, Bridoux V, Zacharopoulou C, Daraï E, et al. Conservative sur-

gery versus colorectal resection in deep endometriosis infiltrating the rectum: a randomized trial. Hum Reprod. 2018;33(1):47–57.
24. Roman H, Darwish B, Bridoux V, Huet E, Coget J, Chati R, et al. Multiple nodule removal in multifocal colorectal endometriosis instead of 'en bloc' large colorectal resection. Gynecol Obstet Fertil. 2016;44(2):121–4.
25. Soriano D, Schonman R, Nadu A, Lebovitz O, Schiff E, Seidman DS, et al. Multidisciplinary team approach to management of severe endometriosis affecting the ureter: long-term outcome data and treatment algorithm. J Minim Invasive Gynecol. 2011;18(4):483–8.
26. Froc E, Dubernard G, Bendifallah S, Hermouet E, Rubod-Dit-Guillet C, Canis M, et al. Clinical characteristics of urinary tract endometriosis: a one-year national series of 232 patients from 31 endometriosis expert centers (by the FRIENDS group). Eur J Obstet Gynecol Reprod Biol. 2021;264:155–61.
27. Keckstein J, Saridogan E, Ulrich UA, Sillem M, Oppelt P, Schweppe KW, et al. The #Enzian classification: a comprehensive non-invasive and surgical description system for endometriosis. Acta Obstet Gynecol Scand. 2021;100:1165.
28. Haas D, Chvatal R, Habelsberger A, Wurm P, Schimetta W, Oppelt P. Comparison of revised American fertility society and ENZIAN staging: a critical evaluation of classifications of endometriosis on the basis of our patient population. Fertil Steril. 2011;95(5):1574–8.
29. Haas D, Chvatal R, Habelsberger A, Schimetta W, Wayand W, Shamiyeh A, et al. Preoperative planning of surgery for deeply infiltrating endometriosis using the ENZIAN classification. Eur J Obstet Gynecol Reprod Biol. 2013;166(1):99–103.
30. Poupon C, Owen C, Arfi A, Cohen J, Bendifallah S, Daraï E. Nomogram predicting the likelihood of complications after surgery for deep endometriosis without bowel involvement. Eur J Obstetr Gynecol Reprod Biol X. 2019;3:100028.
31. Thomassin-Naggara I, Monroc M, Chauveau B, Fauconnier A, Verpillat P, Dabi Y, et al. Multicenter external validation of the deep pelvic endometriosis index magnetic resonance imaging score. JAMA Netw Open. 2023;6(5):e2311686.
32. Tomassetti C, Bafort C, Meuleman C, Welkenhuysen M, Fieuws S, D'Hooghe T. Reproducibility of the endometriosis fertility index: a prospective inter−/intra-rater agreement study. BJOG. 2020;127(1):107–14.
33. Roman H. Disc excision using Transanal circular stapler for deep endometriosis of the rectum in 10 steps. J Minim Invasive Gynecol. 2021;28(1):14–5.
34. Alborzi S, Roman H, Askary E, Poordast T, Shahraki MH, Alborzi S, et al. Colorectal endometriosis: diagnosis, surgical strategies and post-operative complications. Front Surg. 2022;9:978326.
35. Kostov S, Slavchev S, Dzhenkov D, Mitev D, Yordanov A. Avascular spaces of the female pelvis—clinical applications in obstetrics and gynecology. J Clin Med. 2020;9(5):1460.
36. Ceccaroni M, Clarizia R, Tebache L. Role and technique of nerve-sparing surgery in deep endometriosis. J Endometriosis Pelvic Pain Disord. 2016;8(4):141–51.
37. Roman H, Tuech JJ, Huet E, Bridoux V, Khalil H, Hennetier C, et al. Excision versus colorectal resection in deep endometriosis infiltrating the rectum: 5-year follow-up of patients enrolled in a randomized controlled trial. Hum Reprod. 2019;34(12):2362–71.
38. Abo C, Bendifallah S, Jayot A, Nyangoh Timoh K, Tuech J-J, Roman H, et al. Discoid resection for colorectal endometriosis: results from a prospective cohort from two French tertiary referral centres. Colorectal Dis. 2019;21(11):1312–20.
39. Roman H, Puscasiu L, Lempicki M, Huet E, Chati R, Bridoux V, et al. Colorectal endometriosis responsible for bowel occlusion or subocclusion in women with pregnancy intention: is the policy of primary in vitro fertilization always safe? J Minim Invasive Gynecol. 2015;22(6):1059–67.
40. D'Ancona G, Merlot B, Denost Q, Roman H. Robotic assisted rectal disk excision: the 3 cm-diameter cut off may be abandoned. Fertil Steril. 2023;119(5):886–8.
41. Namazov A, Kathurusinghe S, Marabha J, Merlot B, Forestier D, Hennetier C, et al. Double disk excision of large deep endometriosis nodules infiltrating the low and mid rectum: a pilot study of 20 cases. J Minim Invasive Gynecol. 2020;27(7):1482–9.
42. Bokor A, Hudelist G, Dobó N, Dauser B, Farella M, Brubel R, et al. Low anterior resection syndrome following different surgical approaches for low rectal endometriosis: a retrospective multicenter study. Acta Obstet Gynecol Scand. 2021;100(5):860–7.
43. Bendifallah S, Puchar A, Vesale E, Moawad G, Daraï E, Roman H. Surgical outcomes after colorectal surgery for endometriosis: a systematic review and meta-analysis. J Minim Invasive Gynecol. 2021;28(3):453–66.
44. Chapron C, Chiodo I, Leconte M, Amsellem-Ouazana D, Chopin N, Borghese B, et al. Severe ureteral endometriosis: the intrinsic type is not so rare after complete surgical exeresis of deep endometriotic lesions. Fertil Steril. 2010;93(7):2115–20.
45. da Cunha FL, Arcoverde FVL, Andres MP, Gomes DC, Bautzer CRD, Abrao MS, et al. Laparoscopic treatment of ureteral endometriosis: a systematic review. J Minim Invasive Gynecol. 2021;28(4):779–87.
46. Nezhat C, Lavie O, Lemyre M, Unal E, Nezhat CH, Nezhat F. Robot-assisted laparoscopic surgery in gynecology: scientific dream or reality? Fertil Steril. 2009;91(6):2620–2.
47. Raimondo D, Borghese G, Mabrouk M, Arena A, Ambrosio M, Del Forno S, et al. Use of Indocyanine green for intraoperative perfusion assessment in women with ureteral endometriosis: a preliminary study. J Minim Invasive Gynecol. 2021;28(1):42–9.

48. Crestani A, Dennis T, Roman H. Excision of a deep endometriosis nodule of the bladder (with video). J Visc Surg. 2023;160:74.
49. Roman H, Arambage K, Pasquier G, Resch B, Huet E. Combined cystoscopic and laparoscopic approach in deep endometriosis of the bladder. J Minim Invasive Gynecol. 2014;21(6):978–9.
50. Roman H, Braund S, Hennetier C, Celhay O, Pasquier G, Kade S, et al. Combined cystoscopic-abdominal versus abdominal-only route for complete excision of large deep endometriosis nodules infiltrating the supratrigonal area of the bladder: a comparative study. J Minim Invasive Gynecol. 2024;31(4):295–303.
51. D'Ancona G, Merlot B, Verrelli L, Boulos S, Dennis T, Roman H. Robotic management of isolated endometriosis of sciatic nerve: a reproducible approach that can guide through the labyrinth of pelvic neuroanatomy. Fertil Steril. 2023;120(3, Part 2):703–5.
52. Lucarini A, Guida AM, Orville M, Panis Y. Indocyanine green fluorescence angiography could reduce the risk of anastomotic leakage in rectal cancer surgery: a systematic review and meta-analysis of randomized controlled trials. Colorectal Dis. 2024;26(3):408–16.
53. Sibiude J, Santulli P, Marcellin L, Borghese B, Dousset B, Chapron C. Association of history of surgery for endometriosis with severity of deeply infiltrating endometriosis. Obstet Gynecol. 2014;124(4):709–17.

Correction to: Techniques and Reporting of the Imaging Techniques and Classifications: MR Imaging

Isabelle Thomassin-Naggara, Rana Al Rouhban, and Lucia Manganaro

Correction to:
Chapter 15 in: I. Thomassin-Naggara (ed.), *Imaging of Endometriosis: A Comparative Guide of US, MRI and Surgery*, https://doi.org/10.1007/978-3-031-82750-1_15

The original version of this chapter "Techniques and Reporting of the Imaging Techniques and Classifications: MR Imaging" was published with an incorrect caption and related alternate text (viewable by clicking the figure without hovering over) for the figure on page 297. This has now been corrected.

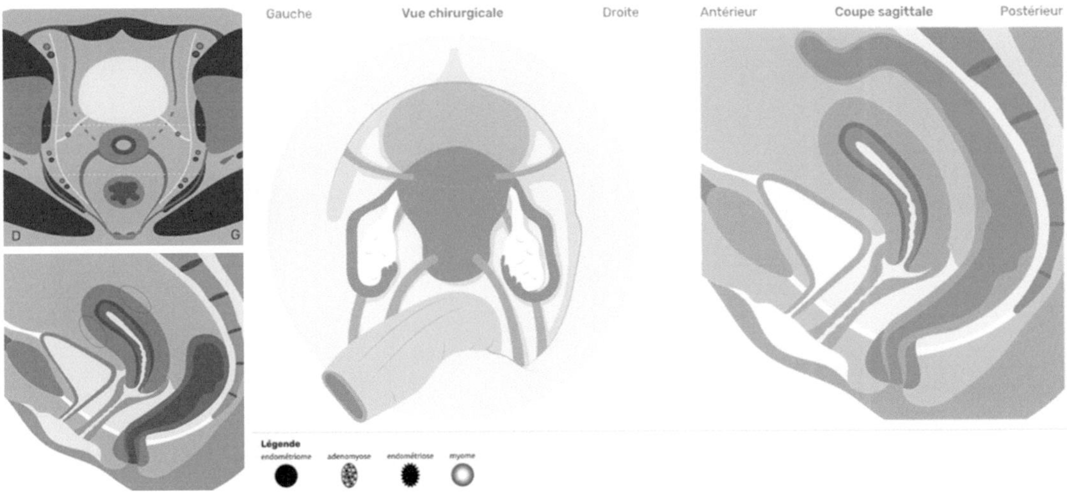

Examples of drawings including axial and sagittal sections and surgical views. These drawings are useful at the end of the MRI report to improve patient understanding (Source: Keydiag)

The updated version of this chapter can be found at https://doi.org/10.1007/978-3-031-82750-1_15

I. Thomassin-Naggara (ed.), *Imaging of Endometriosis: A Comparative Guide of US, MRI and Surgery*, https://doi.org/10.1007/978-3-031-82750-1_17

MIX
Papier aus verantwortungsvollen Quellen
Paper from responsible sources
FSC® C105338

If you have any concerns about our products,
you can contact us on
ProductSafety@springernature.com

In case Publisher is established outside the EU,
the EU authorized representative is:
Springer Nature Customer Service Center GmbH
Europaplatz 3, 69115 Heidelberg, Germany

Printed by Libri Plureos GmbH
in Hamburg, Germany